Psychiatric Nursing

made Incredibly Easy!

Third Edition

Clinical Editors

Cherie R. Rebar, PHD, MBA, RN, COI

Carolyn Gersch, PHD, RN, CNE

Nicole M. Heimgartner, DNP, RN, COI

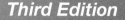 Wolters Kluwer

Philadelphia · Baltimore · New York · Lc
Buenos Aires · Hong Kong · Sydney · Tokyo

Acquisitions Editor: Nicole Dernoski/Michael Kerns
Development Editor: Maria M. McAvey
Senior Editorial Coordinator: Lindsay Ries
Production Project Manager: Barton Dudlick
Design Coordinator: Elaine Kasmer
Manufacturing Coordinator: Kathleen Brown
Marketing Manager: Linda Wetmore
Prepress Vendor: S4Carlisle Publishing Services

Third edition

9 8 7 6 5 4 3

Printed in the United States of America

Library of Congress Cataloging-in-Publication Data

Names: Rebar, Cherie R., editor. | Gersch, Carolyn J., editor. |
   Heimgartner, Nicole M., editor.
Title: Psychiatric nursing made incredibly easy! / clinical editors, Cherie
   Rebar, PhD, MBA, RN, COI, Carolyn Gersch, PhD, RN, CNE, Nicole M.
   Heimgartner, DNP, RN, COI.
Other titles: Psychiatric nursing made incredibly easy! (Lippincott
   Williams & Wilkins)
Description: Third edition. | Philadelphia: Wolters Kluwer, [2020] |
   Series: Mie | Includes bibliographical references and index. | Summary:
   "Welcome to the third edition of Psychiatric Nursing Made Incredibly
   Easy!"—Provided by publisher.
Identifiers: LCCN 2020005642 | ISBN 9781975144340 (paperback)
Subjects: LCSH: Psychiatric nursing.
Classification: LCC RC440 .P764 2020 | DDC 616.89/0231—dc23
LC record available at https://lccn.loc.gov/2020005642

shop.lww.com

Dedication

We dedicate this book to patients, advocates, and providers of care who work to replace the stigma associated with mental health needs with discussion, collaboration, and acceptance.

Thank you!

Cherie R. Rebar, PHD, MBA, RN, COI

Carolyn Gersch, PHD, RN, CNE

Nicole M. Heimgartner, DNP, RN, COI

Contributors

Lorraine Chiappetta, MSN, RN
Washtenaw Community College
Ann Arbor, Michigan

Beverly Cobb, PHD, APRN-CNP
Kettering Behavioral Medicine Center
Kettering, Ohio

Keelin Cromar, MSN, RN
Mississippi Gulf Coast College
Gulfport, Mississippi

Ashley M. Cunningham, PMHNP-BC, MSN, RN
Nurse Practitioner
Cincinnati Children's Hospital Medical
    Center
Cincinnati, Ohio

Angela DelGrande, PHD, PMHNP-BC, CNS
PMHNP Residency Director at New
    Mexico VAMC
University of New Mexico College of
    Nursing
Albuquerque, New Mexico

Brayden Nicole Kameg, DNP, RN, CARN
University of Pittsburgh
Pittsburgh, Pennsylvania

Jennifer Lamb, PMHNP-BC
VA Roseburg Healthcare System
Roseburg, Oregon
Southern Oregon University
Ashland, Oregon

Tara Latimore, MSN, RN
Ohio Institute of Allied Health
Dayton, Ohio

Tiffany Losekamp, MSN, CNE, CHSE
Wittenberg University
Springfield, Ohio

Katie Pimentel, BSN, RN-BC
The Queen's Medical Center
Honolulu, Hawaii

Summer Thompson, MSN, APRN, PMHNP-BC
University of California San Francisco
San Francisco, California

Tamara Thorn, MS, FNP-BC, PMHNP-BC
Co-owner
Greater Dayton Behavioral Health
Kettering, Ohio

Bernadine Tippit, BSN, RN
UF Health Jacksonville
Jacksonville, Florida

Lisa Weldon, PMHNP-BC
Progressive Psychiatric Services, PLLC
Manchester, New Hampshire

Karen Werder, PHD, PMHNP-BC
Sonoma State University
Rohnert Park, California

Previous edition contributors

Dorit Breiter, DNP, ARAP, PMHNP-BC

Barbara Broome, RN, PHD, CNS

Chien Yin Cepeda, RN

Virginia Conley, PHD, APRN, CS, FNP, PMHNP

Linda Carman Copel, RN, PHD, CS, DAPA

William J. Lorman, PHD, MSN, PMHNP-BC, CARN-AP

Elizabeth Lynch, MS, PMHNP-BC

Gilda Mark, APRN

Dana Murphy-Parker, MS, CRNP, PMHNP-BC

Donna Sabella, MD, BSN, PHD, MSN

Janet Somlyay, APRN, PMHNP

Matthew Sorenson, RN, PHD

Kathleen R. Tusaie, RNCS, PHD

Preface

Welcome to the third edition of *Psychiatric Nursing Made Incredibly Easy!* We are pleased to offer you this important contribution to the field of psychiatric–mental health nursing that provides important fundamental knowledge of and care related to various psychiatric-mental health concerns. As a profession, nursing continues to lead the way in understanding mental health needs and interventions that treat the whole person. This book offers a valuable overview of psychiatric–mental health conditions and has been structured to help nurses in all settings to provide patients with the best possible care.

This revised and updated edition has been carefully aligned to follow the logistic layout of the *Diagnostic and Statistical Manual of Mental Disorders*, 5th Edition (*DSM-5*) in order of diagnoses presented. Special focus has been given to covering a broader lifespan implication, with an emphasis on early recognition of symptoms so that diagnoses can be made sooner and a plan of care can be designed. Information has been provided regarding the current opioid crisis, with pertinent screening tools and interventions included to help the nurse identify concerns at any point of care.

Organized into 19 chapters, *Psychiatric Nursing Made Incredibly Easy!* covers patient and family advocacy, health promotion and teaching, psychopharmacology, interprofessional collaboration, and ethical and legal perspectives of mental health care. Nurse Joy and Nurse Jake emphasize concepts, and quick scan tables, flowcharts, and illustrations help to enhance the reader's understanding of material. For students studying for the NCLEX examination, a new *Practice Makes Perfect* section has been incorporated into this edition. Specific icons found within the book define the following:

Advice from the experts—offers tips and how-to's from experienced psychiatric nurses.

Myth busters—distinguishes facts from myths about people with mental health concerns and focuses on the proper care approaches.

Bridging the gap—offers overviews of unique beliefs and needs within specific groups.

Meds matters—focuses on the psychopharmacologic and/or alternative remedies for psychiatric concerns.

We hope that you will find this edition of *Psychiatric Nursing Made Incredibly Easy!* to be an effective professional resource that helps to inform your practice.

Cherie R. Rebar, PHD, MBA, RN, COI

Carolyn Gersch, PHD, RN, CNE

Nicole M. Heimgartner, DNP, RN, COI
Educational Strategists, Connect: RN2ED
Beavercreek, Ohio

Contents

Chapter 1

Introduction to psychiatric nursing

Just the facts

In this chapter, you'll learn:

♦ the nurse's role in caring for patients with psychiatric conditions

♦ ways to enhance therapeutic communication with patients

♦ therapies used to treat psychiatric conditions

♦ components of the nursing assessment of the patient with psychiatric conditions

♦ ethical and legal issues in caring for patients with psychiatric conditions.

A look at psychiatric nursing

Like all people, patients with psychiatric conditions use all medical settings. These patients use medical clinics for wellness and follow-up care and are susceptible to medical illness or injury that require hospitalizations. Any patient in any medical setting may be distressed because of their illness or confused as a result of a long hospitalization. Anxiety, depression, and confusion are commonly seen in the general population. With the increase in longevity, dementia is more common.

To work effectively with any patient, it is essential to consider not only the physical concerns but also the psychological issues that may, or may not, be reported.

Goal: More beautiful minds

According to the Department of Health and Human Services (2014), mental health and substance use disorder spending is projected to increase from $171.7 billion in 2009 to $280.5 billion in 2020. Understanding of psychiatric

> You don't need to work on a psychiatric unit to encounter patients with psychiatric conditions.

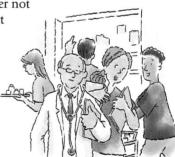

1

illness has grown significantly over the past decade and the link between physical and mental health is better understood. Additionally, the care for patients with psychiatric conditions has evolved from inpatient hospitalization to outpatient community-based programs. Advocacy programs, assertive community treatment programs, and assisted outpatient treatment programs provide follow-up care and monitoring of patients with psychiatric conditions in the community. Programs are available to provide support and education regarding numerous situations or circumstances, including substance use programs, bereavement support, victims of violence groups, and shelters.

Real situations that make us think

Psychiatric concerns are more reported now than ever before. We have seen a number of tragedies reported in the media related to shootings in schools, universities, and community settings caused by untreated or poorly monitored individuals with psychiatric conditions. These tragedies remind us of the seriousness of untreated illness. Additionally, many books on coping and mindfulness have become best sellers. Advertisements on television tout the latest antidepressant or other medication that is available to control symptoms of anxiety, pain, or sadness.

Upgrading our understanding

Through research, our understanding of neurobiology has improved exponentially. This growth in knowledge has expanded the awareness of the physiologic foundation of neurologic function and its relation to mental illness. Genetic testing can be used to improve our understanding of how medications impact our brains based on individual DNA. With this increase in knowledge, diagnosis and treatment of psychiatric illness have improved, particularly in the use of drug therapy (Stahl, 2013). It is essential for psychiatric and mental health nurses to remain current with the changing developments in diagnosis, treatment, and neurobiology.

Scientists are learning more and more about what makes our minds tick.

Holism in the house

Our education as nurses, and particularly in psychiatry, teaches us to look holistically at our patients. We know through research and nursing practice experience that emotional stability and resiliency improve outcomes in recovery from both medical and psychiatric illness. Psychiatric consultations are now more readily ordered when health care professionals observe and recognize symptoms early in the process of delivering care.

Links between stress and disease

Hans Selye, a pioneer in stress research, found a link between the environment and biological response. He noted that emotional and physical stress cause a pattern of responses that, unless treated, lead to infection, illness, disease, and eventually even death. Selye called this set of responses the *general adaptation syndrome* and identified three stages—alarm reaction, resistance, and exhaustion.

Alarm reaction

During this stage, any type of physical or mental trauma triggers immediate biological responses designed to counter the stress. These responses depress the immune system, which lowers resistance and makes the person more susceptible to infection and disease. Unless the stress is severe or prolonged, though, the person recovers rapidly.

Resistance

This stage begins when the body starts to adapt to prolonged stress. The immune system shifts into high gear to meet increased demands. At this point, the person becomes more resistant to illness.

However, the perception of a threat lingers, so the body never reaches complete physiologic equilibrium. Instead, it stays aroused, which places stress on body organs and systems.

Because adaptation appears to work initially, a person in the resistance stage may become complacent and assume some immunity to the effects of stress, failing to take steps for stress reduction.

Exhaustion

With chronic stress, adaptive mechanisms eventually wear down and the body can no longer meet the demands of stress. Immunity and resistance decline dramatically and illness is likely to set in. The point at which exhaustion occurs differs among individuals.

Interrupting the stress response

Selye's work laid the foundation for the use of relaxation techniques in interrupting the stress response, thereby reducing susceptibility to illness and disease (Townsend, 2014).

Social factors

Today, researchers continue to explore the continuing increase of mental illness. They have identified increased stressors related to the changes in family dynamics. Our exposure to national trauma on September 11, 2001, and subsequent military conflicts have contributed to military personnel and veterans struggling with posttraumatic stress and depression related to the trauma, injury, and loss. Financial uncertainty, social isolation, and personal losses experienced by individuals continue to challenge the mental health care system to respond quickly and appropriately to the ever-expanding needs. (See *Links between stress and disease.*)

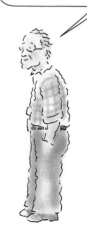

Older adults can sometime experience isolation, which can lead to depression.

Angst through the ages

Psychiatric conditions affect all socioeconomic populations, all ages, and both genders. According to the National Institute of Health (2019), suicide was the second leading cause of death for individuals between 10 and 34 years of age and the fourth highest for individuals

Understanding the *DSM-5*

The APA's *DSM-5* defines a mental disorder as a clinically significant behavioral or psychological syndrome or pattern associated with at least one of the following criteria:

* current distress (a painful symptom)
* disability (an impairment in one or more important areas of functioning)
* a significantly greater risk of suffering, death, pain, and disability
* an important loss of freedom.

The syndrome or pattern must not be merely an expected, culturally sanctioned response—such as grief over the death of a loved one. Whatever its original cause, it must currently be considered a sign of behavioral, psychological, or biological dysfunction.

The structure of the *DSM-5* is based on three sections. Section 1 describes the "Basics" of the new text in understanding the structure and use of the *DSM-5*. Section 2 describes the "Diagnostic Criteria and Codes" and uses a chapter structure to define criteria for illness combining like disorders based on symptoms. Section 3 describes "Emerging Measures and Models" to provide a road map for future development based on research leading to better understanding of the interrelationship of physical and cognitive function.

The hope of the *DSM-5* is that it will be more useful not only for psychiatrists but also for primary care physicians as a reference to assist patients (Kupfer et al., 2013).

between 35 and 54 years of age in 2017. Substance use is reported even in young children. Alcohol and substance misuse and dependence are increasing, whereas services have challenges keeping up with access.

Classifying mental disorders

To successfully understand patients and respond to their needs, it is important to understand the language of psychiatry. The American Psychiatric Association (APA) developed a classification system to provide guidelines to diagnose psychiatric illness. This classification system has been updated over the years, most recently in 2013, with the recent edition of the *Diagnostic and Statistical Manual of Mental Disorders*, 5th Edition (*DSM-5*). This latest edition is focused on viewing patients in a holistic and multidimensional manner so that their needs are more appropriately addressed (Kupfer, Kuhl, & Regier, 2013). (See *Understanding the DSM-5*.) The restructuring of the chapters and outline are designed to better address lifespan considerations, developmental variations in symptom presentations, and cultural perspectives (Kupfer, 2014).

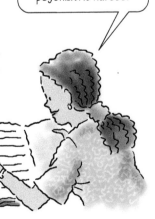

The *DSM-5* is a must-read for all psychiatric nurses.

Role of psychiatric nurses

Psychiatric nursing is recognized by the American Nurses Association (ANA) as a specialized area of nursing practice. Psychiatric nursing incorporates the science of nursing based on clinical assessment skills and nursing diagnoses with the art of "therapeutic use of self" in establishing a professional, therapeutic relationship based on empathy. Psychiatric nurses continue to perform in the traditional role of nurses with the administration of prescribed treatments, monitoring the efficacy of those treatments, and educating patients. Additionally, psychiatric nurses engage patients and families in conversation based on therapeutic models to improve understanding of their illness and to improve function.

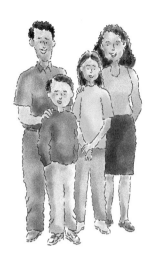

Psychiatric nursing is present in all health care settings such as inpatient, outpatient, community health care centers, mental health clinics, and visiting nurse services. Practice is as diverse as the settings. Therapeutic relationships are present in all nursing interactions as are the principles of psychiatric nursing. (See *The versatile nurse*.)

To work with patients with mental health conditions, a psychiatric nurse brings calm to the storm. Our patients bring challenges as complicated and distinct as the individual. The creativity and compassion of our interactions help establish the therapeutic relationship from which healing can occur (Townsend, 2017).

The versatile nurse

The psychiatric nurse will have one or many of the following roles depending on his or her skills, educational background, and experience:

- staff nurse/nurse leader
- primary provider of care
- administrator
- consultant
- in-service educator
- clinical practitioner
- researcher
- program evaluator
- liaison between the patient and other health care team members
- patient advocate.

Nurse: Know thyself

To effectively work as a psychiatric nurse, we must become aware of our own biases and beliefs. Taking an inventory of what drives us to make the decisions that we make allows us to more fully understand ourselves. Although it is impossible to completely separate from our core beliefs, it is essential to set aside our biases and accept the fact that our patients may feel differently than we do and ultimately make different decisions than we would. Giving patients the autonomy to which they are entitled reinforces our duty as nurses to provide accurate health information from which they can choose or decline.

Knowing yourself will help you care more effectively for patients with mental health conditions.

Scope of practice

The nurse practice act of each state is enacted by the state legislature and describes the scope of practice for all nurses working within their borders. It is important to familiarize yourself with your nurse practice act so that you work based on those laws. Other common standards of practice include:

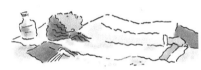

- professional practice standards
- education and experience
- certification
- practice setting
- personal initiative.

Nurse practice acts

Each state regulates the scope of a nurse's practice through the nurse practice act. This act regulates and defines nurse practice for that state. It sets the minimum standards for entry into the practice of nursing, outlines the scope of practice for the nurse, and describes the requirements for advanced practice nurses. Additionally, it sets the requirements for licensure, license renewal, and any other conditions necessary for practice within the state. It is important to become familiar with your individual nurse practice act so that your practice follows the laws of your state.

Professional practice standards

Although nursing practice is regulated by each state, professional practice standards developed by the ANA provide guidelines for practice and performance in an effort to assist in establishing some uniformity in care. The ANA initially developed these standards in 1973 and updated them in partnership with the

American Psychiatric Nurses Association (APNA) and the International Society of Psychiatric Mental Health Nurses (ISPN) most recently in 2014. (See *ANA standards of care for psychiatric and mental health nursing*, pages 8 and 9.)

Education and experience

Integrating behavioral health care into primary care practice has become more common and is creating opportunities for expanding the practice of psychiatric nurses. To answer this need, the psychiatric mental health nurse practitioner (PMHNP), currently a master's or doctoral prepared advanced practice nurse certified in psychiatry, has been added to many clinical, hospital, and community mental health clinics. Because of the changes to our health care system, growing demands for mental health care will continue to expand the need for the PMHNP to new practice areas and new levels of doctoral education.

Certification

Organizations and places of employment are requiring and/or encouraging psychiatric nurses to become certified as experts in their field. ANA and the American Nurses Credentialing Center (American Nurses Credentialing Center; 2014) provide certification testing. To qualify for certification, a psychiatric nurse must meet certain standards set by the credentialing agency as an indication of nursing competence. Some of the standards include length of time in practice, evidence of continued education in psychiatric nursing, recommendations from peers, and passing of an examination. Certification can be obtained as a Psychiatric Mental Health Registered Nurse (PMH-RN) or PMHNP.

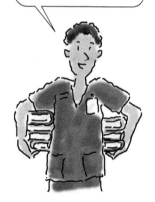

Acing the written test goes a long way toward gaining ANA certification.

Practice setting

Each practice setting shapes the type of care based on the philosophy and focus of the organization. In addition to the state's nurse practice acts, the administration's policies provide guidelines for treatment and the parameters for the practice of the psychiatric nurse. This philosophy outlines the approach to care and the guidelines provide insight to the patient as well as the caregiver of what is expected within the practice.

Personal initiative

Each psychiatric nurse chooses how to perform within his or her scope of practice. He or she is prompted by educational experiences, awareness of biases and belief systems, ability to engage in therapeutic relationships, and clinical competence.

ANA standards of care for psychiatric and mental health nursing

In 1973, the ANA issued standards designed to improve the quality of care provided by psychiatric and mental health nurses. Last revised in 2014, these standards apply to generalists and specialists working in any setting in which psychiatric and mental health nursing is practiced.

Listed below are the standards of care and standards of professional performance, along with rationales. *Note:* Standards 5c through 5h apply only to the advanced practice registered nurse in psychiatric and mental health (APRN-PMH).

Standards of care

Standards of care pertain to professional nursing activities demonstrated through the nursing process. The standards encompass assessment, diagnosis, outcome identification, planning, implementation, and evaluation.

The nursing process is the foundation of clinical decision making and encompasses all significant action taken by nurses in providing psychiatric and mental health care to all patients.

Standard 1: Assessment

The psychiatric mental health registered nurse collects and synthesizes comprehensive health data that are pertinent to the health care consumer's health and/or situation.

Rationale: Collection of comprehensive patient information—which requires linguistically and culturally effective communication skills, interviewing, behavioral observation, database record review, and comprehensive assessment of the patient and relevant systems—enables the psychiatric and mental health nurse to make sound clinical judgments and plan appropriate interventions.

Standard 2: Diagnosis

The psychiatric mental health registered nurse analyzes the assessment data to determine diagnoses, problems, and areas of focus for care and treatment, including level of risk.

Rationale: The basis for providing psychiatric and mental health nursing care is thorough assessment, recognition and identification of patterns of response to actual or potential psychiatric illnesses, mental health problems, and potential comorbid physical illnesses.

Standard 3: Outcome identification

The psychiatric mental health registered nurse identifies expected outcomes and the health care consumer's goals for a plan individualized to the health care consumer or to the situation.

Rationale: Within the context of providing nursing care, the ultimate goal is to partner with the patient to improve health status and outcomes.

Standard 4: Planning

The psychiatric mental health registered nurse develops a plan that prescribes strategies and alternatives to assist the health care consumer in attainment of expected outcomes.

Rationale: A plan of care is used to guide therapeutic intervention, systematically document progress, and work with the patient toward planned outcomes.

Standard 5: Implementation

The psychiatric mental health registered nurse implements the identified plan.

Rationale: Nurses use a wide range of interventions when implementing the plan of care. These interventions are designed to prevent mental and physical illness and to promote, maintain, and restore mental and physical health. They select interventions according to their practice level. At the basic level, nurses may select counseling, milieu therapy, self-care activities, psychobiological interventions, health teaching, case management, health promotion and maintenance, crisis intervention, community-based care, psychiatric home health care, telehealth, and various other approaches to meet the patient's mental health needs.

ANA standards of care for psychiatric and mental health nursing *(continued)*

Standard 5a: Coordination of care
The psychiatric mental health registered nurse coordinates care delivery.

Standard 5b: Health teaching and health promotion
The psychiatric mental health registered nurse employs strategies to promote health and a safe environment.

Standard 5c: Consultation
The psychiatric mental health advanced practice registered nurse provides consultation to influence the identified plan, enhance the abilities of other clinicians to provide services for health care consumers, and effect change.

Standard 5d: Prescriptive authority and treatment
The psychiatric mental health advanced practice registered nurse uses prescriptive authority, procedures, referrals, treatments, and therapies in accordance with state and federal laws and regulations.

Standard 5e: Pharmacologic, biological, and integrative therapies
The psychiatric mental health advanced practice registered nurse incorporates knowledge of pharmacologic, biological, and complementary interventions with applied clinical skills to restore the health care consumer's health and prevent further disability.

Standard 5f: Milieu therapy
The psychiatric mental health advanced practice registered nurse provides; structures; and maintains a safe, therapeutic, recovery-oriented environment in collaboration with health care consumers, families, and other health care clinicians.

Standard 5g: Therapeutic relationship and counseling
The psychiatric mental health advanced practice registered nurse uses the therapeutic relationship and counseling interventions to assist health care consumers in their individual recovery journeys by improving and regaining their previous coping abilities, fostering mental health, and preventing mental disorder and disability.

Standard 5h: Psychotherapy
The psychiatric mental health advanced practice registered nurse conducts individual, couples, group, and family psychotherapy using evidence-based psychotherapeutic frameworks and the nurse-client therapeutic relationship.

Standard 6
The PMH registered nurse evaluates progress toward attainment of expected outcomes.

From American Nurses Association. (2014). *Psychiatric-mental health nursing: Scope and standards of practice* (2nd ed.). Silver Spring, MD: Author.

Theoretical basis of psychiatric nursing

Psychiatric nursing, as is true of all nursing specialties, is based on theoretical concepts and best practice supported by evidence. (See *Theoretical models of behavior*, pages 10 and 11.)

Theoretical models of behavior

Learning about the various models of human behavior gives you a better understanding of psychiatric disorders. These models are summarized below.

Remember, though, that human behavior isn't fully understood, so no model or theory is considered right or wrong or better or worse than any other. Commonly, psychiatric nurses use an eclectic approach, drawing on several theoretical models to inform practice.

Psychoanalytic model (Freud)

According to the psychoanalytic model, the personality consists of the:

- id, encompassing the primitive instincts and energies underlying all psychic activity
- ego, the conscious part of the personality and the part that most immediately controls thought and behavior
- superego, the conscience.

During childhood, development occurs in five psychosexual stages—oral, anal, phallic, latency, and genital. Deviations in behavior result from unsuccessful task accomplishment during earlier developmental stages. Freud also proposed that behavior is motivated by anxiety, the cornerstone of psychopathology.

Understanding the psychosexual stages of childhood provides a framework for the nurse to understand adult behaviors. Also, the nurse can promote effective parenting by teaching parents about the child's needs during each psychosexual stage.

Interpersonal model (Sullivan, Peplau)

The interpersonal model holds that human development results from interpersonal relationships and that behavior is motivated by avoidance of anxiety and attainment of satisfaction.

Peplau drew on Sullivan's original theory to propose an interpersonal nursing theory, which advanced the practice of psychiatric nursing by defining it as an interpersonal process. She proposed that:

- nurses must promote the nurse-patient relationship to build trust and foster healthy behavior
- therapeutic use of self promotes healing
- the therapeutic relationship is directed toward meeting the patient's needs.

Social model (Caplan, Szasz)

The social model proposes that the entire sociocultural environment influences mental health. Deviant behavior is defined by the culture in which a person lives. Undesirable or abnormal behavior in one society may be considered normal in another. In addition, social conditions and interactions predispose people to mental illness.

Existential model (Frankl, Perls, May)

The existential model centers on a person's present experiences rather than past ones. It holds that alienation from the self causes deviant behavior and that people can make free choices about which behaviors to display.

Based on the existential model of behavior, nursing developed the concept that the nurse works to restore the patient to a state of "full life" from a state of "self-alienation."

Nursing model (Rogers, Orem, Sister Roy, Peplau)

The nursing model emphasizes the person as a biopsychosocial being. This holistic approach focuses on caring rather than curing and promotes collaboration between the nurse and the patient. It establishes the nursing process as the basis for providing care.

According to the nursing model, the patient's needs direct the therapeutic relationship and the patient's reactions to nursing interventions guide future interventions.

Medical model

The medical model holds that disease is the cause of deviant behavior. It focuses on diagnosis and treatment of the disease. Application of the medical model to mental illness has led to identification of neurochemicals as possible causes of deviant behavior. The medical model also accepts socioenvironmental influences as potential causes of deviant behavior.

Theoretical models of behavior *(continued)*

Communication models (Berne, Bandler, Grindler)

Communication theory proposes that all human behavior is a form of communication and that the meaning of behavior depends on the clarity of communication between sender and receiver. Unclear communication produces anxiety, which results in behavior deviations.

The communication pattern used with individuals, families, and social and work groups identifies the causes of the behavioral deviation. When communication improves, so does behavior.

Nurses draw on the communication model when they teach patients effective communication techniques.

Behavioral model (Skinner, Wolpe, Eysenck)

According to the behavioral model, all behavior—including mental illness—is learned. Unlike other models, which focus on the patient's emotions, behavioral theory focuses on the patient's actions.

Behaviorists believe that behavior that's rewarded will persist. Desired behaviors can be learned through rewards and negative behaviors can be eliminated through punishment. Thus, people can learn to behave in socially desirable ways.

Humanistic model (Maslow)

In the humanistic model, understanding human behavior requires familiarity with a hierarchy that has six levels of need.

- Level 1: physiologic survival (food, oxygen, and rest)
- Level 2: safety, security, and self-preservation
- Level 3: love and belonging (developing fulfilling relationships)
- Level 4: esteem and recognition (feeling like a worthwhile, contributing member of society, appreciating one's own uniqueness)
- Level 5: self-actualization (self-fulfillment)
- Level 6: truth, harmony, beauty, and spirituality.

Nursing draws from the humanistic model by striving to meet patients' lower level needs before higher level ones. By performing a needs assessment, the nurse determines appropriate intervention strategies to help patients meet their needs (Townsend, 2017).

Nurse–patient relationship

In order to be successful in working with any patient, it is necessary to develop a therapeutic relationship with him or her. This relationship is based on trust, empathy, and caring. It is through your words and actions, as well as your silence, that you communicate to the patient that he or she is important and you are open to his or her needs.

A therapeutic relationship is one focused on the betterment of the patient. It is based on a purpose that leads toward a goal with a set time frame. It is a relationship in which both the patient and the nurse set the agenda—it is not done for the patient; it is a collaborative effort with him or her. It flows through four identifiable stages. (See *Phases of the nurse-patient relationship,* page 12.)

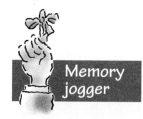

Memory jogger

To encourage your patient to trust you, think of the mnemonic TRUST.

Try expression

Reflection

Use silence

Set limits

Time with the patient

Phases of the nurse-patient relationship

The phases of a therapeutic relationship include the preinteraction, orientation, working, and termination phases.

Preinteraction phase

During the preinteraction phase—which may last a few seconds or several weeks—the nurse assesses the patient for unresolved problems. The patient may not be actively involved at this point.

Orientation (introductory) phase

The orientation (getting-to-know-you) phase sets the tone for the relationship. Introductions are made and each person's roles are defined. Trust begins to develop.

Usually, the nurse initiates this phase, setting the limits of the professional relationship and establishing the focus for conversation based on assessment data.

Then the nurse and patient may make an agreement, write a contract, or discuss and establish goals. Be aware that some patients may be resistant during this phase, testing your true intent or denying that they have a problem.

Working (exploration) phase

During the working phase, the nurse and patient explore and evaluate problems and work toward achieving set goals. The nurse may take on the role of listener and facilitator, with the patient participating actively. The patient is free to examine problems while trying to gain insight or find solutions.

Termination (resolution) phase

During the termination phase, the nurse reviews and summarizes the patient's progress. Together, the nurse and patient determine if goals have been met—and, if not, why not.

Then the nurse formally ends the relationship, being sure to acknowledge the patient's feelings about termination. Be aware that the patient may feel hurt or angry at the nurse's "abandonment" (Townsend, 2017).

Effective communication

Effective, therapeutic communication is essential in psychiatric nursing. Verbal and nonverbal communication involve sending and receiving messages. "Body language" sends volumes of information both to and from your patient. It is important to be aware of the messages that you send.

Verbal communication

Communication exists in spoken, written, or unspoken language as in "body language." Nurses rely on multiple forms of communication to provide information to patients. We often educate our patients on appropriate behaviors or treatment options and provide written documents to educate them on treatment upon discharge from the hospital.

Minimizing obstacles

It is important to remember that patients have biases and beliefs just as we do. In order to communicate effectively, it is important to understand cultural, ethnic, religious, and educational biases that are potential obstacles. Your sensitivity to your patient's beliefs can improve your ability to connect with your patient. (See *Factors that influence verbal communication.*)

Cutting through the fog

Developing a therapeutic relationship with a patient with a mental health condition can be challenging. Thought disorders, dementias, and mood dysregulation can impact the patient's ability to engage therapeutically. (See *Reducing communication barriers*, page 14.)

¿Habla usted inglés?

Not all patients speak the same language as the nurse. The Joint Commission (TJC) requires that hospitals provide interpreters to assist patients with communication. Many hospitals have interpreters among staff or use "language lines" when interpreters are not available. Sign language interpreters assist with hearing-impaired patients and various equipment, that is, paper and pencils and text telephone (TTY) machines, facilitate communication with these patients.

Patient patterns

It is important to listen to not only what the patient is saying but how the patient is saying it. Speech patterns, intensity of speech, and logic of the conversation provide a wealth of information about your patient and his or her health.

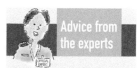

Advice from the experts

Factors that influence verbal communication

Various factors can hinder effective communication between the nurse and the patient. Be sure to consider the patient's
- native language
- culture or nationality
- sexual orientation or gender identity
- age and developmental considerations
- roles and responsibilities
- social background or status
- space and territoriality
- physical, mental, and emotional state
- values
- environment.

Nonverbal communication

We send messages to each other through our gestures, facial expression, posture, eye contact, clothing, touch, and appearance. In fact, most communication is nonverbal. Our body language communicates acceptance, joy, interest, as well as rejection, fear, and discontent.

Body talk

It is essential to be aware of how we approach our patients as much as we are aware of how our patient approaches us. We must monitor our body language to indicate that we are approachable, interested, and accepting of our patients.

Reducing communication barriers

Acknowledging and reducing communication barriers can promote a more effective relationship with psychiatric patients.

Language difficulties or differences

Use words appropriate to the patient's educational level. Avoid terms that he or she is unlikely to understand.

Be aware of words that may have more than one meaning. To some patients, for instance, the word "bad" may also be slang for "good."

If the patient speaks a foreign language or uses an ethnic dialect, obtain an interpreter to help you communicate. However, remember that a third person's presence may make the patient less willing to share his or her feelings.

Impaired hearing

If the patient can't hear you clearly, he or she may misinterpret your questions or responses. Check whether he or she is wearing a hearing aid. If so, is it turned on? If not, can the patient read lips? If possible, face the patient and speak clearly and slowly, using common words. Keep your questions short, simple, and direct.

If the patient has a severe hearing impairment, he or she may have to communicate in writing or you may need to collect information from his or her family or friends.

With aging, the ability to hear high-pitched tones deteriorates first. For older adults, speaking in low-pitched tones may be helpful.

Inappropriate responses

Avoid appearing to discount the patient's feelings, as by changing the subject abruptly. Otherwise, the patient may get the impression that you're disinterested, anxious, annoyed, or you're judging him or her.

Thought disorders

If the patient's thought patterns are incoherent or irrelevant, he or she may be unable to interpret messages correctly, focus on the interview, or provide appropriate responses. When assessing, ask simple questions about concrete topics and clarify responses. Encourage the patient to express himself or herself clearly.

Paranoid thinking

Approach a patient who is paranoid in a nonthreatening way. Avoid touching, which may be misinterpreted as an attempt to enact harm. Also, keep in mind that a patient who is paranoid may not mean the things that he or she says.

Hallucinations

A patient who is hallucinating can't hear or respond appropriately. Show concern but don't reinforce hallucinatory perceptions.

Be as specific as possible when giving commands. For instance, if the patient says he or she is hearing voices, tell the patient to stop listening to the voices and listen to you instead.

Delusions

A patient with delusion defends irrational beliefs or ideas despite factual evidence to the contrary. Some delusions may be so bizarre that you'll recognize them immediately. Others may be hard to identify.

Don't condemn or agree with delusional beliefs, and don't dismiss a statement because you think it's delusional. Instead, gently emphasize reality without arguing.

Delirium

A patient with delirium experiences disorientation, hallucinations, and confusion. Misinterpretation and inappropriate responses commonly result. Talk directly, ask simple questions, and offer frequent reassurances. Delirium is reversible.

Dementia

The patient with dementia (irreversible deterioration of mental capacity) may experience changes in memory and thought patterns. Language may become distorted or slurred.

When interviewing, minimize distractions. Use simple, concise language. Avoid making statements that could be easily misinterpreted.

Using silence

Silence is an important tool for open communication. It allows a patient the time and space to communicate, think, evaluate, and process the challenges that brought them to you. Remember, even with silence, it is important to remain present in the conversation. Using body language sends the message that you are listening and engaged in the conversation.

Listening attentively

Engaging your patient using eye contact, touch (when appropriate), and gestures sends the message that you are actively listening to what he or she has to say. Responding appropriately confirms that you value and accept your patient.

Checking for congruence

One of the roles of a psychiatric nurse is to assess patients for congruence of mood—how a patient describes their feelings—and affect—how a patient physically appears. If a patient is describing a distressing occurrence, the nurse would assess for the appropriate affect—the patient might appear sad and may be tearful during the conversation. Conversely, if the patient describes something happy or exciting, his or her affect should reflect this with a smile or a pleasant demeanor. If this is not what is observed, the patient is described as incongruent with mood.

Therapeutic communication

The use of self is the psychiatric nurses' tool. It is the development of the therapeutic relationship between the nurse and the patient. This relationship allows the nurse to complete assessments and patient teaching, facilitate therapeutic conversations, and listen attentively to patient concerns. It encourages the development of insight and allows patients to evaluate and develop problem-solving strategies. Therapeutic relationships are established through therapeutic communication. Techniques that help to establish a therapeutic relationship include open-ended questions, validating feelings, reframing feelings and events, clarifying, refocusing, collaborating ideas, and providing information.

Blunderin' and bunglin'

Alternatively, communication that is nontherapeutic may impede and slow a patient's ability to engage in a trusting relationship with psychiatric nursing staff. (See *Nontherapeutic ways of communicating*, page 16.)

Nontherapeutic ways of communicating

Nontherapeutic techniques hinder an effective nurse-patient relationship. Avoid the following pitfalls when interacting with patients.

Attacking or defending
- Getting angry or arguing with the patient
- Challenging the patient's beliefs
- Being defensive.

Casting judgment
- Judging or criticizing the patient
- Giving approval or disapproval.

Interrogating (or demanding)
- Asking the patient "why" questions
- Asking excessive, inappropriate, or leading questions
- Probing sensitive areas or making the patient feel uncomfortable.

Minimizing
- Stereotyping the patient
- Not listening
- Not taking the patient's beliefs seriously
- Failing to maintain eye contact
- Changing the subject inappropriately
- Working on a task while the patient is talking to you
- Letting your mind wander during a conversation
- Using clichés.

Giving advice
- Giving advice
- Offering false reassurance.

Pressuring
- Trying to talk the patient into accepting treatment.

Excessive talking
- Talking on and on
- Not letting the patient respond
- Repeating a point you just made
- Interpreting or speculating on the dynamics of patient problems
- Making inappropriate comments.

Rushing
- Responding to the patient before he or she finishes speaking
- Finishing sentences for the patient.

Taking sides
- Joining attacks led by the patient
- Participating in criticism of staff members.

Using open-ended questions or statements

Asking open-ended questions allows your patient to provide information. It requires engagement in the conversation rather than a "yes" or "no" answer. Examples include "Tell me more about that" and "How do you think you could have handled this differently?"

Conversational cul-de-sacs

Close-ended questions, questions that can be answered with a yes or no response, cut off conversation and provide little meaningful information.

Validating

The practice of validating reviews and restates what a patient has reported and allows the patient to correct any misunderstanding. It also assures the patient that he or she has been heard and understood. It also encourages your patient to continue his or her story and provides you with more insight into what is of concern to him or her.

Clarifying

At times, a patient may give confusing or contradictory information. Asking the patient to explain what he or she means allows your patient to clarify what is being described. Responses such as "I don't understand what you're telling me. Would you tell me about this again?" allow you to evaluate your patient's thought process, fosters the therapeutic relationship, and provides more detailed information in understanding what is of concern to your patient.

Sharing impressions

It is important to review what you have heard and reflect back your impression of what your patient is thinking and feeling. Encourage your patient to correct any misunderstanding that may have occurred. A response such as "Tell me if this is what you are saying" conveys that you are listening and wish to fully understand your patient's thoughts and feelings.

Share—don't challenge

Sharing, like restating, allows your patient to correct any confusions or misunderstandings and provides insight into his or her thoughts and feelings. It is important to monitor your response to share not challenge your patient.

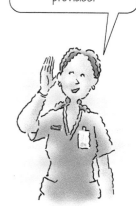

Ask the patient to clarify any confusing or vague information that he or she provides.

Restating

Restating, as with validating, reviews the information that your patient has shared but summarizes the information in your own words to confirm that you understand what he or she has said. This allows your patient to correct any misunderstanding, reinforces that you are interested in listening, encourages continued conversation, and may open an opportunity to provide education on a particular issue. An example of restating includes "If I understand you correctly, you are saying that you don't like taking medication several times a day."

Focusing

At times, patients can be disorganized and confused. Helping a patient to focus by asking a question such as "Can you tell me more about what is bothering you?" allows your patient to address a particular situation.

Providing information

Psychiatric nurses educate patients regarding medications, interventions, and treatment options. Providing information in a way that patients can understand based on their level of health literacy supports a therapeutic alliance and provides meaningful guidance to help them manage their condition. Be cautious not to provide advice while providing education (Townsend, 2017).

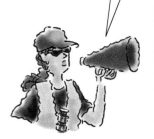

Allow the patient to make his or her own choices; practice listening rather than directing.

Assessment

Assessment is the basis of the nursing process. Psychiatric nursing, like other nursing specialties, is an evidence-based practice that involves evaluating our patients physically, emotionally, and psychosocially to identify assets and deficits. It is essential in initiating and evaluating treatment strategies and broadly informs nursing practice.

Testing—one, two, three

Accurate assessment techniques provide important updates on the physical, emotional, and behavioral changes of our patients. Appropriate screening and assessment tools and scales (e.g., Patient Health Questionnaire-9 [PHQ-9], Mood Disorder Questionnaire [MDQ], and World Health Organization Disability Assessment Schedule 2.0) are helpful in evaluating changes in a patient's presentation over periods of time.

Nursing interview in psychiatric mental health nursing

A systematic interview gathers broad information that helps you to:
1. assess the patient's psychological functioning
2. identify the underlying or precipitating cause of the patient's current concern
3. understand the patient's coping methods and their effect on psychosocial growth
4. formulate the care plan
5. gauge progress and the effectiveness of treatments.

What's the point?

It is important to help patients understand the importance of gathering information in a systematic way to identify concerns. We must also communicate the benefits of addressing those concerns in an organized and appropriate manner.

General guidelines

In patient interviews, nurses ask a lot of personal and sensitive information. It is important to follow guidelines to ensure privacy.

Ensure privacy

Under the federal Health Insurance Portability and Accountability Act of 1996 (HIPAA) law, it is essential to maintain a patient's confidentiality and protect his or her information from being shared unnecessarily. Interviews should be completed in a private, albeit safe, setting that will limit interruptions and provide a calm environment (U.S. Department of Health and Human Services, 2015).

Just the two of us

It is important that your patient understands that his or her privacy will be protected. Allow your patient to express who he or she feels should be involved during the interview process. There are many sensitive topics (e.g., sexual or substance activity) which he or she may be reluctant to share with family members present. It is appropriate to professionally ask them to leave the area while addressing those issues.

Show support and sensitivity

Patients with mental health conditions express themselves in many different ways. It is not uncommon to meet disorganized, psychotic, hypertalkative, withdrawn, or angry patients. Many are unable to explain why they need treatment. It is important to make your patient feel safe and calm so that you are able to obtain an understanding of the concern through careful questioning, listening to responses, and objectively evaluating what you have learned. (See *Interview do's and don'ts*, page 20.)

Use reliable information sources

Some patients are "unreliable reporters" because of their psychotic or emotional presentation at the time of their first interview. It is important to identify collateral sources that know the patient well and are able to provide a better understanding of the history of the patient's concern. It is necessary, however, to obtain permission from our patients prior to interviewing the identified resources.

Consider the patient's culture

It is important to recognize that patients are from diverse backgrounds and cultures. Being aware of bias is essential to avoid misunderstandings and foster acceptance of all patients. (See *Abnormal—or just unfamiliar?*, page 21, and *Culture and conduct*, page 22.)

Interview do's and don'ts

When interviewing patients with mental health conditions, follow these guidelines.

Do set clear goals

An assessment interview is a systematic approach to obtain a history of the present illness (concern), prior episodes of psychiatric treatment, the presentation of symptoms—depressive or psychotic, history of self-harmful behaviors—suicidal thoughts or plans, prior suicide attempts, self-harmful behaviors of cutting or burning, etc. These are important to evaluate for every patient.

Do heed unspoken signals

Listening and observing each patient provide important clues in evaluating the health of your patient. Is the conversation organized and logical? Is speech rapid and pressured? Is he or she hyperverbal or with speech latency? Does the patient provide a lot of detail or seem dismissive? Does he or she appear anxious or depressed? Is he or she dismissive, anxious, grandiose, or depressed? How does the patient describe his or her mood, and does that mood description match your objective assessment (mood/affect congruity)?

Do check yourself

Patients often trigger an emotional response from their provider, such as aggression causing a fear response or anxiousness causing an anxiety response. These feelings of countertransference may occur when a patient sparks an underlying emotional feeling in the provider of care. It is important to be aware of your response to patients to avoid any interference in your ability to work therapeutically and professionally.

Don't rush

Take your time completing the interview. This is a time to gain information and, just as importantly, to establish a therapeutic relationship with your patient.

Don't make assumptions

It is important to ask questions about how situations affected your patient and what meaning he or she gives to each of those events. For one patient, the death of a beloved pet may trigger feelings of deep loss, sadness, and guilt, whereas for another, the response may be of anger and frustration. The importance of the event depends on how each patient internalizes his or her loss. It is dangerous to assume that because we feel a certain way, everyone else also feels that way.

Don't judge the patient

It is important to understand yourself and your biases so that you do not impose these beliefs on your patient. Remaining professional and "nonjudgmental" is essential to developing a therapeutic relationship. Your patient may have different beliefs than you have, but it is the appropriateness and logic of those beliefs that matter, not whether they share the same thinking as you.

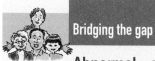

Bridging the gap

Abnormal—or just unfamiliar?

Cultural awareness is very important when working with psychiatric patients. Identifying cultural beliefs early in the assessment avoids confusion and mislabeling of symptoms. It is important to include consultants when evaluating unusual or unclear cultural beliefs. For example, Latina/o immigrants may avoid seeking mental health treatment due to embarrassment and fear of social discrimination. Psychological distress may instead be expressed as physical symptoms. Mental illness is highly stigmatized in many Asian cultures, with a belief that family prestige may be marred for seeking help for depression, anxiety, or other personal issues (Sue & Sue, 2016). It is important for the nurse to understand the underlying cultural beliefs that may support the patient's fears.

Beginning the interview

Introduce yourself and explain the process and purpose of the interview. This often eliminates confusion and reduces the anxiety of your patient. Ask your patient how he or she would like to be addressed, and take the time to answer questions to begin the process of developing a therapeutic relationship.

Listening post

To put your patient at ease, speak in a private—but safe—area, keep a safe distance, sit so that you face the patient and make eye contact, talk in a calm and professional manner, and explain the process. For example, you may state "I'm going to be writing this information down because it is important that we understand what is happening as you describe it." Encourage your patient to provide pertinent details of onset, symptoms, prior treatment, etc.

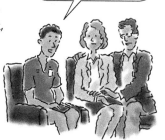

Can you tell me about Mr. Smith? He gave me permission to talk with you, and I'd like to understand what has been happening.

Biographic data

Determine the patient's age, sex, ethnic origin, primary language, birthplace, religion, and marital status.

Socioeconomic data

Asking your patient for their highest degree/grade completed, employment status, source of income, housing, relationship status, and relationship with family and friends allows you to evaluate your patient's resources, support systems, and outside interests. Increased socioeconomic stressors may increase symptoms of illness.

Primary concern

Quote what the patient reports prompted him or her to seek treatment. What symptoms were they having, and what made them

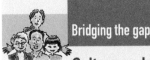

Bridging the gap

Culture and conduct

Culture and conduct
Be aware that several cultures respond differently to stressors. It is important to evaluate a patient's response with an awareness of cultural differences.

Shame and stigma
Mental illness continues to carry a social stigma. Many patients feel shame because of their illness. Some cultures hide their mentally ill family members and rebuff questions about them.

Spiritual balance
Treatment options may be affected by a patient's cultural beliefs. Some cultures may rely on spiritual or traditional remedies when making treatment decisions rather than Western treatment options.

decide that today was the day to seek care? For example, a patient may report "I was feeling more depressed and anxious that usual." Be aware that some patients do not report having mental illness, others deny problems, and some are unclear of why they are seeking treatment.

History of present illness
The history explores the primary concern addressing:
1. onset of symptoms—gradually or sudden onset
2. types of symptoms—auditory/visual hallucinations, paranoia, delusions, etc.
3. whether this is the first time the patient has experienced these symptoms or if he or she has experienced them in the past
4. how severe the symptoms are—mild, moderate, or severe
5. whether there is a trigger for the symptoms
6. if the symptoms get better or worse with medication, treatment, and/or lifestyle changes
7. whether the symptoms affect activity of daily living/employment
8. if there are any unusual/bizarre presentations

You sure there's no problem?
During your assessment, it is important to evaluate any medical issues that a patient may have. Many medical problems mimic psychiatric concerns, such as hypothyroidism/depression, hyperglycemia/psychosis, etc. Many severe or chronic illnesses may cause an onset of depression or anxiety. Some medications, such as steroids, can cause an onset of psychosis (West & Kenedi, 2014).

Great expectations

It is important for each patient to be part of the treatment plan. The patient may have expectations about what he or she would like to accomplish through treatment; for instance, the patient may want to be free from auditory/visual hallucinations and delusions or achieve a stable mood. The more involved a patient in setting goals for treatment, the more likely he or she will work to achieve them.

Personal history

Was the patient born following a normal pregnancy that was full term? Did he or she hit all of the normal milestones? How did the family cope with change? Are there cultural traditions that are honored by the family? Are there any particular generational coping strategies? What was his or her family like? For example, who comprised the family? What were relationships in the family like? How many siblings does he or she have, and where does the patient fall in birth order? What is the highest grade level or degree that the patient has achieved? Does the patient work? What leisure activities or exercise does he or she enjoy? Does the patient have a legal history?

Mental health history

This is a review of all past mental health treatment, including any history of inpatient or outpatient treatment, symptoms of illness, number of hospitalizations, medication trials, and any periods of full remission of symptoms; history and treatment for suicidal/homicidal ideation, suicide attempts, self-harmful behaviors—cutting/burning, and violence; and any history of alcohol, tobacco, or substance use or misuse, including amount, last use, and route.

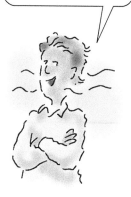

Go ahead. Ask me about my talents and accomplishments.

Reluctant responders

Many patients are reluctant to answer, or they provide incomplete answers to the questions that we ask. Remind patients that it is important to provide complete information to avoid problems such as dangerous withdrawal symptoms. Many patients feel alone or weak related to the stigma attached to psychiatric disease. Providing empathetic support to patients helps them to see these problems as an illness with available treatment rather than a character flaw.

Psychosocial history

A psychosocial history includes the patient's spiritual and cultural beliefs and practices, coping skills, diet, lifestyle, committed relationships, social networks, and sleep patterns.

Upheaval index

Reviewing difficult life changes and how these changes affected the patient gives insight into coping strategies. Learning how the patient managed significant change, such as a recent marriage, birth of a child, divorce, acclimating to a new job or job loss, illness, or death of a loved one, gives insight into resiliency. Ask about coping methods, support systems, and resources used to gain a full understanding of how the patient reacts in stressful circumstances.

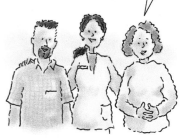

Inquire about coping with life events such as a recent marriage or divorce.

It's all relative

Some mental health disorders may have a genetic component. Because of this, it is important to ask about relatives with diagnosed or suspected mental health disorders. Additionally, if a family member has been treated successfully for a mental health disorder, the medication/treatment used to stabilize that family member may be effective in stabilizing the patient. Becoming aware of substance or alcohol problems within the family may indicate a potential problem for misuse. Even if this is not a problem at this time, it may provide an opportunity to educate your patient on the increased risk of misuse because of a family history of abuse. Successful family suicides or suicide attempts is a significant red flag for potential suicide risk for your patient. Additionally, child misuse and violence often follow in families and need to be evaluated.

Medication history

Many medical disorders can mimic mental health disorders. It is important to evaluate the patient for physical disorders, particularly diabetes mellitus or thyroid disorders. These disorders require a full evaluation because a perceived "psychiatric disorder" may be one of organic origin. Stabilize the medical problem and the psychiatric symptoms disappear. Additionally, be aware that many medications, including over-the-counter nutritional and herbal supplements, can impact mental health and cause drug-drug interactions and need to be reported (Gerberg, Muskin, & Brown, 2017).

Review the patient's medication history for therapeutic drug effects and adverse reactions.

Compliance check

It is important to have a complete list of all of the patient's prescribed medications (including over-the-counter nutritional and herbal supplements), a history of treatment adherence, and notation of any side effects that were experienced from medication. Additionally, under TJC guidelines, medication reconciliation of home medications is completed on admission to, and discharge from, the hospital. Throughout the hospitalization and on discharge, medication education and review is provided to the patient and written documentation is provided for reference.

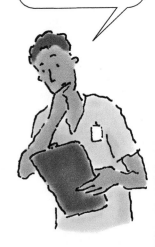

Physical illnesses

Many chronic medical conditions may mimic mental health symptoms. It is important to have a full review of systems and physical examination complete upon admission to rule out psychotic changes related to a medical condition. Some symptoms commonly associated with medical conditions, as well as psychiatric conditions, include disorientation, thought distortions, and mood dysregulation. Kidney or liver failure, infection, thyroid disease, metabolic disorders, or increased intracranial pressure are often to blame.

Mental status evaluation

The mental status examination (MSE) is an objective review of a patient's cognitive functioning. MSE is a structured, objective approach to describe the physical and cognitive function through multiple areas on a given day.

The areas of review with normal findings are:

1. appearance: appears stated age, no acute distress, dressed appropriately for weather and season
2. attitude: calm, cooperative
3. speech: normal rate, volume, rhythm, tone
4. orientation: alert and oriented to date, time, location, and circumstance
5. motor: no psychomotor agitation/retardation
6. mood: "I'm good."
7. affect: full range and congruent with mood
8. thought process: linear, logical, goal directed
9. thought content: denies auditory/visual hallucinations, denies suicidal/homicidal ideation, denies paranoid thoughts and delusions, and no thought distortions evident
10. insight: appropriate
11. judgment: appropriate
12. eye contact: appropriate.

Master of the MSE?

Nurses frequently complete MSEs to observe for changes from the patient's baseline. Careful observation of a patient helps to determine when to change the plan of nursing care.

Level of consciousness

Evaluating a patient's level of consciousness (LOC)—a basic brain function—assesses the amount of stimulation necessary to arouse a patient. Some medical and mental health disorders present with a reduced LOC, such as catatonia. Additionally, changes in LOC may indicate a change in condition, a change in liver function, acid-base imbalances, new or changing medical conditions, or a serious side effect from mediation that requires an immediate evaluation or a rapid response.

General appearance

A patient's general appearance gives physical clues to help evaluate mental status. As in the MSE, a patient's appearance is measured

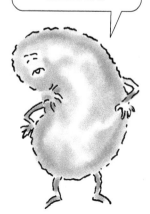

Oh dear. Kidney failure can cause an altered LOC.

against what is considered normal. When evaluating a patient's physical appearance, it is important to answer the following questions:

1. Is the patient dressed appropriately according to age, sex, and season?
2. Is the patient dressed in clean clothing?
3. Is the patient appropriately groomed, with clean hair, nails, and teeth?
4. Does the patient use cosmetics appropriately?

If your patient is disheveled with inappropriate clothing, poorly groomed, with excessive or bizarre makeup, it may indicate an increase in psychiatric symptoms or destabilization of mood.

Touchy subjects

It is important to measure a patient's height and weight on admission. Many medications can affect the metabolic rate, so baseline measurements are essential to monitor change. Assessing the color, condition of the skin, and any physical impairments or deformities provides clues to physical health. Unpleasant odors may indicate poor hygiene or infection.

Slouches, slumps, and substances

Assessing a patient's gait and posture on admission is important to evaluate for physical deformities, mood dysregulation, or fatigue. Changes in gait may indicate a patient is using substances or alcohol and may need to be monitored for withdrawal and other safety concerns. Poor posture or gait may place a patient at a higher risk for falling and safety precautions may need to be implemented. A shuffling, lurching, or unsteady gait may indicate neurologic problems.

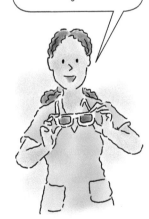

Are the glasses merely a fashion statement—or a way to avoid eye contact?

Facial facts

Assess your patient's facial expression and response. Is he or she alert with an appropriate affect? Are eyes tracking appropriately? Do pupils respond appropriately and of equal size? Does he or she avoid eye contact? Unequal pupils can indicate head trauma with an undiagnosed subdural hematoma.

Reality check

Assess your patient's understanding of his or her psychiatric symptoms and what brought him or her to the hospital. It is important to compare the patient's understanding with your observations. Document incongruities.

Behavior

Assess your patient's attitude and presentation. What is the patient's mood? Does he or she report feeling happy, sad, or euphoric? Is he or she hyperactive, restless, or calm? Is he or she cooperative, irritable, or mute? Are there any reports of inappropriate hypersexual or violent behaviors? Does he or she interact appropriately with staff and peers? Document your findings.

Gestures

Evaluate any gestures noted. Are gestures appropriate or inappropriate? Is he or she gesturing as if interacting with someone? If so, your patient may be experiencing auditory or visual hallucinations.

Mannerisms

Does your patient have any rhythmic, repetitive mannerisms? Could these be tics or tremors? Are they restless movements, fidgety, pacing—tardive dyskinesia or akathisia?

Attitude

Evaluate the patient's attitude. Is he or she calm and cooperative or aggressive, hostile, or violent?

Activity level

An increased level of activity, decreased sleep, restlessness, and increased anxiety, coupled with rapid and pressured speech, may indicate a bipolar manic episode. A decrease in activity, increased sleeping, poor interaction with staff and peers, poor appetite, and poverty of speech may indicate an episode of depression.

Speech

Assessing speech patterns, content, rate, volume, rhythm, and tone gives clues to a patient's level of function. This is also assessed in the MSE. It is important to note the characteristics of speech patterns to determine whether they reflect:
- illogical choice of topics
- irrelevant or illogical replies to questions
- speech defects, such as stuttering
- excessively fast or slow speech
- sudden interruptions
- excessive volume or barely audible speech
- altered vocal tone and modulation
- slurring
- excessive number of words (overproductive speech)
- minimal, monosyllabic responses (underproductive speech).

Sign language

Multiple modalities are available for hearing-impaired patients while in the hospital. American Sign Language interpreters, TTY machines, call relay services, etc., are available by appointment and by telephone. It is important to determine if a patient is hearing impaired or if his or her behavior is related to a psychotic event.

Time warp?

Does your patient struggle with poverty or latency of speech? This should be noted and evaluated.

Where's the logic?

Assess speech characteristics to evaluate changes in thought process. These alterations should be evaluated and noted:
- illogical or irrelevant replies to questions
- minimal or monosyllabic responses
- convoluted or excessively detailed speech
- repetitious speech patterns
- flight of ideas
- sudden silence for no apparent reason.

Mood and affect

To assess a patient's mood, ask a patient how he or she is feeling in concrete terms. Mood is a prevalent feeling but may change over the course of the day. Manic patients exhibit labile moods reporting alternating happiness and sadness throughout the day. An affect, on the other hand, is what is objectively observed: happiness = laughter, smiling, whereas sadness = depressed, tearfulness. The relationship between mood and affect is described as mood congruence—does the mood match the affect?

Mood control

Mood changes may indicate a physiologic problem as well as a psychiatric problem. Acid/base levels, dehydration, alcohol, substance, stress, and medication side effects as well as mania may cause mood lability. Mood lability can be associated with poor sleep, hyperactive behaviors, periods of happiness, and irritability. Inconsistencies of mood or mood incongruity may be observable during these periods and should be documented as such. These inconsistencies need to be evaluated and monitored to rule out metabolic or endocrine problems.

Flighty or flat?

Assess and monitor for indicators of mood fluctuations:
- lability of affect—rapid, dramatic fluctuation in the range of emotions
- flat affect—an unresponsive range of emotion, which may signify schizophrenia or Parkinson disease
- inappropriate affect—inconsistency between affect and mood, as when the patient smiles when discussing an anger-provoking situation.

Intellectual performance

Intellectual ability, the ability to reason abstractly, make judgments, and problem solve, is affected in emotionally unstable patients. Multiple tests have been developed to evaluate the distressed patient. These simple tests also identify organic mental syndrome. The Mini-Mental State Examination (MMSE) provides an easy assessment tool to evaluate intellectual performance:

1. Orientation: person, place, time, and circumstance
2. Immediate/delayed recall: List three items and have your patient repeat them immediately and again in 5 to 10 minutes.
3. Remote memory: Assess the ability of the patient to recall distant events that were important in his or her life and can be collaborated.
4. Attention level: Evaluate the ability to concentrate and complete a task over a reasonable period of time. If a patient is found to have a short attention span, simple directions may assist in maintaining a patient's independence.
5. Comprehension: Evaluate the ability to read, grasp the content, recall, and explain a news or magazine article.
6. Concept formation: Ask your patient to explain the proverb "Birds of a feather flock together."
    a. Aspire for the abstract: If he or she is able to report that people who think or behave the same way often are found together, the patient is exhibiting abstract thinking.
    b. Confoundingly concrete: If the patient reports that birds fly in a group, then he or she is demonstrating concrete thinking—found in organic mental syndrome, mental retardation, severe anxiety, or schizophrenia.

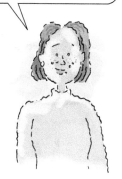

I'm only 12, but I'm old enough to think abstractly.

General knowledge

To evaluate "common knowledge," it is appropriate to ask questions such as "Who is the president of ..." or "What day of the week is it?"

Judgment

To evaluate a patient's understanding of illness and the ability to make appropriate decisions, it is important to assess judgment. While reviewing educational material on your patient's illness, you can ask "How do you know that some of the symptoms may be coming back and you need to call your doctor?" An appropriate response for a bipolar patient might be "I'm not sleeping as well. Instead of sleeping 7 hours per night, I'm only able to sleep 5 hours."

Insight

To evaluate the insight of your patient, it is appropriate to ask "What do you think is causing the problem with your sleeping pattern?" An expected response would be, "I had a stomach virus for 1 day and may not have taken all of my medication."

Degrees of insight

Assessing degrees of insight is important to understand risks to your patient and the need for further education. For example, a patient with bipolar disorder may blame his or her inability to take a morning dose of lithium to skipping breakfast and not wanting to take lithium on an empty stomach. Continuing to educate this patient may help to improve medication adherence. A lack of insight is commonly seen in patients with psychosis.

All in the interpretation

There is an ongoing debate of the impact of "nature versus nurture" when considering psychiatric illness. Many experts believe that both impact mood and function. Psychoanalysts and psychopharmacologists often view mental illness as a combination of unresolved conflict as a result of a real or perceived loss that may cause change within the neurobiology of the brain. For instance, posttraumatic stress disorder is the result of a real or perceived life-threatening event that changes the neurobiology in the brain on how this memory is encoded and the physiologic response to an event that triggers the memory. Both psychoanalytic and psychopharmacologic approaches work together to understand the underlying trigger through therapy and decrease the physiologic response via medication to control the symptoms of this disorder.

Sensory perception disorders

Sensory perceptions are described as hallucinations or illusions. Hallucinations are perceptions that appear real but occur in a patient's mind, whereas illusions are a distortion of how the brain analyzes sensory information.

Hallucinations can be auditory, visual, tactile, olfactory, or gustatory. Auditory and visual hallucinations are often reported in psychiatric disorders, whereas tactile, olfactory, or gustatory hallucinations are more commonly observed in organic disorders.

Illusions can occur with a misinterpretation of any of the senses, but the most common are "optical illusions." "Heat mirages" are a common type of illusion experienced by people who drive on a hot, dry, black highway. Illusions are not necessarily a psychiatric disorder.

Patients with a variety of psychotic disorders report auditory and/or visual hallucinations that can lead to disorganized and illogical behaviors. Patients in severe alcohol withdrawal may experience auditory, visual, tactile, or olfactory hallucinations that resolve over time. At times, patients report command auditory hallucinations (CAHs) that tell them to do certain things. CAH can be as benign as walking in a particular pattern or as serious as jumping from a bridge or stabbing someone with a knife.

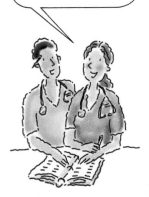

If the patient suggests something that is not grounded in reality, the nurse will assess the patient for hallucinations.

Thought content/thought process

During your assessment, it is important to note any thought distortions that become apparent. Is conversation linear, logical, and goal directed? Does he or she perseverate about a particular thought or idea, report auditory or visual hallucinations, and/or report paranoid thoughts of being followed or monitored?

Delusions

Delusions are fixed, false beliefs that have no basis, or a tangential basis, in reality. Grandiose delusions such as "You work for me. I own this hospital and I'll fire you if you don't do what I want" or religious delusions such as "God sent me to tell people about the coming flood. He gave me special powers" are commonly seen in patients with schizophrenia.

Check the references

Ideas of reference are those in which a patient interprets an innocuous event to be of personal significance. For example, a patient may believe that a television newscaster is reporting news directly about the patient himself or herself. The terms *ideas of reference* and *delusions of reference* are often used interchangeably.

Obsessions and compulsions

Obsessive and compulsive behaviors can create havoc in a patient's life. Obsessions, the thought or preoccupation with a particular aspect of life, may lead to compulsions to act on the obsession. For example, an obsession about safety may lead to constantly checking that the doors are locked or the gas is turned off on the stove. The creation of these rituals can severely impact activities of daily life. It requires considerable effort, often coupled with therapy and medication, to control these obsessions and compulsions.

Morbid thoughts and preoccupations

Assess the patient for:
1. suicidal, self-destructive, violent, or superstitious thoughts
2. recurring dreams
3. distorted perceptions of reality
4. feelings of worthlessness.

Sexual effects

Remember that sexual orientation and beliefs are unique to each patient. It is important to evaluate changes in libido. This can provide important insight into an emotional assessment. A nonjudgmental approach to sexual concerns, or other sensitive topics, allows patients to engage in what can be perceived as an awkward discussion. Be aware of your own biases or discomfort when addressing sexuality with a patient.

Competence

Does your patient have insight into his or her illness and need for treatment? Does he or she have any appreciation of the problems that exist, or may develop, from a lack of treatment? Are his or her thoughts based in reality, and is he or she aware of the effects of personal behaviors?

Be careful about competence

Assume that your patient is competent unless his or her thoughts or behavior strongly suggest otherwise. Ultimately, it is a judge's responsibility to evaluate and rule on competency and, if necessary, to assign a guardian.

Defense mechanisms

Defense mechanisms are coping strategies used to reduce stress and to protect ourselves. We all use these strategies when we are in challenging situations. These strategies can be adaptive or maladaptive and are often unconscious responses.

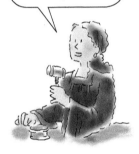

Only a judge can declare a person incompetent.

Name that defense mechanism

Defense mechanisms include denial, regression, displacement, projection, reaction formation, and fantasy. It is important to evaluate patients' use of defense mechanisms.

(For common defense mechanisms you may encounter, see *Defining defense mechanisms*.)

Potential for self-destructive behavior

It is essential to evaluate patients for self-harmful behaviors. Asking the patient if he or she is suicidal will not cause the patient to become suicidal but provides important information about risk for self-injury. It is important to be aware that not all self-harmful behaviors necessarily mean that a patient is suicidal. Some patients engage in behaviors, such as cutting, burning, or mutilation, which they report help them to "feel" through the release of endorphins or reduce what they perceive as overwhelming distress.

Suicidal behavior

Some suicidal patients report that they would rather be dead than to continue with the ongoing pain of depression or other mental illnesses. If we are able to reduce the symptoms of their illness through medication and therapy, we may empower them to better manage their symptoms. Remember, patients with depression struggle to find positives in their life, whereas patients with schizophrenia may have command hallucinations telling them to harm themselves and patients with bipolar disorder may behave impulsively. Recognizing the risk of suicide can be challenging and it is better to err on the side of caution

Defining defense mechanisms

People use defense, or coping, mechanisms to relieve anxiety. The definitions below will help you determine whether a patient is using one or more of these mechanisms.

Acting out
Acting out refers to repeating certain actions to ward off anxiety without weighing the possible consequences of those actions.

Compensation
Also called *substitution*, compensation involves trying to make up for feelings of inadequacy or frustration in one area by excelling or overindulging in another.

Denial
A person in denial protects himself or herself from reality—especially the unpleasant aspects of life—by refusing to perceive, acknowledge, or face it.

Displacement
In displacement, the person redirects impulses (commonly anger) from the real target (because that target is too dangerous) to a safer but innocent person. For example, a patient may yell at a nurse after becoming angry with his or her mother for not calling. The nurse is the "safer, innocent" person, whereas the mother is the "real target."

Fantasy
Fantasy refers to creation of unrealistic or improbable situations as a way of escaping from daily pressures and responsibilities or to relieve boredom. For instance, a person may daydream excessively, watch TV for hours on end, or imagine being highly successful when actually feeling unsuccessful. Fantasy helps the patient feel better momentarily.

Identification
In identification, the person unconsciously adopts the personality characteristics, attitudes, values, and behavior of someone else (such as a hero that is emulated and admired) as a way to allay anxiety.

Intellectualization
Also called *isolation*, intellectualization refers to hiding one's emotional responses or problems under a façade of big words and pretending there's no problem.

Introjection
A person interjects when he or she adopts someone else's values and standards without exploring whether they are personally fitting.

Projection
In projection, the person attributes his or her own unacceptable thoughts, feelings, and impulses to others.

Rationalization
Rationalization occurs when a person substitutes acceptable reasons for the real or actual reasons that are motivating his or her behavior. The rationalizing patient makes excuses for shortcomings and avoids self-condemnation, disappointments, and criticism.

Reaction formation
In reaction formation, the person behaves the opposite of the way he or she actually feels. For instance, a loved one may be treated with hatred, whereas a hated enemy is treated with kindness.

Regression
Under stress, a person may regress by returning to the behaviors used in an earlier, more comfortable time in life.

Repression
Repression refers to unconsciously blocking out painful or unacceptable thoughts and feelings, leaving them to operate in the subconscious.

Sublimation
In sublimation, a person consciously transforms personally or socially unacceptable drives into constructive ambitions and actions. For instance, a person who lost a friend to alcohol misuse may channel his or her anger into organizing a local chapter of Alcoholics Anonymous.

Undoing
In undoing, the person tries to undo the harm he or she feels he or she has inflicted on another. A patient who says something bad about a friend may try to undo the harm by saying nice things about the friend or by being kind and apologizing.

Withdrawal
Withdrawal refers to growing emotionally uninvolved by pulling back and being passive.

Recognizing and responding to suicidal patients

Assess your patient for the following indications of suicidal ideation (thoughts of suicide):

- withdrawal from others (social isolation)
- signs and symptoms of depression—crying, sadness, fatigue, helplessness, poor concentration, reduced interest in sex and other pleasurable activities, constipation, and weight loss
- overwhelming anxiety (the most common trigger for a suicide attempt)
- saying farewell to friends and family
- putting affairs in order
- giving away possessions
- conveying covert suicide messages and death wishes
- making overt suicidal statements, such as "I'd be better off dead."

Responding to a suicide threat

If you believe the patient intends to attempt suicide, assess the seriousness of the intent and the immediacy of the risk. A patient with a chosen method and who plans to commit suicide in the next 48 to 72 hours should be considered a high risk.

Tell the patient you're concerned, and urge him or her to avoid self-destructive behavior until the staff has an opportunity to help. Then consult with the treatment team about arranging for psychiatric hospitalization or a safe equivalent such as having someone be present with the patient at home.

Safety precautions

If you believe the patient is at high risk for suicide, initiate the following safety precautions:

- Provide a safe environment. Check for and correct any conditions that pose a danger. Look for exposed pipes, windows without safety glass, and access to the roof or open balconies.
- Remove dangerous objects—belts, razors, suspenders, light cords, glass, knives, scissors, nail files, and clippers.
- Supervise the patient when shaving, taking medication, or using the bathroom.
- Make the patient's specific restrictions clear to staff members.
- Plan for observation of the patient. Do not leave a patient at risk alone.
- Clarify day staff and night staff responsibilities.

Stay close

Helping the patient build appropriate emotional ties to others is the ultimate means of preventing suicide. Besides observing the patient, maintain personal contact with him or her. Encourage continuity of care and consistency of primary nurses.

When to keep secrets

A patient may ask you to keep his or her suicidal thoughts confidential. Remember that such requests are ambivalent—a suicidal patient typically wants to escape the pain of life but also wants to live.

Tell the patient you can't keep secrets that endanger life or conflict with treatment. You have a duty to keep the patient safe and ensure the best care (Townsend, 2017).

when creating an environment of safety. With any change in presentation, or an increase of symptoms of helplessness, hopelessness, or worthlessness, a suicide assessment should be completed immediately. (See *Recognizing and responding to suicidal patients.*)

Crisis control

If you have identified a patient at risk for suicide, it is essential to provide a safe environment to protect him or her from self-harm. With treatment, it is anticipated that this patient will be able to identify people important in his or her life and positive reasons for continuing to live. Unfortunately, we are not always able to save everyone.

Personality and projective tests

There are many assessment tools used to evaluate potential problems with patients. Several that are commonly used include the MMSE, Beck Depression Inventory, Hamilton Depression Scale (Ham D), Bipolar Depression Rating Scale (BDRS), Assessment of Involuntary Movement Score (AIMS), and the CAGE questionnaire. Psychological testing provides additional information that gives insight into intellectual functioning, focusing problems, or personality-related issues. Some of these screening tools are performed routinely during nursing assessments; however, many are scored and evaluated by the provider.

Physical examination

As discussed earlier, many physical illnesses present with similar symptoms as psychiatric illness. It is important that each patient is fully evaluated with a complete physical examination—including diagnostic studies—prior to any diagnosis.

Diagnosis

As nurses, we do not provide psychiatric or medical diagnoses, but we do choose applicable nursing diagnoses based on our evaluation and assessment. These nursing diagnoses assist us in planning effective care.

Planning

As an integral part of the treatment team, nurses are involved in creating and implementing a plan of care (see *Who's who on the interprofessional care team*, page 36). This plan is based on nursing diagnoses, the patient's diagnosis that is determined by the provider, and orders given by the provider. It is important to prioritize goals based on the severity of the problem—safety is always a priority—and how significant the impact is on the patient's life.

Effective planning must:
- focus on specific patient needs
- consider the patient's strengths and weaknesses

Who's who on the interprofessional care team

Professionals from varying disciplines and backgrounds may be involved in the care of patients with mental health disorders. The chart below identifies the education and responsibilities of each member of the interdisciplinary team.

Team member	Education	Responsibilities
Physician	Medical doctor or doctor of osteopathy, with a residency in psychiatry	Diagnosis and treatment of mental disorders
Psychologist	Master of science (MS) or doctor of philosophy (PhD)	Diagnosis of mental disorders, psychological testing, psychological treatments such as psychotherapy
Social worker	MS	Diagnosis of mental disorders; psychosocial therapies such as family, couple; also linked with community resources
Counselor	MS or PhD	Counseling
Occupational therapist	MS or occupational therapy doctorate (OTD)	Functional independence in tasks of living
Recreational therapist	Bachelor of science (BS)	Leisure-related activities
Nutritionist	MS	Nutritional therapy, education, maintaining balanced diet
Speech therapist	MS	Communication disorders
Expressive therapist (visual, musical, dance)	Master of arts (MA)	Expressive therapy through art, music, or dance
Pastoral counselor	Master of theology (or equivalent); ecclesiastical endorsement by faith group	Determination of spiritual and faith assets of each patient in the healing process
Vocational counselor	BS	Evaluation of student abilities, interests, talents, and personality characteristics so that they can develop realistic academic and career goals
Nurse generalist	Bachelor of science in nursing (BSN)	Provision of nursing care to patients in inpatient settings, offering direct and indirect care through the nurse-patient relationship
Clinical specialist	Master of science in nursing (MSN)	Provision of individual, family, and group psychotherapy in inpatient, outpatient, and community health settings and in private practice
Advanced practice nurse	MSN or doctor of nursing practice (DNP); certification in specialty (e.g., psychiatric nurse practitioner)	Provision of psychiatric mental health consultation to other nurses, patients, and families in the hospital setting

- encourage the patient to help set achievable goals and participate in his or her own care
- include feasible interventions
- be within the scope of applicable nursing practice acts.

Care plan

A care plan provides the structure for consistency of patient care. It is a document created by the interdisciplinary team that is reviewed and acknowledged by the patient that identifies problems, goals, and treatment strategies. It is the baseline for documentation and provides a benchmark for improvement of the patient. Each care plan is reviewed and revised based on a patient's progress.

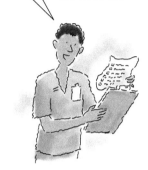

The care plan isn't a mere formality. It helps ensure continuity of care.

Goals

Each goal must:
- relate directly the identified problem
- be measurable and realistic
- be stated as a desired outcome as a result of multidisciplinary care
- reflect the agreement of the patient and family
- be stated in a way that the patient and family can understand (Townsend, 2017).

Implementation

The treatment plan is implemented on admission and continues throughout treatment. The patient and family are involved in the development and application of the plan. They are included in the ongoing review and revisions of the plan in order to best meet the needs of the patient. Each plan is individualized based on continued assessments and evaluations to provide effective care. It is the goal of every treatment plan to provide a decrease or elimination of symptoms so that each patient will be safely discharged and achieve an optimal level of function.

Treatments

There is a vast array of treatments available for patients. The cornerstone of treatment remains medication and therapy based on individual needs. Nurses work with a diverse community and many treatments are available to address particular issues including psychiatric illnesses, drug/alcohol withdrawal and detoxification, traumatic brain injury, and cognitive loss.

Drug therapy

Medications target particular symptoms by affecting neurotransmitters in the brain. These medications are carefully titrated to therapeutic levels to avoid uncomfortable or serious side effects and must be carefully monitored for efficacy, adverse effects, and adherence. Education about medication therapy is an ongoing role of the psychiatric nurse.

Types of psychotherapy

The therapist may act as a neutral observer or active participant. The success of therapy depends largely on patient-therapist compatibility, treatment goals, and the patient's commitment to therapy.

Individual therapy

Individual therapy involves a series of counseling sessions, which may be short- or long term. After working with the patient to establish appropriate goals, the therapist mediates the patient's disturbed behavior patterns to promote personality growth and development.

Group therapy

Guided by a psychotherapist, a group of people (ideally 4 to 10) experiencing similar emotional problems meet to discuss their concerns. The duration of group therapy may vary from a few weeks for acute conditions requiring hospitalization to several years for chronic conditions. Group therapy can be especially useful in treating addictions.

Cognitive therapy

According to cognitive theory, depression stems from low self-esteem and a belief that the future is bleak and hopeless. The goal of cognitive therapy is to identify and change the patient's negative generalizations and expectations—and thereby reduce depression, distress, and other emotional problems.

The therapist assigns homework, such as making lists of pleasurable activities to reduce or replace automatic negative thoughts and conclusions.

Family therapy

Family therapy aims to alter relationships within the family and change the problematic behavior of one or more members. Useful in treating childhood or adolescent adjustment disorders, marital discord, and abusive situations, family therapy may be short- or long term.

Crisis intervention

Crisis intervention seeks to help patients develop adequate coping skills to resolve an immediate problem. The crisis may be developmental (such as a marriage or the death of a family member) or situational (such as a natural disaster or an illness).

Therapy focuses on helping the patient resume the precrisis functional level. It usually involves just the patient and therapist but sometimes includes family members. It may consist of one session or of multiple sessions over several months.

Counseling and other therapies

Nurses are an important part of the interdisciplinary health care team. Psychologists; psychiatrists; and occupational, recreational, and art therapists may all be involved in patient care.

Psychotherapy

Psychologists, psychiatrists, and licensed social workers provide treatment through a broad range of therapeutic approaches designed to engage patients in identifying and modifying maladaptive attitudes, feelings, or behaviors. Psychologists are also involved in psychological testing that reflects underlying problems that impact treatment and treatment plan modifications. (See *Types of psychotherapy*.)

What is behavior therapy?

Behavioral therapy is appropriate for children and adults and may be used for individual or group therapy. It is used to change patterns of behavior, and multiple therapeutic modalities fall under its umbrella, including assertiveness training, aversion therapy, desensitization, flooding, positive conditioning, response prevention, thought stopping, thought switching, and token economy.

Assertiveness training

Assertiveness training increases self-esteem by encouraging patients to appropriately stand up for themselves while respecting the rights of others (Townsend, 2017). It teaches the patient ways to express feelings, ideas, and wishes without feeling guilty or demeaning others.

You can help the patient by providing examples of appropriate behavior and role modeling responses that are assertive rather than nonassertive, aggressive, or passive-aggressive.

Aversion therapy

In aversion therapy, a technique based on classical and operant conditioning, an unwanted stimulus is used to change unwanted habits (Halter, 2018). For example, a patient who abuses alcohol may be prescribed disulfiram, which makes the individual extremely ill if they ingest alcohol (Halter, 2018).

Systematic desensitization

The treatment of choice for phobias, desensitization involves teaching the patient techniques that promote relaxation and then slowly introducing exposure to the thing that is feared (Halter, 2018). For example, a patient who has a fear of flying in airplanes may be taught deep breathing and other relaxation techniques and then gradually introduced to a series of stimuli related to flying (e.g., visualization of an airplane; thinking about walking onto the plane to be seated; and eventually taking an actual flight).

During desensitization therapy, provide the patient with reassurance and review relaxation techniques. Monitor responses to each anxiety-producing situation and emphasize that the patient need not proceed to the next one until he or she feels ready.

Implosion therapy

Also called *flooding*, implosion therapy involves direct exposure to an anxiety-producing situation. However, instead of using relaxation techniques (as in systematic desensitization), this approach is based on the assumption that fast, direct confrontation helps the patient overcome fear (Townsend, 2017).

Implosion therapy is contraindicated in patients who have fragile psyches and for those who may have medical conditions (e.g., heart dysrhythmias) that could be exacerbated during treatment (Townsend, 2017).

Operant conditioning

Operant conditioning involves behavioral modification based on a system of positive or negative reinforcement (Halter, 2018). Positive reinforcement encourages behavior to occur more frequently, whereas negative reinforcement discourages behavior from occurring.

Thought stopping

Thought stopping helps the patient control inappropriate expressions of feelings by saying a phrase such as "stop" and then redirecting attention on another activity or thought. It can be helpful to teach the patient to visualize an actual stop sign when saying "stop" (Boyd, 2018).

Token economy

Using token economy, selected acceptable patient behavior is rewarded by giving out tokens, which the patient uses to "buy" a privilege or object, such as television viewing time, or special snacks (Boyd, 2018).

During this type of treatment, monitor the patient's behavior and provide or withhold rewards consistently and promptly (Boyd, 2018).

Behavior therapy

Behavioral therapy identifies problematic behaviors presumed to be learned and used in response to "triggers." Several therapeutic models look at the maladaptive responses, attempt to identify the trigger, and then challenge the response with the goal of changing the maladaptive behavior. Cognitive behavioral therapy (CBT) and dialectical behavioral therapy (DBT) are widely used therapeutic models to address problematic behaviors. (See *What is behavior therapy*, page 39.)

Milieu therapy

Controlling the therapeutic environment is the core of milieu therapy. The therapeutic milieu is more than the physical area of the unit. It is the community that is established by the staff and patients to promote a calm, healing environment. This occurs on locked or unlocked inpatient units as well as in outpatient treatment sites. It is one of many tools used to foster recovery through appropriate behavior. It requires the shared responsibility of staff and patients in their roles in conforming to the rules and policies of the community to maintain a therapeutic environment.

Out of uniform

Frequently, staff that care for patients with psychiatric concerns wears street clothing rather than uniforms while working in mental health settings. This provides an environment that feels "normal" instead of "clinical."

Detoxification

Many patients have primary or co-occurring problems with drugs or alcohol. Programs that are designed to safely withdraw patients from drugs or alcohol use frequent monitoring and medication to avoid uncomfortable and/or life-threatening complications of detoxification. These inpatient or outpatient programs provide a safe alternative to a "cold turkey" self-withdrawal following long-term substance misuse. During and following medical monitoring of withdrawal, therapy is offered to help patients understand the risks associated with continued substance use, and referrals for ongoing treatment are provided.

Drugs and dual diagnosis

Substance misuse and/or dependence continues to be an ever-increasing problem, and psychiatric illness does not preclude a patient from using alcohol or illicit drugs. These items are easy to obtain and readily available; are highly addictive; and may cause significant, permanent damage to the brain tissue. *Dual diagnosis also known as co-occurring disorders* is a term that is used to describe individuals with psychiatric conditions who have coexisting problems with alcohol or drug use, which over 7.9 million people in the United States experience (National Association on Mental Illness [NAMI], 2017).

Patients with dual diagnosis are less likely to follow treatment plans than those without mental health disorders (National Institute of Drug Abuse, 2018) and may be at higher risk for impulsive, violent, and suicidal acts (NAMI, 2017).

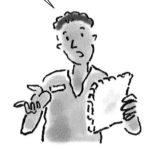

Many patients experience both mental health disorders and substance misuse.

Electroconvulsive therapy

Electroconvulsive therapy (ECT) has been used successfully to provide relief for patients with severe major depression or bipolar disorder that has not responded to other treatment methods (American Psychiatric Association [APA], 2016). ECT remains controversial as a result of preconceived beliefs and misinformation. It is important that nurses understand the risks and benefits of ECT to properly educate and support patients who choose this treatment option.

APA practice guidelines provide recommendations for the use of ECT, including education on the procedure with written and signed consent.

Procedure

ECT is performed in the operating room using general anesthesia. Small electrodes are placed on the head, either bilaterally or unilaterally, and a brief electrical stimulation of the brain induces seizure activity (Videbeck, 2017). ECT is typically administered two to three times per week for approximately 6 to 12 treatments, depending on the patient's symptom severity and responsiveness to treatment. Sustained improvement in depressive symptoms is often noted after a minimum of six treatments (Videbeck, 2017).

The most common side effects of ECT that occur the day of treatment are similar to those experienced after a grand mal seizure and include headache, fatigue, confusion, and short-term memory loss (Videbeck, 2017). Patients may also report persistent short-term memory loss and difficulty learning or remembering short-term events following ECT. Short-term memory loss typically resolves within a few months.

Can't explain it

Although ECT is not completely understood, it is thought that the electrical impulse causes a neurochemical change in the brain that is effective, over time, in assisting to control symptoms.

Evaluation

Through continued assessment, the nurse can evaluate the effectiveness of treatment. Assessment and evaluation are processes that are ongoing and provide continued information on the patient's progress. Additionally, they provide needed data when reviewing and revising the plan of care to best meet the needs and expectations of the patient.

Documentation

Documenting interactions and observations completely, accurately, and in a timely manner is the legal and ethical responsibility of the nurse. It is essential for continuity of care as well as confirming that nurses have completed the necessary treatments ordered for patients. Documentation should objectively address assessments, the plan of care, interventions, and the patient's progress toward meeting identified goals.

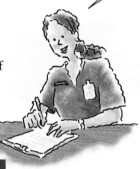

Documentation provides legal proof of the nature and quality of patient care.

Legal duty
It is the legal duty of health care providers to document the details of the care provided to the patient. Unclear, insufficient, or subjective documentation may result in a denial of reimbursement for services provided or provide grounds for liability of the nurse, other providers of care, and/or facility for inadequate or improper care.

Trends and concerns in psychiatric care

In the American health care setting, there has been a steady decrease over the decades since the 1970s in the number of patients that have been admitted and maintained at the various state hospitals as care has moved back into the community setting. Americans experience parity in the care of patients with mental health disorders. Reimbursement and funding dollars are often controlled by insurance companies that use case management algorithms designed to move patients to a lower level of care as soon as possible. Because of this, improved collaboration between inpatient, outpatient, community, residential, and ancillary services must improve.

Deinstitutionalization

Following the exposure of abuse to patients hospitalized in psychiatric facilities in the 1960s and 1970s, and with the advent of medications that better controlled the symptoms of psychiatric ill-nesses, state institutions discharged patients with psychiatric condi-tions more quickly. These discharged patients were to receive care within their communities in residential housing and outpatient treatment centers. Unfortunately, the quantity of services was not adequate for the number of patients that needed them. This failure has led to homelessness for some and the criminalization of mental health disorders for others.

Shame and stigma

Stigma and shame remain the most significant barriers to treatment for patients with psychiatric conditions. Advocacy groups continue to work to create public awareness and understanding for this vulnera-ble population while providing support and resources for the patient and family.

Legal and ethical issues

Professional standards established by the ANA describe the legal and ethical issues that structure the role of the psychiatric nurse. Professional psychiatric nurses must meet the same standards of "reasonable and prudent behavior" as deemed acceptable of other professional psychiatric nurses with the same experience and educa-tion preforming in the same capacity. Additionally, the nurse practice act of each state outlines the legal obligations of all nurses working with patients.

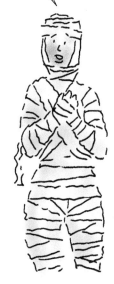

What's wrong with this picture? Caregivers can't restrict the liberty of a patient with mental health disorder.

Rights of the mentally ill and developmentally disabled

The U.S. Constitution protects the rights of all citizens. Patients with psychiatric conditions or developmentally disabled citizens cannot be denied rights because of disability or dependency. A violation of rights, even unknowingly, could result in serious legal penalties.

Life and liberty

Patients with psychiatric conditions and developmentally disabled patients have a right to life, liberty, and control of their lives as much as they are able. Unless a patient represents a danger to self or others, impeding a patient's liberty and controlling his or her behavior is illegal. The protection of the freedoms for vulnerable populations is the result of historic abuses imposed on individuals within these populations and the commitment to prevent this from happening again.

Right to treatment

The Constitution has been interpreted by the courts and establishes the right to appropriate, humane treatment for patients via all available treatment options.

Discrimination elimination

The Americans with Disabilities Act of 1990 (revised in 2009) guarantees parity for the disabled citizen by providing clear, comprehensive standards to eliminate discrimination against people who have disabilities. The term *disability* included impairments that are both physical and mental in nature.

Mental health patient's bill of rights

A universal bill of rights for patients with a mental health disorder was established in the Mental Health Systems Act of 1980. Congress outlined that treatment will be provided:

- by adequate staff
- in the least restrictive setting
- in privacy
- in a facility that provides a comfortable bed, an adequate diet, and recreational facilities
- with the patient's informed consent before unusual treatment
- with payment for work done in the facility, outside of program activities
- according to an individual treatment plan.

Keeping the patient informed

Nurses caring for a patient with a mental health condition must assess and evaluate what the patient knows about his or her illness and the need for treatment. Discharge planning begins at the admission. Enlisting the patient in development of a treatment plan encourages him or her to consider important elements in maintaining health and may improve "buy in" while discharge preparations take place. If the patient is unwilling or unable to participate in formulating a comprehensive plan, it is important to document specific barriers.

Right to refuse treatment

Most patients are able to make informed decisions to refuse or postpone treatment if that is their choice. These patients are considered competent to make health care decisions for themselves. If a patient chooses to refuse or postpone treatment within the hospital setting, he or she is stated to be making decisions "against medical advice."

Order from the court

In some cases, the health care provider or treatment team may determine that a patient presents a danger to self or others and requires medication, treatment, and a continued inpatient hospitalization. The laws governing retention of a patient against the patient's wishes vary from state to state. It is important to familiarize yourself with the laws in your specific state regarding this process. In most states, to retain a patient against his or her will, the hospital must petition the court to "hear" the argument from the hospital to retain the patient and listen to the patient explain the reason that he or she should be released from the hospital. If the court agrees with the hospital, then the patient will remain "committed" to the hospital for a specified period of time for treatment. If, however, the court agrees with the patient, the court will issue an order for the patient to be released from the hospital.

Rights of minors

It is essential for a hospital or facility to establish legal guardianship immediately upon the admission of a mentally ill or developmentally disabled minor. Generally, the minor is accompanied by a parent or an appointed legal guardian on admission.

Parental waiver

If the parents have surrendered responsibility for their minor child to an institution and the institution has provided the appropriate documentation to support this, the hospital may be responsible for decisions related to the care of the minor child.

Right to informed consent

It is not the nurses' responsibility to obtain informed consent from a patient; that responsibility falls to the primary provider of care. It is, however, the nurses' responsibility to provide important, pertinent information; clarify questions about the consent; and document any concerns the patient may identify. If a patient has additional questions regarding the actual treatment or procedure to be performed, the nurse must have the primary provider of care return to talk further with the patient. If the nurse answers "no" to any of the following questions, the mental health care team must be notified prior to initiating any treatment, so that clarification regarding the consent process can be further discussed.

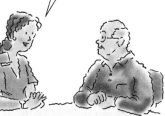

Let's discuss your understanding of the procedure you're about to undergo.

- Can this patient consent in the same way as another patient to treatment?
- Does this patient have a complete understanding of the risks, benefits, or alternatives of this treatment?
- Is this patient able to give informed consent?

Satisfying answers

It is the responsibility of the treatment team to provide complete information to the patient or the legal guardian so that they can make an informed decision. Because of the relationship that a nurse has with his or her patient, the nurse is often involved in answering questions, providing resources, and evaluating how well the patient or legal guardian understands the treatment option. The nurse may then enlist specific members of the health care team to address any confusion that may remain.

Who is liable?

It is important to remember that the role as a nurse is to advocate for patients. If informed consent is not obtained and the nurse chooses to participate in the procedure, the nurse—along with the primary provider of care and/or the facility—could be held liable. In many states, that statute may be until the minor becomes an adult (e.g., age 18). Obtaining consent or partitioning the courts for treatment over objection protects your patient as well as you, your team, and the facility.

Consent to medical research

Drastic, extreme, or questionable forms of treatment prompt many complicated questions and ethical considerations. Hospitals and organizations rely on their institutional review board (IRB) to review the risks, benefits, and needs of any patient that may be considered for these treatments that are part of research studies. Individuals should participate only when the potential benefits outweigh the risks and should be considered for a clinical trial. Patients or their guardians must fully understand the risks and benefits of any treatment and sign consent to participate in the study.

Ask the Feds

There are strict state and federal regulations that direct how clinical trials are implemented and require great care with the inclusion of mentally ill patients in a trial.

Right to privacy

Each of us has a right against unwarranted and unwanted intrusion into our personal lives. However, patients may have this right violated when health care providers carelessly discuss their private information in public areas. Be mindful of your environment, and protect your patient's privacy.

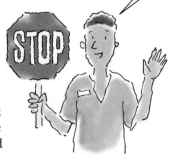

You must protect your patient's privacy and teach him or her about privacy rights.

Codes and bills

The federal HIPAA regulations, the American Hospital Association's Patient's Bill of Rights, and the ANA code of ethics provide information on how you share information, to whom you share information, and your responsibility in preserving your patient's right to keep personal health information private. In our role as health care providers, we are often informed of private, sensitive information and it is incumbent upon us to protect this information from unwanted disclosure. All records concerning care must be kept confidential unless the patient agrees to their disclosure. Remember that HIPAA is the law!

Teaching patients about privacy rights

As an advocate for patients, it is our responsibility as a nurse to behave in a professional, ethical manner as described by the nurse practice act of our state as well as other guidelines mentioned earlier. In this role, we rigorously protect our patient's privacy and educate the patient on his or her rights to privacy, not only while receiving treatment but also to personal medical records once treatment has been concluded. Within these rights, a patient is able to refuse the release of information, even to his or her family. Picture taking of a patient is prohibited in mental health facilities to avoid inadvertently including other patients in the picture and accidently breaching other patients' rights of confidentiality.

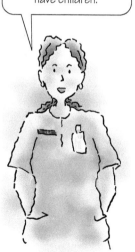

Patients with a mental health disorder have the right to marry and have children.

When you must disclose

The HIPAA regulations require that hospitals maintain confidentiality of their patient except in four instances:
1. suspected child abuse
2. criminal cases
3. government requests
4. when the public has a right to know.

Reproductive and sexual rights

Reproductive and sexual rights of the mentally ill patients have been upheld by the U.S. Supreme Court. These rights include the right to:
1. marry
2. have children
3. use contraception, abortion, or sterilization, if desired
4. follow a lifestyle of their own choosing.

Legal guardianship

If the developmentally disabled or mentally ill patient is an adult, it is important for the facility to determine if this patient has or requires a legal guardian. The legal guardian should be identified in the patient's chart. The legal guardian may be a spouse, parent, or someone appointed by the courts and it is important for the facility to be aware of the contact information.

When parents have been found unfit or unable to care for their children by the courts, a legal guardian will be appointed to accept responsibility for the care of the minor. If, however, the courts have appointed no guardian, the state will act in this role.

Can't seem to agree

Disagreements about a patient's care may occur between the patient and a legal guardian. If that occurs, it is essential to alert the appropriate channels within the facility.

Competence

Just because a patient has a mental health condition, it does not mean that they are incompetent or lack capacity to consent to treatment. Sometimes, however, members of the interdisciplinary team question the competence of a patient even if the patient has not been judged to be legally incompetent. Sometimes, illness may cause temporary mental incompetence. In this situation, it is important to consult state laws to determine who is able to make health care decisions for the patient. Frequently, it is a family member or relative that would make these decisions, but if there is no relative legally designated, willing, or able to make these decisions, a court must authorize treatment or appoint someone to make these decisions.

Restraints and seclusion

Seclusion and restraints are used only to prevent a patient from injuring self or others and only when other less restrictive methods have failed.

Restraints are a short intervention, often coupled with medication, and/or used in an emergency to maintain safety. Seclusion and restraints are not used for punishment or convenience but are meant to allow a patient to be in a safe place and regain control.

Restraint policies

The use of seclusion and restraints is governed by facility policies and accrediting body guidelines, such as those from TJC. The orders are time limited with the patient on continuous observation with frequent documentation. Patients are assessed

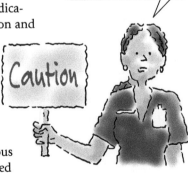

If you must restrain a patient, use the minimal amount of restraint necessary.

Caution

on a schedule for food, fluids, toileting, and safety. Seclusion or restraints are discontinued as quickly as the patient is able to regain control and agrees to remain in control.

Orders from the primary provider of care

Many states require an order from a licensed independent practitioner (LIP) prior to the application of the restraints. However, several states continue to allow an emergency application of restraints to be followed by an order as soon as possible following the application of the restraints. The use of restraints is time limited, and monitoring per TJC guidelines is required.

Quick quiz

1. Who developed the system for classifying and diagnosing mental health disorders?
    A. American Nurses Association.
    B. American Psychiatric Association.
    C. State boards of nursing.
    D. American Medical Association.

Answer: B. The American Psychiatric Association established the currently used system of classifying and diagnosing mental disorders. The latest version, published in *DSM-5*, emphasizes observable data and deemphasizes subjective and theoretical impressions.

2. Which assessment data are not included in the MMSE?
    A. level of consciousness.
    B. mood, affect, and perceptions.
    C. medication side effects.
    D. activities of daily living.

Answer: C. The MMSE examines the patient's LOC, general appearance, behavior, speech, mood and affect, perceptions, intellectual performance, judgment, insight, and thought content.

3. Which nursing statement reflects the nontherapeutic communication technique of minimizing?
    A. "If I were you, I would take this medication."
    B. "Don't feel badly. Everything will work out fine."
    C. "Why do you feel so depressed all of the time?"
    D. "I think your sister is right about how bad of a temper that you have."

Answer: B. A reflects "giving advice," C reflects "interrogating," and D reflects "taking sides." B minimizes the patient's feelings by telling them that everything will be fine.

4. How will the nurse document a preoccupation that is acted out?
   A. an obsession.
   B. a compulsion.
   C. a delusion.
   D. a hallucination.

Answer: B. A compulsion is a repetitive behavior that the patient feels compelled to perform in response to an obsession.

Scoring

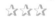 If you answered all four items correctly, superb! Your psychiatric sagacity is spectacular!

 If you answered three items correctly, well done! You're obviously all psyched up about psychiatric disorders.

If you answered fewer than three items correctly, don't despair! You have plenty of time to digest the material in this *Incredibly Easy* resource!

Selected references

American Nurses Association. (2014). *Psychiatric-mental health nursing: Scope and standards of practice* (2nd ed.). Author.

American Nurses Credentialing Center. (2014). http://www.nursecredentialing.org/

American Psychiatric Association. (2013). *Diagnostic and statistical manual of mental disorders* (5th ed.). Author.

American Psychiatric Association. (2016, January). *What is electroconvulsive therapy (ECT)*. https://www.psychiatry.org/patients-families/ect

American with Disabilities Act of 1990. P.L 110-325. https://www.ada.gov/pubs/adastatute08.pdf

Boyd, M. (Ed.). (2018). *Psychiatric nursing: Contemporary practice* (6th ed.). Wolters Kluwer.

Gerbarg, P. L., Muskin, P. R., & Brown, R. P. (Eds.). (2017). *Complementary and integrative treatments in psychiatric practice*. American Psychiatric Association. https://www.proquest.com/products-services/ebooks/ebooks-main.html

Halter, M. (Ed.). (2018). *Varcarolis' foundations of psychiatric-mental health nursing: A clinical approach* (8th ed.). Elsevier.

Kupfer, D. (2014). DSM-5: New opportunities and challenges for teaching and training. *Academic Psychiatry, 38*(1), 58–60. https://doi.org/10.1007/s40596-013-0002-x

Kupfer, D. J., Kuhl, E. A., & Regier, D. A. (2013). DSM-5—The future arrived. *Journal of the American Medical Association, 309*, 1691–1692.

National Association on Mental Illness. (2017, August). *Dual diagnosis: Substance abuse and mental illness*. https://www.nami.org/Learn-More/Mental-Health-Conditions/Related-Conditions/Dual-Diagnosis

National Institute of Drug Abuse. (2018, February). *Common comorbidities with substance use disorders*. https://www.drugabuse.gov/publications/research-reports/common-comorbidities-substance-use-disorders/introduction

National Institute of Mental Health. (2019, April). *Mental health information: Suicide statistics.* https://www.nimh.nih.gov/health/statistics/suicide.shtml#part_154968

Stahl, S. M. (2013). *Stahl's essential psychopharmacology: Neuroscientific basis and practical applications* (4th ed.). Cambridge University Press.

Sue, D. W., & Sue, D. (2016). Counseling the culturally diverse: Theory and practice, (7th ed.). Hoboken, NJ: Wiley. https://www.proquest.com/products-services/ebooks/ebooks-main.html

Townsend, M. C. (2017). *Essentials of psychiatric mental health nursing: Concepts of care in evidence-based practice.* (7th ed.) F.A. Davis.

U.S. Department of Health & Human Services. (2014). *Projections of national expenditures for treatment of mental and substance use disorders, 2010-2020.* https://store.samhsa.gov/system/files/sma14-4883.pdf

U.S. Department of Health and Human Services. (2015). *Health information privacy.* http://www.hhs.gov/ocr/privacy/index.html

Videbeck, S. (2017). *Psychiatric-mental health nursing* (7th ed.). Lippincott Williams & Wilkins.

West, S., & Kenedi, C. (2014). Strategies to prevent the neuropsychiatric side-effects of corticosteroids: A case report and review of the literature. *Current Opinion in Organ Transplantation, 19*(2), 201–208.

Chapter 2

Neurodevelopmental disorders

Just the facts

In this chapter, you'll learn:

♦ what constitutes a neurodevelopmental disorder

♦ signs and symptoms of neurodevelopmental disorders in children

♦ treatment options for children and adolescents with neurodevelopmental disorders.

What is a neurodevelopmental disorder?

Neurodevelopmental disorders involve an impairment in communication, behavior, cognition, and motor skills (American Psychiatric Association [APA], 2013). These conditions usually have an onset in a child's early developmental period.

Attention deficit hyperactivity disorder

A neurobiological disorder, attention deficit hyperactivity disorder (ADHD) is characterized by a pattern of inattention, hyperactivity, and impulsivity that is more severe than normally observed in children at the same developmental level. ADHD often co-occurs with other disorders, so all children identified at risk should also be screened for behavior or conduct problems, learning disorders, anxiety, and depression. On average, 8% to 11% of school-age children have ADHD (Krull, 2019).

Children evaluated for ADHD must have presenting symptoms before the age of 12 and experience them in two or more settings (e.g., home, school, with others, during activities) (APA, 2013). Diagnosis can be made by a health care provider who identifies the patient's behavior as primarily inattentive, primarily hyperactive, or combined (Centers for Disease Control and Prevention [CDC], 2019a).

Paying attention?

Approximately 6.1 million children in the United States have been diagnosed with ADHD (Danielson et al., 2018).

Gender preference: Males

Although ADHD affects males and females, males are more likely to be diagnosed with this disorder (Danielson et al., 2018). This does not mean that more males actually have ADHD; however, it does reflect that they are more likely to be diagnosed with it. Theories regarding this phenomenon include that males may be more likely to present with disruptive, hyperactive behavior (vs. females, who may present more often with inattentive, yet less disruptive, symptoms) that therefore requires earlier intervention.

Causes

The underlying cause for ADHD is not fully understood. Brain imaging studies in people with ADHD show some structural differences that may be related to functional impairment (Bukstein, 2018). Research shows that the disorder has genetic components, with an estimated heritability of 76% based on twin studies (Bukstein, 2018).

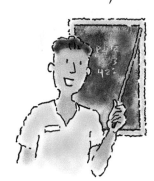

On average, 8% to 11% of school-age children have ADHD.

Risk factors

Some scientists believe the following conditions may predispose a child to ADHD (National Institute of Mental Health, 2019):

- genetics
- environmental exposure to toxins (e.g., lead) at a young age
- maternal use of drugs, alcohol, or cigarettes while pregnant
- maternal exposure to environmental poisons while pregnant
- prematurity or low birth weight
- brain injury.

Signs and symptoms

Signs and symptoms of ADHD are classified as "inattention" or "hyperactivity and impulsivity" (APA, 2013). These types of symptoms can intensify when the child is bored, in an unstructured situation, or required to concentrate or focus on a task for an extended period.

Inattention

Children with ADHD have a short attention span, may appear to not listen, and have difficulty keeping their minds on a specific task (unless tremendously interested in it). They get bored easily, tiring of tasks they do not enjoy after just a few minutes.

Difficulty concentrating

Although children with ADHD may give effortless attention to the things they enjoy, they have difficulty concentrating and focusing deliberate, conscious attention on organizing and completing a task or learning something new. Inattention causes them to disengage, lose things, be forgetful, and make careless mistakes. They may not pay attention to necessary details, fail to finish tasks, and have trouble with organization. Easily distracted, they may be reluctant to engage in tasks that call for sustained mental effort. (See *Is ADHD related to psychosis?*)

Impulsiveness

Children with ADHD have trouble controlling immediate reactions. They are often observed acting before they think. For example, the child with ADHD may not wait for a person to ask a complete question; they may blurt out remarks or answer a question before the person has finished asking it.

Difficulty waiting

Waiting for their turn or things they want can be challenging for children with ADHD. When upset, they may grab another child's toy or strike out physically to obtain what is desired at that moment.

Hyperactivity

Children with ADHD may appear to be always in motion. In school, it is common to notice this child fidgeting or squirming in their seat, roaming around the room, or talking excessively. They often have difficulty engaging in quiet activities and may find it very challenging to sit through a class.

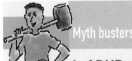
Myth busters

Is ADHD related to psychosis?

Myths and misinformation can cause needless worry in caregivers of children with ADHD. One myth involves the reputed link between ADHD and psychosis.
Myth: Children with ADHD can easily become psychotic.
Reality: Children with ADHD may seem disorganized because of their impulsiveness and distractibility. Research shows that although psychosis and ADHD can be comorbid conditions, this is also true of many psychiatric disorders. It should not be automatically assumed that the child with ADHD will have psychosis.

Diagnosis

The child should receive a complete medical and neurologic examination, along with hearing and vision screening. Laboratory tests such as a blood lead level may be ordered. Behavior rating scales, such as Vanderbilt Assessment Scale, can be exceptionally helpful in diagnosis (National Institute for Children's Health Quality, 2002). A psychiatric evaluation should be performed to assess intellectual ability, academic achievement, and potential learning disorder problems. Sometimes, speech and language evaluations are also necessary.

Pathway to the diagnosis

Caregivers frequently report that the child who may have ADHD was very active as a toddler. Symptoms including hyperactivity and inattention usually become more visible in the early elementary school years, although children as young as 4 can be evaluated (Wolraich et al., 2019). During adolescence, the outward signs of hyperactivity diminish and turn inward to feelings of restlessness, annoyance, and impatience. It is important to note that children with serious inattention-type symptoms tend to have academic difficulty and problems with peers and daily school activities. Adolescents with ADHD often experience emotional dysregulation which negatively impacts social relationships (Bunford et al., 2018).

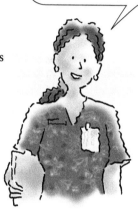

During adolescence, the outward signs of hyperactivity diminish and turn inward to feelings of restlessness, annoyance, and impatience.

Treatment

Treatment focuses on coordinating the child's psychological and physiologic needs. Drugs like methylphenidate (Concerta) or lisdexamfetamine dimesylate (Vyvanse) help to ease inattention, impulsiveness, and hyperactivity. Psychotherapy can reduce ADHD symptoms and teach the child and family ways to modify behaviors. (See *Pharmacologic options for treating ADHD*, pages 56–59.)

The child also may benefit from an individualized educational plan (IEP), constructed with special services that support and build strengths and minimize problems stemming from identified vulnerabilities.

Nursing interventions

These interventions are appropriate for a child with ADHD:

- Create and maintain a safe, calm environment that minimizes stimulation and distractions, and helps the child remain in control.

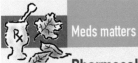

Pharmacologic options for treating ADHD

Central nervous system stimulants and nonstimulants have been used effectively to control symptoms of ADHD in both children and adults—lisdexamfetamine dimesylate (Vyvanse), methylphenidate (Concerta), atomoxetine (Strattera), and guanfacine (Intuniv). For many patients, these drugs dramatically reduce hyperactivity and improve their ability to focus, learn, and work.

Drug	Adverse reactions		Contraindications
Lisdexamfetamine dimesylate (Vyvanse)	• Anorexia • Anxiety • Decreased appetite • Gastrointestinal (GI) pain or upset • Growth suppression or weight loss • Insomnia • Psychosis or manic symptoms in patients with no prior history of such • Xerostomia		• Use of monoamine oxidase (MAO) inhibitor therapy within previous 14 days (may cause a hypertensive crisis) • Cardiac abnormalities (cardiomyopathy, structural abnormalities, heart arrhythmias, coronary artery disease) • Glaucoma • Pregnancy and breastfeeding
Methylphenidate (Concerta, Ritalin)	• Anorexia • Palpitations • Growth suppression or weight loss • GI pain or upset • Insomnia • Xerostomia • Tremors	• Headache • Insomnia • Transient motor tics • Mild blood pressure elevation • Social withdrawal • Rebound hyperactivity or irritability • Metallic taste • Blurred vision	• Use of MAO inhibitor therapy within previous 14 days (may cause a hypertensive crisis) • Tourette disorder • Motor tics • Cardiac abnormalities (cardiomyopathy, structural abnormalities, heart arrhythmias, coronary artery disease) • Glaucoma • Severe anxiety or agitation
Guanfacine (Intuniv)	• Dizziness • Insomnia • Irritability, confusion, or agitation • Nightmares • Depression • GI pain or upset • Rash • Syncope • Rebound effect • Xerostomia	• Weight gain • Blood pressure alterations • Headache • Vision disturbance • Increased urination • Enuresis • Rhinitis	• Children younger than 6 years • Cardiovascular disease • Cardiac abnormalities (hypotension, orthostatic hypotension, bradycardia, heart block) • Impaired renal function • Impaired liver function • Pregnancy • History of syncope

Nursing interventions

- Administer early in the day to avoid insomnia.
- Teach to swallow without chewing or crushing.
- Discuss concurrent use of prescription and over-the-counter (OTC) drugs with child's primary health care provider.
- Monitor height and weight regularly.
- Monitor sleep patterns.
- Be aware that stimulant drugs have the potential for dependency and misuse.
- Use of caffeine can increase stimulant effect.
- Teach caregivers about having the child continue medication over vacations and holidays.

- Give oral dose with meals to minimize anorexia.
- Apply Ritalin patch directly upon opening pouch to a dry, clean hip area and use on alternate hips daily while assessing skin integrity.
- Administer at least 6 hours before bedtime or 8 hours if extended release.
- Monitor growth and development regularly. Weigh the child two to three times weekly.
- Monitor vital signs.
- Monitor for tics.
- Teach caregivers about having the child continue medication over vacations and holidays.
- Be aware that stimulant drugs have the potential for dependency and misuse.

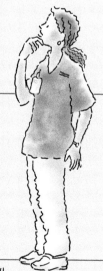

- Give with food in the evening to minimize daytime sleepiness.
- Take extended-release tablets with liquids like water or milk but not with a high-fat meal.
- Tell caregivers that therapeutic effects take 3 to 4 weeks to appear.
- Monitor for signs of dehydration or overheating.
- Discuss concurrent use of OTC drugs with the child's primary health care provider.
- Teach caregivers about having the child continue medication over vacations and holidays.
- Instruct caregivers not to abruptly stop the drug, but to wean off of it under the health care provider's directions.

(continued)

Pharmacologic options for treating ADHD *(continued)*

Drug	Adverse reactions		Contraindications
Atomoxetine (Strattera)	• Anorexia • Diaphoresis • Weight loss • GI pain or upset • Mood swings with crying • Xerostomia • Skin rash	• Urinary hesitancy or retention • Orthostatic hypertension • Headache • Muscle pain • Dermatitis • Irritability • Hypersensitivity reactions • Insomnia • Elevated liver enzymes • Jaundice	• Children younger than 6 years • Cardiac structural abnormalities, cardiomyopathy, arrhythmias • Glaucoma • Impaired cardiac function • Impaired liver function • Pheochromocytoma • Use of MAO inhibitor therapy within previous 14 days (may cause a hypertensive crisis) • Pregnancy

- Develop a trusting and accepting relationship with the child.
- Encourage the child to talk about problems, difficulties, and feelings.
- Assess potential for risk of injury related to hyperactivity and gross motor behaviors.

Learn acceptable behaviors

- Help the child differentiate between acceptable and unacceptable behaviors.
- Discuss disruptive behaviors, patterns of losing control, and the consequences of these behaviors.
- Teach the child ways to make positive choices and select appropriate ways of behaving.
- Monitor the child's activities and assist the child to learn to set limits, stay calm, and take opportunities to control undesirable behaviors.

Subdue the symptoms

- Schedule frequent breaks to help the child control impulsiveness and minimize hyperactive behavior.
- Teach caregivers that hunger, thirst, fatigue, the need to urinate, and other physical needs may trigger hyperactivity.

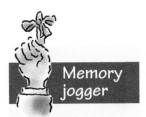

Memory jogger

The word **PEPS** can help you recall the major treatment components for ADHD.

Psychotherapy

Education

Pharmacology

Strengths

Nursing interventions

- Warning: This drug may increase risk of suicide ideation in children and adolescents.
- Monitor client very closely for depression or suicidal thoughts.
- Give single dose in morning or give half the dose in the morning and the other half in early evening.
- Give with food to minimize anorexia and GI upset.
- Monitor growth and development regularly.
- Tell caregivers that therapeutic effects take 3 to 4 weeks to appear.
- Monitor vital signs.
- Discuss concurrent use of OTC drugs with the child's primary health care provider.
- Know that higher doses decrease seizure threshold.
- Teach caregivers about having the child continue medication over vacations and holidays.
- Be aware that stimulant drugs have the potential for dependency and misuse.

- Instruct caregivers on the use of problem solving, time-outs, and natural consequences.
- Encourage caregivers to communicate with the children's school for an educational evaluation and development of a plan for needed services and accommodations (e.g., untimed tests, review sessions, repeating or reviewing assignment instructions, tutoring).
- Teach caregivers to implement a healthy meal and snack plan, as poor nutrition may exacerbate ADHD symptoms.

Ease impulsivity

- Help the child learn how to take turns, wait in line, and follow rules.
- Work with the child to divide tasks into doable steps in order to experience success in meeting identified goals.
- Encourage opportunities to participate in activities with peers.
- Provide the child with positive feedback for improvement and with encouragement to take steps to manage behaviors.

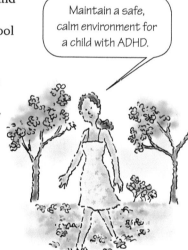

Maintain a safe, calm environment for a child with ADHD.

Autism spectrum disorder

Autism spectrum disorder (ASD) is a developmental disability that impacts social abilities, communication, and behavior (CDC, 2019b). It is usually diagnosed by the age of 2 and lasts throughout life. The health care provider will assess the child's responses to the environment and impairments in language, communication, and social interaction. Severity is determined based on the degree of social impairment and restricted, repetitive behaviors (Autism Speaks, n.d.). The provider will note the child's responses to the environment and impairments in language, communication, and social interaction. Individuals with ASD range in functional ability from highly functional to those who need constant care and support.

There are three levels of severity for ASD (Autism Speaks, n.d.):

- Level 1: requires support
- Level 2: requires substantial support
- Level 3: requires very substantial support.

At a loss for words

Typically, the child with autism displays a rigid thinking pattern (Autism Speaks, n.d.). He or she may have learning difficulties, intellectual differences, and challenges understanding and using language. The child may withdraw or appear to retreat into a personal fantasy world. People with autism often have trouble understanding the feelings of others and the world around them. Behaviors that are repetitive (e.g., rocking, body swaying) and self-injurious (e.g., head banging, biting self) may be demonstrated. Symptoms must be present in the early developmental stages and must significantly affect social, occupational, or other types of function (Autism Speaks, n.d.).

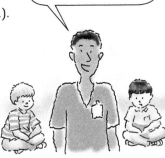

The child may withdraw or appear to retreat into a personal fantasy world.

Interpersonal challenges

A child with ASD may appear removed from others, may be averse to affection or physical touch, and refrain from engaging in social interactions. He or she may show a preference for inanimate objects rather than human companionship or friendships with others and may grow attached to such objects.

Five boys for every girl

This disorder occurs four times more frequently in boys than in girls, with 1 in every 59 children in the United States being diagnosed with an ASD (Baio et al., 2018). If girls do not have noticeable intellectual impairment or language delays, they may go unrecognized for a longer period of time.

Causes

No known cause for ASD exists. Some studies suggest it may stem from abnormalities in brain structure or function. Brain scans show differences in brain shape and structure in children with ASD.

Other possible causes of ASD include genetic or chromosomal predisposition, environmental factors, and environmental exposure (CDC, 2019b).

Signs and symptoms

Symptoms of ASD may be noted during infancy into the early toddler years. It is most commonly discovered when caregivers notice their child doesn't continue to develop as expected, becomes withdrawn or aggressive, or loses language skills already acquired. Sometimes, the child appears to develop normally until about age 2 and then regresses rapidly.

Mysterious crying

Young children with ASD may have impaired language development and difficulty expressing their needs. They may laugh or cry for no apparent reason. Even those who gain rudimentary language skills may not be able to communicate effectively.

Signs and symptoms

Other signs and symptoms of ASD include:
- abnormal speech patterns, such as echolalia (repeating words or phrases spoken by others)
- lack of intonation and expression in speech
- repetitive rocking motions
- hand flapping or body swaying
- dislike of changes in daily activities and routines
- self-injurious behaviors, such as head banging, hitting, or biting
- unusual fascination with inanimate objects, such as fans and air conditioners
- dislike of touching and cuddling
- frequent outbursts and tantrums
- little or no eye contact with others
- increased or decreased sensitivity to pain
- no fear of danger.

Diagnosis

Usually, most children with ASD are diagnosed by ages 2 to 3. However, no definitive diagnostic tool exists. Several other conditions, such as Rett syndrome and selective mutism, may resemble the disorder; the health care provider may use these as differentials until a firm diagnosis is made.

Narrowing the field

After ruling out other disorders (such as neurologic disorders, hearing loss, speech problems, and intellectual development disorder), a comprehensive evaluation is performed by an interprofessional team composed of a psychologist, neurologist, psychiatrist, speech therapist, and other professionals (National Institute of Neurological Disorders and Stroke, 2019).

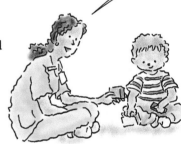

ASD is usually diagnosed by ages 2 to 3.

A team strategy

The interprofessional team uses various methods to identify the disorder. Multiple developmental screening tools are used to assess behaviors and developmental status. Tests may be ordered for certain genetic and neurologic problems. Caregivers are interviewed to elicit information about the child's behavior and early development and may be asked to videotape the child's behavior at home.

Screening for developmental problems

Developmental screening may reveal behaviors that suggest ASD, such as (Autism Speaks, 2019):
- limited or no eye contact by 6 months
- failure to babble or point/reach by age 12 months
- failure to say single words by age 16 months
- failure to say two-word phrases by age 24 months
- persistent preference for solitude; resistance to routine changes at any age
- loss of language or social skills at any age. (See *Screening tools for ASD*.)

Check the tape

Reviewing family videos, photos, and baby scrapbooks may help caregivers document when the child reached certain developmental milestones and when signs of ASD began to appear.

Screening tools for ASD

Although no single behavioral or communication test can detect ASD, several screening instruments can be used as aids in diagnosing ASD (Autism Speaks, 2019).

Modified Checklist for ASD in Toddlers (M-CHAT) (Robins et al., 2001)
This scale screens for ASD in children age 18 months. This is a short questionnaire that can help the caregiver determine if a professional should be consulted for further evaluation.

Autism Spectrum Screening Questionnaire (ASSQ) (Ehlers et al., 1999)
This 27-item screening scale is completed by lay informants regarding symptoms associated with ASD.

Screening tool for ASD in 2-year-olds (STAT) (Stone et al., 2000)
This scale uses direct observation to study behavioral features in children younger than age 2. It identifies three skill areas important in diagnosing ASD: play, motor imitation, and joint attention.

Diagnostic criteria

After evaluation and testing, the interprofessional team may arrive at a diagnosis based on clear evidence of:
- poor or limited social relationships
- underdeveloped communication skills
- repetitive behaviors, activities, and interests.

Treatment

A combination of early intervention, special education, family support, and, in some cases, medication may help some children with ASD to lead more functional lives. Early intervention and special education programs may increase the child's capacity to learn, communicate, and relate to others. This approach also may reduce the impaired social relationships, communication problems, and restricted activities and behaviors.

Biochemical boosts

Although no drug has been shown to treat the underlying disorder of ASD, the Food and Drug Administration (FDA) has approved risperidone (Risperdal) and aripiprazole (Abilify) for autism-related irritability. Short-term use of stimulants such as methylphenidate has been shown in limited research to reduce inattentiveness, impulsivity, and overactivity in some children with ASD (Sturman et al., 2017).

However, stimulant drugs also may increase the child's internal preoccupation, stereotypical behavior, and social withdrawal.

Other classes of drugs may be considered to manage symptoms such as compulsive behavior, irritability, and withdrawal.

Comfort through coping

Counseling can help the family better understand the disorder and assist them with coping strategies and behavior modification therapies. In some situations, home care is available to assist with the child's physical or behavioral management. If the child's disruptive behavior persists, alternative residential placement may be necessary.

Intellect, talent, and education

Intellectual differences are noted in people with ASD. Many children with ASD are good at drawing and using computers. Some children with ASD benefit from attending special schools that use behavior modification, whereas educational mainstreaming is preferable for others.

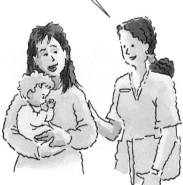

ASD symptoms start during the toddler period. Caregivers need to be watchful of developmental delays and regression in social skills or language.

Nursing interventions

These nursing interventions are appropriate for a child with ASD:
- Supervise the child and establish safe environments at home, school, and in the community.
- Monitor the use of language carefully by effectively choosing appropriate words, as the child is likely to interpret words concretely.
- Be in tune with the child's nonverbal communication because the child may express needs this way.
- Offer emotional support and information to the caregivers. Suggest support groups as a resource.
- Promote effective communication by teaching caregivers to learn about the child's communication style and verbal and nonverbal habits.

Routines and regularity

- Teach the child self-care slowly over time, using simple, concrete, and visual instructions based on what is reasonable for the child to accomplish.
- Teach the caregivers to maintain a regular, predictable daily routine, with consistent times for waking, dressing, eating, attending school, and going to bed.
- Suggest that caregivers use a picture board, especially if the child is a visual learner, showing the activities that will occur during the day to help make transitions more easily.
- If the child's routine must be changed, instruct caregivers to prepare the child for the changes.

Decrease temper tantrums

- Teach caregivers to learn triggers to aggression and avoid situations known to stimulate outbursts.
- Teach caregivers how to recognize behaviors that precede temper tantrums, such as increased hand flapping or irritability, and intervene accordingly.
- Help caregivers devise a plan to improve behavior by giving tangible rewards for desired behavior.

Strive for safety

- Instruct caregivers on ways to make the home safer (e.g., by installing locks and gates so the child can't wander unsupervised).
- If the child's behavior is self-injurious, teach caregivers ways to prevent injury by providing helmets and protective padding.
- Instruct caregivers to intervene to stop anxiety from escalating and offer diversionary activities.
- Inform caregivers that punishment may worsen self-injurious behavior.

Communication disorders

Communication disorders are characterized by ongoing difficulty in the use of language as well as the development of language skills. Per the *Diagnostic and Statistical Manual of Mental Disorders*, 5th Edition (*DSM-5*), communication involves any verbal or nonverbal behavior that ultimately influences attitudes or behaviors of another person (APA, 2013, p. 41). Language includes the actual form, function, and use of symbols to communicate (APA, 2013).

Risk factors for communication disorders

The main risk factor associated with communication disorders is a familial history of a communication disorder.

Specific types of communication disorders

Language disorder

Language disorder includes difficulty in acquiring and using spoken, written, or nonverbal language (APA, 2013).

Speech sound disorder

Speech sound disorder involves ongoing difficulty with speech sound production that interferes with, or prevents, verbal communication (APA, 2013).

Childhood-onset fluency disorder

This disorder, often called "stuttering," involves disturbances in fluency and timing of speech (APA, 2013).

Social (pragmatic) communication disorder

Social pragmatic communication disorder involves ongoing difficulty in social use of verbal and nonverbal communication (APA, 2013).

Nursing interventions for communication disorders

- Give the individual time to express themselves fully.
- Identify the ways in which the individual best communicates, such as through sign language or communication board, and use this modality.
- Collaborate with speech services for individuals with a language impairment.
- Encourage group therapy with others to help work on social communication skills (American Speech-Language-Hearing Association, 2019a).

Intellectual disability (intellectual developmental disorder)

Intellectual disability (ID) is a developmental disorder that is defined by limitations in general mental abilities and in performing usual activities of daily living. There are associated deficits in communication, social skills, self-care, and adaptive behavior.

ID affects approximately 7% of children aged 3 to 17 in the United States (CDC, 2017). Its onset occurs before age 18. Early intervention for babies and toddlers is recommended.

Learning process

Children with ID may take longer to speak, walk, and develop the skills to dress and feed themselves. They also may have difficulty learning while in school. They can learn; however, it takes them longer periods of time to master a skill. Challenges arise from the child's inability to handle the expected activities of daily living appropriate for age and culture.

Degrees of impairment

The degree of impairment for children with ID is based on severity and classified as mild, moderate, severe, or profound. (See *Severity levels for persons with ID*, page 68 and 69.)

Causes

Research shows that ID has prenatal, perinatal, and postnatal origins (American Speech-Language-Hearing Association, 2019b):

Prenatal

- Genetic components
- Metabolism differences
- Brain malformation (e.g., microcephaly)
- Maternal disease (e.g., placental disease)
- Environmental components (e.g., alcohol, drugs, toxins)

Perinatal

- Labor and delivery events that lead to neonatal encephalopathy
- Anoxia experienced at birth

Postnatal

- Hypoxic ischemic injury
- Traumatic brain injury
- Infection
- Seizure disorders
- Demyelinating disorders
- Severe social deprivation
- Exposure to toxins (e.g., lead, mercury)

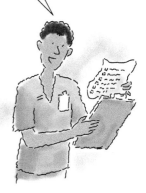

Children with ID may take longer to speak, walk, and develop the skills to dress and feed themselves.

Signs and symptoms

Family members may suspect ID if the child's motor, language, and self-help skills fail to develop or are developing much more slowly than those of the child's peers.

Typical indications of ID include:

- failure to achieve developmental milestones
- deficiencies in cognitive functioning such as inability to follow commands or directions
- failure to achieve intellectual developmental markers
- reduced ability to learn or to meet academic demands
- expressive or receptive language problems
- psychomotor skill deficits
- difficulty performing self-care activities
- neurologic impairments
- medical problems such as seizures
- negativity and low self-esteem

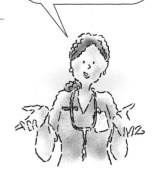

Maternal disease is one possible cause of ID.

Severity levels for persons with ID

The functioning level of a person with an ID varies with the degree of severity.

	Self-care ability	Conceptual	Social	Practical
Mild	May be able to live somewhat independently with monitoring or assistance with life changes, challenges, or stressors (such as personal illness or the death of a loved one).	Requires academic support to learn age-appropriate skills.	Can learn and use social skills in structured settings, although may be immature for age.	Can develop skills to achieve independence; may need assistance with health care, nutrition, finances.
Moderate	Requires supervision and needs to be monitored when performing certain independent activities.	Noticeably lags behind peers in conceptual and academic skills. Needs substantial academic support.	Speech limitations and difficulty following expected social norms may impede peer relationships, yet communication is possible with simple spoken language.	Can develop skills to care for self with assistance; may be employable in a supportive environment.
Severe	Requires complete supervision but may be able to perform simple hygiene skills, such as brushing teeth and washing hands.	Has little understanding of concepts such as written language or time. Requires extensive support.	Limited verbal skills are present; very basic single words, phrases, or gestures may be made to convey needs.	Trainable in basic activities of daily life; requires significant support and supervision.
Profound	Requires constant assistance and supervision.	May benefit only mildly from academic or vocational training yet may master simple self-care skills.	May understand some symbolic communication; does not use words yet may express self nonverbally.	Dependent upon others for support for all activities of daily living.

Severity levels for persons with ID

Adaptive skills used to define and determine severity of ID.

Adaptive domain	Skills
Conceptual	These skills include language, reading, and writing (literacy); money, time, and number concepts (mathematics); reasoning; memory; self-direction; and judgment in novel situations.
Social	These skills include interpersonal social communication, empathy, ability to relate to peers as friends, social problem solving, social responsibility, and self-esteem. Gullibility, the ability to follow rules, and avoiding victimization may also be included.

Severity levels for persons with ID *(continued)*

Adaptive domain	Skills
Practical	These skills include activities of personal care or daily living, such as eating, dressing, mobility, and toileting. Additional skills may include following a schedule or routine, using a telephone, managing money, preparing meals, occupational skills, and abilities in transportation/travel, health care, and safety.

A diagnosis of ID requires impaired intellectual and adaptive functioning in at least one of these domains. Impairment in ID generally affects participation in multiple settings (home, community, and/or school) and requires support. The severity of ID is defined according to the level of adaptive impairment and the level of supports needed.

Adapted from the following sources:
1. American Psychiatric Association. (2013). Intellectual disability (intellectual developmental disorder). In *Diagnostic and statistical manual of mental disorders* (5th ed.). Author.
2. American Association of Intellectual and Developmental Disabilities. Definition of ID. http://aaidd.org/intellectual-disability/definition

- irritability when frustrated or upset
- depression or labile moods
- acting-out behavior
- persistence of infantile behavior
- lack of curiosity.

Just a quiet child?

Disruptions or limitations in adaptive behaviors reflect the severity of ID. For example, a child with mild ID may show lack of curiosity and quiet behavior, yet may be somewhat self-sufficient, whereas a child with severe ID may have limited independent functioning that may persist throughout life.

Diagnosis

Diagnosis can be made by a health care provider after a comprehensive personal and family medical history is taken, a complete physical examination is completed, and thorough developmental assessment and intelligence testing has been undertaken. Various screening tests are used to help formulate a diagnosis. These may include screenings for hearing, speech, language, communication, and swallowing, as well as standardized assessments, parent-teacher surveys, and observational techniques (American Speech-Language-Hearing Association, 2019).

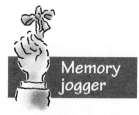

Memory jogger

To remember the major signs of ID, think of the five **D**s.

Decreased cognitive and intellectual functioning

Deficits in psychomotor skills

Difficulties in performing self-care activities

Degrees of neurologic impairment

Depressed or labile mood

The child should also be examined for underlying organic problems, including neurologic, chromosomal, and metabolic disorders. When discovered early, conditions such as hyperthyroidism and phenylketonuria (PKU) can be treated and the progression of disability can be stopped or, in some cases, partially reversed. If brain injury or another neurologic cause is suspected, the child may be referred to a neurologist or neuropsychologist for testing.

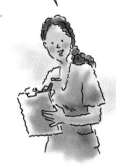

Screening tests measure the child's intellectual functioning and adaptive behaviors.

Treatment

Treatment focuses on coordinating the child's psychological and physiologic needs. Drugs are rarely indicated unless the child has an overlapping psychiatric disorder.

Key components of treatment for persons with ID include:

- behavior management
- environmental supervision
- monitoring of the child's developmental needs and problems
- programs that maximize speech, language, cognitive, psychomotor, social, self-care, and occupational skills
- ongoing evaluation for overlapping psychiatric disorders, such as depression, bipolar disorder, and ADHD
- family therapy to help caregivers develop coping skills and deal with guilt or anger.

Basic skills training

Many states have early intervention programs for children younger than age 3 with ID. Day schools may be available to train the child in basic skills, such as bathing and feeding. Extracurricular activities and social programs help the child gain self-esteem and learn social behaviors.

Independent living

Training in independent living and job skills typically starts in early adulthood (depending on the degree of disability). Many persons with mild disability can gain the skills they need to live independently and hold a job. Persons with moderate to profound disability usually need supervised community living. (See *Settings for those with ID*.)

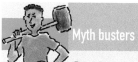

Myth busters

Settings for those with ID

It is often assumed that people with ID have to live in institutions.
Myth: Most people with ID live in institutional settings.
Reality: Since the advocacy movement of the 1970s, only persons with the most severe and profound ID are institutionalized (National Council on Disability, 2012).

Nursing interventions

These nursing interventions are appropriate for a person with ID:

- Determine the child's strengths and abilities and develop a plan of care to maintain and enhance capabilities.
- Teach the child adaptive skills, such as eating, dressing, grooming, and toileting.
- Demonstrate and help practice self-care skills.
- Monitor the child's developmental levels and initiate supportive interventions, such as speech, language, or occupational skills, as needed.
- Provide for safety needs in a consistent, supervised environment.
- Prevent self-injury, and be prepared to intervene if self-injury occurs.
- Teach about natural and normal feelings and emotions, and societal norms and behaviors.
- Monitor for physical or emotional distress.
- Modify the behavior by teaching and role-modeling how to redirect energy.
- Keep communication brief, simple, and consistent.
- Maintain adequate environmental stimulation.
- Set supportive limits on activities.
- Work to establish satisfactory communication and social interaction patterns.
- Work to maintain and enhance positive feelings about self and daily accomplishments.
- Teach caregivers to be patient and hopeful as they work with the child to develop skills for as much independence as possible.

Motor disorders

Developmental coordination disorder

Children with developmental coordination disorder experience a delay in motor skills that govern handwriting or coloring, walking, catching, using scissors, or riding a bike (APA, 2013).

Stereotypic movement disorder

Stereotypic movement disorder involves repetitive, purposeless motor behavior such as hand shaking, hitting own body, self-biting, body rocking, or hand waving that interferes with daily functioning (APA, 2013). It is understood that simple stereotypic movements like rocking, for example, are common in early development (APA, 2013).

Males are affected more with tic disorders than females.

Tic disorders

A tic is a sudden, rapid, recurrent, nonrhythmic motor movement or vocalization (APA, 2013). Simple tics may take the form of eye blinking, shoulder shrugging, extremity extension, sniffing, grunting, throat clearing, whereas complex tics include saying obscenities or making gestures, echopraxia, or echolalia. Males are affected more than females by a 4:1 ratio (APA, 2013). Treatment of tic disorder includes medications such as antidopaminergic drugs, alpha-adrenergic agonists, botulinum toxin injection, habit-reversal training, and behavioral intervention (Jankovic, 2019).

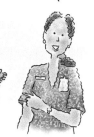

Nursing interventions

These nursing interventions are appropriate for a person with tic disorder:
- Allow the patient to focus on one thing at a time to avoid overstimulation.
- Help the patient become aware of feelings or sensations that may precede onset of tic.
- Teach about natural and normal feelings and emotions, and societal norms and behaviors.
- Provide the caregiver of a child with tic disorder with resources that are geared to prevent bullying.

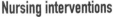

Quick quiz

1. The nurse is educating the caregiver of a high-functioning child who was recently diagnosed with autism. Which caregiver statement indicates that teaching has been effective?
    A. "My child will get well soon."
    B. "I will try to hug my child more."
    C. "I have caused my child to be this way."
    D. "I will create a daily schedule for our family to use."

Answer: D. Children with ASD respond more favorably to a predictable schedule.

2. Which teaching will the nurse include regarding administration of methylphenidate ER (Concerta) to an 8-year-old client?
    A. Administer at any time of day.
    B. Ask the provider who prescribed the drug.
    C. Give at least 8 hours prior to child's bedtime.
    D. Provide at lunch so food assists with absorption.

Answer: C. Stimulant medications should be administered at least 8 hours prior to child's bedtime. The stimulant medication can affect the child's sleep if given too late in the day.

3. The nurse is teaching the caregiver of a child with ID. Which caregiver statement demonstrates that teaching has been effective?
    A. "Better schools will help improve my child's abilities."
    B. "I am glad that there are medications to treat my child's condition."
    C. "My child will need support mechanisms in order to learn to the best of their ability."
    D. "There are no resources available that can help me with my child and their functioning."

Answer: C: Support mechanisms can help the child learn and function to the best of their intellectual ability.

4. A caregiver tells the nurse that a 4-year-old client stutters. Which disorder does the nurse anticipate?
    A. Language disorder
    B. Speech sound disorder
    C. Childhood-onset fluency disorder
    D. Social (pragmatic communication) disorder

Answer: C. Stuttering involves disturbances in fluency and timing of speech and is termed "Childhood-onset fluency disorder" (APA, 2013).

5. The nurse is preparing to administer lisdexamfetamine dimesylate (Vyvanse) to a client who received a monoamine oxidase inhibitor (MAOI) 7 days prior. What is the appropriate nursing action?

    A. Hold the drug and notify the health care provider.

    B. Contact the pharmacy to substitute guanfacine (Intuniv).

    C. Obtain a baseline blood pressure and administer the drug.

    D. Wait until at least the eighth day after the MAOI to give lisdexamfetamine dimesylate (Vyvanse).

Answer: A. Most drugs approved to tread ADHD should not be given within 14 days of taking an MAOI, due to the risk for hypertensive crisis.

Scoring

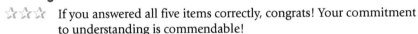 If you answered all five items correctly, congrats! Your commitment to understanding is commendable!

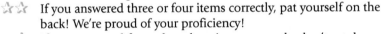 If you answered three or four items correctly, pat yourself on the back! We're proud of your proficiency!

If you answered fewer than three items correctly, don't get depressed! Review the chapter and pay close attention!

Selected references

American Psychiatric Association. (2013). *Diagnostic and statistical manual of mental disorders* (5th ed.). Author.

American Speech-Language-Hearing Association. (2019). *Intellectual disability.* https://www.asha.org/PRPSpecificTopic.aspx?folderid=8589942540&section=Causes

Autism Speaks. (2019). *Learn the signs of autism.* https://www.autismspeaks.org/learn-signs-autism

Autism Speaks. (n.d.). *DSM-5 diagnostic criteria.* https://www.autismspeaks.org/autism-diagnosis-criteria-dsm5

Baio, J., Wiggins, L., Christensen, D. L., Maenner, M. J., Daniels, J., Warren, Z., Kurzius-Spencer, M., Zahorodny, W., Robinson Rosenberg, C., White, T., Durkin, M. S., Imm, P., Nikolaou, L., Yeargin-Allsopp, M., Lee, L. C., Harrington, R., Lopez, M., Fitzgerald, R. T., Hewitt, A., … Dowling, N. F. (2018). Prevalence of autism spectrum disorder among children aged 8 years—Autism and Developmental Disabilities Monitoring Network, 11 Sites, United States, 2014. *MMWR. Surveillance Summaries, 67*(SS-6), 1–23. http://doi.org/10.15585/mmwr.ss6706a1

Bukstein, O. (2018). Attention deficit hyperactivity disorder in adults: Epidemiology, pathogenesis, clinical features, course, assessment, and diagnosis. *UpToDate.* https://www.uptodate.com/contents/attention-deficit-hyperactivity-disorder-in-adults-epidemiology-pathogenesis-clinical-features-course-assessment-and-diagnosis#H2002692884

Bunford, N., Evans, S. W., & Langberg, J. M. (2018). Emotion dysregulation is associated with social impairment among young adolescents with ADHD. *Journal of Attention Disorders, 22*(1), 66–82.

Centers for Disease Control and Prevention. (2017). *Estimated prevalence of children with diagnosed developmental disabilities in the United States, 2014–2016.* https://www.cdc.gov/nchs/products/databriefs/db291.htm

Centers for Disease Control and Prevention. (2019a). *Symptoms and diagnosis of ADHD.* https://www.cdc.gov/ncbddd/adhd/diagnosis.html

Centers for Disease Control and Prevention. (2019b). *What is autism spectrum disorder?* www.cdc.gov/ncbddd/autism/facts.html

Danielson, M. L., Bitsko, R. H., Ghandour, R. M., Holbrook, J. R., Kogan, M. D., & Blumberg, S. J. (2018). Prevalence of parent-reported ADHD diagnosis and associated treatment among U.S. children and adolescents, 2016. *Journal of Clinical Child and Adolescent Psychology, 47*(2), 199–212.

Ehlers, S., Gillberg, C., & Wing, L. (1999). A screening questionnaire for Asperger syndrome and other high-functioning autism spectrum disorders in school age children. *Journal of autism and Developmental Disorders, 29*(2), 129–141.

Jankovic, J. (2019). Tourette syndrome: Management. In UpToDate, Nordli, D. (Ed.), Waltham, MA. https://www.uptodate.com/contents/tourette-syndrome-management

Krull, K. (2019). Attention deficit hyperactivity disorder in children and adolescents: Epidemiology and pathogenesis. *UpToDate.* https://www.uptodate.com/contents/attention-deficit-hyperactivity-disorder-in-children-and-adolescents-epidemiology-and-pathogenesis

National Council on Disability. (2012). *Deinstitutionalization: Unfinished business.* https://ncd.gov/rawmedia_repository/NCD_UnfinishedBusiness_Paper_FINAL508.pdf

National Institute for Children's Health Quality. (2002). *NICHQ Vanderbilt assessment scales.* https://www.nichq.org/sites/default/files/resource-file/NICHQ_Vanderbilt_Assessment_Scales.pdf

National Institute of Mental Health. (2019). *Attention-deficit/hyperactivity disorder.* https://www.nimh.nih.gov/health/topics/attention-deficit-hyperactivity-disorder-adhd/index.shtml

National Institute of Neurological Disorders and Stroke. (2019). *Autism spectrum disorder fact sheet.* https://www.ninds.nih.gov/Disorders/Patient-Caregiver-Education/Fact-Sheets/Autism-Spectrum-Disorder-Fact-Sheet

Robins, D. L., Fein, D., Barton, M. L., & Green, J. A. (2001). The modified checklist for autism in toddlers: An initial study investigating the early detection of autism and pervasive developmental disorders. *Journal of Autism and Developmental Disorders, 31*(2), 131–144. http://doi.org/10.1023/a:1010738829569

Shprecher, D., & Kurlan, R. (2009). The management of tics. *Movement Disorders, 24*(1), 15–24. http://doi.org/10.1002/mds.22378

Stone, W. L., Coonrod, E. E., & Ousley, O. Y. (2000). Brief report: Screening tool for autism in two-year-olds (STAT): Development and preliminary data. *Journal of Autism and Developmental Disorders, 30*(6), 607–612. http://doi.org/10.1023/a:1005647629002

Sturman, N., Deckx, L., & van Driel, M. (2017). Methylphenidate for children and adolescents with autism spectrum disorder. *Cochrane Database of Systematic Reviews*, (11), CD011144. http://doi.org/10.1002/14651858.CD011144.pub2

Wolraich, M., Hagan, J. F., Allan, C., Chan, E., Davison, D., Earls, M., Evans, S. W., Flinn, S. K., Froehlich, T., Frost, J., Holbrook, J. R., Lehmann, C. U., Lessin, H. R., Okechukwu, K., Pierce, K. L., Winner, J. D., & Zurhellen, W. (2019). Clinical practice guideline for the diagnosis, evaluation, and treatment of attention-deficit/hyperactivity disorder in children and adolescents. *Pediatrics, 144*(4), e20192528. https://doi.org/10.1542/peds.2019-2528

Chapter 3

Schizophrenia spectrum and other psychotic disorders

Just the facts

In this chapter, you'll learn:

♦ symptoms of schizophrenia spectrum and other psychotic disorders

♦ theories on the cause of schizophrenia spectrum and other psychotic disorders

♦ assessment, diagnosis, and treatment of patients with schizophrenia spectrum and other psychiatric disorders

♦ nursing interventions for patients with schizophrenia spectrum and other psychotic disorders.

The schizophrenia spectrum refers to a group of severe, chronic, and disabling psychiatric disorders marked by withdrawal from reality, illogical thinking, delusions and hallucinations, and other emotional, behavioral, or intellectual disturbances. These disturbances may affect everything, from speech, affect, and perception to psychomotor behavior, interpersonal relationships, and sense of self.

Patients with schizophrenia or another disorder on the schizophrenia spectrum may have trouble distinguishing reality from fantasy. Their speech and behavior may frighten or mystify those around them. There are numerous diagnoses encompassed within this category, including schizotypal disorder, brief psychotic disorder, schizophreniform disorder, catatonia, catatonic disorder due to another medical condition, and unspecified catatonia. For purposes of this reference, focus is placed on three of the most common diagnoses within the spectrum: schizophrenia, delusional disorder, and schizoaffective disorder.

A look at schizophrenia

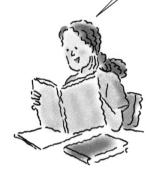

It says here that patients with schizophrenia have trouble distinguishing reality from fantasy.

Statistically speaking...

Schizophrenia affects more than 21 million people worldwide, and individuals with schizophrenia are two to three times more likely to die early than the general population (WHO, 2018). Schizophrenia is a debilitating and chronic disease and is one of the most economically and emotionally costly of all mental disorders on individuals, caregivers, and society. (See *The truth about schizophrenia and violence*, page 80.)

Functional fade-out

The patient's overall degree of disability depends mainly on the severity of cognitive impairment. Symptoms may impair the individual's ability to hold a job, stay in school, maintain relationships, and even perform self-care. It is not uncommon for a patient with schizophrenia to be found unemployable, socially isolated, and estranged from family and friends.

Life interrupted

People with schizophrenia do not often seek initial treatment on their own. Because of impaired thought processes and perceptual problems, they may deny that they need help and resist seeking health care.

Many people with schizophrenia often neglect personal hygiene and ignore (or are not aware of) their health needs. As a result, their life expectancy is about 10 years shorter than that of the general population. Approximately 4.9% of people with schizophrenia commit suicide (National Institute on Mental Health [NIMH], 2018).

Risk of suicide is high among young males with schizophrenia who have comorbid substance use, and those who have been newly diagnosed after a psychotic break, which is often associated with feelings of hopelessness and depression.

Symptom start-up

Although sudden onset of full-blown schizophrenia symptoms may occur, the majority of people with schizophrenia develop signs and symptoms in a more gradual and insidious fashion. Many individuals begin by experiencing prodromal symptoms such as development of depressive symptoms, gradual isolation from friends and family, cognitive alteration, and personality changes in late adolescent years. The first psychotic episode for males usually occurs by 18 to 25 years of age, whereas females tend to have a later onset between 25 and 35 years of age (Fischer & Buchanan, 2019).

Prognosis

The prognosis for patients with schizophrenia worsens with the occurrence of each acute episode. Few of these patients experience just a single psychotic episode. Some individuals suffer through periods of exacerbations and remissions. Between periods of exacerbation, some patients may have no disability, whereas others need continuous institutional care. The course of the disease becomes increasingly debilitating, with deteriorating symptoms experienced upon each occurrence.

Although there is no cure for schizophrenia, early intervention is the best way to improve changes of managing the illness. Discoveries into possible causes and brain-imaging techniques continue, as researchers attempt to gain further insight into therapeutic advances.

Risk factors

Risk factors are genetic and environmental in nature, and substance use increases the chance for poorer outcomes. Schizophrenia is more prevalent among individuals who live in urban areas (Fischer & Buchanan, 2019). It is also more common among single persons. This may reflect the effects of the illness or its impact on the person's social functioning.

It is commonly associated with co-occurring conditions such as depressive disorders, anxiety, and/or substance misuse (Fischer & Buchanan, 2019). People with schizophrenia who misuse drugs (other than tobacco) are associated with poorer outcomes and functioning. Substance use may contribute to nonadherence to prescribed medication, increased psychotic symptoms, repeated illness relapses, frequent hospitalizations, declining function, loss of social support, and increased risk for suicide.

Unfortunately, many people with schizophrenia also misuse substances—which certainly doesn't aid recovery. The prognosis for patients with schizoaffective disorder is difficult to determine due to lack of research, but is suggested to be more positive than that of schizophrenia but not as good as that of a mood disorder alone.

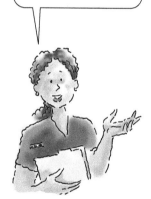

Possible causes of schizophrenia

Schizophrenia is a complex illness whose precise cause is unknown. Researchers believe that a combination of genetics, brain chemistry, and the environment contributes to the disorder (Fischer & Buchanan, 2019).

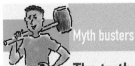

Myth busters

The truth about schizophrenia and violence

Are people with schizophrenia harmless victims of mental illness or unpredictable perpetrators of violence?

Myth: People with schizophrenia are more violent than other people.

Reality: People with schizophrenia are not usually violent. Although some threaten violence and have minor aggressive outbursts, few are far less likely to behave violently than individuals who misuse substances.

Nonetheless, a patient with schizophrenia who obeys hallucinatory voices telling him or her to attack someone poses a real danger. In rare cases, a patient with schizophrenia who is depressed, isolated, or paranoid attacks or kills someone he or she views as the cause of his or her problems.

Genetic factors

Experts have long known that schizophrenia runs in families. In monozygotic twins, 40% to 50% of people will develop the condition; in dizygotic twins, the rate is 10% to 15% (Fischer & Buchanan, 2019).

Predictable—not!

Most likely, multiple genes are involved in creating a predisposition to schizophrenia (called "polygenic"). Other factors, such as prenatal infections, perinatal complications, and certain stressors, seem to influence disease development (Fischer & Buchanan, 2019). To date, researchers have not been able to isolate exactly how the genetic predisposition is transmitted and they cannot predict whether a given person will develop the disease. (See *Vulnerability theories.*)

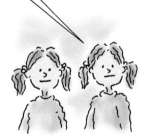

If one of us develops schizophrenia, the other one stands a 50% chance of getting it.

Biochemical theories

Scientists strongly suspect that people with schizophrenia have abnormalities in the brain's *neurotransmitters*—particularly dopamine, acetylcholine, gamma-amino-butyric acid (GABA), and glutamate (Fischer & Buchanan, 2019).

Dopamine theory

According to the dopamine hypothesis of schizophrenia, the disease results when the dopamine system in the brain is disturbed. Hyperactivity of dopaminergic activity in the limbic regions of the

Vulnerability theories

Some experts believe that schizophrenia occurs when a biologically susceptible person experiences an environmental stressor. According to certain vulnerability theories, a stressful event (such as the death of a loved one, job loss, or divorce) can trigger symptom onset in a vulnerable person.

Forebodings

What causes this vulnerability in the first place? Some researchers hypothesize (Fischer & Buchanan, 2019; NIMH, n.d.):
- genetic predisposition
- viral infections of the central nervous system
- malnutrition prior to birth
- birth complications
- illness or complications during pregnancy, delivery, or the neonatal period.

Developmental neurobiologists suspect that schizophrenia results from faulty connections formed by neurons during fetal development. These errors may lie dormant until puberty, when the brain changes that occur normally at this time may interact adversely with the faulty connections. A study by Selten and Termorshuizen (2017) suggest that exposure to influenza during first trimester of pregnancy increases the risk for schizophrenia. Researchers continue to attempt to prenatal factors that influence the apparent abnormality.

brain results in positive symptoms such as hallucinations, agitation, delusional thinking, and grandiosity. Hypoactivity of dopaminergic activity in the prefrontal cortex is thought to result in negative symptoms such as flattened affect, anhedonia, and defects in executive functions.

Acetylcholine theory

Some researchers hypothesize that nicotine, which stimulates some acetylcholine receptors, attempts to correct neurochemical imbalances in people with schizophrenia (Fischer & Buchanan, 2019). This observation has been made after studying smoking behaviors in patients with schizophrenia.

GABA theory

GABAergic interneurons are necessary for regulation of prefrontal cortical function; it is thought that these interneurons are dysfunctional in people with schizophrenia (Fischer & Buchanan, 2019).

Glutamate theory

Some cognitive symptoms of schizophrenia may be associated with abnormalities of glutamate—a neurotransmitter involved in dopamine breakdown as well as learning and memory impairment. The

Psychophysiologic markers of schizophrenia

Schizophrenia is known to affect eye movements.

Not-so-smooth pursuit

When tracking a moving object, such as a baseball in flight, the human eye uses a movement called *smooth pursuit*. The neuromuscular system produces pursuit movement by adjusting the moving eyeball's velocity to that of the object being viewed. This allows a stable image to be reflected onto the retina.

In people with schizophrenia, smooth pursuit eye movements are interrupted inappropriately by rapid eye movements, such as those used to read or look around. Although this genetically driven abnormality doesn't directly relate to the cause or effects of schizophrenia, it may serve as a genetic marker and a predictor of possible disease development.

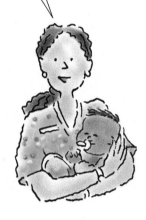

An infant whose mother had the flu during the first trimester of pregnancy has an increased risk for developing schizophrenia.

glutamate theory assumes that hypofunction of the *N*-methyl-D-aspartate (NMDA) glutamate receptor leads to schizophrenic symptoms (Fischer & Buchanan, 2019).

Structural brain abnormalities

For more than three decades, neuroimaging has been used to study brain dysfunction in patients with schizophrenia and other psychiatric illnesses (Chiapponi et al., 2018). Findings associated with schizophrenia include cortical and subcortical, structural, and microstructural anomalies (Chiapponi et al., 2018).

Assessment

Although behaviors and functional deficiencies may vary widely among patients—and even in the same patient at different times—some characteristic signs and symptoms usually are present upon assessment.

To assess a patient for schizophrenia, a comprehensive history is gathered, and a physical examination is conducted. It is often necessary to obtain information from family, friends, teachers, and others who know the patient well, because many people with schizophrenia may have cognitive alterations that prevent insight on their illness, perceptions, emotions, and behavior. Keep in mind that assessment findings will depend partly on the disease subtype, prevailing symptom type, and illness phase. (See *Recognizing schizophrenia.*)

Recognizing schizophrenia

During the assessment interview, you may note characteristic signs and symptoms in a patient with schizophrenia.

Speech abnormalities
The patient's speech may include:
- clang associations—words that rhyme or sound alike, used in an illogical, nonsensical manner (e.g., "It's the rain, train, pain")
- echolalia—meaningless repetition of words or phrases
- flight of ideas—rapid succession of incomplete ideas that aren't connected by logic or rationality
- word salad—illogical or random word groupings (e.g., "She had a star, barn, plant")
- neologisms—bizarre words that have meaning only for the patient.

Thought distortions
Stay alert for evidence of:
- overly concrete thinking—inability to form or understand abstract thoughts
- delusions—false ideas or beliefs accepted as real by the patient

- hallucinations—false sensory perceptions with no basis in reality
- thought blocking—sudden interruption in the train of thought
- magical thinking—a belief that thoughts or wishes can control other people or events.

Social interactions
Note whether the patient exhibits:
- poor interpersonal relationships
- withdrawal and apathy—disinterest in objects, people, or surroundings.

Other findings
In some people with schizophrenia, you may also assess:
- regression—return to an earlier developmental stage
- ambivalence—coexisting strong positive and negative feelings, leading to emotional conflict
- echopraxia—involuntary repetition of movements observed in others.

Symptom categories

Many clinicians refer to positive, negative, and disorganized symptoms of schizophrenia. In most patients, one of these symptom clusters predominates. (See *Tall tales about schizophrenia*, page 84.)

Positive symptoms
Positive symptoms are not present in most individuals but are found in patients with schizophrenia. They include primarily delusions, hallucinations, disordered speech and thoughts, and alterations in behavior (Varcarolis, 2018).

Keep in mind that in this context, "positive" does not mean "good." Quite the contrary—positive symptoms are psychotic and show that there is a disconnection between actual reality and the patient's perception of reality.

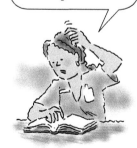

How odd ... they're called positive symptoms but that doesn't mean they are "good."

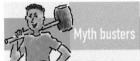

Myth busters

Tall tales about schizophrenia

The behavior of people with schizophrenia can be frightening and puzzling to individuals who are not familiar with this condition. This can lead to misconceptions about the disease. Two of these misconceptions are addressed below.

Myth: The agitated psychomotor behavior of some patients with schizophrenia reflects excessive energy, which causes them to engage in violent acts.

Reality: People with schizophrenia frequently show a lack of energy and have difficulty performing activities of daily living and interacting with other people.

Myth: A person with schizophrenia may experience either hallucinations or delusions, but not both.

Reality: Individuals who experience positive symptoms of schizophrenia may experience both hallucinations and delusions—especially delusions of paranoia or persecution.

Delusions

Delusions are erroneous beliefs that usually grow out of misinterpretations of experience. They may cause the patient to think that someone is reading his or her thoughts, involved in a conspiracy against him or her, or monitoring him or her—or that he or she can control the minds of other people.

Delusional distinctions

Delusions fall into several categories.

A patient with a *persecutory* delusion thinks that he or she is being tormented, followed, tricked, or spied on. This patient may believe that they are being singled out for harm (Varcarolis, 2018).

A patient with a *reference* delusion may think that passages in books, newspapers, television shows, song lyrics, or other environmental cues are directed at him or her.

In delusions of *thought withdrawal* or *thought insertion,* the patient believes that others can read his or her mind, that his or her thoughts are being transmitted to others, or that outside forces are imposing thoughts or impulses on him or her.

A patient with *grandiose* delusions considers themselves a major figure, like a politician or a religious figure.

Other types of delusions include (Varcarolis, 2018):

- *erotomanic*—the patient's erroneous belief that another person romantically desires him or her

- *nihilistic*—the patient's erroneous belief that a catastrophe is about to occur (e.g., a natural disaster)
- *somatic*—the patient's erroneous belief that his or her body is changing (e.g., "my lungs are rotting inside my body")
- *control*—the patient's erroneous belief that another person, group, or force controls thoughts, feelings, or behaviors (e.g., aluminum foil blocks the alien transmissions).

Hallucinations

The most common feature of schizophrenia is hallucinations, which involve auditory (hearing voices or sounds), visual (seeing persons or things), olfactory (smelling odors), gustatory (experiencing tastes), or tactile (feeling sensations) (Varcarolis, 2018). For example, the patient may "hear" voices commenting on his or her behavior, conversing with one another, or making critical and abusive comments.

Disordered speech and thoughts

Disorganized symptoms include speech abnormalities, thought disorders, and altered behaviors.

- *Speech abnormalities* may include incoherent speech and frequent derailment from the topic at hand.
- *Thought disorder* refers to confused thinking and speech, ranging from mildly disorganized speech to incoherent ramblings. The person may make loose associations, jumping from one idea to another, and wander further and further from the original topic. He or she may have trouble carrying on conversations with others.
- *Altered behavior* may include (Varcarolis, 2018):
  - catatonia—increase or decrease in movement rate and amount
  - waxy flexibility—maintaining a posture inappropriately (e.g., raising an arm and leaving it there)
  - motor retardation or agitation—pronounced slowing or increasing of movement
  - stereotyped behaviors—repetitive behaviors that serve no purpose
  - echopraxia—mimicking another person's movements
  - negativism—resisting or opposing requests of others
  - impaired impulse control—difficulty resisting one's own impulses
  - gesturing or posturing—assuming unusual positions or facial expressions
  - boundary impairment—impairment in understanding one's own boundaries (e.g., invading the personal space of another).

Negative symptoms

Negative (deficit) symptoms reflect the absence of normal characteristics. They include apathy, avolition, affect, alogia (poverty of speech), anhedonia, and asociality.

- *Apathy* refers to a lack of interest in people, things, and activities.
- *Avolition* impairs the motivation and ability of the person to start and follow through with activities.
- *Affect* refers to the expression of emotions. Patients with schizophrenia often demonstrate flattening of the emotions, referred to as a "blunt affect." The person's face may appear immobile and inexpressive. As schizophrenia progresses, the blunted affect may grow more pronounced. (Keep in mind that inability to *show* emotions does not mean inability to *feel* emotions.)
- *Alogia*, also known as *poverty of speech*, refers to speech that is brief and lacks content. The person may give terse replies to questions, creating the impression of inner emptiness.
- *Anhedonia* is diminished capacity to experience pleasure.
- *Asociality* refers to avoidance of relationships. A person with schizophrenia may withdraw socially because of depression. He or she may feel relatively safe when alone or may be completely caught up in personal feelings and fears, or it may be difficult to manage the company of others.

Impact on the family

Schizophrenia profoundly affects the patient's family. Although the patient needs the understanding and support of family members, his or her behavior may frighten and frustrate loved ones.

Family members may be uninformed about schizophrenia and its management. Few families are adequately prepared to deal with the stressors caused by chronic schizophrenia, which include personality decompensation, hospitalizations, and medication nonadherence.

Disease phases

Schizophrenia usually progresses in distinct phases—prodromal, acute, stabilization, and maintenance/residual (Varcarolis, 2018). The symptoms and length of each phase may vary.

Prodromal phase

During the *prodromal phase*, which may arise months or years before the first hospitalization, the person shows a clear change from his or her previous level of functioning.

A low profile

The person may withdraw from friends, hobbies, and other interests and may exhibit peculiar behavior, neglect personal hygiene and grooming, and lack energy and initiative. Work or school performance may deteriorate.

Acute phase

During the *acute phase* (commonly triggered by a stressful event), the person has acute psychotic symptoms, such as hallucinations, delusions, incoherence, or catatonic behavior. (See *What is catatonia, as in DSM-5?*) Functional deficits worsen. Hospitalization may be needed.

Number of acute episodes

Some patients with schizophrenia have just one acute episode and no more. Others have repeated, acute exacerbations of the active phase. With each acute episode, the prognosis worsens.

Stabilization

Symptoms experienced in the acute phase begin to diminish or stabilize. Outpatient care or a partial hospitalization program may be helpful.

Residual phase

During the *residual phase*, which follows the stabilization phase, symptoms resemble those of the prodromal phase. Positive symptoms usually discontinue, whereas negative symptoms such as blunted affect and impaired role functioning may be more pronounced.

During the residual phase, the illness pattern may become established, disability levels may stabilize, or late improvements may appear.

Remissions

Although few people with schizophrenia return to their full pre-illness functioning level, some full remissions have occurred (Varcarolis, 2018).

What is catatonia

Catatonia refers to abnormal and bizarre psychomotor disturbance that may involve decreased motor activity such as immobility or increased motor activity such as agitation or echopraxia (American Psychiatric Association [APA], 2013).

Disease course

The course of schizophrenia varies among patients and depends largely on adherence with prescribed antipsychotic drug regimen.

Mild course

The person with a mild disease course is usually stable. This person always adheres to drug treatment, has just one or two major relapses by age 45, and experiences only a few mild symptoms.

Moderate course

Typically, the person with a moderate disease course takes drugs as prescribed most of the time but isn't fully adherent to the treatment plan. The person has several major relapses by age 45 and has experienced increased symptoms during stressful periods. Between relapses, symptoms persist.

Severe, unstable course

The person with a severe disease course doesn't adhere to the prescribed drug regimen. He or she has frequent relapses and is stable only for brief periods between relapses. The person experiences bothersome symptoms and needs help with activities of daily living. There is also the likelihood of coexisting other problems (such as substance misuse) that make recovery more difficult.

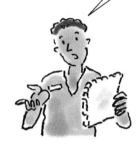

The patient has stopped taking the prescribed medications ... he or she may be destined for a difficult disease course.

Symptoms over time

During the first years of the illness, the person's level of functioning may deteriorate. Social and work skills may decline, cognitive deficits grow more pronounced, and self-care neglect may worsen progressively. Also, negative symptoms may grow more severe.

In the most common disease course, acute episodes are followed by residual impairment. During the first few years of schizophrenia, impairment between episodes commonly increases. For many patients, a plateau is reached.

Diagnosis

A mental status examination, psychiatric history, and careful clinical observation form the basis for diagnosing schizophrenia.

For a thorough evaluation, the patient should undergo physical and psychiatric examinations to rule out other possible causes of symptoms—including physical disorders, substance-induced psychosis, and primary mood disorders with psychotic features.

The stamp of authority

Official diagnosis, determined by the health care provider, is based on the criteria indicated in the *Diagnostic and Statistical Manual of Mental Disorders*, 5th Edition (*DSM-5*).

Diagnostic test results

There are no diagnostic tests that definitively confirm schizophrenia. Because other disorders such as vitamin deficiencies, uremia, thyrotoxicosis, and electrolyte imbalances can cause symptoms that mimic schizophrenia, other tests may be done to rule out these types of conditions.

Computed tomography (CT) scans and a ventricular-brain ratio (VBR) analysis may show structural brain abnormalities that suggest schizophrenia. A meta-analysis regarding brain structure in patients with schizophrenia shows that there is a significantly greater variability in putamen, temporal lobe, and thalamus volumes when compared with patients without schizophrenia (Brugger & Howes, 2017).

General treatment

Antipsychotic drugs (sometimes called *neuroleptics*) are the mainstay of treatment.

Value of early treatment
People with schizophrenia who develop psychotic symptoms may wait months to years before they present for medical care. The interval between symptom onset and the first treatment correlates with the speed and quality of the initial treatment response and severity of negative symptoms. Patients treated soon after being diagnosed are more likely to respond more quickly and fully than those who do not begin drug therapy until later in the disease course.

Mixed modalities

Although psychopharmacology remains the foundation of treatment of schizophrenia, a more holistic and comprehensive treatment plan requires the integration of other treatment modalities such as:
- psychosocial treatment and rehabilitation
- compliance promotion programs
- vocational counseling
- psychotherapy
- appropriate use of community resources.
    Certain people with schizophrenia may also be candidates for electroconvulsive therapy (ECT) (Sanghani et al., 2018).

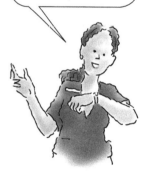

The sooner a patient with schizophrenia begins treatment, the faster and more fully he or she is likely to respond.

Treatment goals

Treatment goals for the patient with schizophrenia include:
- reducing the severity of psychotic symptoms
- preventing recurrences of acute episodes and associated functional decline
- meeting the patient's physical, psychosocial, developmental, cultural, and spiritual needs
- helping the patient function at the highest level possible. (See *Myths about dependence*, page 90.)

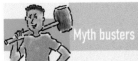

Myth busters

Myths about dependence

People may think that individuals with schizophrenia are unable to manage every-day life.

Myth: People with schizophrenia are incapable of making life decisions and need help of a legal guardian.

Reality: Although some people with schizophrenia need guidance through certain periods, only a small minority depend on others fully to make decisions and for care at all times.

Drug therapy

Antipsychotic drugs control symptoms adequately in most people with schizophrenia. The wide choice of drug treatment options available today has improved patients' chances for remission and recovery.

Just say no to dopamine

Antipsychotic drugs appear to work at least in part by blocking post-synaptic dopamine receptors. These drugs have multiple benefits, including:

- reducing positive symptoms, such as hallucinations and delusions
- easing thought disorders
- relieving anxiety and agitation
- maximizing the patient's level of functioning.

Antipsychotic drug categories

Two categories of antipsychotics are available—conventional (typical) antipsychotics and atypical antipsychotics.

Conventional (typical) antipsychotics

In the past, conventional (typical) antipsychotics were traditionally used to treat patients with schizophrenia. Because of their potential for adverse effects and the availability of atypical antipsychotics, they have not been the first-line treatment of choice for the past decade. (See *Adverse effects of antipsychotic drugs*.) However, patients who do well on them without experiencing troublesome effects may be advised by their health care provider to continue taking them.

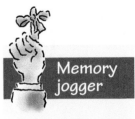

Memory jogger

The word **PRESSURE** can help you remember the treatment goals for a patient with schizophrenia.

Psychiatric medications administered properly and monitored

Realistic perceptions and self-expectations developed

Environmental situations managed effectively

Safety needs addressed

Self-care performed adequately

Use of community resources on an ongoing basis

Relationships developed and sustained

Establishment and maintenance of family involvement in care

Adverse effects of antipsychotic drugs

Patients with schizophrenia must take antipsychotic drugs for a long time—usually for life. Unfortunately, some of these drugs may cause unpleasant side effects.

Sedative, anticholinergic, and extrapyramidal effects

High-potency conventional (typical) antipsychotics (such as haloperidol) can cause some sedation and anticholinergic effects, such as rapid pulse, dry mouth, inability to urinate, and constipation.

These drugs carry a high incidence of extrapyramidal (motor) effects. The most common motor effects are dystonia, parkinsonism, and akathisia.

• *Dystonia* refers to prolonged, repetitive muscle contractions that may cause twisting or jerking movements—especially of the neck, mouth, and tongue.

• Drug-induced *parkinsonism* results in bradykinesia (abnormally slow movements), muscle rigidity, shuffling gait, stooped posture, flat facial affect, tremors, and drooling. It may emerge 1 week to several months after drug treatment begins.

• *Akathisia* causes restlessness, pacing, and an inability to rest or sit still.

Intermediate-potency conventional (typical) antipsychotics have a moderate incidence of extrapyramidal effects. Low-potency agents (such as chlorpromazine) are highly sedative and anticholinergic but cause few extrapyramidal effects.

Orthostatic hypotension

Low-potency antipsychotics may cause orthostatic hypotension (low blood pressure when standing).

Tardive dyskinesia

Antipsychotics may cause tardive dyskinesia—a disorder characterized by repetitive, involuntary, purposeless movements. Signs and symptoms include grimacing, rapid eye blinking, tongue protrusion and smacking, lip puckering or pursing, and rapid movements of the hands, arms, legs, and trunk.

Symptoms may resolve, or be permanent, after the patient stops taking the antipsychotic drug.

Neuroleptic malignant syndrome

Although infrequent, antipsychotic drugs can cause neuroleptic malignant syndrome. This life-threatening condition leads to fever, extremely rigid muscles, and altered consciousness. It may occur hours to months after drug therapy starts or the dosage is increased.

Examples of conventional (typical) antipsychotics include the following. Some have trade names, whereas others are only available as a generic preparation.

• chlorpromazine
• fluphenazine
• haloperidol (Haldol)
• loxapine
• molindone
• perphenazine
• pimozide
• thiothixene
• trifluoperazine.

Atypical antipsychotics

The advent of atypical antipsychotics in the 1990s gave new hope to many people with schizophrenia. These drugs are referred to as *atypical* because they work differently than conventional antipsychotics by reducing negative symptoms of schizophrenia, and they are much less likely to cause extrapyramidal side effects.

Clozapine

Clozapine was the first atypical antipsychotic. It has proven to be effective in many patients who do not respond to conventional (typical) antipsychotics. The drug controls a wider range of signs and symptoms than conventional (typical) agents and causes few or no adverse motor effects.

Agranulocytosis and other adversities

Clozapine carries the risk of serious side effects such as agranulocytosis—a potentially fatal blood disorder marked by a low white blood cell count and pronounced neutrophil depletion. Patients receiving it should undergo routine blood monitoring to detect the disorder. When caught early, agranulocytosis can be reversible.

Cardiomyopathy and myocarditis are two other rare but potentially serious conditions that may result from using clozapine. Older patients with dementia-related psychosis should be administered atypical antipsychotics *with extreme caution* due to risk of cardiovascular complications. Other adverse effects include drowsiness, sedation, hypotension, weight gain, excessive salivation, hyperglycemia, tachycardia, dizziness, and seizures.

Other atypical antipsychotics

Atypical antipsychotics being used in the market include:
- aripiprazole (Abilify)
- asenapine (Saphris)
- brexpiprazole (Rexulti)
- cariprazine (Vraylar)
- clozapine (Clozaril)
- iloperidone (Fanapt)
- lurasidone (Latuda)
- olanzapine (Zyprexa)
- olanzapine/fluoxetine hydrochloride (Symbyax) (combination antipsychotic and selective serotonin reuptake inhibitor)
- paliperidone (Invega)
- quetiapine (Seroquel)
- risperidone (Risperdal)
- ziprasidone (Geodon).

Depending on the specific drug, the health care provider will prescribe a trial period. Most drugs take effect within several weeks, although clozapine may take up to 12 weeks. For acute treatment, rapid symptom resolution is the goal. For maintenance, patients should receive the lowest dose that is sufficient to prevent relapse.

Atypicals' advantages

Atypical antipsychotics offer many benefits. They:
- have a selective affinity for brain regions involved in schizophrenia symptoms
- relieve positive symptoms
- may improve negative symptoms more effectively than typical antipsychotics
- enhance the brain's serotonin levels while stabilizing dopamine levels
- may improve neurocognitive deficits
- are more effective in treating refractory schizophrenia (in particular, clozapine)
- are less likely to cause motor adverse effects
- produce little or no prolactin elevation (a possible adverse effect of typical antipsychotics).

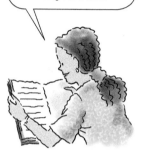

Better symptom coverage, fewer adverse effects, higher serotonin levels—atypical antipsychotics offer many benefits.

But ...

The use of atypical antipsychotics has been associated with the development of metabolic syndrome, which includes dyslipidemia, obesity, hypertension, and non-insulin-dependent diabetes. Monitor metabolic parameters prior to and during treatment with antipsychotics to reduce the risk of other health issues.

Drug depots—injectable medication

Commonly referred to as *depot formulations*, a number of long-acting injectable (LAI) antipsychotics are available. These are administered intramuscularly, and the drug then gradually releases over time. Injectable antipsychotics may require administration on a biweekly or monthly basis. At time of writing, formulation is available for (Lauriello & Campbell, 2019):
- aripiprazole extended release (aripiprazole LAI)
- aripiprazole lauroxil (aripiprazole lauroxil LAI)
- fluphenazine decanoate (fluphenazine LAI)
- haloperidol decanoate (haloperidol LAI)
- olanzapine pamoate (olanzapine LAI)
- paliperidone palmitate, 4-week (paliperidone LAI)
- paliperidone palmitate, 12-week (paliperidone 12-week LAI)
- risperidone microspheres (risperidone LAI)
- risperidone extended-release subcutaneous injection (risperidone SQ LAI).

The key benefit of using injectable formulation is better medication adherence. People with schizophrenia who have difficulty remembering to take medication daily, or those who do not adhere to the treatment plan, can benefit from receiving drug therapy in this manner. Other benefits include maintenance of stable drug levels in

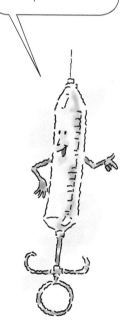

Injectable antipsychotics can improve medication adherence, reduce relapse, and prevent hospitalization.

the body, prevention or delay of relapse and subsequent acute hospitalizations, and better monitoring of patient compliance.

Other drugs
Antidepressants and anxiolytics may be used to treat associated signs and symptoms in some patients. Mood-stabilizing agents may be given to manage negative symptoms.

Psychosocial treatment and rehabilitation

Besides antipsychotic drugs, patients need support to manage their illness and the isolation, stigma, and fear that often accompany it. Psychosocial treatment, rehabilitation services, and special living arrangements to aid in the various stages of recovery can be helpful. (See *Home is where the help is.*)

Psychosocial treatment
The key components of psychosocial treatment for patients with schizophrenia include:
- patient and family teaching about the disease and its treatment
- collaborative decision-making opportunities
- monitoring of drug therapy and symptoms
- social services assistance with obtaining prescribed drugs and resources
- supervision of financial resources, as needed
- training and assistance with activities of daily living
- peer support and self-help groups
- psychotherapy.

Psychotherapy
Used as a singular method of treatment, individual or group psychotherapy has little value in managing schizophrenia. However, adjunctive psychotherapy provides emotional support, reinforces health-promoting behaviors, aids adjustment to the illness, and helps patients make the most of their abilities. Typically, psychotherapy is used during the maintenance phase or during the stabilization phase that follows an acute episode.

Go it alone or hang with a group?
The focus of individual therapy is reality-based and supportive. Group therapy helps patients to encourage socialization, develop coping skills, and resolve interpersonal conflicts.

Family therapy
Because schizophrenia may be disruptive to the family, all family members may benefit from psychotherapy. This type of therapy can

Home is where the help is

A stable place to live is an important component of treating schizophrenia. Depending on the patient's geographic location, different types of residential options may be available.

Brief respite or crisis homes

Brief respite or crisis homes are intensive residential programs with on-site clinical staff who can provide 24-hour supervision and treatment. These homes may be a good choice for patients experiencing acute episodes or during the stabilization phase that follows an acute episode. For patients experiencing relapse, these homes may help them avoid the need for hospitalization.

Transitional group homes

Transitional group homes are structured programs that typically offer in-house daily training in living skills and 24-hour coverage by paraprofessionals. They help stabilize patients after acute episodes or after a stay in a hospital or brief respite home.

Foster or boarding homes

Foster or boarding homes are supportive group living situations run by laypersons. Usually, the staff provides supervision during the day, with one staff member sleeping over at night. These homes may be recommended for patients in long-term recovery and maintenance.

Supported or supervised apartments

Supported or supervised apartments usually have a specially trained on-site residential manager who provides support, assistance, and supervision. Alternatively, a mental health professional may provide these services.

These apartments are useful for patients in long-term recovery and maintenance. They help the patient remain autonomous while providing sufficient care to minimize the chance of relapse and the need for inpatient hospitalization.

Family living

For some patients, living with family members may be an acceptable long-term arrangement. For others, it may be needed only during acute episodes. Support and advocacy groups can provide families with information and support.

Independent living

During long-term recovery and maintenance, independent living is recommended for most patients. Of course, this may be impossible during acute episodes and for patients with a more severe disease course.

reduce guilt and disappointment, foster acceptance of the patient and behavior, and teach the family stress-management skills. For patients who live with their families, psychoeducational family interventions can reduce the relapse rate.

Rehabilitation

Rehabilitation may be particularly important for patients who need to develop their job skills, want to work, and have only a few symptoms.

A range of rehab

During the long-term recovery and maintenance phases of the illness, three types of rehabilitation programs may be used.

1. *Cognitive* rehabilitation programs help patients develop and improve cognitive processes (e.g., attention, memory, function, social cognition) (Morin & Franck, 2017).

2. *Psychiatric* rehabilitation teaches patients the skills needed to define and achieve their personal goals regarding education, work, socialization, and living arrangements.
3. *Vocational* rehabilitation involves a strict focus on work assessment and training to help patients prepare for full-time employment.

Preserving the people's rights
Remember that patients with schizophrenia have the same rights as other hospitalized patients.

Nursing interventions
These nursing interventions are appropriate when caring for a patient with schizophrenia.
- Convey a nonjudgmental attitude to help establish a trusting and therapeutic relationship.
- If the patient is able, engage in shared decision-making regarding the plan of care. This gives the patient an opportunity to be meaningfully involved in his or her own well-being (Mahone et al., 2016).
- Teach about the importance of adherence to medication and the plan of care. Depending on the patient's level of function, work with members of the interprofessional team to coordinate care in the community setting.

Role-play and reinforce
- Role model appropriate communication and behaviors.
- Depending on the patient's level of function, teach problem-solving and communication skills. Provide role-playing opportunities to become comfortable and more self-confident when using these new skills.
- Reinforce the patient's acceptable behavior and positive behavior changes.
- Work with the patient and family to address concerns and improve communication skills.

Schizophrenia in children
Although schizophrenia usually presents during adolescence, there are rare instances where the symptoms begin during childhood. It is imperative that health care providers be mindful of other medical or organic conditions that may produce symptoms that mimic the symptoms of schizophrenia. The social norm and the individual child's stage of development should be considered in the assessment of symptoms in ruling out other developmental disorders. In children, hallucinations are more common than delusions (Skehan & Dvir, 2019). Treatment course will vary depending on the age of the child at diagnosis and the extent of symptoms.

Memory jogger

RIGHTS **Preserving the people's rights**
Remember that patients with schizophrenia have the same rights as

other hospitalized patients.

Refusal of nonemergency treatment

Individualized care

Grievances addressed as they occur

Health alternatives given

Treatment obtained in the least restrictive setting

Security of the patient's civil rights

Schizophrenia in older adults

Late-onset schizophrenia (LOS) is defined as onset of symptoms after age 40 (Varcarolis, 2018) and very-late-onset schizophrenia-like psychosis (VLOSLP) consists of onset after age 60 (Howard et al., 2018). More women than men are diagnosed with a later onset (Fischer & Buchanan, 2019). Risk of suicide in this population is high. Medication management for older adults with schizophrenia may be more conservative to factor in the aging body's diminished ability to metabolize and excrete drugs. Dosage of medication is often adjusted lower to decrease incidence of fall, sedation, confusion, orthostatic hypotension, and toxicity.

A look at delusional disorder

Delusional disorder is characterized by at least 1 month of delusions without the presence of other psychotic symptoms (APA, 2013). A patient with delusional disorder has difficulty recognizing reality and has false beliefs despite evidence of the contrary.

Statistically speaking …

In the United States, 0.02% of Americans are diagnosed with delusional disorder (APA, 2013). More women than men are diagnosed with this condition.

Life interrupted

Unlike schizophrenia, patients with delusions often do not have problems with day-to-day functioning; their cognitive function often appears intact, as they are alert and oriented and attentive to other elements of function with the exception of the delusion (Manschreck, 2019). However, when a patient becomes excessively preoccupied with their delusions and their ability to function independently decompensates, professional intervention may be required for stabilization.

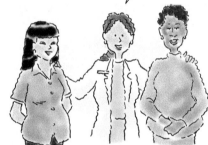

More women than men are diagnosed with delusional disorder.

Symptom start-up

Symptoms of delusional disorder may be difficult to define if the delusions are nonbizarre and somewhat believable. Patients with delusional disorder may have difficulty accepting their thoughts as irrational, regardless of being informed otherwise. Individuals may also present with a depressed, irritable, or angry mood depending on the context of their delusions (Manschreck, 2019).

Prognosis

Delusional disorder may subside or last for months. Research shows that approximately two-third of patients experience this as a life-long condition, whereas approximately one-third enter into a remission (Manschreck, 2019). The prognosis for delusional disorder is unfavorable mainly because patients believe their delusions are real, and therefore may not wish to enter into any kind of treatment.

Impact on the family

Living with someone who has delusional disorder may become challenging, especially if family and loved ones are not educated well on the symptoms, treatment, and how to obtain necessary support to cope. For example, a patient with a delusional belief that their spouse is allegedly having an affair with another person may create marital stress that eventually leads to divorce.

Possible causes of delusional disorder

The actual cause of delusional disorder is unknown, and research is limited. Researchers believe that a family history of paranoid personality disorder and sensory impairment may contribute to development of this condition (Manschreck, 2019).

Assessment

A mental status assessment may determine pertinent information regarding the patient's level of cognition, current mood, insight, and judgment in regard to the false beliefs, speech, and general appearance, and behaviors. Safety is critical when assessing a patient for delusional disorder or any other mental health concern by ensuring the patient is not in any imminent danger to self or others through expression of suicidal thoughts or homicidal ideation.

Symptoms

The presentation of a patient with delusional disorder is usually unremarkable, with exception of their false beliefs. The delusions are usually identified within a specific theme or subtype delusion. Delusion subtypes are included in "Delusional Distinctions."

Diagnosis

Diagnosing delusional disorder can be challenging. The health care provider will rule out other causes of symptoms prior to making the diagnosis. Assessment of medical, psychiatric, and family history (including current medication regimen) may provide insight to the patient's symptoms. Baseline blood work and urinalysis may be ordered to rule out other physiologic causes. A urine drug screen may rule out if delusions are a result of alcohol and drug use. A CT or MRI may be ordered to rule out neurologic issues.

The Global Assessment of Functioning Scale, which can be used for any patient with a mental health concern, can be used to determine a patient's ability to perform activities of daily living and to function independently.

Diagnostic test results

There is no definitive test to diagnose delusional disorder. Recurring admissions to the hospital because of exacerbation of symptoms and close monitoring may provide the health care provider and treatment team an insight into the patient's patterns of behavior, allowing for more accurate diagnosis.

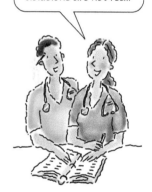

Usually patients with delusional disorder are unaware that their delusions are not real.

General treatment

Usually patients with delusional disorder have limited or poor insight into their illness, are unaware that their delusions are not real, and do not believe that they need treatment. Establishing a rapport and trusting therapeutic relationship is key to a better treatment outcome. A combination of drug therapy and psychotherapy may be used to treat the condition.

Treatment goals

The goal of treatment is to improve the patient's quality of life and prevent symptoms from exacerbating. A patient's readiness to learn will influence the effectiveness of teaching and adherence to the treatment plan. Symptoms may be managed by use of medications; however, the chance of adherence is low because of poor insight and judgment into the delusional thought process. Cognitive behavioral therapy (CBT) can also be beneficial.

Drug therapy

There are no drugs that are indicated to treat delusional disorder; rather, primary pharmacologic treatment with atypical antipsychotics such as aripiprazole or ziprasidone can be used. Any trial of medication must be monitored closely, because patients with this disorder often remain in denial about their diagnosis.

Cognitive behavioral therapy

Outpatient CBT is most commonly used to treat a patient with delusional disorder. With the high risk of nonadherence to any treatment plan, it is critical a rapport and therapeutic trust relationship be established between the patient and therapist before addressing the patient's delusions. The outcome of the patient's response to psychotherapy may be more positive if the initial focus begins with addressing the patient's goals in life and then shifting into a more gradual focus on addressing delusional thoughts and behaviors. This allows the patient to recognize and change disruptive thoughts and behaviors into positive thoughts and behaviors.

Support groups and family therapy may allow the family and patient to gain more insight into the delusions, how to effectively cope when addressing reality versus nonreality-based thinking, and allow for a more supportive environment in which the patient can live.

Nursing interventions

These nursing interventions are appropriate when caring for a patient with delusional disorder (Varcarolis, 2018):

- Convey a nonjudgmental attitude to help establish a trusting and therapeutic relationship.
- Do not debate the delusional content; however, do validate that the patient's perception of delusion is real.
- Do not dwell on delusions; refocus into reality as often as possible.
- Help the patient identify triggers that bring on delusions.
- Focus on the feelings that the delusion(s) bring, and attempt to help patient manage those.

A look at schizoaffective disorder

Schizoaffective disorder is a chronic mental health condition characterized by symptoms of schizophrenia and a mood disorder (National Alliance on Mental Illness [NAMI], 2020). The main symptoms include hallucinations and/or delusions, and disorganized thinking, with depression or mania.

Statistically speaking ...

The prevalence of schizoaffective disorder is hard to determine due to changes in diagnostic criteria over recent years and limited studies. It is estimated to be at only 0.3% (NAMI, 2019). Schizoaffective disorder affects men and women equally, although men usually develop the illness at an earlier age (NAMI, 2019).

Life interrupted

Just like people with schizophrenia, individuals with schizoaffective disorder function at different levels. This disorder, although much less studied than schizophrenia, appears to be able to be managed effectively with medication and therapy if the patient is adherent to treatment (NAMI, 2019).

Symptom start-up

Presenting symptoms may range from mild to severe, in which case the patient may then require hospitalization to stabilize symptoms. Symptoms include a combination of hallucinations, delusions, disorganized thought process, and depression or acute mania (NAMI, 2019).

Prognosis

Delusional disorder may subside or last for months. Research shows that approximately 2/3 of patients experience this as a life-long condition, while approximately 1/3 enter into a remission (Manschreck, 2019). The prognosis for delusional disorder is unfavorable mainly because patients believe their delusions are real, and therefore may not wish to enter into any kind of treatment.

Impact on the family

Living with someone who has delusional disorder may become challenging, especially if family and loved ones are not educated well on the symptoms, treatment, and how to obtain necessary support to cope. For example, a patient with a delusional belief that their spouse is allegedly having an affair with another person may create marital stress that eventually leads to divorce.

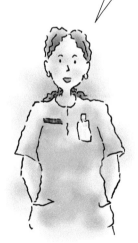

Some symptoms of schizoaffective disorder are hallucinations and delusions.

Possible causes of schizoaffective disorder

The actual cause of schizoaffective disorder is unknown. As with other psychiatric conditions, it is thought to be the result of numerous factors, including genetics, brain structure, and environmental factors.

Assessment

Assessment for schizoaffective disorder follows a similar course to assessment for schizophrenia. In addition to assessing symptoms of hallucinations, delusions, and disordered thinking, the health care provider will also evaluate the patient's mood for depression or mania.

General treatment

Schizoaffective disorder is usually treated with a combination of drugs and psychotherapy. How well the patient responds to the treatment depends on the severity and duration of symptoms, and the patient's adherence to the plan of care. Hospitalization may be necessary if depressive or manic symptoms are severe, the patient expresses thoughts of suicide or harm to others, cannot verbalize a safety plan, or is unable to function independently.

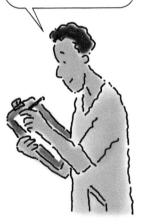

A combination of antipsychotic and antidepressant drugs is used to treat schizoaffective disorder.

Drug therapy

A combination of antipsychotic and antidepressant drugs is used to treat schizoaffective disorder. Atypical antipsychotics are generally preferred due to their lower profile for adverse reactions, with the addition of selective serotonin reuptake inhibitor (SSRI) due to their low risk of cardiac dysrhythmias.

Psychosocial treatment

Psychosocial treatment for schizoaffective disorder resembles what is recommended for patients with schizophrenia—psychotherapy and family therapy.

Nursing interventions

The same nursing interventions included for patients with schizophrenia are appropriate when caring for a patient with schizoaffective disorder. In addition, because of the mood component of this disorder, monitor the patient for suicidal or homicidal ideation, and create a plan of action in case the patient develops feelings of harm toward self or others.

Quick quiz

1. How will the nurse document the assessment finding of a patient with schizophrenia who displays flattened emotions?
    A. Anhedonia
    B. Asociality
    C. Blunted affect
    D. Regression

Answer: C. Blunted affect is the flattening of emotions. The person's face may be immobile and inexpressive, with poor eye contact. This assessment finding is common in patients with schizophrenia.

2. The nurse is caring for a patient who professes to be the president of the United States. How will the nurse document this finding?
    A. Delusion
    B. Illusion
    C. Hallucination
    D. Magical thinking

Answer: A. Delusions are false ideas or beliefs accepted as real by the patient. Among people with schizophrenia, delusions of grandeur, persecution, and reference are common.

3. The nurse has received a report that a patient with schizophrenia is displaying neologisms. What patient statement is reflective of this abnormality?
    A. "That is a parf and a parner."
    B. "Dogs dogs dogs dogs dogs dogs."
    C. "My friend has a flower, power, tower."
    D. "I'm hungry; let's fly a kite and read the news."

Answer: A. Neologisms are bizarre words that have meaning only for the patient. Repeating words or phrases meaninglessly is reflective of echolalia. Clang associations are made by words that rhyme or sound alike but are used illogically. Flight of ideas includes rapid successful of incomplete ideas that aren't connected logically.

4. A patient with schizophrenia who began taking haloperidol 1 week ago reports signs of tardive dyskinesia. What assessment finding does the nurse anticipate?
    A. Lip puckering
    B. Pill-rolling of the fingers
    C. Posing in awkward positions
    D. Sensation of ants crawling on the body

Answer: A. Tardive dyskinesia is a disorder characterized by repetitive, involuntary, purposeless movements. Signs and symptoms include grimacing, rapid eye blinking, tongue protrusion and smacking, lip puckering or pursing, and rapid movements of the hands, arms, legs, and trunk. Pill-rolling is indicative of parkinsonism. Positing in awkward positions is associated with waxy flexibility. The sensation of ants crawling on the body is reflective of a hallucination.

5.   The nurse is preparing to care for a patient with schizophrenia experiencing positive symptoms. Which assessment finding does the nurse anticipate?
   A.   Anhedonia
   B.   Flattened affect
   C.   Disordered speech
   D.   Defects in executive function

Answer: A. Examples of positive symptoms associated with schizophrenia include hallucinations, delusions, and disordered speech. A flattened affect, anhedonia, and defects in executive function are negative symptoms.

Scoring

   If you answered all five items correctly, spectacular! We hereby declare that you have superior savvy in understanding schizophrenia!

   If you answered three or four items correctly, good show! Continue to develop your understanding of schizophrenia.

   If you answered fewer than three items correctly, just give it another go!

Selected references

American Psychiatric Association. (2013). *Diagnostic and statistical manual of mental disorders* (5th ed.). Arlington, VA: Author.

Arnedo, J., Svrakic, D. M., del Val, C., Romero-Zaliz, R., Hernández-Cuervo, H., Fanous, A. H., Pato, M. T., Pato, C. N., de Erausquin, G. A., Cloninger, C. R., & Zwir, I. (2014). Uncovering the hidden risk architecture of the schizophrenias: Confirmation in three independent genome-wide association studies. *The American Journal of Psychiatry, 172*(2), 139–153. http://ajp.psychiatryonline.org/doi/abs/10.1176/appi.ajp.2014.14040435?journalCode=ajp

Brugger, S., & Howes, O. (2017). Heterogeneity and homogeneity of regional brain structure in schizophrenia. *JAMA Psychiatry, 74*(11), 1104–1111.

Chiapponi, C., De Rossi, P., Piras, F., Gili, T., & Spalletta, G. (2018). Brain morphometry: Schizophrenia. In G. Spalletta, F. Piras, & T. Gili (Eds.), *Brain morphometry* (pp. 323–338). Humana Press.

Cleveland Clinic. (2018). *Delusional disorder.* https://my.cleveland clinic.org/health/diseases/9599-delusional-disorder

Fischer, B., & Buchanan, R. (2019). Schizophrenia in adults: Epidemiology and pathogenesis. *UpToDate.* https://www.uptodate.com/contents/schizophrenia-in-adults-epidemiology-and-pathogenesis

Harvard Health. (2019). *Delusional disorder: What is it?* https://www.health.harvard.edu/a_to_z/delusional-disorder-a-to-z

Howard, R., Cort, E., Bradley, R., Harper, E., Kelly, L., Bentham, P., Ritchie, C., Reeves, S., Fawzi, W., Livingston, G., Sommerlad, A., Oomman, S., Nazir, E., Nilforooshan, R., Barber, R., Fox, C., Macharouthu, A. V., Ramachandra, P., Pattan, V., … Gray, R. (2018). Antipsychotic treatment of very-late onset schizophrenia-like psychosis (ATLAS): A randomized, controlled, double-blind trial. *The Lancet: Psychiatry, 5*(7), 553–563.

Lauriello, J., & Campbell, A. (2019). Pharmacotherapy for schizophrenia: Long-acting injectable antipsychotic drugs. *UpToDate.* https://www.uptodate.com/contents/pharmacotherapy-for-schizophrenia-long-acting-injectable-antipsychotic-drugs

Mahone, I., Maphis, C., & Snow, D. (2016). Effective strategies for nurses empowering clients with schizophrenia: Medication use as a tool in recovery. *Issues in Mental Health Nursing, 37*(5), 372–379.

Manschreck, T. (2019). Delusional disorder. *UpToDate.* https://www.uptodate.com/contents/delusional-disorder

Morin, L., & Franck, N. (2017). Rehabilitation interventions to promote recovery from schizophrenia: A systematic review. *Frontiers in Psychiatry, 8*, 100.

National Alliance on Mental Illness. (2020). *Schizoaffective disorder.* https://www.nami.org/learn-more/mental-health-conditions/schizoaffective-disorder

National Institute on Mental Health. (2013). *NIH-funded study adds to evidence of overlap with schizophrenia.* https://www.nih.gov/news-events/news-releases/flu-pregnancy-may-quadruple-childs-risk-bipolar-disorder

National Institute on Mental Health. (2016). *Mental health medications.* https://www.nimh.nih.gov/health/topics/mental-health-medications/index.shtml

National Institute on Mental Health. (2018). *Schizophrenia.* https://www.nimh.nih.gov/health/statistics/schizophrenia.shtml#part_154881

National Institute on Mental Health. (n.d.). *What is schizophrenia?* https://www.nimh.nih.gov/health/publications/schizophrenia/index.shtml

National Institutes of Health. (2019). *Delusional disorder.* https://ghr.nlm.nih.gov/condition/schizoaffective-disorder

Sanghani, S., Petrides, G., & Kellner, C. (2018). Electroconvulsive therapy (ECT) in schizophrenia: A review of recent literature. *Current Opinion in Psychiatry, 31*(3), 213–222.

Selten, J. P., & Termorshuizen, F. (2017). The serological evidence for maternal influenza as risk factor for psychosis in offspring is insufficient: Critical review and meta-analysis. *Schizophrenia Research, 183*, 2–9.

Skehan, B., & Dvir, Y. (2019). Schizophrenia in children and adolescents: Epidemiology, pathogenesis, clinical manifestations, course, assessment, and diagnosis. *UpToDate.* https://www.uptodate.com/contents/schizophrenia-in-children-and-adolescents-epidemiology-pathogenesis-clinical-manifestations-course-assessment-and-diagnosis

Tusaie, K., & Fitzpatrick, J. (2013). *Advanced practice psychiatric nursing.* Springer Publishing Company.

Vannorsdall, T., & Schretlin, D. (2013). Late-onset schizophrenia. In L. D. Ravdin & H. L. Katzen (Eds.), *Handbook on the neuropsychology of aging and dementia: Clinical handbooks in neuropsychology* (pp. 487–500). Springer.

Varcarolis, M. (2018). *Foundations of psychiatric-mental health nursing* (8th ed.). Elsevier.

World Health Organization. (2018). *Schizophrenia.* https://www.who.int/news-room/fact-sheets/detail/schizophrenia

Chapter 4

Bipolar and related disorders

Just the facts

In this chapter, you'll learn:

◆ effects of mood disorders on functioning

◆ proposed causes of mood disorders

◆ how to assess a patient's suicide risk

◆ types of bipolar and related disorders

◆ assessment and interventions for patients with bipolar and related disorders.

A look at mood disorders

Mood disorders are disturbances in the regulation of mood, behavior, and affect that go beyond the normal fluctuations that most people experience. In the United States, an estimated 21.4% of adults experience a mood disorder at some time in their lives (National Institute of Mental Health [NIMH], 2017). Throughout the world, mood disorders are one of the leading causes of disability.

This chapter discusses bipolar and related disorders. Chapter 5 discusses depressive disorders. These potentially disabling mood disorders can affect every aspect of a person's life—thought processes, emotions, behaviors, and even physical health. Many people with mood disorders have coexisting medical and psychiatric diagnoses.

Mood and affect

Mood refers to a pervading feeling, or an emotional state (NIMH, 2017). When someone has a mood disorder, their mood becomes so intense and persistent that it interferes with their social and psychological functioning. Mood is one element of the mental status examination that is historical and not typically able to be observed except in situational encounters.

Special affects

Affect refers to the outward expression of emotion attached to ideas—including but not limited to facial expression and vocal modulation. Variations in affect are called the *range of emotional expression*.

Patients with mood disorders may exhibit various abnormalities in affect, such as:

- blunted affect—a severe reduction in the intensity of outward emotional expression
- flat affect—a complete or almost complete absence of outward emotional expression
- constricted affect (not restricted)—a reduction in the intensity of outward emotional expression
- inappropriate affect—an affect that doesn't match the situation or the content of the verbalized message (e.g., laughing when talking about someone who died)
- labile affect—a rapid and easily changing affective expression unrelated to external events or stimuli.

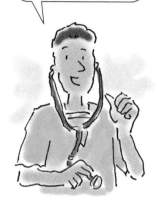

I don't have a flat affect because I like to smile.

Causes

Theories regarding the causes of mood disorders involve genetic, biological, and psychological factors.

Genetic factors

Children, parents, and siblings of people diagnosed with severe depression are more likely to suffer from depression than the general population. A genome-wide meta-analysis shows that there are important relationship between genetic risk factors that predispose individuals to major depressive disorders (Wray et al., 2018).

Biological factors

Biological research into the roots of mood disorder focuses on deficiencies or abnormalities in the brain's chemical messengers— neurotransmitters such as norepinephrine, serotonin, dopamine, and acetylcholine. The success of drugs that affect neurotransmitter levels in treating mood disorders supports the theory that these illnesses have biological roots. A research study published in the *Journal of Neuroscience* also showed that out of 24 women, the hippocampus was 9% to 13% smaller in women who were depressed than in those who were not depressed. The more depressive episodes a woman had, the smaller the hippocampus (Harvard Medical School, 2017).

Psychological theories

Cognitive, behavioral, and psychoanalytic theories also offer explanations for mood disorders.

Cognitive theory

Cognitive theory suggests that people who experience depression process information in a characteristically negative way in terms of selective abstraction, overgeneralization, and negative self-attributions (Beck et al., 1979, in Leahy, 2002).

Behavioral theory

According to the learned helplessness theory, people may become depressed after a negative event, such as a loved one's death or loss of a job, if the event makes them feel helpless. The perceived lack of control over life events dampens motivation, self-esteem, and initiative. Lack of social support, coupled with ineffective stress management and problem-solving skills, increases the risk of depression after stressful events.

Psychoanalytic theory

According to psychoanalytic theory, depression results from a harsh superego (the *conscience* of the unconscious mind) and feelings of loss. Loss—especially at an early age—makes a child more susceptible to depression later in life.

Signs and symptoms of a mood disorder

Mood and affect

Symptoms of a mood disorder will vary, depending on the patient's underlying diagnosis. A patient with bipolar disorder in a manic phase may exude a mood of euphoria, whereas a patient with major depressive disorder may exhibit a sad or morose mood. Specific symptoms will be explored within each discussed disorder.

Caring for patients with mood disorders

Caring for patients with mood disorders requires an understanding of the following elements:

- Mood disorders may cause somatic (physical) symptoms, so they may be mistaken for physical illnesses.
- The patient may neglect self-care because of lowered motivation and energy levels.
- Mood disorders may alter family and social relationships and lead to frustration, anger, and guilt. As a result, the patient may be the victim or perpetrator of abuse.
- If the patient is unable to work because of the mood disorder, financial hardship may occur.
- A patient with a mood disorder is at an increased risk for suicide.

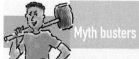

Bipolar disorder and psychotic symptoms

There is question about whether individuals with bipolar disorder experience psychosis.

Myth: Patients with bipolar disorder never experience psychotic symptoms.

Reality: Some patients with bipolar disorder do experience hallucinations and/or delusions. The *Diagnostic and Statistical Manual of Mental Disorders*, 5th Edition (*DSM-5*) has a specific code for this diagnosis (determined by the health care provider) that is termed "bipolar disorder with psychotic features."

Bipolar disorders

Bipolar disorders are mood disorders marked by severe, pathologic mood swings. Typically, the patient experiences extreme highs (mania or hypomania) with alternating extreme lows (depression). Interspersed between the highs and lows are periods of normal mood.

Variations can occur in the pattern of highs and lows. For instance, some people experience only acute episodes of mania.

Many people with moods

About 2.8% of the U.S. adult population experience bipolar disorder (National Alliance on Mental Illness, 2017). The disorder affects men and women equally. (See *Bipolar disorder and psychotic symptoms*.)

Onset usually occurs around the age of 18 to 20 years old, although earlier presentations have been documented (Stovall, 2020). Many patients with bipolar disorder have difficulties in work performance and psychosocial functioning.

Classification

Bipolar disorder is classified in three ways (American Psychiatric Association [APA], 2013):

- *Bipolar I disorder* is the classic and most severe form of the disorder. The patient has manic episodes or mixed episodes (with symptoms of both mania and depression) that alternate with major depressive episodes. The depressive phase may immediately precede or follow a manic phase, or it may be separated from the manic phase by months or years.

- In *bipolar II disorder*, the patient doesn't experience severe mania but instead has milder episodes of hypomania that alternate with depressive episodes.
- In *cyclothymic disorder*, the patient has a history of numerous hypomanic episodes intermingled with numerous depressive episodes that don't meet the criteria for major depressive episodes.

Episodes and residuals

Most patients with bipolar disorder have recurring episodes of mania and depression across the life span, with symptom-free periods between episodes. Many patients experience residual symptoms and some have chronic, unremitting symptoms despite treatment.

Mania and hypomania

The highs of bipolar disorder may involve mania or hypomania. *Mania* is characterized by poor judgment and a lack of insight, as well as:

An increase in ....
- Agitation
- Elation
- Euphoria
- Hyperactivity (hyperexcitability)
- Impulsivity
- Rapid thought and speech
- Sexuality

A decrease in ....
- Attention span
- Awareness of illness
- Eating (too busy to eat)
- Sleep

Not quite so manic

Hypomania refers to an expansive, elevated, or agitated mood that resembles mania but is less intense and lacks psychotic symptoms. For some patients, hypomania doesn't cause problems in social activities or work. In fact, it may feel good, bringing high energy, confidence, and enhanced social functioning and productivity.

You call that progress?

For others, however, hypomanic episodes can be troublesome. Without proper treatment, these episodes may progress to severe mania or switch to depression.

Psychotic symptoms

Some patients with bipolar disorder have severe episodes of mania or depression that involve psychotic symptoms such as hallucinations (hearing, seeing, touching, smelling, or tasting things that

> I may be high right now, but I'm not manic.

aren't actually there) or delusions (false beliefs not influenced by logical reasoning or explained by a person's usual cultural concepts). Although these symptoms resemble schizophrenia, remember that bipolar disorder does not always involve psychosis. Even when it does, this disorder is characterized by other features in addition to psychosis. (For information on schizophrenia, see Chapter 3.)

Side effects

The impulsive behavior that takes place during a manic episode may have far-reaching emotional and social consequences such as relationship difficulty, joblessness, bankruptcy, and promiscuity. Hyperactivity and sleep disturbances may lead to exhaustion and poor nutrition.

People with bipolar disorders often experience an increase in risky sexual behaviors during a manic episode, and therefore, run the risk of acquiring sexually transmitted infections (STIs) and having unwanted pregnancies.

Bipolar disorder also increases the risk for suicide. A suicide attempt may occur impulsively during a manic episode or in a depressive episode. The risk for suicide in this population is 20- to 30-fold higher than in the average population (Plans et al., 2019).

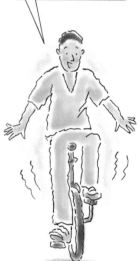

For someone with rapid-cycling bipolar disorder, mood swings come fast and furious.

Rapid cycling

Some patients who have bipolar disorder experience rapid cycling. In this variant, four or more distinct periods of depression, mania, hypomania, or mixed states occur within a 12-month period (APA, 2013). Periods of normal mood may be brief or even absent. Rapid cycling tends to develop later in the course of the illness.

Pedaling as fast as they can

The more rapid the cycling, the more numerous the mood swings. Some sufferers experience multiple illness episodes within a single week. Some ultra-rapid cyclers have several mood swings in a single day.

Experts believe that any bipolar patient can *switch* to a rapid-cycling pattern—but most return to their normal bipolar pattern in time.

Causes

The precise cause of bipolar disorder isn't known. However, genetic, biochemical, and psychological factors are thought to play a role.

Genetic factors

Twin, family, and adoption studies strongly suggest that bipolar disorder has a genetic component. First-degree relatives of a person with bipolar disorder are more likely than the general population to develop the disorder, although researchers have not yet determined why some families seem to have a higher risk of inheriting the condition than others (U.S. National Library of Medicine, 2019).

Biochemical factors

Experts think bipolar disorder stems at least in part from neurotransmitter abnormalities or imbalances. Some studies suggest the illness involves sensitivity of receptors on nerve cells.

Precipitating events

Stressful life events, such as a serious loss, chronic illness, or financial problems, may trigger a bipolar episode in persons who are predisposed to the disorder. Other conditions associated with bipolar disorder include substance misuse and traumatic head injury (U.S. National Library of Medicine, 2019). However, bipolar episodes can occur with no obvious trigger.

Signs and symptoms

Assessment findings in patients with bipolar disorder vary with the illness phase.

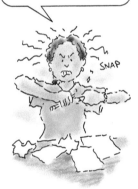

Some people get super irritable during the manic phase.

During the manic phase

Signs and symptoms that may appear during the manic phase include those listed under *Mania and hypomania*, page 110.

When experiencing severe mania, the patient may have delusions, paranoid thinking, and an inflated sense of self-esteem ranging from uncritical self-confidence to marked grandiosity.

During the depressive phase

During a depressive episode, the patient may report or exhibit:

- low self-esteem
- overwhelming inertia
- social withdrawal
- feelings of hopelessness, apathy, or self-reproach
- difficulty concentrating or thinking clearly (without obvious disorientation or intellectual impairment)
- psychomotor retardation (sluggish physical movements and activity)
- slowing of speech and responses
- sexual dysfunction
- sleep disturbances
- decreased muscle tone

- weight loss
- slow gait
- constipation.

Diagnosis

The diagnosis of bipolar disorder is confirmed if the patient meets the criteria in *DSM-5*. The health care provider will determine whether the patient has bipolar I disorder, bipolar II disorder, or cyclothymic disorder.

Treatment

Treatment of bipolar disorder requires drug therapy. Lithium is highly effective in both preventing and relieving manic episodes. It curbs accelerated thought processes and hyperactive behavior without the sedating effect of antipsychotic drugs. Lithium may also prevent the recurrence of depressive episodes, although it's ineffective in treating acute depression.

Not much wiggle room

Lithium has a narrow margin of safety and can easily cause toxicity. Treatment must begin cautiously with a low dose, which is adjusted slowly as needed. The patient must maintain therapeutic blood levels for 7 to 10 days before the desired effects appear, so the doctor may prescribe antipsychotic drugs in the interim for symptomatic relief. (See *Lithium alert*, page 114.)

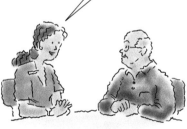

Lithium can be tricky because of its narrow margin of safety.

Other drugs

The doctor may prescribe valproic acid (Depakote) for patients who cycle rapidly, or for patients who can't tolerate lithium. Carbamazepine (Tegretol) has also been shown to be useful in treating mania.

Flip–flop effect

Antidepressants are occasionally prescribed to treat depressive symptoms. They must be used with extreme caution, however, because they may trigger a manic episode in patients with a bipolar disorder.

Nursing interventions

Appropriate nursing interventions vary with the phase of the bipolar disorder.

Advice from the experts

Lithium alert

For a patient who's receiving lithium, routine blood level monitoring is crucial because of the medication's narrow therapeutic margin. Lithium shouldn't be used if the patient can't have regular blood tests. In addition, because lithium is excreted by the kidneys, it shouldn't be given to patients with renal impairment.

Blood levels should be checked 8 to 12 hours after the first dose, two or three times weekly for the first month, and then weekly to monthly during maintenance therapy.

Patient teaching

• Instruct the patient to maintain a fluid intake of 2,500 to 3,000 mL/day to promote adequate lithium excretion.
• Inform the patient that the lithium may cause sodium depletion, especially during initial therapy, until consistent blood levels are achieved. Instruct the patient not to make dietary changes that might alter sodium intake because this might reduce lithium elimination and increase the toxicity risk.
• Inform the patient that increasing salt intake may increase lithium excretion, which could lead to the return of mood symptoms. Teach to maintain adequate salt and water intake and to eat a normal, well-balanced diet. Remind the patient that sodium loss (which can result from diarrhea, illness, extreme sweating, or other conditions) may alter lithium levels.
• Teach the patient and family to watch for evidence of toxicity—diarrhea, vomiting, tremors, drowsiness, muscle weakness, and ataxia. Instruct patients to withhold one dose and call the doctor if toxic symptoms occur, but not to stop taking the drug abruptly.

During a manic episode

• Provide for the patient's physical needs during this time of energy abundance. Involve the patient in activities that require safe gross motor movements.
• Encourage the patient to eat. He or she may be inclined to jump up and walk around the room after every mouthful but will sit down again if you remind him or her. If the patient can't sit still long enough to finish a meal, offer high-calorie, nutritious finger foods, sandwiches, and cheese and crackers to supplement his or her diet.
• Suggest short daytime naps and help with personal hygiene. As symptoms subside, encourage the patient to assume responsibility for personal care.
• Provide diversionary activities suited to a short attention span. Set boundaries and reinforce these so that the patient does not become overextended.

Mission: Harmony

• Maintain a calm environment and protect the patient from overstimulation (e.g., large groups, loud noises, and bright colors).
• Provide therapeutic emotional support and set realistic goals for behavior.

- Tactfully divert the conversation if the patient becomes inappropriately involved with other patients or staff.
- Avoid reinforcing socially inappropriate or suggestive comments.

Limit setting and listening

- In a calm, clear, therapeutic manner, set limits for demanding, hyperactive, manipulative, and acting-out behaviors. Redirect testing or argumentative behaviors.
- Listen to requests attentively and with a neutral attitude, but avoid power struggles if the patient pressures you for an immediate answer. Explain that you'll seriously consider the request and respond later.
- Collaborate with other staff members to provide consistent responses to the patient's behaviors.
- Anticipate the need for excessive verbalization.

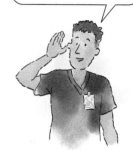

Listen to the patient's requests with a neutral attitude.

No acting out

- Watch for early signs of frustration, such as when anger escalates from verbal threats to hitting an object.
- Tell the patient firmly that threats and hitting are unacceptable and indicate that help may be needed to control behavior. Inform the patient that the staff will help with movement to a quiet area and with control of behavior so the patient will not impose a danger to self or others. Staff members who have practiced as a team can work effectively to prevent acting-out behavior or to remove the patient from the vicinity if necessary.
- Alert the care team promptly when acting-out behavior escalates. It's safer to have help available before you need it than to try to assist on your own a patient who is anxious or frightened.
- When the incident ends and the patient is calm and in control, discuss feelings with the patient and teach ways of coping to prevent recurrence.

Minding medications

- Advise the patient to take lithium with food or after meals to avoid stomach upset.
- Because lithium may impair mental and physical function, caution the patient against driving or operating dangerous equipment.
- Encourage to stay well hydrated because lithium is excreted via the kidneys. (See *Lithium Alert*.)

During a depressive episode
- Provide for the patient's physical needs. If the patient is too depressed to provide self-care, help with personal hygiene.
- Encourage eating, or feed the patient if necessary. If the patient is constipated, add high-fiber foods to the diet; offer small, frequent meals; and encourage appropriate types and amounts of physical activity.
- To help the patient sleep, teach methods of sleep hygiene, provide a calm environment, and encourage a predictable evening routine.

Provide pick-me-ups

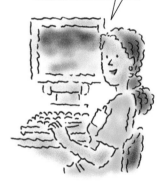

Be sure to assess and document the severity, duration, and other features of the patient's pain.

- Keep in mind that a patient who is in the depressed phase of a bipolar disorder needs continual positive reinforcement to improve self-esteem. Provide a structured routine, including activities to boost confidence and promote interaction with others (e.g., group therapy). Reassure the patient that the depression will lift as you work together on medication management and therapy.
- Assume an active role in communicating. Encourage the patient to talk, or to write down feelings if he or she is having trouble expressing them. Listen attentively and respectfully. If the patient seems sluggish, give adequate time to formulate thoughts. Document your observations and conversations to assist in evaluating the patient's condition.
- Avoid overwhelming the patient with expectations.

Injury aversion

- To prevent self-injury or suicide, remove all harmful objects (such as glass, belts, rope, shoelaces, paper clips, bobby pins, alcohol-based hand sanitizer) from the patient's environment.
- Institute suicide precautions per facility policy.
- Observe the patient closely and strictly supervise medication administration.

Medication teaching

- Teach information contained in "Lithium alert" if the patient has been prescribed this drug.
- Teach the importance of continuing the medication regimen even if he or she feels better.
- If the patient is taking an antidepressant, assess for signs and symptoms of mania.

Cyclothymic disorder

In cyclothymic disorder, short periods of mild depression alternate with short periods of hypomania. Between the depressive and manic episodes, brief periods of normal mood occur. According to *DSM-5*, the patient does not exceed 2 consecutive months without symptoms of depression or hypomania (APA, 2013).

In many persons with cyclothymic disorder, manic episodes emerge over a few days to weeks, although onset within hours is possible.

Mood indigo

Both the depressive and hypomanic episodes of cyclothymic disorder are shorter and less severe than those in bipolar I or II disorder. Also, delusions don't occur, and few patients require hospitalization. In essence, cyclothymic disorder may be diagnosed when the patient experiences these symptoms, but does not meet the criteria for major depression, mania, or true hypomania (Suppes, 2019). Nonetheless, these mood swings may impair social and occupational functioning.

Damage and instability

Hypomanic periods of cyclothymic disorder may enhance a person's achievement in business and artistic endeavors but also may damage interpersonal and social relationships. The frequency of mood shifts may lead to an uneven work and academic history, impulsive and frequent changes of residence, repeated romantic or marital breakups, and/or an episodic pattern of alcohol and drug misuse.

Signs and symptoms

General features of cyclothymia include:
- inconsistency in maintaining enthusiasm for new projects
- a pattern of pulling close and then pushing away in interpersonal relationships
- abrupt changes in personality from cheerful, confident, and energetic to sad, blue, or mean.

Symptoms by phase

The patient experiencing the hypomanic phase may report or exhibit symptoms that are similar to, but not as vibrant as, those experienced by a patient with bipolar disorder in the manic phase. During the depressive phase, signs and symptoms resemble those experienced by a patient with bipolar disorder in the depressive phase, yet not as pronounced.

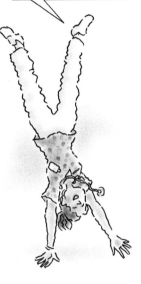

Physical restlessness is a possible sign of hypomania.

Causes

As with bipolar disorder, genetic factors are thought to influence the development of cyclothymic disorder.

Diagnosis

The health care provider makes the diagnosis on the basis of subjective and objective assessments, and in relationship to the *DSM-5* criteria (APA, 2013).

Treatment

No medications are specifically FDA-approved to treat cyclothymia; however, the health care provider may recommend mood stabilizers to manage mood fluctuations. Antidepressants are not recommended due to the increased risk of triggering manic symptoms. Other pharmacologic options for cyclothymic disorder include:

- lithium carbonate (Lithobid)
- carbamazepine (Tegretol)
- lamotrigine (Lamictal)
- valproic acid (Depakote)
- verapamil (Calan SR)

Other therapies may include individual psychotherapy, and couple or family therapy, which can help patients deal with personal and relationship problems that may arise due to this disorder.

Nursing interventions

Nursing interventions for patients with cyclothymic disorder mirror interventions that are appropriate for patients with bipolar I or bipolar II disorder. It may also be helpful to encourage vocational opportunities that allow flexible work hours.

Quick quiz

1. A patient with bipolar II disorder is smiling, laughing, and engaging well with staff at the nurse's station, and then informs the nurse, "My day isn't good; I feel suicidal and want to hurt myself." How will the nurse document this affect?
    A. Flat
    B. Labile
    C. Blunted
    D. Inappropriate

Answer: D. The patient is not displaying the emotion that is appropriate and consistent to having a bad day and feeling suicidal with an intent to harm self.

2. Which factor does the nurse identify as a possible trigger for a manic episode in a patient with bipolar disorder?
    A. Hypertension
    B. Hyperthyroidism
    C. Taking antimanic drugs
    D. Taking antidepressant drugs

Answer: D. In a patient with bipolar disorder, the use of antidepressant drugs can trigger a manic event.

3. When teaching a patient with bipolar disorder, how will the nurse describe *rapid cycling*?
    A. No depressive episodes; only manic episodes in a year
    B. One or more episodes of depression or mania in 1 year
    C. Two or more episodes of depression or mania in 1 year
    D. Four or more episodes of depression or mania in 1 year

Answer: D. Rapid cycling in a bipolar disorder reflects four or more episodes of depression or mania occurring within a 1-year period.

4. Upon admission, the nurse requires the patient with bipolar disorder to turn over any belts, shoestrings, neckties, and sweatshirt ties. When the patient asks, "Why do I have to give you all these things," what is the appropriate nursing response?
    A. "This is our unit's protocol."
    B. "My job requires me to take these from you."
    C. "Why do you need these while you are on the unit?"
    D. "All patients turn over these items to keep everyone safe from harm."

Answer: D. It is important to communicate openly and honestly. The nurse will tell the patient that everyone turns these over to create a safe environment. Telling the patient that this is protocol, or a job requirement, does not address the patient's question. Asking why the patient needs these items does not address the question, nor does it change the fact that these must be turned over.

5. What teaching will the nurse provide to a patient who has been prescribed lithium?
   A. Restrict sodium
   B. Monitor carbohydrate intake
   C. Maintain a daily fluid intake of 2,500 mL
   D. Decrease the amount of consumed daily protein

Answer: C. A patient taking lithium must maintain a high fluid intake. Restricting sodium is not advised; the patient does not need to monitor carbohydrate intake or decrease daily proteins while on lithium.

Scoring

  If you answered all five items correctly, your performance was excellent!

  If you answered three or four items correctly, your insight into mood disorders is expanding.

If you answered fewer than three items correctly, don't be sad. Just read the chapter and try again!

Selected references

American Psychiatric Association. (2013). *Diagnostic and statistical manual of mental disorders* (5th ed.). Author.

Beck, A. T. (1979). Cognitive models of depression. In R. L. Leahy & E. T. Dowd (Eds.) 2002, *Clinical advances in cognitive psychotherapy: Theory and application* (pp. 29–61). Springer Publishing Company.

Harvard Medical School. (2017). *What causes depression? Onset of depression more complex than a brain chemical imbalance.* https://www.health.harvard.edu/mind-and-mood/what-causes-depression

National Institute of Mental Health. (2017). *Any mood disorder.* Retrieved from https://www.nami.org/learn-more/mental-health-conditions/bipolar-disorder

Plans, L., Barrot, C., Nieto, E., Rios, J., Schulze, T. G., Papiol, S., Mitjans, M., Vieta, E., & Benabarre, A. (2019). Association between completed suicide and bipolar disorder: A systematic review of the literature. *Journal of Affective Disorders, 242,* 111–122.

Stovall, J. (2020). Bipolar disorder in adults: Epidemiology and pathogenesis. https://www.uptodate.com/contents/bipolar-disorder-in-adults-epidemiology-and-pathogenesis

Suppes, T. (2019). Bipolar disorder in adults: Assessment and diagnosis. *UpToDate.* https://www.uptodate.com/contents/bipolar-disorder-in-adults-assessment-and-diagnosis

U.S. National Library of Medicine. (2019). Bipolar disorder. *Genetics Home Reference.* https://ghr.nlm.nih.gov/condition/bipolar-disorder#inheritance

Wray, N. R., Ripke, S., Mattheisen, M., Trzaskowski, M., Byrne, E. M., Abdellaoui, A., Adams, M. J., Agerbo, E., Air, T. M., Andlauer, T. M. F., Bacanu, S.-A., Bækvad-Hansen, M., Beekman, A. F. T., Bigdeli, T. B., Binder, E. B., Blackwood, D. R. H., Bryois, J., Buttenschøn, H. N., Bybjerg-Grauholm, J., ... Sullivan, P. F. (2018). Genome-wide association analyses identify 44 risk variants and refine the genetic architecture of major depression. *Nature Genetics, 50*(5), 668.

Chapter 5

Depressive disorders

Just the facts

In this chapter, you'll learn:

◆ types of depressive disorders

◆ effects of depressive disorders on functioning

◆ how to mitigate suicide risk in patients with depressive disorders

◆ assessment and interventions for patients with depressive disorders.

A look at depressive disorders

People have good days and bad days and days in between. Everyone feels sad, lonely, overwhelmed, and tired occasionally, especially during stressful times (Videbeck, 2017). These feelings are normal and resolve within a short period of time. However, persistent feelings of sadness (depression) can affect every aspect of a person's life—thought processes, emotions, behaviors, and physical health. These persistent feelings can impair judgment and lead to negative views of the world (Boyd, 2018). Depression is a symptom of depressive disorders.

The American Psychiatric Association (APA, 2013) describes eight different types of depressive disorders. In this chapter, we will be focusing on two depressive disorders: major depressive disorder and persistent depressive disorder (dysthymia). The other six depressive disorders are briefly described. (See *Depressive disorders*, page 122.)

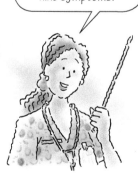

Mild depressive disorder has five symptoms, moderate depressive disorder has six to seven symptoms, and severe depressive disorder has eight to nine symptoms.

Major depressive disorder

Major depressive disorder (also called *unipolar major depression*) is a syndrome of a persistent sad mood lasting 2 weeks or longer with other accompanying symptoms (Hasin et al., 2018) that include:
• feelings of guilt, helplessness, hopelessness, or worthlessness
• poor concentration
• sleep disturbances: insomnia or hypersomnia

Depressive disorders

Depressive disorders recognized by the APA are described here. Major depressive disorder and persistent depressive disorder are described in more detail in the chapter.

Disruptive mood dysregulation disorder
• Characteristics of this disorder involve outbursts of temper disproportionate to the situation and inconsistent with the individual's developmental level and irritable mood, with symptoms lasting longer than 12 months.

Premenstrual dysphoric disorder
• Characteristics of this disorder involve mood swings, increased sensitivity, marked irritability, marked depressed mood, marked anxiety, and feelings of being on edge that occur the week before menses, with symptoms starting to resolve the week following the onset of menses.

Substance/medication-induced depressive disorder
• Characteristics of this disorder involve the use or withdrawal of a substance or medication that results in a persistent change in mood and a lack of interest or pleasure in life activities.

Depressive disorder due to another medical condition
• Characteristics of this disorder involve a persistent depressed state resulting from the pathophysiology of a medical condition that causes marked distress in most aspects of life, such as work and relationships. The symptoms usually occur within 1 month of the onset of the medical condition.

Other specified depressive disorder
• Characteristics of this disorder involve symptoms that do not meet full criteria for the depressive disorders listed earlier. For example, the individual experiences recurrent brief episodes of depression.

Unspecified depressive disorder
• Characteristics of this disorder involve symptoms that cause marked distress or impairment of daily activities. The symptoms do not fully meet any of the criteria for the depressive disorders listed earlier because of lack of assessment information such as situations in an emergency department.

Adapted from American Psychiatric Association. (2013). *Diagnostic and statistical manual of mental disorders, DSM-5* (5th ed.). Author; Boyd, M. (2018). *Psychiatric nursing: Contemporary practice* (6th ed.). Wolters Kluwer; Videbeck, S. (2017). *Psychiatric-mental health nursing* (7th ed). Wolters Kluwer.

- lethargy
- appetite loss
- anhedonia (inability to feel pleasure)
- loss of mood reactivity (failure to feel a mood uplift in response to something positive)
- thoughts of death or suicide.

Major depression often goes undiagnosed, and those who have it commonly receive inadequate treatment.

Beyond sad to bad

In major depressive disorder, sad feelings go beyond—and last longer than—"normal" sadness or grief. Also, some symptoms of severe depression, such as disinterest in pleasurable activities, hopelessness, and loss of mood reactivity, rarely accompany "normal" sadness.

In harm's way

Major depression can profoundly alter a person's social, family, and occupational functioning. The number of individuals worldwide with depression has increased significantly in the last two decades (Cipriana et al., 2018). Suicide—the most serious complication—can occur if feelings of worthlessness, guilt, and hopelessness are so overwhelming that the person no longer considers life worth living.

Nearly 4% of adults report having serious thoughts of suicide, with the highest number occurring between ages 18 and 25 (Nguyen et al., 2018). In the United States, the most common mental disorder is major depressive disorder (National Institute of Mental Health [NIMH], 2019).

Depression and the United States

At some time in their lives, 15% of the adult population in the United States experience major depressive disorder, with women experiencing depression at almost twice the rate as men (NIMH, 2019). The median age of depression onset is 32.5 years, and individuals may have recurrences throughout their lifetime. Recurrences may follow a prolonged symptom-free period or may occur sporadically. For some people, they come in clusters. For others, recurrences grow more frequent with age.

More than 50% of patients who have one episode go on to have at least two more. An untreated episode can last from 1 month to a year—or even longer.

Causes

Genetic, biochemical, physical, psychological, and social factors have been implicated in major depression. The relationship between psychological stress, stressful life events, and depression onset is unclear. However, the patient history often reveals a specific personal loss or severe stress. According to one theory, the stressor interacts with the person's predisposition to provoke major depression.

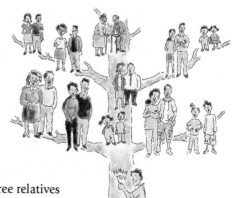

Genetic basis

Depression is more common in people with first-degree relatives with the disorder, indicating a genetic vulnerability. The risk of major depression is two to four times higher than the general population for individuals who have first-degree relatives with major depression (APA, 2013).

The p factor

Researchers have found high comorbidity rates among patients with psychiatric mental health disorders including depressive disorders. A general genetic factor (p factor) has been identified that provides underlying evidence for these correlations (Selzam et al., 2018).

Biochemical defects

The neural networks of the brain's prefrontal cortex and basal ganglia may be the primary defect sites in major depressive disorder.

The neuroendocrine and hypothalamic-pituitary-adrenal regulation systems may also be involved in the development of depression. Differences in biological rhythms may also play a role, as seen by changes in circadian rhythms and various neurochemical and neurohormonal factors. Depression involves altered functioning of neurotransmitters, including monoamines (serotonin, dopamine, norepinephrine), gamma-aminobutyric acid (GABA), and glutamate (Krishnan, 2019).

Finally, some researchers are homing in on abnormal cortisol levels as a factor in depression. In the dexamethasone suppression test, about 50% of patients with depression fail to suppress cortisol levels.

Organic causes

Health care professionals must distinguish major depression from depression caused by a specific event or a recognizable organic condition. Depression can result from a wide range of physical disorders (see *Depressive disorders: Depressive disorder due to another medical condition*, page 122), including:

- metabolic disturbances, such as hypothyroidism, diabetes mellitus, and vitamin D deficiencies
- endocrine disorders, such as diabetes and Cushing disease
- neurologic diseases, such as Parkinson disease, traumatic brain injury, and Alzheimer disease
- cancer (especially of the pancreas)
- infectious disorders, such as neurosyphilis and HIV
- cardiovascular disorders, such as heart failure
- inflammatory disorders, such as degenerative arthritis, irritable bowel syndrome
- gastrointestinal disorders, such as irritable bowel syndrome
- genitourinary problems, such as incontinence
- collagen vascular diseases, such as lupus
- anemias (Krishnan, 2019).

Medications that can cause depression

Drugs prescribed for certain medical and psychiatric conditions can cause depression. (See *Depressive disorders: Substance/medication-induced depressive disorder*, page 122.) Examples include:

- antihypertensives
- psychotropics
- antiparkinsonian drugs
- opioids and nonnarcotic analgesics
- numerous cardiovascular medications
- antidiabetic medications
- antimicrobials
- steroids (especially glucocorticoids)
- chemotherapeutic agents
- cimetidine.

Alcohol use may also contribute to depression.

Signs and symptoms

During the assessment interview, a patient with major depression may seem unhappy or apathetic. The patient may report such changes or deficits in:

- feeling "down in the dumps"
- attention span
- task shifting (ability to shifts tasks)
- executive function (ability to problem solve and reasoning)
- memory
- increased or decreased appetite
- sleep disturbances (e.g., insomnia or early awakening)
- disinterest in sex
- difficulty concentrating or thinking clearly
- easy distractibility
- indecisiveness
- low self-esteem
- poor coping
- constipation or diarrhea
- suicidal ideation (Lyness, 2019).

During the physical examination, you may note agitation (such as hand wringing or restlessness) or psychomotor retardation (slow movements). With severe depression, the patient may have delusions of persecution or guilt, which can have an immobilizing effect.

Psychosocial clues

The psychosocial history may reveal life problems or losses that may explain or contribute to depression. Or, the medical history may implicate a physical disorder or use of a prescription drug or other substance that can cause depression.

A danger to oneself

Stay alert for clues to suicidal thoughts, a preoccupation with death, or previous suicide attempts. Many patients are reluctant to verbalize suicidal thoughts unless prompted, so you may need to assess the patient's suicide risk by asking direct questions. Use the SAD PER-SONS Scale to determine the patient's suicide risk (Juhnke, 1994). (See *Memory jogger.*)

Scoring system: 1 point for each positive answer.
Score risk
0 to 2: No real problems, keep watch
3 to 4: Send home, but check frequently

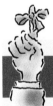

Memory jogger

Can't remember the things that may predispose a patient to suicide? Use the **SAD PERSONS** Scale to guide you.

Sex—females are more likely to attempt suicide, but males are more likely to choose a more deadly means

Age—15 to 24 years and 75 and older are high-risk groups

Depression

Previous attempts

Ethanol and other drug use

Rational thinking loss

Social support lacking

Organized plan—the more specific the plan, the greater the risk

No spouse

Sickness

Juhnke, G. A. (1994). SAD PERSONS Scale review. *Measurement and Evaluation in Counseling and Development, 27*(1), 325–327.

5 to 6: Consider hospitalization, involuntarily or voluntarily, depending on your level of assurance that patient will return for another session
7 to 10: Definitely hospitalize involuntarily or voluntarily.

A patient who has specific suicide plans or significant risk factors (such as a history of a suicide attempt, profound hopelessness, concurrent medical illness, substance misuse, or social isolation) should be referred to a mental health specialist for immediate care. (See *Obstacles to detecting depression*, page 128.)

Is path warm

Another mnemonic for patient assessment in determining suicide risk is IS PATH WARM (Juhnke et al., 2007).

Suicide Ideation:
- Does the patient report active suicidal ideation or written about suicide or death?
- Does the patient report the desire to commit suicide?
- Does the patient voice a desire to purchase a gun (or other means) with the intention of using it to commit suicide?
- Does the patient voice the intention to commit suicide with a gun, or other means currently in possession or can gain access to?

Substance use:
- Does the patient use alcohol or other drugs excessively, or has begun using alcohol or other drugs?

Purposelessness:
- Does the patient voice a lack or loss of purpose in life?
- Does the patient see little or no sense or reason for continued living?

Anger:
- Does the patient express feelings of rage or uncontrolled anger?
- Does the patient seek revenge against others whom he or she has perceived to have wronged him or her, or are at fault for his or her current concerns or problems?

Trapped:
- Does the patient feel trapped?
- Does the patient believe there is no way out of the current situation?
- Does the patient believe death is preferable to a pained life?
- Does the patient believe that no other choices exist except living the pained life or death?

Obstacles to detecting depression

Always consider the patient's cultural background and values when assessing for signs and symptoms of depression. In most parts of world, depression and other mood disorders are viewed as social or moral problems—not as mental health problems appropriate to discuss with health care providers.

Even in the United States, some ethnic groups are less likely to seek and use treatment (Hudson et al., 2018).

Hopelessness:
- Does the patient have a negative sense of self, others, and his or her future?
- Does the future appear hopeless with little chance for positive change?

Withdrawing:
- Does the patient indicate a desire to withdraw from significant others, family, friends, and society?
- Has the patient already begun withdrawing?

Anxiety:
- Does the patient feel anxious, agitated, or unable to sleep?
- Does the patient report an inability to relax?
- Does the patient report sleeping all the time?

Recklessness:
- Does the patient act recklessly or engage in risky activities, seemingly without thinking or considering potential consequences?

Mood change:
- Does the patient report experiencing dramatic mood shifts or states?

Diagnosis

The health care provider may complete a physical examination and laboratory evaluation to determine possible underlying or contributing factors. The health care provider will administer psychological tests, such as the Patient Health Questionnaire (PHQ-9) or the Beck Depression Inventory, to determine symptom onset, severity, duration, and progression.

The diagnosis of major depressive disorder (or unipolar depressive disorder) is confirmed if the patient exhibits symptoms lasting 2 or more weeks (APA, 2013).

Treatment

The primary treatments for major depressive disorder are pharmacologic therapy, psychotherapy, and electroconvulsive therapy (ECT). Treatment is considered effective if the patient has positive outcomes. (See *Memory jogger*.)

Evidence-based treatment of mild to moderate depression includes:

- treatment of coexisting anxiety
- advice on sleep hygiene
- active monitoring
- low-intensity psychosocial interventions (cognitive-behavioral therapy [CBT], computerized cognitive-behavioral therapy [CCBT])
- group CBT
- antidepressant medication treatment in limited cases
- advice against using St. John's wort if taking antidepressant medications.

Evidence-based treatment of moderate and severe depression includes:

- antidepressant drug treatment, such as selective serotonin reuptake inhibitors (SSRIs)
- high-intensity psychological intervention (CBT, interpersonal therapy, behavioral activation, behavioral couples therapy)
- combined antidepressant medication and high-intensity psychological intervention
- counseling
- short-term psychodynamic psychotherapy
- choice of antidepressant medication other than SSRIs
  - serotonin and norepinephrine reuptake inhibitors (SNRIs), for example, venlafaxine (Effexor) and duloxetine (Cymbalta)
  - tricyclic antidepressants (TCAs), for example, amitriptyline (Elavil)
- assessing during the initial phase of medication treatment, for example, suicide risk, side effects
- treatment choice based on depression subtypes and personal characteristics

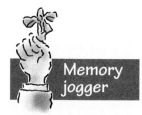

Memory jogger

For a depressed patient, positive OUTCOMES include:

Overwhelming feelings of grief and loss are processed

Uses problem-solving and reasoning skills to handle stressors

Talks with others willingly and appropriately

Cognitive distortions are decreased or eliminated

Overcomes thoughts of physically harming self

Maintains a positive sense of self

Eats nutritionally balanced meals and snacks

Sleeps 6 to 8 hours each night

- enhanced care for depression: referral to specialist mental health services
- switching antidepressants
- combining and augmenting medications, for example, addition of lithium, an antipsychotic, another antidepressant
- continuation and relapse prevention.

Evidence-based management of complex and severe depression includes:
- referral to specialist mental health services
- inpatient care
- crisis resolution
- home treatment teams
- pharmacologic management of depression with psychotic symptoms
- noninvasive neuromodulation therapies
  - ECT (See *Electroconvulsive therapy*, page 134.)
  - Repeated (or repetitive) transcranial magnetic stimulation (rTMS)
    - Alternating currents are passed through a coil placed on the patient's scalp, resulting in the depolarization of neurons in the surface cortex.
    - Must use effective parameters, especially for treatment of unipolar depression, after antidepressants have been tried (Holtzheimer, 2019).

Pharmacologic therapy

Medication is the most effective means of achieving remission and preventing relapse. Combining medication with psychotherapy can improve the treatment outcome by helping the patient cope with low self-esteem and demoralization.

Types of antidepressants
Generally, antidepressant drugs work by modifying the activity of relevant neurotransmitter pathways. These agents fall into several categories:
- SSRIs
- TCAs
- SNRIs
- monoamine oxidase inhibitors (MAOIs)
- atypical antidepressants
- other antidepressants.

No ideal antidepressant exists for all patients. The health care provider must consider the patient's metabolism, possible adverse effects, agents that have been effective with family members, and potential for toxicity (if suicidal overdose is a concern).

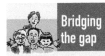

Bridging the gap

Matching the treatment to the culture

No matter what the diagnosis, always consider your patient's cultural and religious background. Some patients, for instance, may have cultural or religious reasons for not complying with the prescribed medication regimen. When this occurs, consider possible alternative treatments.

Meds matters

Pharmacologic therapy for depressive disorders

This chart highlights several of the drugs used to treat depressive disorders.

Drug	Adverse effects	Contraindications	Nursing considerations
Selective serotonin reuptake inhibitor			
Fluoxetine (Prozac)	• Dry mouth • Insomnia • Nausea • Nervousness • Rash • Vertigo • Weight loss	• Within 14 days of taking a monoamine oxidase inhibitor (MAOI)	• Know that medication is usually given in the morning with or without food. • Assess patient for weight loss if nausea occurs. • Know that patient should wait 5 weeks after stopping fluoxetine before starting an MAOI. • Tell patient to avoid alcoholic beverages. • Instruct patient to report adverse effects, especially rash or itching.
Serotonin norepinephrine reuptake inhibitor			
Venlafaxine (Effexor)	• Nausea and vomiting • Diarrhea • Appetite changes • Weight changes • Dry mouth • Dizziness • Headache • Vision changes • Decreased sex drive • Insomnia	• Do not use within 7 days before or 14 days after using an MAOI • Not approved for children under 18 years of age • Herbal therapies and many medications cause interactions • Opioid, NSAIDs • Diabetes • History of seizures • Thyroid disorders • Hyponatremia • Pregnancy	• Monitor for mood and behavioral changes, especially when taking this medication for the first time. • Teach patient not to stop taking medication without health care provider's knowledge. • Teach patient about side effects/adverse reactions and to report: blurred or tunnel vision, eye pain or halos around lights, easy bruising or bleeding, cough, chest tightness, dyspnea, seizures, mood or behavioral changes, anxiety, panic attacks, agitation, feeling hostile, or thoughts about suicide. • Teach patient to avoid driving or operating heavy machinery until effect of drug is known.
Monoamine oxidase inhibitor			
Isocarboxazid (Marplan)	• Blurred vision • Constipation • Dry mouth • Drowsiness or insomnia • Fatigue	• Cardiovascular or cerebrovascular disease • Confusion, uncooperativeness	• Monitor patient's blood pressure every 2 to 4 hours during initial therapy. Instruct patient to change positions slowly. • Assess for signs and symptoms of hypertensive crisis.

(*continued*)

Pharmacologic therapy for depressive disorders *(continued)*

Drug	Adverse effects	Contraindications	Nursing considerations
	• Hepatic dysfunction (jaundice, malaise, right upper abdominal quadrant pain, change in stool color or consistency) • Hypertensive crisis • Hypomania • Muscle twitching • Orthostatic hypotension • Skin rash • Vertigo • Weakness • Weight gain	• Elderly or debilitated patients • Glaucoma • Heart failure • History of severe headaches • Impaired renal function • Liver disease • Paranoid schizophrenia • Pregnancy	• Monitor fluid intake and output. • Assess patient for suicidal risk. • Caution patient not to ingest foods and beverages containing tyramine, caffeine, or tryptophan. Warn the patient that ingesting tyramine can cause a hypertensive crisis. Give patient a list of foods and beverages that contain such substances. • Instruct patient to avoid meperidine (Demerol), epinephrine, local anesthetics, decongestants, cough medicines, diet pills, and most over-the-counter agents. • Teach patient to wear medical identification jewelry. • Advise patient to go to emergency department immediately if hypertensive crisis develops.

Tricyclic antidepressant

Drug	Adverse effects	Contraindications	Nursing considerations
Amitriptyline (Elavil) Imipramine (Tofranil)	• Agranulocytosis • Arrhythmias • Blurred vision • Bone marrow depression • Constipation • Dry mouth • Esophageal reflux • Galactorrhea • Hallucinations • Heart failure • Increased or decreased libido • Jaundice and fatigue • Mania • Myocardial infarction (MI) • Orthostatic hypotension or hypertension • Palpitations • Shock • Slowed intracardiac conduction • Urinary hesitancy • Weight gain	• Concomitant use of MAOIs • Recent MI • Renal or hepatic disease	• Supervise patient's drug ingestion. • Monitor blood pressure and pulse for signs of orthostatic hypotension. • Monitor liver function and complete blood counts. • Institute suicide precautions as needed. • Know that special monitoring is required if patient poses a suicide risk or has a history of angle-closure glaucoma or seizure disorder. • Instruct patient to change positions slowly. • Tell patient to avoid driving or hazardous machinery if drowsiness occurs. • Instruct patient to avoid alcohol and over-the-counter agents unless the health care provider approves. • Inform patient that the drug may take up to 4 weeks to become effective.

NSAID, nonsteroidal anti-inflammatory drug.

Whichever drug is prescribed, the patient's response should be re-evaluated after the first 2 months of therapy, with dosage changes made as needed. After remission, drug therapy should continue for at least 6 to 9 months. (See *Matching the treatment to the culture*, page 130.)

Selective serotonin reuptake inhibitors

SSRIs include citalopram (Celexa), fluoxetine (Prozac), fluvoxamine (Luvox), paroxetine (Paxil), escitalopram (Lexapro), and sertraline (Zoloft). These agents inhibit serotonin reuptake and may inhibit the reuptake of other neurotransmitters as well.

SSRIs have become the first-choice treatment for most patients. They lack most of the disturbing adverse effects associated with TCAs and MAOIs.

Serotonin/norepinephrine reuptake inhibitors

SNRIs, such as venlafaxine (Effexor), inhibit serotonin and norepinephrine uptake. These drugs are generally used as second-line agents for patients with major depressive disorder.

Atypical antidepressants

Atypical antidepressants include bupropion (Wellbutrin) and mirtazapine (Remeron). These medications' mechanisms of action aren't well understood. Bupropion (Wellbutrin) is thought to inhibit reuptake of serotonin, norepinephrine, and dopamine to varying degrees. Mirtazapine (Remeron) is thought to inhibit serotonin and norepinephrine reuptake while blocking two specific serotonin receptors.

Although effective in certain patients, atypical antidepressants generally are used as second-line agents.

Tricyclic antidepressants

An older class of antidepressants, TCAs inhibit the reuptake of norepinephrine, serotonin, and dopamine and cause a gradual decline in beta-adrenergic receptors.

Specific TCAs include:
- amitriptyline (Elavil)
- amoxapine (Asendin)
- desipramine (Norpramin)
- doxepin (Sinequan)
- imipramine (Tofranil)
- nortriptyline (Pamelor)
- trimipramine (Surmontil).

Although TCAs can be effective, they may cause intolerable adverse effects. TCA overdose can quickly be lethal. For this reason, most TCAs have a black box warning for prescribers indicating

TCA therapy may cause some people to have suicidal thoughts or commit suicide.

Consequently, they generally are not used as first-line agents.

Monoamine oxidase inhibitors

MAOIs, such as phenelzine (Nardil), increase norepinephrine, serotonin, and dopamine levels by inhibiting MAO, an enzyme that inactivates them. They may have additional actions that contribute to their antidepressant effect.

MAOIs may be prescribed for patients with atypical depression (e.g., depression marked by an increased appetite and increased sleep rather than anorexia and insomnia) or for patients who don't respond to TCAs.

Although often effective, MAOIs carry a high risk of adverse effects and dangerous interactions with various foods and medications. Consequently, they're rarely used today—although conservative doses may be combined with a TCA for patients refractory to either type of drug alone.

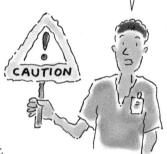

MAOIs can cause serious adverse effects and dangerous interactions with foods and other drugs.

FYI on MAOIs

If the patient is taking an MAOI, emphasize the avoidance of foods that contain tyramine, caffeine, or tryptophan. Warn that ingesting tyramine can cause a hypertensive crisis. Give the patient a list of foods and beverages that contain these substances, which include aged cheeses, sour cream, beer, Chianti, sherry, pickled herring, liver, canned figs, raisins, bananas, avocados, chocolate, soy sauce, fava beans, yeast extracts, meat tenderizers, coffee, and colas.

Electroconvulsive therapy

In ECT, a tiny electrical current is applied to the patient's brain through electrodes—one placed on each side of the skull. The current produces a seizure lasting from 30 seconds to 1 minute. ECT is recommended primarily for the treatment of severe major depression, in the context of either unipolar or bipolar disorders. The procedure is performed while the patient is under general anesthesia (Kellner, 2018).

A quicker picker-upper

Although controversial, ECT sometimes is used to treat severe depression when psychotherapy and medication aren't effective or when ECT poses a lower risk than other treatments. ECT produces faster results than antidepressant drugs.

Get ready

The patient fasts for 6 to 8 hours before ECT. Just before the session, dentures, glasses, hearing aids, contact lenses, and hairpins are removed and the patient is asked to void. The patient may be given a variety of medications before the procedure, including:

- atropine or glycopyrrolate to reduce secretions, prevent aspiration, and reduce the risk of bradycardia
- a short-acting general anesthetic
- a muscle relaxant
- oxygen.

The patient is connected to devices that monitor brain waves (electroencephalogram), heart rhythm (electrocardiogram), and arterial oxygen saturation. Vital signs (heart rate, blood pressure, and temperature), blood oxygen saturation, end-tidal carbon dioxide levels, and electromyogram (to record the duration of the motor component of the seizure) are monitored during ECT (Kellner, 2018).

Then a 1-second electrical current is applied to the brain through the electrodes. The current produces a brief seizure.

In a typical course of treatment for major depression, the patient receives two or three ECT treatments a week, for a total of 6 to 12 treatments. Contraindications include recent myocardial infarction, a history of stroke, and intracranial lesions. Special considerations are needed if the patient is pregnant (Kellner, 2018).

Psychotherapy

Short-term psychotherapy can aid in relieving major depression. Many psychiatrists believe the best results occur from combining individual, family, or group psychotherapy with medication.

After the acute episode of depression resolves, a patient with a history of recurrent depression may be maintained on a low dose of an antidepressant drug as a preventive measure.

A quicker picker-upper

Although controversial, ECT sometimes is used to treat severe depression when psychotherapy and medication aren't effective or when ECT poses a lower risk than other treatments, ECT produces faster results than antidepressant drugs (see "Meds matters", "Pharmacologic therapy for depressive disorders".)

Nursing interventions

These nursing interventions may be appropriate for a patient with major depression.

- Provide for the patient's physical needs. If the patient is too depressed to perform self-care, help with personal hygiene. Encourage the patient to eat or feed if necessary. If constipated, add

high-fiber foods to the patient's diet; offer small, frequent meals; and encourage physical activity and fluid intake. Give warm milk or back rubs at bedtime to improve sleep.
- Record all observations and conversations with the patient. They're valuable in evaluating the response to treatment.
- Plan activities for times when the patient's energy level peaks.

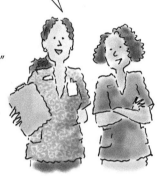

For a patient with depression, plan activities for times when the patient's energy level peaks.

Connection and communication
- Assume an active role in initiating communication.
- Share your observations of the patient's behavior. You might say, "You're sitting all by yourself, looking sad. Is that how you feel?"
- The patient may think and react sluggishly, so speak slowly and allow ample time for response.
- Avoid feigned cheerfulness, but don't hesitate to laugh and point out the value of humor.
- Encourage the patient to talk about and write down feelings. Show that the individual is important by listening attentively and respectfully, avoiding interruptions, and remaining nonjudgmental.

Structure and socialization
- Provide a structured routine, including noncompetitive activities, to build the patient's self-confidence and promote interaction with others. Urge socialization and joining group activities.
- Try to spend some time with the patient each day to decrease isolation. Avoid long periods of silence, which tend to increase anxiety.

Self-help suggestions
- Reassure the patient that expressing feelings, engaging in pleasurable activities, and improving grooming and hygiene help to decrease depression.
- Teach the patient about depression. Emphasize that effective methods are available to relieve symptoms.
- Help with recognition of distorted perceptions and link them to depression. Once depressive thought patterns are recognized, the patient can begin to substitute self-affirming thoughts.

Inklings of suicide
- Ask the patient about having thoughts of death or suicide. Such thoughts signal an immediate need for consultation and assessment. Failure to detect suicidal thoughts early may encourage a suicide attempt.
- Be aware that the suicide risk rises as depression lifts. (See *Recognizing suicide potential.*)

Recognizing suicide potential

A patient with a mood disorder may be at risk for attempting suicide. Stay alert for:
• overwhelming anxiety (the most frequent trigger for a suicide attempt)
• withdrawal and social isolation
• saying farewell to friends and family
• putting affairs in order
• giving away prized possessions
• sending covert suicide messages and death wishes
• expressing obvious suicidal thoughts ("I'd be better off dead")
• describing a suicide plan
• hoarding medications
• talking about death and a feeling of futility
• behavior changes, especially as depression begins to subside.

Taking action
If you think your patient is at risk for suicide, take these steps:

• Keep communication lines open. Maintaining personal contact may help the suicidal patient feel less alone or without resources or hope. Continuity of care and consistency of primary nurses also can help the patient maintain emotional ties to others—the ultimate technique for preventing suicide.
• To ensure a safe environment, check for dangerous conditions, such as exposed pipes, windows without safety glass, and access to the roof or open balconies.
• Remove belts; sharp objects such as razors, knives, nail files, and clippers; suspenders; light cords; and glass from the patient's room.
• Make sure an acutely suicidal patient is observed around the clock. Stay alert when the patient uses a sharp object (as when shaving), takes medications, or uses the bathroom (to prevent hanging or other injury). Assign the patient a room near the nurses' station and with another patient.

Medication edification

- If the patient is taking an antidepressant, stress the need for adherence and review adverse reactions. For drugs that produce strong anticholinergic effects (such as amitriptyline [Elavil]), suggest using sugarless gum or hard candy to relieve dry mouth. For sedating antidepressants (such as amitriptyline), warn the patient to avoid activities that require alertness, including driving and operating mechanical equipment.
- Monitor the patient for seizures as some antidepressants lower the seizure threshold.
- Inform the patient that antidepressants may take several weeks to produce the desired effect.
- Caution the patient taking a TCA or an SSRI to avoid drinking alcoholic beverages or taking other central nervous system depressants during therapy.

Persistent depressive disorder (Dysthymia)

Persistent depressive disorder, or dysthymia, refers to mild depression that lasts at least 2 years in adults or 1 year in children. The depression is mild or moderate, and most patients may not be certain when they first became depressed.

Despite its mildness, dysthymic disorder may impair functioning at home, in school, or at work. However, hospitalization rarely is needed unless suicidal intent is present.

Dysthymic disorder may affect up to 2% of the population. It's twice as common in women as in men and more prevalent among the poor and unmarried.

Depressed? Who—me?

This disorder often goes unrecognized by those experiencing it, as well as by their family and friends. Dysthymic persons may not consider themselves depressed. Because of the mild symptoms—which may be physical rather than emotional—patients typically see a mental health professional only if dysthymia progresses to major depression.

Even when recognized, dysthymia is hard to treat. Recovery is slower if the condition becomes chronic and goes untreated.

Additional agonies

Many patients with dysthymia have a coexisting psychiatric or medical disorder, such as heart disease, cancer, diabetes, or another psychiatric disorder (e.g., substance misuse or an anxiety disorder).

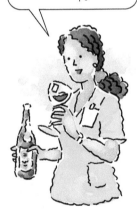

Alcohol should be avoided for a patient during TCA or SSRI therapy.

Causes

Biological, psychological, and medical factors may play a role in dysthymic disorder. Patients with dysthymic disorder may have below-normal serotonin levels, so it's likely that serotonin is involved in development of this disorder.

As with many other psychiatric disorders, personality problems and multiple stressors, combined with inadequate coping skills, may increase a person's vulnerability to this disorder.

Signs and symptoms

Signs and symptoms of dysthymic disorder include:
- persistent sad, anxious, or empty mood
- loss of interest in activities previously enjoyed
- increased feelings of guilt, helplessness, or hopelessness

- weight or appetite changes
- sleep difficulties
- poor school or work performance
- social withdrawal
- conflicts with family and friends
- increased restlessness and irritability
- poor concentration
- inability to make decisions
- reduced energy level
- thoughts of death or suicide or suicide attempts
- physical symptoms, such as headache or backache.

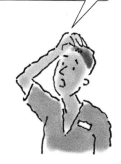

A patient who's under a lot of stress and lacks the skills to cope may be destined for dysthymia.

Diagnosis

The patient may be diagnosed with dysthymic disorder after a careful psychiatric examination and medical history are performed by a psychiatrist or other mental health professional.

Treatment

Short-term psychotherapy teaches the patient more constructive ways of communicating with family, friends, and coworkers. It also allows ongoing assessment of suicidal ideation and suicide risk.

Behavioral therapy may be used to reeducate the patient in social skills. Group therapy can help the patient to change maladaptive social functioning.

Pharmacologic treatment of dysthymic disorder may involve antidepressants, such as SSRIs or TCAs. Patients who exhibit pessimism, disinterest, and low self-esteem typically respond to antidepressant drugs.

Nursing interventions

These nursing interventions may be appropriate for a patient with dysthymic disorder.

- Provide supportive measures, such as reassurance, warmth, availability, and acceptance—even if the patient becomes hostile.
- Teach the patient about the illness and prescribed antidepressant medication.
- Urge the patient to engage in activities that enhance his or her sense of accomplishment.
- Encourage positive health habits, such as eating well-balanced meals, avoiding drugs and alcohol (which can worsen depression), and getting physical exercise (which can lift mood).
- Encourage the use of effective coping skills.

Quick quiz

1. Which statement best describes unipolar depressive disorder?
    A. Sadness following a death of a family member
    B. Persistent feeling of sadness lasting longer than 2 weeks
    C. A mood disorder that mostly occurs in older adults
    D. Neurologic changes associated with physical conditions

Answer: B. Major depressive disorder (also called unipolar major depression) is a syndrome of a persistent sad mood lasting 2 weeks or longer with other accompanying symptoms.

2. Which assessment tool is used to assess suicidal risk?
    A. MMSE
    B. SAD PERSONS Scale
    C. Beck Depression Inventory
    D. Patient Health Questionnaire (PHQ-9)

Answer: B. The SAD PERSONS Scale is used to determine suicide risk. The mnemonic stands for sex, age, depression, previous attempts, ethanol and other drugs, rational thinking loss, social support lacking, organized plan, no spouse, and sickness.

3. A patient is undergoing ECT. Which nursing action is appropriate?
    A. Place dentures in the patient's mouth.
    B. Use the IS PATH WARM to assess patient.
    C. Teach patient to fast 6 to 8 hours prior to procedure.
    D. Wrap patient in warm bath blankets 20 minutes before treatment.

Answer: C. The patient fasts for 6 to 8 hours before ECT. Just before the session, dentures, glasses, hearing aids, contact lenses, and hairpins are removed and the patient is asked to void.

4. The patient is taking an MAOI. Which will the nurse teach the patient to avoid?
    A. Pork
    B. Apples
    C. Cheese
    D. Spinach

Answer: C. Emphasize the avoidance of foods that contain tyramine, caffeine, or tryptophan. Warn that ingesting tyramine can cause a hypertensive crisis. Give the patient a list of foods and beverages that contain these substances, which include aged cheeses, sour cream, beer, Chianti, sherry, pickled herring, liver, canned figs, raisins, bananas, avocados, chocolate, soy sauce, fava beans, yeast extracts, meat tenderizers, coffee, and colas.

Scoring

☆☆☆   If you answered all four items correctly, superb! You are doing GREAT!

☆☆   If you answered three items correctly, well done! Keep up the good work!

☆   If you answered fewer than three items correctly, don't despair! Review and increase your knowledge!

Selected references

American Psychiatric Association. (2013). *Diagnostic and statistical manual of mental disorders, DSM-5* (5th ed.). Author.

Boyd, M. (2018). *Psychiatric nursing: Contemporary practice* (6th ed.). Wolters Kluwer.

Cipriani, A., Furukawa, T., Salanti, G., Chaimani, A., Atkinson, L., Ogawa, Y., Leucht, S., Ruhe, H. G., Turner, E. H., Higgins, J. P. T., Egger, M., Takeshima, N., Hayasaka, Y., Imai, H., Shinohara, K., Tajika, A., Ioannidis, J. P. A., & Geddes, J. R. (2018). Comparative efficacy and acceptability of 21 antidepressant drugs for the acute treatment of adults with major depressive disorder: A systematic review and network meta-analysis. *The Lancet, 391*, 1357–1366. https://doi.org/10.1016/S0140-6736(17)32802-7

Hasin, D., Sarvet, A., Meyers, J., Saha, T., Ruan, J., Stohl, M., & Grant, B. (2018). Epidemiology of adult DSM-5 major depressive disorder and it specifiers in the United States. *Journal of American Medical Association, 75*(4), 336. https://doi.org/10.1001/jamapsychiatry.2017.4602

Holtzheimer, P. (2019). Unipolar depression in adults: Indications, efficacy, and safety of transcranial magnetic stimulation (TMS). *UpToDate*. https://www.uptodate.com/contents/unipolar-depression-in-adults-indications-efficacy-and-safety-of-transcranial-magnetic-stimulation-tms

Hudson, D., Eaton, J., Banks, A., Sewell, W., & Neighbors, H. (2018). "Down in the sewers": Perceptions of depression and depression care among African American men. *American Journal of Men's Health, 12*(1), 126–137. https://doi.org/10.1177/1557988316654864

Juhnke, G. A. (1994). SAD PERSONS Scale review. *Measurement and Evaluation in Counseling and Development, 27*(1), 325–327.

Juhnke, G. A., Granello, P. F., & Lebrón-Striker, M. A. (2007). IS PATH WARM? A suicide assessment mnemonic for counselors (ACAPCD-03). American Counseling Association.

Kellner, C. (2018). Technique for performing electroconvulsive therapy (ECT) in adults. *UpToDate*. https://www.uptodate.com/contents/technique-for-performing-electroconvulsive-therapy-ect-in-adults

Krishnan, R. (2019). Unipolar depression in adults: Epidemiology, pathogenesis, and neurobiology. *UpToDate*. https://www.uptodate.com/contents/unipolar-depression-in-adults-epidemiology-pathogenesis-and-neurobiology

Lyness, J. (2019). Unipolar depression in adults: Clinical features. *UpToDate*. https://www.uptodate.com/contents/unipolar-depression-in-adults-clinical-features

National Institute of Mental Health. (2019). *Major depression.* https://www.nimh.nih.gov/health/statistics/major-depression.shtml

Nguyen, T., Hellbuyck, M., & Halpern, M. (2018). The state of mental health in America, 2018. *Suicide Prevention Resource Center.* https://www.sprc.org/resources-programs/state-mental-health-america-2018

Selzam, S., Coleman, J., Caspi, A., Moffiett, T., & Plomin, R. (2018). A polygenic p factor for major psychiatric disorders. *Translational Psychiatry, 8,* 205. https://doi.org/10.1038/s41398-018-0217-4

Videbeck, S. (2017). *Psychiatric-mental health nursing* (7th ed.). Wolters Kluwer.

Chapter 6

Anxiety disorders

Just the facts

In this chapter, you'll learn:

♦ effects of anxiety

♦ how anxiety disorders impair functioning

♦ risk factors and proposed causes of anxiety disorders

♦ risk for suicide for those with anxiety disorders

♦ assessment and intervention for patients with an anxiety disorder.

A look at anxiety disorders

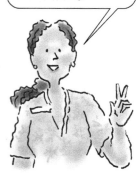

Anxiety disorders are a group of conditions marked by two core symptoms: fear and worry.

Anxiety disorders are a group of conditions marked by two core symptoms: extreme fear and worry. Those with anxiety experience disturbances of thinking, mood, behavior, and physiologic activity. Their fear and worry are difficult to control. Many feel anxious most of the time, with no apparent reason.

The anxiety may be so uncomfortable that they stop doing certain everyday activities to avoid the feeling of dread. Some have terrifying bouts of intense anxiety that immobilize them. To relieve overwhelming feelings of anxiety, impending catastrophe, guilt, shame, helplessness, or worthlessness, sufferers may cling to maladaptive behaviors, which only make their symptoms worse.

The anatomy of anxiety

From time to time, everyone experiences worry, uncertainty, or apprehension—particularly when confronting a stressful event such as a job interview or a first date. Mild or moderate anxiety rarely threatens one's coping ability. In fact, it can motivate us to try new things and take risks. In that sense, it's useful and productive.

The degree of anxiety experienced and the ability to perceive it accurately and channel it appropriately determine if the anxiety will help or hinder the person's level of functioning. Someone who perceives anxiety as severe will feel threatened—and either avoid it or become overwhelmed by it.

Anxiety prevalence

Anxiety disorders are the most common mental health disorders in the United States from childhood, adolescence, and adulthood (Essau et al., 2018). Globally, it is estimated that 3.6% of the population has an anxiety disorder (World Health Organization, 2017), with women twice as affected as men (Baldwin, 2019). Although the number of individuals officially diagnosed is high, it is suggested that the numbers of those who have undiagnosed anxiety may be even higher. Treatment for anxiety disorder is readily available and, in most cases, very successful in restoring a productive and fulfilling life to those with anxiety.

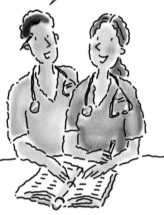

In patients with anxiety disorders, stay alert for other psychiatric and medical conditions.

Over and above anxiety

Anxiety disorders are often accompanied by other psychiatric conditions, especially mood disorders and substance misuse—as well as medical disorders (Baldwin, 2019). Health care providers must stay alert for this possibility. Many of the symptoms of anxiety disorders are similar to symptoms of major depression. (See *Plain talk about anxiety disorders.*)

Causes

Anxiety disorders are thought to result from a combination of genetic, biochemical, neuroanatomic, and psychological factors—plus life experiences. Specific causes for each disorder will be discussed with that disorder.

Genetic factors

Research shows that some anxiety disorders are inherited. Many of them—including panic disorder, obsessive-compulsive disorder (OCD), generalized anxiety disorder (GAD), and major phobias—run in families. Research continues to find genetic influences on inheritance and predisposition to anxiety in varying degrees (Cheesman et al., 2019).

Researchers are looking for specific genetic factors that might explain or contribute to an inherited risk. Some studies are focusing on defective genes that regulate specific chemical messengers in the brain (neurotransmitters), such as serotonin, dopamine, norepinephrine, glutamate, and gamma-aminobutyric acid (GABA).

Biochemical factors

Some experts believe that people with anxiety disorders have a biological vulnerability to stress, which makes them more susceptible to environmental stimuli. Neurotransmitter (see previous list)

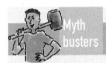

Plain talk about anxiety disorders

Here's a reality check to help the nurse stay on course when caring for patients with anxiety disorders.
Myth: All anxiety disorders cause psychological symptoms, but only panic attacks cause physiologic symptoms.
Reality: Both physiologic and psychological symptoms accompany all levels of anxiety, from mild to severe.

imbalances may also contribute to anxiety disorders. Researchers suggest it is the effects of neurotransmitters contributing to the complex phenomena of emotions that are the basis for everyday behavior (Pantic, 2019).

Neuroanatomic factors

Brain structures known collectively as the limbic system play a role in regulating emotion. The most notable structures comprising the limbic system include the hippocampus (responsible for emotional memory), the amygdala (integrates emotions physiologically and behaviorally), the hypothalamus (organizes behaviors such as fight or flight), and the thalamus (relays sensory impulses to the cerebral cortex). Scientists are using functional magnetic resonance imaging (fMRI), positron emission tomography, single-photon emission computed tomography (SPECT), electroencephalography (EEG), and other functional brain imaging studies to locate the brain areas or abnormalities associated with anxiety responses. Linder et al. (2018) noted structural changes, such as a reduction in the communication between the amygdala and the orbitofrontal cortex, in individuals with anxiety disorders.

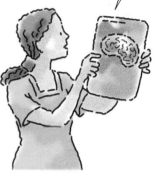

MRI scans have found brain abnormalities in some patients with anxiety disorders.

The other component of anxiety disorders is worry. Excessive worry that is difficult to control will, over time, trigger stress hormones such as cortisol. Anxiety can release cortisol, and in a cyclical relationship, excess cortisol causes anxiety. Worry and stress also release adrenaline, which causes many of the symptoms associated with anxiety.

Psychological factors

Some theories suggest that certain anxiety disorders arise when unconscious defense mechanisms become overwhelmed and dysfunctional. Interpersonal and/or intrapsychic conflicts also contribute to anxiety.

Fear in the family

The family's role in phobias is also under investigation. Several studies show a strong correlation between a parent's fears and those of their children. In other words, a child "learns" fears by observing the parent's fearful reaction to an object or situation.

Traumatic life events

Traumatic events can trigger anxiety disorders, such as posttraumatic stress disorder (PTSD) (see Chapter 8). Panic disorders have also been associated with anxiety following separation and loss.

Some experts, however, believe that only someone who is vulnerable because of psychological, genetic, or biochemical factors will

Advice from the experts

Differentiating fear, anxiety, worry, and panic

When assessing patients for anxiety disorders, keep in mind the key differences among fear, anxiety, worry, and panic:

• Fear is a response to external stimuli. The emotional responses are regulated by connections between the amygdala and two specific areas of the prefrontal cortex, the anterior cingulate cortex and the orbitofrontal cortex.

• Anxiety is a response to internal conflict that may influence behavior even after the cause of the anxiety is removed.

• Worry is a maladaptive response to decrease anxiety triggered by events that are not within the individual's control, resulting in negative emotions and anxiety (Ellard et al., 2017). It may include anxious misery, apprehensive expectation, catastrophic thinking, and obsessions.

• Panic is an extreme level of anxiety characterized by sudden, overwhelming feelings of impending doom.

develop an anxiety disorder in response to trauma. Some people may even have a biological propensity for specific phobias (such as a fear of snakes) that is triggered by a single exposure.

Medical conditions

Some anxiety symptoms are associated with particular medical conditions. For example, someone who has a hyperthyroid condition or adrenal disorder may have symptoms that mimic an anxiety disorder. Withdrawal of certain medications, as well as alcohol, can promote symptoms of anxiety. Many health conditions, such as hormone imbalances, thyroid malfunctioning, diabetes, asthma, digestive disorders, vertigo, sleep apnea, and heart disease, can lead to feelings of anxiety. However, it is important to distinguish symptoms of anxiety as they relate to an underlying medical problem versus symptoms of anxiety as they relate to anxiety disorder. Anxiety disorder is diagnosed when the symptoms are persistent and excessive (Baldwin, 2019).

Risk factors

• Female gender
• Physical comorbidity
• Depression or other psychiatric disorder.

Panic disorder

Panic disorder represents anxiety in its most severe form. In this disorder, patients have recurrent, unexpected panic attacks that cause intense apprehension and feelings of impending doom. Between attacks, the patient persistently worries about having additional panic attacks and the consequences of the attacks and may change personal behaviors because of the attacks. The frequency of panic attacks and the high level of anxiety may cause functional impairments. Note that panic attacks can occur in the context of other mental disorders or medical conditions and should then be described as a specifier, that is, PTSD, with panic attacks, rather than panic disorder.

Panic attacks

Panic attacks occur suddenly, with no warning. They usually build to peak intensity within 10 to 15 minutes and rarely last longer than 30 minutes. However, repeated attacks may continue to recur for hours.

During the panic episode, patients may fear dying, going crazy, or losing control of emotions or behavior. The patient may have a strong urge to escape or flee the place where the panic attack began.

The frequency and severity of panic attacks vary from one person to the next. Attacks may arise once a week or in clusters separated by months. Because they occur spontaneously—without exposure to a known anxiety-producing situation—the patient worries about when the next one will occur and may restrict routine activities in an attempt to avoid a panic episode.

Panic tally

Roughly 4.7% of the U.S. general population experiences panic disorder at some time in their lives. The prevalence of panic disorder gradually increases in adolescence and peaks in adulthood and is twice as common in women versus men (Roy-Byrne, 2019).

Affliction overlap

For many sufferers, panic disorder is complicated by major depressive disorder. The tendency to self-medicate with alcohol or antianxiety drugs may result in alcoholism and substance misuse disorders. Many patients with panic disorder also have additional anxiety disorders—including social phobia, GAD, specific phobia, and OCD (Roy-Byrne, 2019).

Risk for suicide

According to the American Psychiatric Association (2013), panic attacks and a diagnosis of panic disorder are related to higher rates of suicide attempts and suicidal ideations. This risk increases in patients with a comorbid diagnosis of a mood disorder, personality disorders, or alcohol misuse.

Causes

Although intense stress or a sudden loss may trigger panic disorder, the underlying cause of the disorder involves a combination of genetic, biochemical, and other factors.

Genetic factors

Panic disorder tends to run in families, with higher rates of panic disorder in patients who have first-degree relatives with the disorder. It also occurs to a much higher degree in identical twins (Roy-Byrne, 2019).

Neurobiology

Specific areas in the amygdala are neural triggers for panic attacks. The activated amygdala stimulates the sympathetic nervous system and the hypothalamic-pituitary-adrenal axis. There is thought that some individuals have an inherited susceptibility to symptoms of panic when the person is exposed to internal or external stressors.

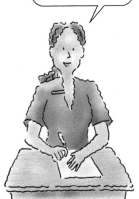

Panic disorder tends to run in families.

Some researchers believe that people with panic disorder may have a heightened sensitivity to somatic (physical) symptoms. This sensitivity, in turn, may trigger the autonomic system, which sets off a series of events leading to a panic attack.

Risk factors

Such physical illnesses as asthma, cardiovascular disease, and gastrointestinal (GI) disorders may predispose a person to panic disorder by causing fear. The first experience of one of these conditions may be so frightening that it causes a panic attack. Intensely stressful life events or multiple stressors can contribute to panic disorder. Smoking and negative experiences with illicit drugs represent risks for panic attacks and panic disorder. Childhood adversity increases the risk of panic disorder developing as an adult.

Symptoms of panic attack

Abrupt onset and intense discomfort that builds to a peak rapidly within 10 minutes, panic episodes include symptoms that can be categorized as somatic (physical) and cognitive.

Somatic symptoms include:
- Hyperventilation
- Palpitations
- Pounding heart
- Dizziness/faintness
- Hot flushes or cold chills
- Chest pain/pressure
- Shortness of breath, smothering
- Trembling or shaking
- Numbness or tingling
- Nausea and stomach discomfort.

Cognitive symptoms include:
- Dread
- Impending doom, that something bad is going to happen
- Depersonalization or detachment
- Derealization (feeling that things aren't real)
- Fear of dying
- Fear of losing control.

  Patients sometimes go to a hospital emergency department or seek some other type of urgent assistance out of concern for acute physical symptoms they experience and a fear of dying.

Diagnosis

Because some physical conditions and drug effects can mimic panic disorder, the health care provider may order tests to rule out an organic or pharmacologic basis for symptoms. For example, urine and serum toxicology tests can rule out the presence of psychoactive substances capable of triggering panic attacks, such as barbiturates, caffeine, and amphetamines.

Treatment

Panic disorder is highly treatable with a combination of patient teaching, cognitive or behavioral therapies, and relaxation techniques. Biofeedback can also be of help to these patients. Some patients also require medication.

Patient teaching
Teaching the patient about the disorder and its physiologic effects can help the individual overcome it. Many patients experience some relief simply by understanding exactly what panic disorder is and how many others suffer from it.

Cognitive therapy

Cognitive restructuring through cognitive-behavioral therapy (CBT) can be helpful for patients who worry that their panic attacks mean they're going crazy or are about to have a heart attack. This method teaches them to replace those negative thoughts with more realistic, positive ways of viewing the attacks. It also helps them identify and evaluate the thoughts that precede anxiety and then restructure them to gain a more realistic perception.

Trigger talk

Through cognitive therapy, the patient can identify possible triggers for the panic attacks, such as a particular thought or situation or even a slight change in the heartbeat. Once the patient understands that the panic attack is separate and independent of the trigger, that trigger starts to lose some of its power to induce an attack.

Panic interrupted

In a technique called *interoceptive conditioning* (or *panic control treatment*), a therapist guides the patient through repeated exposure to the sensations experienced during a panic attack (such as palpitations or dizziness). The feared sensations may be produced using such methods as controlled hyperventilation or physical exertion (such as running up a flight of stairs to cause tachycardia). Through this approach, the patient learns that these sensations need not progress to a full-blown attack.

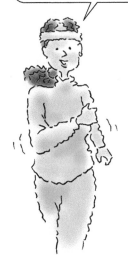

Baby steps

Behavioral therapy also can help the patient deal with the situational avoidance associated with panic attacks. In one behavioral technique called *systematic desensitization,* a trained therapist helps the patient break down a fearful situation into small, manageable steps. The patient then performs the steps one at a time until he or she can master the most difficult step.

Relaxation techniques

Relaxation techniques help the patient cope with a panic attack by easing physical symptoms and directing the patient's attention elsewhere. These techniques include:

- deep breathing exercises, which also reduce the risk of hyperventilation (a contributing factor for anxiety)
- progressive relaxation, which involves conscious tightening and relaxation of the skeletal muscles in a sequential fashion
- positive visualization or guided imagery, in which the patient elicits peaceful mental images or some other purposeful thought or action, promoting feelings of relaxation, renewed hope, and a sense of being in control of a stressful situation
- listening to calming music.

Biofeedback

Biofeedback is a technique in which an individual learns how to control physiologic reactions to stress in order to avert a panic attack. This is done with a computer application and equipment, which monitors heart rate variability.

Pharmacologic therapy

Evidence from clinical trials shows efficacy of pharmacologic interventions with antidepressants:

- Selective serotonin reuptake inhibitors (SSRIs) such as citalopram (Celexa), escitalopram (Cipralex or Lexapro), fluoxetine (Prozac), sertraline (Zoloft), fluvoxamine (Luvox), paroxetine (Paxil)
- Serotonin norepinephrine reuptake inhibitors (SNRIs) such as venlafaxine (Effexor) and duloxetine (Cymbalta)
- Tricyclic antidepressants (TCAs) such as imipramine (Tofranil) and clomipramine (Anafranil).

For some patients, the health care provider may prescribe antianxiety drugs (e.g., benzodiazepines) such as lorazepam (Ativan) with an antidepressant to promote rapid stabilization of panic symptoms until the onset of therapeutic action of the antidepressants (in several weeks).

Novel drugs for treatment-resistant panic disorder include mirtazapine (Remeron) (an atypical noradrenergic and specific serotonergic antidepressant), reboxetine (Edronax), nefazodone (Serzone), and low-dose risperidone (Risperdal) (an atypical antipsychotic agent) (Zulfarina et al., 2019).

Some patients also benefit from beta blockers such as propranolol (Atenolol) and alpha-2 receptor agonists such as clonidine (Catapres), as they suppress the somatic manifestations that can occur with anxiety.

Nursing interventions

These nursing interventions may be appropriate for patients with panic disorder.

During a panic attack

- Stay with the patient until the attack subsides. If left alone, the patient may grow even more anxious.
- If the patient loses control, guide the patient to a smaller, quieter area.

Just breathe

- Instructing the patient to take slow breaths can help to prevent hyperventilation. Breathing in and out slowly and deeply with the patient can help to shift thoughts away from the distressing symptoms.

Serenity now

- Maintain a calm, serene approach so as not to transfer anxiety to the patient.
- Speak in short, simple sentences, and slowly give the patient one direction at a time. Avoid giving lengthy explanations and asking too many questions.

Out with the extraneous

- Reduce external stimuli, such as groups of people, as this can increase anxiety. Excessive stimuli may be overwhelming. Dim lights if necessary.
- Provide a safe environment, and prevent harm to the patient or others.

Express emotions

- Encourage the patient to express feelings and to cry, if necessary.
- Administer medication (such as antianxiety medication) as prescribed by the health care provider.

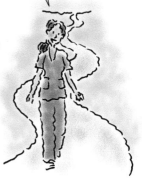

Keep a patient experiencing a panic attack away from crowds, bright lights, and noise.

Between panic attacks

- Teach relaxation techniques.
- Determine things that increase anxiety, such as caffeine, and teach the patient how to avoid those substances.
- Encourage the patient to discuss fears. Help the patient identify situations or events that trigger the attacks.
- Ask questions to clarify and dispute illogical thinking:
  1. What evidence do you have?
  2. Explain the logic in that thinking.
  3. Are you basing that conclusion on fact or feeling?
  4. What's the worst thing that can happen? (Halter, 2017, p. 286)
- Discuss alternative coping mechanisms and use positive self-talk, such as "I can control my anxiety" to replace negative self-talk.
- Monitor therapeutic and adverse effects of prescribed medications. Teach the patient how to recognize adverse effects and when to use medication for panic attacks and/or anxiety.
- Instruct the patient to notify the health care provider before discontinuing medication because abrupt withdrawal could cause severe symptoms.
- Make appropriate referrals to a mental health professional.

Agoraphobia

Agoraphobia is an abnormal and out-of-proportion anxiety or fear about being in places or situations from which escape might be difficult or embarrassing (McCabe, 2019). Patients with agoraphobia worry they won't be able to get somewhere safe and may fear they'll have a panic attack or panic symptoms (such as dizziness, vomiting, loss of control, or difficulty breathing). Eventually, they begin to avoid situations where they feel uncomfortable.

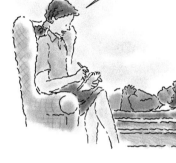

Without treatment, agoraphobia may get worse.

Holed up at home

Without treatment, agoraphobia may get worse. In extreme cases, the person becomes a prisoner in the home, too fearful to leave the "safe" zone. In less severe cases, the individual is able to engage in activities or travel if a trusted companion goes along.

Many experts view agoraphobia as an adverse behavioral outcome of repeated panic attacks and the subsequent worry, preoccupation, and avoidance. However, agoraphobia sometimes occurs without a history of panic disorder. (See *Panic disorder*, page 147.)

Scary territory

Among agoraphobic patients, common fears include large public spaces (such as parks, malls, theaters, and supermarkets), crowds, and places where the person feels trapped (such as airplanes or driving in rush-hour traffic or on a bridge). Most patients can verbalize fears and where they fear it, although some know only that they have a sense of dread.

The facts

Women are more commonly diagnosed with agoraphobia than men (McCabe, 2019). Patients with agoraphobia commonly have other anxiety disorders, depression, and up to one-third of those with agoraphobia have substance use disorder (McCabe, 2019).

Causes

The exact cause of agoraphobia isn't known. Theories include biochemical imbalances (especially related to neurotransmitters) and environmental factors. The disorder may run in families, suggesting a genetic basis.

Personality factors such as introversion, anxiety sensitivity, dependent personality traits, lack of perceived control, and low self-efficacy have all been associated with agoraphobia. In addition, cognitive factors include fear of having an illness, bodily preoccupation, and fear that the individual will be trapped or unable to cope due to a physical limitation (McCabe, 2019).

Signs and symptoms

The patient's avoidance of the feared situation significantly impairs daily functioning, including the ability to work and care for one's self independently. Patients may have other family members do routine shopping and errands to allow the individual to stay within the safe confines of home.

The patient may report or exhibit:

- fear and avoidance of open spaces or public places
- fear or anxiety of enclosed spaces such as theaters or airplanes
- fear of standing in line or being in a crowd
- fear of being outside the home
- concern that help might not be available in public places.

If the patient also has panic disorder, he or she may express concern that a panic attack in public will lead to embarrassment or the inability to escape. (For symptoms of a panic attack, see *Panic disorder*.)

Diagnosis

Agoraphobia is diagnosed when the patient exhibits the signs and symptoms associated with agoraphobia. It is important to note that this is a separate diagnosis from panic disorder. Agoraphobia can exist as an isolated diagnosis or in conjunction with the diagnosis of panic disorder.

Treatment

Treatment usually includes both medication and behavioral therapy. The health care provider may prescribe an SSRI, such as paroxetine (Paxil), or an SNRI, such as duloxetine hydrochloride (Cymbalta). To treat a panic attack in progress, the patient may receive a benzodiazepine, such as alprazolam (Xanax). Treatment is similar to the treatment of panic disorder.

The overexposure cure

One treatment for agoraphobia is desensitization, which gradually exposes the patient to the situation that triggers fear and avoidance. Recently, this has included exposure to internal stimuli (e.g., rapid heart, increased respiratory rate), which can precipitate symptoms. Such exposure helps the patient learn to cope with the situation and break the mental connection between the situation and anxiety. The patient may receive antianxiety medications to reduce anxiety during desensitization sessions.

Implosive therapy has also been used in the treatment of agoraphobia. The patient is presented with anxiety-provoking imagery, which depicts the fear as vividly as possible. This technique is frequently used in conjunction with flooding where a patient is desensitized by being repeatedly exposed to the trigger without breaks until the anxiety subsides.

Patients may also benefit from relaxation techniques and also psychotherapy in which the patient discusses underlying emotional conflicts with a therapist or support group.

Nursing interventions

For a patient with agoraphobia, these nursing interventions may be appropriate.

- Encourage the patient to discuss the feared object or situation.
- Collaborate with the patient and interprofessional team to develop and implement a systematic desensitization program that exposes the patient gradually to the feared situation in a controlled environment.
- Provide training in assertiveness skills to reduce submissive and fearful responses. Such strategies allow the patient to experiment with new coping skills and encourage the patient to discard ineffective ones.
- Administer antianxiety or antidepressant medications, as prescribed by the health care provider.
- If the patient is taking a medication for anxiety, stress the importance of complying with prescribed therapy. Teach the patient about adverse drug reactions and what needs to be reported to the health care provider.

Generalized anxiety disorder

Occasional anxiety is a normal part of life. However, with GAD, the anxiety and worry are persistent, generalized, and excessive.

Effects of GAD range from mild to severe and incapacitating. Many individuals with GAD self-medicate with alcohol and antianxiety drugs in an effort to relieve anxiety.

Look at the numbers

In the United States, GAD affects an estimated 5% of the general population, occurring more often in women than men and is the most common mental health disorder in older adults (Baldwin, 2019).

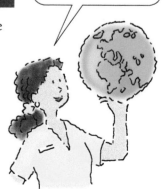

Constant worrying can feel like the weight of the world on your shoulders. It can cause your heart to be unhappy with a chronic elevated heart rate.

Usually, GAD emerges slowly; many people report feeling anxious and nervous since early childhood. Occasionally, it is triggered by a stressful event. GAD tends to be chronic, with periods of exacerbation and remission.

Medley of maladies

Many patients also have other psychiatric disorders, such as social phobia, specific phobia, panic disorder, and depression (Baldwin, 2019).

Untreated, GAD can cause constant, unremitting tension that ultimately results in immunosuppression, leaving the patient more susceptible to physical health conditions. GAD has been commonly associated with physiologic conditions, such as increased blood pressure and heart disease.

> With GAD the anxiety and worry are persistent, generalized, and excessive.

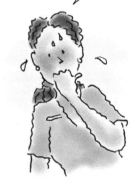

Causes

The exact cause of GAD is unknown. As with other anxiety disorders, genetic, biochemical, psychosocial, and other factors are suspected.

Genetic factors

GAD has a moderate genetic risk of approximately 30%, and these genetic factors are closely related to other anxiety and mood disorders (Gottschalk & Domschke, 2017).

Biochemical abnormalities

Imbalances in serotonin, norepinephrine, glutamate, and GABA may play a key role in susceptibility to GAD. Serotonin seems to be vital to feelings of well-being, whereas GABA helps prevent nerve cells from overfiring. Glutamate is an excitatory neurotransmitter. Serotonin is a key neurotransmitter that innervates the amygdala as well as other parts of the brain such as the prefrontal cortex and thalamus, which regulates fear and worry.

Psychosocial and environmental factors

Children of anxious parents may learn to see the world as dangerous and uncontrollable, predisposing them to GAD. Experts believe that adults with GAD have had higher incidences of undesirable or traumatic experiences in childhood (Baldwin, 2019). Children with specific behaviors such as a tendency to be timid and shy in new experiences are more likely to have GAD than others who do not exhibit these behaviors (Baldwin, 2019).

Death of a loved one, illness, job loss, or divorce can increase a person's stress level and may trigger anxiety or stress responses. However, experts believe stress is merely a trigger for GAD, not the cause.

Risk factors

Several risk factors for the development of GAD include:
- Female gender
- Low socioeconomic status
- Recent or current adverse life events
- Chronic physical and mental disorders
- Parental loss or separation
- History of mental conditions in parents (Baldwin, 2019).

Signs and symptoms

Signs and symptoms of GAD fall into three general categories—excessive physiologic arousal, distorted cognitive processes, and poor coping.

Excessive physiologic arousal

With excessive physiologic arousal, the patient may report or exhibit:
- shortness of breath
- tachycardia or palpitations
- dry mouth
- sweating
- nausea or diarrhea
- inability to relax
- muscle tension, aches, and spasms
- irritability
- fatigue
- restlessness
- trembling
- headache
- cold, clammy hands
- insomnia.

Distorted cognitive processes

Signs and symptoms of distorted cognitive processes include:
- poor concentration
- unrealistic assessment of problems
- excessive anxiety and worry over minor matters
- fears of grave misfortune or death.

Poor coping
A patient with poor coping may exhibit:
- avoidance
- procrastination
- poor problem-solving skills.

Diagnosis

Because anxiety is the central feature of many mental disorders, the patient should undergo a psychiatric evaluation to rule out phobias, OCD, depression, and acute schizophrenia. GAD is characterized by excessive worry lasting more than 6 months that significantly impairs the patient's ability to function in his or her personal and social life (APA, 2013).

Treatment

Treatment depends on the severity and the needs of the patient. For patients with mild anxiety, monitoring and nonpharmacologic methods are the treatments of choice. Relaxation techniques and biofeedback can decrease arousal. Psychotherapy helps the patient identify and deal with the cause of anxiety, anticipate the patient's reactions, and plan effective responses to deal with anxiety.

Other treatment options include CBT and medications.

Worry ledger

In the cognitive therapy approach, the patient may be taught to record worries and list evidence that justifies or contradicts each one. The patient also learns that "worrying about worry" maintains anxiety and that avoidance and procrastination are ineffective problem-solving techniques.

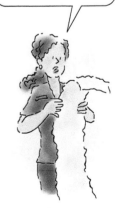

Should I be worried about having such a long list of worries?

Cognitive-behavioral therapy
CBT with pharmacologic therapy is a first-line treatment for GAD. CBT involves modifying problematic coping strategies and cognitive approaches (e.g., reality testing negative thoughts) and also addressing the physiologic aspects of GAD (relaxation strategies) (Craske & Bystritsky, 2019).

Biofeedback training
Biofeedback training eases physical symptoms of anxiety by teaching the patient how to become aware of—and then consciously control—various body functions (including blood pressure, heart and respiratory rates, skin temperature, and perspiration). Using a biofeedback device, the patient learns when changes in these functions occur.

With adequate training, the patient can repeat this response at will, even when not hooked up to the biofeedback device.

Pharmacologic therapy

SSRIs and SNRIs are the preferred medications in the treatment of GAD. First-line medications include SSRIs paroxetine (Paxil), sertraline (Zoloft), citalopram (Celexa), or escitalopram (Lexapro). Fluoxetine (Prozac) and fluvoxamine (Luvox) have also been found to be effective. SNRIs include venlafaxine extended release (Effexor XR) and duloxetine (Cymbalta). These drug classifications have shown the best efficacy and safety outcomes for patients with GAD (Craske & Bystritsky, 2019).

Adjunctive treatment with second-line medications include buspirone (Buspar) and pregabalin (Lyrica). Other medications that have been found to be helpful include benzodiazepines such as lorazepam (Ativan), antidepressants such as mirtazapine (Remeron), and antipsychotic medications such as quetiapine (Seroquel).

Benzodiazepines reduce anxiety by decreasing vigilance and easing somatic symptoms (for instance, muscle tension). These drugs are most effective when used initially to manage symptoms while waiting for other pharmacologic interventions to take effect as medications may take a few weeks to produce an optimal effect.

It takes a while ...

Buspirone (Buspar) causes less sedation and rarely leads to physical dependence or tolerance than benzodiazepines. However, onset of action takes several weeks, so patients should be told to expect a delay in symptom relief. The same applies to SSRIs and SNRIs. Benzodiazepines can be used to assist the patient with the symptoms of GAD until the other medication takes effect (Craske & Bystritsky, 2019).

Nursing interventions

When caring for a patient with GAD, these nursing interventions may be appropriate.

- Stay with the patient when the patient is experiencing anxiety. Remain calm and nonjudgmental. Suggest activities that distract the individual from the anxiety symptoms.
- Encourage the patient to discuss feelings.
- Reduce environmental stimuli.
- Ensure healthy sleep patterns.

Stress-busting strategies

- Teach the patient progressive muscle relaxation, guided imagery, deep breathing, or other relaxation techniques. Besides easing anxiety, these methods reduce the risk of hyperventilation, help the patient focus on something other than the anxiety, and interrupt the flow of negative or stressful thoughts.

- Provide nutritional counseling to reduce stress and promote health. Advise the patient to avoid caffeine, energy drinks, and alcohol, for instance. A well-balanced diet is also important in decreasing stress.
- Instruct the patient in time management skills, such as making lists, setting realistic goals, and grouping tasks in batches to help manage anxiety.
- Make appropriate referrals to a mental health professional. It is very important to address comorbidities, including sleep disturbances, which is a symptom of GAD, but also contributes to increased anxiety when healthy sleep patterns do not occur.

Drug discussions

- Administer medications as prescribed by the health care provider.
- Inform the patient and family that these drugs may cause adverse reactions, such as drowsiness, fatigue, ataxia, blurred vision, slurred speech, tremors, and hypotension. Instruct the patient to not use heavy equipment or drive and to report these side effects to the health care provider.
- Advise the patient not to discontinue medications except with the health care provider's approval because abrupt withdrawal could cause severe symptoms.

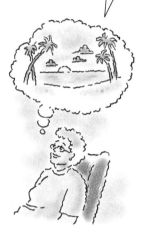

Teach the patient guided imagery or other relaxation techniques.

Social anxiety disorder (social phobia)

Social anxiety disorder (SAD) refers to marked, persistent fear or anxiety in social or performance situations. The anxiety causes the one with social anxiety to avoid these situations whenever possible out of fear of embarrassment, scrutiny, humiliation, or ridicule. Common situations that provoke anxiety include speaking or eating in public and using a public restroom. The hallmark physical response is blushing.

Could you be specific?

Social phobia may be limited to performing (e.g., musicians, athletes) or speaking in public. It can be generalized where the patient has symptoms almost anytime the individual is with other people (e.g., social situations) and being observed (e.g., drinking and eating).

Spotlight shunners

Many people with social phobia are concerned that others will see their anxiety symptoms (such as sweating or blushing) or will judge them to be weak, stupid, or crazy. Some fear fainting, losing bowel or bladder control, or going mentally blank.

Even when around familiar people, they may feel overwhelmed, fearing that others are watching their every move and making negative judgments about them.

Expecting the worst

Socially phobic people may have anticipatory anxiety for days or weeks before the dreaded event. Such anxiety may further handicap the person's performance and heighten embarrassment.

The disorder can be debilitating, preventing the patient from going to work or school on some days. It can cause loss of a job or job promotion out of fear of speaking in public, or result in continual inconvenience—for instance, from fear of using a public lavatory.

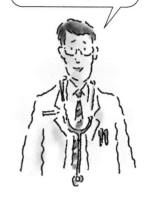

The hallmark physical response of SAD is blushing.

Also of concern

Patients with SAD have higher rates of suicide than the general population (Schneier, 2019).

Numeric rundown

An estimated 3% to 7% of Americans suffer from SAD. More common in women, the disorder typically starts in childhood or adolescence (Schneier, 2019). Median age of onset is mid-teens.

Risk factors

- Female gender
- Family history of SAD
- Shy or timid in early childhood (inhibited temperament) (Schneier, 2019).

Causes

For many people, SAD is linked with the traits of shyness and social inhibition, early childhood adversity, and parental/peer influences. Female gender and a family history of SAD are also linked to this disorder (Schneier, 2019). The interaction of biological and environmental factors can cause a child with a genetic predisposition and expression of high behavioral inhibition to be socially anxious as modeled by parents.

Scientists exploring biological aspects of the disorder believe there may be a physiologic basis for increased sensitivity to autonomic arousal (e.g., increased heart rate, trembling). Neurotransmitters implicated in SAD include serotonin, possibly dopamine, increased glutamate levels, and peripheral oxytocin. Others are investigating the role of the amygdala, a brain structure that controls fear responses. The amygdala plays a role in the hyperactivity of limbic and paralimbic fear circuits. The medial prefrontal cortex may have decreased activation. The hypothalamic-pituitary-adrenal axis may have increased reactivity to social stressors, especially in those with a history of early childhood abuse (Schneier, 2019).

Signs and symptoms

Signs and symptoms of SAD may include:
- fear or avoidance of eating, writing, or speaking in public fear of being stared at, meeting strangers, or being in large groups of people
- pronounced sensitivity to criticism
- low self-esteem
- scholastic underachievement because of test anxiety.

Physical manifestations may include:
- blushing
- profuse sweating
- trembling
- nausea or stomach upset
- difficulty talking.

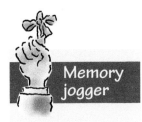

Memory jogger

FEAR can cue you in to signs and symptoms of phobias.

Fear of an object or a situation

Emotional conflict occurring unconsciously

Avoidant behavior demonstrated

Reacts with severe anxiety

Worried about looking worried

Visible signs of SAD, such as blushing or profuse sweating, heighten the patient's fear of disapproval and may become an additional focus of fear. Thus, a vicious cycle may begin: The more the patient worries about experiencing symptoms of SAD, the greater chance of developing symptoms.

Diagnosis

No specific test can diagnose SAD. Diagnosis is based on signs and symptoms associated with SAD.

Treatment

The first-line treatment of SAD is CBT with or without pharmacotherapy. Treatment is selected based on the severity of the disorder, informed patient preference, and treatment availability (Stein & Taylor, 2019).

A mental health professional may use desensitization therapy to gradually reintroduce the feared situation while coaching the patient on relaxation techniques.

Relaxation techniques, such as progressive muscle relaxation, deep breathing exercises, or listening to calming music, may be helpful, too. By role-playing in guided imagery, the patient rehearses ways to relax while confronting a feared object or situation.

A model for behavior

Modeling behavior and assertiveness training also can be valuable. In modeling behavior, the patient observes someone modeling, or demonstrating, appropriate behavior when confronted with the feared situation.

Thought-stopping

A behavioral technique called *negative thought-stopping* can reduce the frequency and duration of disturbing thoughts by interrupting them and substituting competing thoughts. In thought-stopping, the patient is taught to recognize negative thoughts and then use an intense distracting stimulus (such as snapping a rubber band around the wrist) to stop the thought. With practice, the patient can control thoughts without this distracting stimulus.

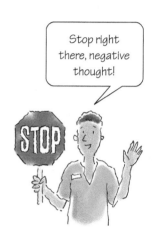

Stop right there, negative thought!

Pharmacologic therapy

SSRIs are the most commonly prescribed medication in the treatment of SAD. Paroxetine (Paxil) was the first SSRI approved by the U.S. Food and Drug Administration (FDA) for the treatment of SAD. Other SSRIs approved by the FDA are fluvoxamine (Luvox), sertraline (Zoloft), and the SNRI venlafaxine XR (Effexor XR). Alpha-2-delta ligands such as gabapentin (Neurontin) and pregabalin (Lyrica) have also been first-line choices.

Beta-adrenergic blockers (e.g., propranolol) are used for performance-type SAD. They are not effective in generalized SAD. Benzodiazepines (e.g., clonazepam [Klonopin], lorazepam [Ativan]) have very limited usefulness for generalized SAD, but some use in performance-type SAD. The sedation and potential for abuse and dependence are very real risks in the use of benzodiazepines.

Nursing interventions

These nursing interventions may be appropriate for patients with SAD.
- No matter how illogical the patient's phobia seems, avoid the urge to trivialize the fears. Remember that the behavior represents an essential coping mechanism. A simplistic pep talk or ridicule may cause more alienation or worsen preexisting low self-esteem.
- Keep in mind that the patient fears criticism. Encourage the individual to interact with others and provide continuous support and positive reinforcement.
- Teach the patient progressive muscle relaxation, guided imagery, or thought-stopping techniques as appropriate.
- Gradual desensitization to the anxiety-provoking situation can be useful.

- Ask the patient how he or she normally copes with the fear. When the patient is able to face the fear, encourage the individual to verbalize and explore personal strengths and resources with you.
- Suggest ways to channel energy and relieve stress, such as running and creative activities.
- Do not allow the patient to withdraw completely. If the patient is being treated as an outpatient, work collaboratively with the patient to suggest small steps to help overcome fears.
- If the patient is taking a medication for anxiety, stress the importance of complying with prescribed therapy. Teach the patient about adverse drug reactions and what needs to be reported to the health care provider.

Specific phobia

In specific phobia (also called *simple phobia*), a person experiences intense, irrational anxiety when exposed to a specific feared object (such as a snake) or situation (such as being in an enclosed space). The exposure can take place either in real life or through images from movies, television, photographs, or the imagination.

For many, the anxiety leads to avoidance or disabling behavior that interferes with activities or even confines them to the home. Anxiety may reach panic levels, especially if there's no apparent escape from the feared thing or situation.

Just can't help feeling that way

Although adults with specific phobias realize their fears are irrational and out of proportion to any actual danger, they still experience severe anxiety or panic attacks when facing (or perhaps even thinking about) the feared object or situation. Most try to avoid the stimulus or endure exposure to the stimulus with great difficulty. Some even make important career or personal decisions to avoid the object of their fears. Many people have multiple specific phobias.

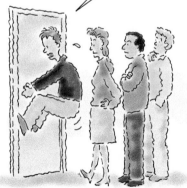

I'm terrified of enclosed spaces! Let me out of here!

Phobia figures

Specific phobias affect about 7.7% to 12.5% of the U.S. population (lifetime rates). They are more common in women than men. Onset occurs in childhood or early adolescence; the age of onset varies with the type of phobia. An example of a specific phobia is demophobia (fear of crowds). Most specific phobias persist for years or even decades. Mean duration of the disorder is 20 years. Phobias tend to be lifelong, if untreated; however, exposure-based treatment allows an excellent prognosis (McCabe, 2019).

Comorbidities associated with specific phobias include other anxiety disorders, mood disorders, and alcohol dependence. Individuals with specific phobias are often phobic of multiple things or situations.

Causes

No one knows what causes specific phobias. Because they seem to run in families (especially those involving blood or injury), researchers suspect that genetic predisposition plays a role. Neurobiological factors that could play a role in specific phobias include hyperactivation in the amygdala and insula (McCabe, 2019).

Other factors that may predispose a person to a specific phobia include:
- experiencing or observing a trauma
- repeated warnings of danger about the feared object or situation
- panic attacks when exposed to the feared object or situation
- disgust sensitivity (the tendency to experience disgust in response to certain stimuli)
- anxiety sensitivity (believing that the physical sensations of anxiety are harmful)
- increased attentional biases to perceived threats.

Role models in fear

Family members may have phobias and the patient may have learned to adopt them. Spontaneous, unexpected panic attacks also appear to play a role in the development of specific phobia. Cognitive and perceptual distortions consistent with the phobia support continuation of the phobia. Direct conditioning, vicarious acquisition, and informational transmission are other factors in the development of a specific phobia. Direct conditioning is "experiencing a traumatic event in the phobic situation such as being hurt or frightened. Vicarious acquisition involves observing someone behave fearfully in the phobic situation or witnessing a traumatic event (e.g., seeing someone being bit by a dog). Informational transmission involves learning to be fearful through information obtained verbally from others or through the media" (McCabe, 2019).

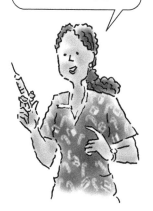

Phobias involving blood or injury tend to run in families.

Suicide risk

Patients with phobias or other anxiety disorder have a higher rate of suicide than those of the general population (American Psychiatric Association, 2013).

Signs and symptoms

The patient experiences severe anxiety when confronted with the feared thing or situation. The object or situation of the phobia is actively avoided or endured with intense anxiety. The fear is out of proportion to the situation; it causes significant distress and impairs functioning in some areas of the person's life.

Diagnosis

Specific phobia diagnosis is considered when the patient has a history of anxiety when exposed to a specific object or situation. This anxiety can also occur with anticipation of the object or situation.

Treatment

First-line treatment is CBT in combination with exposure treatment. Successful treatment usually involves desensitization or exposure therapy in which a mental health professional and a trusted companion gradually expose the patient to the feared object of situation. It can be especially helpful for phobias involving driving, flying, heights, bridges, or elevators.

Other techniques

Relaxation, breathing exercises, and thought-stopping can reduce anxiety symptoms. Role-playing in guided imagery teaches the patient to relax while confronting a feared object or situation.

Pharmacologic therapy

No proven drug treatments for specific phobias exist, but the health care provider may prescribe medications to reduce anxiety symptoms in advance of a phobic situation, such as flying in an airplane. Benzodiazepines (e.g., lorazepam [Ativan]) are most often used in this situation. SSRIs (e.g., sertraline [Zoloft]) have also been effectively used.

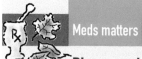

Pharmacologic therapy for anxiety disorders

This chart highlights FDA-approved drugs used to treat anxiety disorders.

Drug	Adverse effects	Contraindications	Nursing considerations
Antihistamine			
Hydroxyzine (Atarax, Vistaril)	• Dry mouth • Sedation • Tremor Rare: • Convulsions • Cardiac arrest (intra-muscular only) • Bronchodilation • Respiratory depression	• Early stages of pregnancy; proven allergy to hydroxyzine	• Dose reduction and close monitoring of elderly patients due to increased risk of confusion and oversedation • Evaluate alertness; sedation may occur (tell patient not to drive or engage in other potentially dangerous activities) • If on a high dose, monitor oral hydration and increase fluids as necessary • No concomitant use of alcohol • If the patient has also been given central nervous system (CNS) depressants, dose reduction will be needed in the depressant and the patient needs to be monitored closely
Antipsychotic			
Trifluoperazine (Stelazine)	• Neuroleptic-induced deficit syndrome • Akathisia • Rash • Priapism • Extrapyramidal symptoms • Galactorrhea	• CNS depression • Presence of blood dyscrasias • Bone marrow depression • Liver disease	• Observe closely for signs of neuroleptic malignant syndrome • Administer cautiously in patients in alcohol withdrawal or seizure history • Respiratory disorders • Glaucoma • Urinary retention • Avoid extreme sunlight and heat exposure • Not to be administered for longer than 12 weeks due to risk of tardive dyskinesia

(continued)

Pharmacologic therapy for anxiety disorders *(continued)*

Drug	Adverse effects	Contraindications	Nursing considerations
Benzodiazepines			
Alprazolam (Xanax) Chlordiazepoxide (Librium) Clonazepam (Klonopin) Clorazepate (Tranxene) Diazepam (Valium) Lorazepam (Ativan) Oxazepam (Serax)	• Ataxia • Confusion • Constipation • Double or blurred vision • Dry mouth • Sedation • Skin reactions (rash, urticaria, photosensitivity) • Vertigo • Weight change	• Acute alcohol intoxication • Acute angle-closure glaucoma or untreated open-angle glaucoma • Coma • Depression or psychosis without anxiety • Pregnancy or breast-feeding • Shock • Within 14 days of taking an MAOI	• Monitor closely after giving each dose because of a possible disinhibitory effect (excitement) rather than calming effect • Administer cautiously in the elderly and in patients with epilepsy, myasthenia gravis, impaired hepatic or renal function, history of substance abuse, or other CNS depressant use • Assess for unexplained bleeding • Monitor liver function and blood counts • Instruct patient to avoid alcohol, antidepressants, and anticonvulsants • Caution patient not to drive or operate hazardous machinery until drowsiness subsides • Stress the importance of avoiding abrupt drug withdrawal
Beta-adrenergic blocking agent			
Propranolol (Inderal) Off-label intervention	• Bradycardia • Dizziness • Emotional lability • Fatigue • Fever • GI disturbances • Heart block • Hypotension • Impaired concentration • Impotence and decreased libido • Mental depression • Skin rash • Shortness of breath • Sore throat • Worsening of angina	• Concomitant use of reserpine, MAOIs, digoxin, calcium channel blockers, theophylline, norepinephrine, or dopamine • Compromised cardiac function • Diabetes • Respiratory disease	• Take patient's apical pulse for 1 full minute after giving dose • Monitor blood pressure. Take blood pressure prior to administration and after administration of medication • Monitor cardiac function (fluid intake and output, daily weight, serum electrolytes) • Assess patient for signs and symptoms of depression • Advise patient not to change dose or stop drug without doctor's approval • Instruct patient to report weight gain of more than 2 lb/week • Inform diabetic patients that drug may mask hypoglycemia symptoms • Instruct patient to take drug with food to minimize GI disturbance • Teach patient which adverse effects to report

Pharmacologic therapy for anxiety disorders *(continued)*

Drug	Adverse effects	Contraindications	Nursing considerations
Serotonin norepinephrine reuptake inhibitors			
Duloxetine (Cymbalta) Venlafaxine (Effexor)	• GI (nausea, diarrhea, decreased appetite, dry mouth, constipation) • Insomnia, sedation, dizziness • Sexual dysfunction • Increase in blood pressure (2 mm Hg) • Urinary retention • Rare seizures • Rare induction of hypomania • Rare activation of suicidal ideations and behavior	• Uncontrolled narrow angle-closure glaucoma • Substantial alcohol use • If patient is taking thioridazine or an MAOI • Proven allergy to duloxetine	• Give in the morning with or without food • Monitor for weight loss if nausea occurs • Instruct patient to avoid alcoholic beverages • Monitor blood pressure • Tell patient to report adverse effects, especially rash or itching • Advise patient that stopping medication abruptly may cause serotonin withdrawal syndrome
Selective serotonin reuptake inhibitors			
Escitalopram (Lexapro) Fluoxetine (Prozac) Fluvoxamine (Luvox) Paroxetine (Paxil) Sertraline (Zoloft)	• Insomnia • Nausea • Nervousness • Vertigo • Sexual dysfunction • Rare activation of suicidal ideations and behavior	• Within 14 days of taking an MAOI	• Give in the morning with or without food • Monitor for weight loss if nausea occurs • Instruct patient to avoid alcoholic beverages • Tell patient to report adverse effects, especially rash or itching • Advise patient that stopping medication abruptly may cause serotonin withdrawal syndrome

(continued)

Pharmacologic therapy for anxiety disorders *(continued)*

Drug	Adverse effects	Contraindications	Nursing considerations
Tricyclic antidepressants			
Clomipramine (Anafranil) Doxepin (Sinequan)	• Agranulocytosis • Arrhythmias • Blurred vision • Bone marrow depression • Constipation • Dry mouth • Esophageal reflux • Galactorrhea • Hallucinations • Heart failure • Increased or decreased libido • Jaundice and fatigue • Mania • MI • Orthostatic hypotension or hypertension • Palpitations • Shock • Slowing of intracardiac conduction • Urinary hesitancy • Weight gain	• Concomitant use of MAOIs • Recent myocardial infarction (MI) • Renal or hepatic disease	• Monitor blood pressure and pulse for signs of orthostatic hypotension • Monitor patients for suicidal thoughts and behaviors • Supervise drug ingestion • Know that special monitoring is required if patient has a history of angle-closure glaucoma or seizure disorder • Monitor for adverse effects • Monitor liver function and complete blood counts • Tell patient to change positions slowly • Instruct patient to avoid driving or hazardous machinery if drowsiness occurs • Teach patient to avoid alcohol and over-the-counter (OTC) agents unless the doctor approves • Inform patient that desired drug effects may take up to 4 weeks to appear
Other antianxiety agent			
Buspirone (Buspar)	• Dizziness • Excitement • Headache • Light-headedness • Nausea • Nervousness	• Concomitant MAOI therapy • Renal or hepatic impairment	• Assist with ambulation if needed. • Instruct patient to inform all health care providers of all prescription, OTC, and recreational drug use • Caution patient against driving or operating machinery until drowsiness subsides • Instruct patient to report adverse effects • Inform the patient that improvement may take 3 to 4 weeks • Advise patient to have liver and kidney tests periodically

GI, gastrointestinal; MAOI, monoamine oxidase inhibitor.

Nursing interventions

These nursing interventions may be appropriate for patients with specific phobia.

- Encourage the patient to discuss the feared object or situation.
- Collaborate with the patient and the interprofessional team to develop and implement a systematic desensitization program in which the patient is systematically exposed to the feared object or situation in a controlled environment.
- Teach the patient assertiveness skills to help reduce submissive, fearful responses. Such strategies enable the patient to experiment with new coping skills and discard coping skills that have not worked in the past.
- Instruct the patient in relaxation and thought-stopping techniques as appropriate.
- To increase self-esteem and reduce anxiety, explain to the patient that the phobia is a way of coping with anxiety.
- Administer medications as ordered.

Quick quiz

1. A patient has acute stress disorder. Which describes the timing of acute stress disorder signs and symptoms?
    A. At least 3 days and last no more than 1 month.
    B. Several months after the traumatic event.
    C. On and off again for years.
    D. Whenever the trigger is experienced.

Answer: A. Acute stress disorder lasts no more than 1 month. If symptoms persist after 1 month, the diagnosis is PTSD.

2. Which condition best reflects fear of situations or places that may be difficult or embarrassing to leave?
    A. Social phobia.
    B. Panic disorder.
    C. Agoraphobia.
    D. GAD.

Answer: C. Agoraphobia is the fear and avoidance of situations or places that may be difficult or embarrassing to leave.

3. A patient has general anxiety disorder. Which signs and symptoms will the nurse anticipate during the assessment?
    A. Dissociation, avoidance, and repeated hand washing.
    B. Onset is shortly after an event, fear of leaving home, and fear of spiders.

    C. Difficulty concentrating, easily fatigued, and occurs for at least 6 months.

    D. Fear of performing a task in public, fear of a specific object, and fear of losing control.

Answer: C. Difficulty concentrating, easily fatigued, and has occurred for at least 6 months are signs and symptoms consistent with general anxiety disorder.

4. The fear of losing one's mind or having a heart attack is most likely to occur in which disorder?

    A. Social phobia.

    B. Panic disorder.

    C. GAD.

    D. Demophobia.

Answer: B. Anxiety severe enough to cause the patient to fear losing his or her mind or having a heart attack occurs with panic disorder. Social phobia, GAD, and demophobia may have a panic component to the patient, but the anxiety is less severe.

Scoring

☆☆☆ If you answered all four items correctly, terrific! You're doing a great job!

☆☆ If you answered three items correctly, relax. You have a basic knowledge of anxiety disorders.

☆ If you answered fewer than three items correctly, just breathe deeply, relax, stop those negative thoughts—and review the chapter for further study.

Selected references

American Psychiatric Association. (2013). *Diagnostic and statistical manual of mental disorders* (5th ed.). Author.

Baldwin, D. (2019). Generalized anxiety disorder: Epidemiology, pathogenesis, clinical manifestations, course, assessment, and diagnosis. *UpToDate.* https://www.uptodate.com/contents/generalized-anxiety-disorder-in-adults-epidemiology-pathogenesis-clinical-manifestations-course-assessment-and-diagnosis

Cheesman, R., Rayner, C., & Eley, T. (2019). The genetic basis of child and adolescent anxiety. In S. N. Compton, M. A. Villabø, & H. Kristensen (Eds.), *Pediatric anxiety disorders* (pp. 17–46). Elsevier.

Craske, M., & Bystritsky, A. (2019). Approach to treating generalized anxiety disorder in adults. *UpToDate.* https://www.uptodate.com/contents/approach-to-treating-generalized-anxiety-disorder-in-adults

Ellard, K., Barlow, D., Whitfield-Gabriele, S., Gabrieli, J., & Deckersbach, T. (2017). Neural correlates of emotion acceptance vs worry or suppression in generalized anxiety disorder. *Social Cognitive and Affective Neuroscience, 12*(6), 1009–1021. https://doi.org/10.1093/scan/nsx025

Essau, C., Lewinson, P., Lim, J., Moon-Ho, R., & Rohde, P. (2018). Incidence, recurrence and comorbidity of anxiety disorders in four major developmental stages. *Journal of Affective Disorders, 228*, 248–253. https://doi.org/10.1016/j.jad.2017.12.014

Gottschalk, M., & Domschke, K. (2017). Genetics of generalized anxiety disorder and related traits. *Dialogues in Clinical Neuroscience, 19*(2), 159–168.

Halter, M. (2017). *Varicolis' foundation of psychiatric mental health nursing: A clinical approach* (8th ed.). Elsevier.

Linder, P., Flodin, P., Larm, P., Budhiraja, M., Savic-Berglund, I., Jokinen, J., Tiihonen, J., & Hodgins, S. (2018). Amygdala-orbitofrontal structural and functional connectivity in females with and without conduct disorders. Scientific Reports, 8(1101). https://doi.org/10.1038/s41598-018-19569-7

McCabe, R. E. (2019). Agoraphobia in adults: Epidemiology, pathogenesis, clinical manifestations, course, and diagnosis. *UpToDate.* https://www.uptodate.com/contents/agoraphobia-in-adults-epidemiology-pathogenesis-clinical-manifestations-course-and-diagnosis

Pantic, I. (2019). Neurophysiological and neurological basis of emotion and mood. In A. Starcevic (Ed.), *Chronic stress and its effect on brain structures and connectivity.* IGI Global.

Roy-Byrne, P. P. (2019). Panic disorder in adults: Epidemiology, pathogenesis, clinical manifestations, course, assessment, and diagnosis. *UpToDate.* https://www.uptodate.com/contents/panic-disorder-in-adults-epidemiology-pathogenesis-clinical-manifestations-course-assessment-and-diagnosis

Schneier, F. R. (2019). Social anxiety disorder in adults: Epidemiology, clinical manifestations, and diagnosis. *UpToDate.* https://www.uptodate.com/contents/social-anxiety-disorder-in-adults-epidemiology-clinical-manifestations-and-diagnosis

Stein, M., & Taylor, C. (2019). Approach to treating social anxiety disorder in adults. *UpToDate.* https://www.uptodate.com/contents/approach-to-treating-social-anxiety-disorder-in-adults

World Health Organization. (2017). *Depression and other common mental disorders: Global health estimates.* https://apps.who.int/iris/bitstream/handle/10665/254610/WHO-MSD-MER-2017.2-eng.pdf

Zulfarina, M. S., Syarifah-Noratiqah, S.-B., Nazrun, S. A., Sharif, R., & Naina-Mohamed, I. (2019, March). Pharmacological therapy in panic disorder: Current guidelines and novel drugs discovery for treatment-resistant patient. *Clinical Psychopharmacology and Neuroscience, 17*(2), 145–154. https://doi.org/10.9758/cpn.2019.17.2.145

Chapter 7

Obsessive-compulsive and related disorders

Just the facts

In this chapter, you will learn:

◆ possible causes of obsessive-compulsive and related disorders

◆ signs and symptoms of obsessive-compulsive and related disorders

◆ assessment methods and nursing interventions for patients with obsessive-compulsive and related disorders.

A look at obsessive-compulsive and related disorders

Obsessive-compulsive disorder

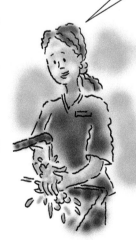

Washing hands excessively can endanger health and safety.

Obsessive-compulsive disorder (OCD) is characterized by unwanted, recurrent, and intrusive thoughts or images (obsessions), which the person tries to alleviate through repetitive behaviors or mental acts (compulsions). The compulsions are meant to reduce anxiety or prevent a dreaded event from happening. The person has rules in the compulsion that are applied in a rigid fashion.

Obsessions and compulsions may be simple or complex and ritualized. Compulsions include both overt behaviors, such as hand washing or checking, and mental acts, such as praying or counting. Although anxiety disorder is closely related to OCD, there are marked differences between these disorders. The Diagnostic and Statistical Manual of Mental Disorders, 5th edition (DSM-5) by the American Psychiatric Association (APA) categorizes OCD and related disorders separately from anxiety disorders (APA, 2013).

Run-on rituals

Obsessive-compulsive behaviors and activities related to OCD may take hours to complete and may consume the majority of the patient's time and energy.

Not surprisingly, OCD causes significant distress and may severely impair occupational and social functioning. Compulsive behaviors can also endanger health and safety. For example, severe dermatitis or a skin infection may result from compulsive hand washing.

But then, who's counting?

OCD affects about 2.3% of the general population (Simpson, 2017). In males, it typically begins in adolescence to young adulthood; in females, it usually begins in young adulthood (Simpson). The onset is usually gradual—over months or years. For most patients, the disorder takes a fluctuating course, with exacerbations linked to stressful events. In some cases, psychosocial functioning steadily deteriorates.

To make matters worse …

Those with OCD often have co-occurring psychiatric diagnoses. Statistically, the most prevalent comorbid condition with OCD is depression (20% to 60%) (Altintaş & Taşkintuna, 2015). In clinical samples, approximately 30% of patients with OCD report a past history of tics. Tic-related OCD has been identified as a separate diagnosis by the *DSM-5* (APA, 2013).

Causes

Genetic, biological, and psychological factors may be involved in OCD development. (See *The strep connection.*)

Genetic factors

Studies indicate that there is a strong genetic component regarding OCD, particularly in cases of pediatric-onset OCD (Simpson, 2017).

The strep connection

During the past few decades, providers and researchers have discovered a alarming relationship between OCD and beta-hemolytic streptococci (strep) infection. Studies have linked the sudden appearance of obsessions, compulsions, and motor or vocal tics with streptococcal throat infection in children.

It is hypothesized that an autoimmune response to the infection occurs. The strep bacteria trick the immune system by looking like host cells. This can cause some antibodies to mistakenly attack the basal ganglia, a brain region involved in movement and motor control.

The pediatric connection

A syndrome involving the dramatic onset of OCD symptoms following a strep infection in children is called *pediatric autoimmune neuropsychiatric disorders associated with streptococcal infections* (PANDAS) (Swedo & Williams, 2017). In some of these children, OCD symptoms respond to prompt antibiotic treatment. The reality of PANDAS continues to be debated within the research world.

(Vogel, 2018)

Biological aspects

Biological evidence for OCD is also strong. Magnetic resonance imaging (MRI) and computed tomography (CT) scans show structural abnormalities in some OCD patients. Positron emission tomography scans found increased glucose metabolism in a particular part of the basal ganglia. The cortico-striato-thalamo-cortical circuit hyperactivity has been implicated in OCD (Zike et al., 2017). Abnormalities in serotonin and dopamine signaling have also been hypothesized to play a role in the development of OCD.

Risk factors

Children who internalize symptoms and have negative emotionality and behavioral inhibition are at higher risk for the development of OCD (APA, 2013). Individuals who experience physical and sexual abuse are also at higher risk (APA, 2013).

Suicide risk

Up to half of patients with OCD are reported to have experienced suicidal thoughts. Individuals with coexisting psychiatric disorders have an increased risk of suicide (APA, 2013).

Signs and symptoms

The content of obsessions and compulsions in patients with OCD varies; however, most fall into a category known as "symptom dimensions" including (Simpson, 2017):

- Cleaning—obsession involves the fear of germs or contamination; cleaning rituals are the compulsion.
- Symmetry—obsession involves order and symmetry; counting is a compulsion.
- Forbidden or taboo thoughts—obsession involves thoughts about aggressive, sexual, or religious content; compulsions are based on the obsessive thought.
- Harm—obsession involves thoughts or images of harm to self or others; compulsion is constant checking to make sure oneself or others are unharmed.

They know it's weird

Most patients with OCD are aware that their obsessions are excessive or irrational and interfere with normal daily activities. In fact, many hide their symptoms out of embarrassment. However, a minority don't perceive their obsessions and compulsions as irrational. (See *Cultural practices and OCD.*)

Bridging the gap

Cultural practices and OCD

Don't mistake certain cultural or religious practices for OCD. For example, in some cultures, people pray repetitively or mourn a loved one's death with intensely ritualized behavior that may seem unusual to an observer. For this reason, always assess the patient within the context of cultural, spiritual, and religious beliefs.

Crucial criteria

Remember—culturally prescribed ritual behavior in itself doesn't signal OCD unless it:
* exceeds cultural norms
* occurs at times and places that others in the culture would deem inappropriate
* interferes with the patient's social role functioning.

Diagnosis

The diagnosis of OCD is confirmed if the patient meets the criteria listed in the *DSM-5* regarding the presence of obsessions and compulsions that interfere with daily living (APA, 2013).

Treatment

Treatment options for OCD include:
* behavioral techniques
* relaxation techniques, such as deep breathing, progressive muscle relaxation, meditation, imagery, or music
* support groups, which decrease the patient's isolation
* partial hospitalization and day treatment programs
* medication.

Behavior therapy

The behavioral technique of exposure and response prevention (ERP) is a type of cognitive-behavioral therapy that is used to treat patients with OCD. This is the treatment of choice for mild to moderate OCD. For moderate to severe OCD, medication and ERP is the treatment of choice. ERP exposes the patient to the object or situation that triggers the obsessions—but then challenges the individual to refrain from engaging in the usual compulsive response. The patient writes down what happens as a result of the behavioral restraint and comes to realize that not performing the ritual doesn't bring distressing outcomes. Eventually, the individual learns to manage his or her intense anxiety until it subsides (International OCD Foundation [IOCDF], 2020b).

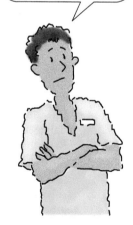

Most patients with OCD are aware that their obsessions are excessive or irrational and interfere with normal daily activities.

ERP therapy proves effective in about half of patients with mild to moderate OCD (Abramowitz et al., 2018). Because of the success of ERP in this population, computer and telephone access therapy—in which OCD patients call in and get computer-generated or in-person ERP therapy—was developed to improve access to this type of therapy.

Pharmacologic therapy

Pharmacologic interventions used in the treatment of OCD include selective serotonin reuptake inhibitors (SSRIs), serotonin-norepinephrine reuptake inhibitors (SNRIs), and tricyclic antidepressants (TCAs). (See *Meds matters*.) SSRIs are the first line of treatment for OCD and have been so for more than 30 years. The Food and Drug Administration (FDA) has approved the use of clomipramine (Anafranil), fluoxetine (Prozac), fluvoxamine (Luvox), paroxetine (Paxil), and sertraline (Zoloft) in the treatment of OCD (Food and Drug Administration, 2019).

Nursing interventions

These nursing interventions are appropriate for patients with OCD (Halter, 2018).

- Perform a self-assessment to identify any bias before working with the patient. It is important to recognize that the behaviors noted in patients with OCD can be frustrating for both nurse and patient.
- During the patient assessment, be aware of patient's mood and demeanor. It is important to remain calm and professional.
- Provide a supportive and nonjudgmental environment for the patient.
- Help the patient to identify obsessions and compulsions, and precursor feelings.
- Use therapeutic communication to encourage the patient to verbalize how they feel.
- Keep the patient's physical health in mind. For example, compulsive hand washing may cause skin breakdown; rituals or preoccupations may cause inadequate food and fluid intake and exhaustion. Provide for basic needs, such as rest, nutrition, and grooming, if the patient becomes involved in ritualistic thoughts and behaviors to the point of self-neglect.
- Collaborate with the interprofessional team including the health care provider, psychiatrist, social worker, and therapist to increase chances of better patient outcomes.

Isn't it tiring?

- Therapeutically observe and nonjudgmentally note certain behaviors. For example, the nurse might say, "I noticed you've made your bed three times today. That must be very tiring for you."
- Help the patient explore feelings associated with the behavior. For example, ask, "What do you think about while you perform your chores?" Listen attentively, offering feedback as necessary.
- Encourage the patient to explore patterns leading to the behavior or recurring problems.

Don't be shocked

- Maintain an accepting/nonjudgmental attitude.
- Don't show shock, amusement, or criticism of the ritualistic behavior.
- Understand that OCD is irrational and will not be changed by logical explanations.

Don't try to block

- Give the patient time to carry out the ritualistic behavior (unless it's dangerous). Be aware that blocking such behavior could increase the anxiety to an intolerable level.
- Allow the patient to have some control over anxiety-provoking situations. Never force the individual to do something.
- Establish reasonable expectations and time limits, and make their purpose clear. Avoid creating situations that increase frustration and provoke anger, which may interfere with treatment.

Diversionary tactics

- Encourage healthy active diversions, such as exercising or playing games, to divert attention from the unwanted thoughts while promoting a pleasurable experience.
- Explain how to channel emotional energy to relieve stress (e.g., through creative endeavors).
- Engage the patient in activities that create positive accomplishments and raise self-esteem and confidence.

Time's up!

- Assist the patient in exploring new ways to solve problems and developing more effective coping skills by setting limits on unacceptable behavior (e.g., by limiting the number of times per day the individual may participate in the compulsive behavior). Gradually shorten the time allowed. For the remainder of the time, help the individual focus on other feelings or problems.

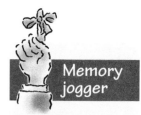

Memory jogger

To help the patient cope with OCD, remember the word COPING.

Concerns and feelings are discussed.

Offer a structured routine that allows time for rituals.

Practice thought-stopping skills.

Initiate a behavioral contract to decrease rituals and reward nonritualistic behaviors.

Nurture effective ways to problem-solve stressful situations.

Get the patient to perform relaxation techniques.

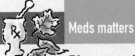

Pharmacologic therapy for obsessive-compulsive and related disorders

This chart highlights FDA-approved drugs used to treat OCD.

Drug	Adverse effects	Contraindications	Nursing considerations
SSRIs			
Fluoxetine (Prozac) Fluvoxamine (Luvox) Paroxetine (Paxil) Sertraline (Zoloft)	• Insomnia • Nausea • Diarrhea • Nervousness • Vertigo • Sleep disturbances • Sexual dysfunction	• Within 14 days of taking a monoamine oxidase inhibitor (MAOI)	• Give in the morning with or without food. • Monitor for weight loss if nausea occurs. • Teach patient to avoid alcoholic beverages. • Teach patient to report adverse effects, especially rash or itching. • Advise that stopping medication abruptly may cause serotonin withdrawal syndrome. • Monitor for suicidal thoughts and behaviors.
TCAs			
Clomipramine (Anafranil)	• Arrhythmias • Blurred vision • Bone marrow depression • Cardiac conduction issues • Constipation • Dry mouth • Hallucinations • Heart failure • Hematologic changes (leukopenia, agranulocytosis) • Jaundice and fatigue • Mania • MI • Orthostatic hypotension or hypertension • Palpitations • Sexual dysfunction • Suicidal ideation • Urinary hesitancy • Weight gain	• Concomitant use of MAOIs • Recent myocardial infarction (MI) • Renal or hepatic disease	• Monitor blood pressure and pulse for signs of orthostatic hypotension and teach to change positions slowly. • Monitor for suicidal thoughts and behaviors. • Know that special monitoring is required if patient has a history of angle-closure glaucoma or seizure disorder. • Monitor liver function and complete blood counts. • Teach to avoid driving or operating hazardous machinery if drowsiness occurs. • Teach to avoid alcohol and over-the-counter (OTC) drugs. • Teach patient that desired drug effects may take up to 4 weeks to appear.

- Identify insight and improved behavior (reduced compulsive behavior and fewer obsessive thoughts). Evaluate behavioral changes by your own and the patient's reports.
- Observe when interventions don't work; reevaluate and recommend alternative strategies.
- Help the patient identify progress and set realistic expectations.
- Encourage the use of healthy coping mechanisms to relieve loneliness and isolation.
- Monitor the patient for suicidal behaviors and thoughts. Hopelessness and helplessness may overwhelm the individual who feels powerless to control their behavior.
- Monitor for desired and adverse effects of prescribed drugs.

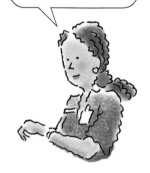

Each time the patient performs an OCD task, shorten the time that he or she may engage in the compulsive behavior.

Body dysmorphic disorder

Body dysmorphic disorder (BDD) is closely related to OCD. This condition is characterized by an upsetting or debilitating fixation with a perceived defect in appearance. Like OCD, patients with BDD practice behaviors to alleviate stress and anxiety related to the obsession. These include mirror checking, excessive grooming, overexercising, or seeking reassurance (APA, 2013). Patients with BDD usually have very poor insight about the reality of their own appearance.

Causes and risk factors

Causes of BDD have not been extensively studied, but it is hypothesized that development of BDD is complex and multifactorial. These factors may be genetic, biological, and/or environmental. Specifically, low serotonin levels are thought to play a role in the development of BDD (Sündermann & Veale, 2017). BDD can manifest as early as age 5, but typically occurs before the age of 18. Women are more likely to have BDD than men (Phillips, 2020).

I'm just teasing!
Teasing and bullying, especially in childhood, have been found to trigger BDD. These adverse childhood experiences lead to low self-esteem and insecurities. Nearly 70% of patients with BDD report some sort of experience with teasing or bullying (Brito et al., 2016).

Signs and symptoms

As with OCD, patients with BDD experience obsessions and compulsions that present in the following ways:
- Mirror checking or avoiding
- Excessive grooming
- Extreme exercise routines

- Constant comparisons with others
- Disguising or concealing appearance
- Surgery seeking (e.g., plastic surgery)
- Picking or touching area of concern
- Persistent reassurance-seeking

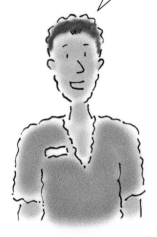

As with OCD, patients with BDD experience obsessions and compulsions.

Diagnosis

The diagnostic criteria for BDD according to the *DSM-5* includes preoccupation with one's perceived flaws or defects in appearance that results in repetitive behaviors and impairs functioning (APA, 2013).

Treatment

Treatment options for BDD include:
- behavioral therapy
- individual or group therapy
- medication.

Time for a change?

Some with BDD seek permanent changes like cosmetic surgery to help alleviate anxiety and obsession. They believe that the change will "fix" the problem and help with coping. However, research suggests the opposite; patients who seek expensive and body-altering treatments do not feel better, and sometimes feel worse (Higgins & Wysong, 2017). Patients often return for subsequent surgeries in an attempt to continue addressing what they perceive to be the problem.

Pharmacologic therapy

Currently, there are no FDA-approved medications for BDD. Because behaviors associated with BDD and OCD are similar, the medication choices are often the same. SSRIs are the first line of medication treatment used for BDD. (See *Meds matters*, page 180.)

Nursing interventions

These nursing interventions are appropriate for patients with BDD (Halter, 2018):
- Perform a self-assessment to identify any bias before working with the patient.
- Be aware of patient's changing moods and demeanor.
- Provide a supportive and nonjudgmental environment for the patient.
- Help the patient to identify obsessions.
- Encourage the patient to communicate how they feel.
- Collaborate with the interprofessional team including the health care provider, psychiatrist, social worker, and therapist to increase chances of better patient outcomes.

Hoarding disorder

Hoarding disorder is classified with OCD and BDD in the *DSM-5* (APA, 2013). All three of these disorders exhibit obsessions and compulsions. Individuals with hoarding disorder have very poor insight about their situation. Those who hoard collect items that may appear useless to others (newspapers, magazines, paper and plastic bags, cardboard boxes, photographs, household supplies, food, clothing, and even animals). The thought of getting rid of these items usually causes distress for the patient, even though the items clutter their living space and can cause a dangerous or unhealthy environment.

Want to see my stamp collection?

There are key differences between a collector and someone who hoards. Collectors often look for specific items and take pride in displaying them. Collectors will organize and maintain their collection. Someone who hoards will often carelessly pile the hoarded items. They may also have delusions about the objects or items.

Causes

Causes for hoarding disorder are not fully understood, although development is thought to involve genetics, brain chemistry, personal beliefs, and life events (Dozier & Ayers, 2017). Research demonstrates that there may be a genetic component to this disorder. Neurobiology studies demonstrate that possible damage to ventromedial prefrontal/anterior cingulate cortices and subcortical limbic structures could be a possible etiology (Mataix-Cols & de la Cruz, 2019).

Wait, there's more!

Psychiatric comorbid conditions are common with hoarding disorder. Approximately 57% to 68% of those who hoard also have major depressive and/or anxiety disorders and up to 20% have OCD (Mataix-Cols & de la Cruz, 2019). Because of poor insight, these patients will often seek treatment related to comorbid disorders instead of hoarding disorder (Halter, 2018).

Signs and symptoms

The following are signs and symptoms of hoarding disorder:
- Accumulating possessions without need or space
- Refusal or inability to throw possessions away
- Lack of organization of possessions
- Anxiety when attempting to get rid of hoarded possessions
- Loss of function
- Loss of living space

- Social isolation
- Health hazards (related to the accumulation)
- Relationship conflict
- Financial problems
- Embarrassment related to home or possessions
- Obsessive or delusional thoughts related to possessions or objects.

Diagnosis

Trained health care providers can administer the following assessment tools to help interpret patient beliefs and feelings (IOCDF, 2020a):
- Saving Inventory-Revised (SIR) (verbal tool) (Frost et al., 2004)
- Hoarding Rating Scale (HRS) (verbal tool) (Tolin et al., 2010)
- Clutter Image Rating Scale (CIRS) (picture-based tool) (Frost et al., 2008).

The diagnostic criteria for hoarding disorder can be found in the *DSM-5* and reflect ongoing difficulty discarding accumulated possessions regardless of value, which causes distress or functional impairment (APA, 2013).

Treatment

Treatment options for hoarding disorder include:
- therapy (cognitive-behavioral therapy, motivational interviewing)
- skills training
- medication.

Pharmacologic therapy

Like BDD, little research exists regarding the efficacy of pharmacotherapy for the treatment of hoarding disorder. SSRIs have traditionally been used for treatment. In recent years, research findings have been split about the efficacy of SSRIs in the treatment of hoarding disorder. In practice, the consensus is that the patient should be treated with therapy and an SSRI for 12 weeks; if the patient does not respond within that time frame, it is up to the provider to decide the next course of treatment (IOCDF, 2020c). (See *Meds matters*, page 180.)

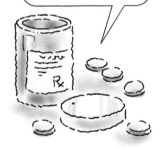

Treatment options for hoarding disorder include therapy, skills training, and/or medication.

Nursing interventions

These nursing interventions are appropriate for patients with hoarding disorder:
- Perform a self-assessment to identify any bias before working with the patient.
- Provide a supportive and nonjudgmental environment for the patient.
- Utilize, as ordered, the HRS, SIR, and CIRS for assessment purposes.

- Ensure safety for both the patient and family members.
- Work with patient and their support system to make plans and interventions.
- Encourage the patient to communicate how they feel and to engage in therapy as prescribed.
- Collaborate with the interprofessional team including the provider, psychiatrist, social worker, and therapist to increase chances of better patient outcomes.

Quick quiz

1.   Which therapy technique has been found to be useful in the treatment of OCD?
  A.   Aversion therapy
  B.   Guided self-help therapy
  C.   Rapid eye movement therapy
  D.   ERP

Answer: D. ERP is the therapeutic treatment of choice for OCD. ERP exposes the patient to the object or situation that triggers the obsessions, yet challenges the individual to refrain from engaging in the usual compulsive response.

2.   The nurse is caring for a 6-year-old patient with new-onset OCD-type behaviors after a strep infection. What will the nurse teach the family?
  A.   The behavior may have been triggered by an immune response.
  B.   OCD is harmless and will go away quickly.
  C.   There is a concern that this condition may be contagious.
  D.   Medication therapy is required for the child to recover.

Answer: A. PANDAS, a syndrome associated with OCD development after a strep infection, has been hypothesized to be caused by an autoimmune response to a strep infection. OCD is not harmless; it can cause distress to the patient as well as caregivers. This condition is not contagious. Medication therapy may be considered, but is not required in the treatment of this disorder.

3.   The nurse is caring for a patient recently diagnosed with OCD. Which first line of treatment does the nurse anticipate will be prescribed?
  A.   Duloxetine
  B.   Fluvoxamine
  C.   Alprazolam
  D.   Clomipramine

Answer: B. Fluvoxamine is an SSRI that is considered a first-line medication treatment for OCD. Duloxetine is an SNRI; alprazolam is a benzodiazepine; and clomipramine is a TCA.

4.   The nurse is caring for a patient being evaluated for BDD. Which statement requires immediate nursing intervention?
   A.   "I am worried that I might have cancer."
   B.   "I lift for 3 hours a day because my muscles are never big enough."
   C.   "I think I could lose a few pounds before the end of the year."
   D.   "My breasts cause me back pain; I would like a reduction."

Answer: B. Excessive exercise can be a sign of BDD. Further nursing intervention via assessment is required when the patient makes this statement. Concern about cancer does not indicate BDD unless the statement is targeted toward the way a patient looks. Observing that a few pounds could be lost is a reasonable statement that does not require immediate nursing intervention. Voicing a physical concern associated with a body structure does not indicate BDD and does not require immediate nursing intervention.

5.   The nurse is caring for a client with hoarding disorder. Which assessment finding does the nurse anticipate?
   A.   Gives away belongings that are meaningful
   B.   Organizes and displays extensive collections of items
   C.   Engages in buying and trading of select types of objects
   D.   Refuses to part with things that are stored within the home

Answer: D. Individuals with hoarding disorder cannot, or refuse to, part with items that are stored in their home. They do not give away meaningful belongings, organize or display collections, or engage in normal buying and trading of items.

Scoring

☆☆☆   If you answered all five items correctly, terrific! No need to keep going over it!

☆☆   If you answered three or four items correctly, just review one more time!

☆   If you answered two or fewer items correctly, no need to panic. Just breathe deeply, relax, stop those negative thoughts—and then read the chapter again!

Selected references

Abramowitz, J. S., Blakey, S. M., Reuman, L., & Buchholz, J. L. (2018). New directions in the cognitive-behavioral treatment of OCD: Theory, research, and practice. *Behavior Therapy, 49*, 311–322. https://doi.org/10.1016/j.beth.2017.09.002

Altintaş, E., & Taşkintuna, N. (2015). Factors associated with depression in obsessive-compulsive disorder: A cross-sectional study. *Archives of Neuropsychiatry (Noro Psikiyatri Arsivi), 52*(4), 346–353. https://doi.org/10.5152/npa.2015.7657

American Psychiatric Association. (2013). *Diagnostic and statistical manual of mental disorders* (5th ed.). Author.

Brito, M. J., Nahas, F. X., Cordas, T. A., Gama, M. G., Sucupira, E. R., & Ramos, T. D. (2016). Prevalence of body dysmorphic disorder symptoms and body weight concerns in patients seeking abdominoplasty. *Aesthetic Surgery Journal, 36,* 324–332.

Dozier, M. E., & Ayers, C. R. (2017). The etiology of hoarding disorder: A review. *Psychopathology, 50,* 291–296. https://doi.org/10.1159/000479235

Food and Drug Administration. (2019). *Drugs@FDA: FDA-approved drugs.* https://www.accessdata.fda.gov/scripts/cder/daf/index.cfm

Frost, R., Steketee, G., & Grisham, J. (2004). Measurement of compulsive hoarding: Saving inventory-revised. *Behavior Research and Therapy, 42*(10), 1163–1182.

Frost, R. O., Steketee, G., Tolin, D. F., & Renaud, S. (2008). Development and validation of the clutter image rating. *Journal of Psychopathology and Behavioral Assessment, 30*(3), 193–203.

Grisham, J. R., Frost, R. O., Steketee, G., Kim, H. J., & Hood, S. (2006). Age of onset of compulsive hoarding. *Journal of Anxiety Disorders, 20*(5), 675–686. https://doi.org/10.1016/j.janxdis.2005.07.004

Halter, M. J. (2018). *Varcarolis' foundations of psychiatric-mental health nursing: A clinical approach* (8th ed.). Elsevier.

Higgins, S., & Wysong, A. (2017). Cosmetic surgery and body dysmorphic disorder: An update. *International Journal of Women's Dermatology, 4*(1), 43–48. https://doi.org/10.1016/j.ijwd.2017.09.007

International OCD Foundation. (2020a). *Clinical assessment: Hoarding disorder.* https://hoarding.iocdf.org/professionals/clinical-assessment/

International OCD Foundation. (2020b). *Exposure and response prevention (ERP).* https://iocdf.org/about-ocd/ocd-treatment/erp/

International OCD Foundation. (2020c). *Treatment of hoarding disorder.* https://hoarding.iocdf.org/professionals/treatment-of-hoarding-disorder/

Mataix-Cols, D., & de la Cruz, L. (2019). Hoarding disorder in adults: Epidemiology, pathogenesis, clinical manifestations, course, assessment, and diagnosis. *UpToDate.* https://www.uptodate.com/contents/hoarding-disorder-in-adults-epidemiology-pathogenesis-clinical-manifestations-course-assessment-and-diagnosis

Phillips, K. A. (2020). Who gets BDD? *International OCD Foundation.* https://bdd.iocdf.org/about-bdd/who-gets/

Simpson, H. (2017). Obsessive-compulsive disorder in adults: Epidemiology, pathogenesis, clinical manifestation, course, and diagnosis. *UpToDate*. https://www.uptodate.com/contents/obsessive-compulsive-disorder-in-adults-epidemiology-pathogenesis-clinical-manifestations-course-and-diagnosis

Sündermann, O., & Veale, D. (2017). Complexity in obsessive-compulsive and body dysmorphic disorder: A functional approach to complex difficulties. *The Cognitive Behaviour Therapist, 10*, E15. https://doi.org/10.1017/S1754470X17000113

Swedo, S., & Williams, K. (2017). PANDAS as a post-Streptococcal autoimmune neuropsychiatric form of OCD. In C. Pittenger (Ed.), *Obsessive-compulsive disorder: Phenomenology, pathophysiology, and treatment* (p. 311). Oxford University Press.

Tolin, D., Stevens, M. C., Villavicencio, A. L., Norberg, M. M., Calhoun, V. D., Frost, R. O., Steketee, G., Rauch, S. L., & Pearlson, G. D. (2012). Neural mechanisms of decision making in hoarding disorder. *Achieves of General Psychiatry, 69*(8), 832–841. https://doi.org/10.1001/archgenpsychiatry.2011.1980

Tolin, D. F., Frost, R. O., & Steketee, G. (2010). A brief interview for assessing compulsive hoarding: The Hoarding rating scale-interview. *Psychiatry Research, 178*, 147–152.

Vogel, L. (2018). Growing consensus on link between strep and obsessive-compulsive disorder. *Canadian Medical Association Journal, 190*(3), E86–E87. https://doi.org/10.1503/cmaj.109-5545

Zaboski, B. A., Merritt, O. A., Schrack, A. P., Gayle, C., Gonzalez, M., Guerrero, L. A., Dueñas, J. A., Soreni, N., & Mathews, C. A. (2019). Hoarding: A meta-analysis of age of onset. *Depression & Anxiety, 36*, 552–564. https://doi.org/10.1002/da.22896

Zike, I. D., Chohan, M. O., Kopelman, J. M., Krasnow, E. N., Flicker, D., Nautiyal, K. M., Bubser, M., Kellendonk, C., Jones, C. K., Stanwood, G., Tanaka, K. F., Moore, H., Ahmari, S. E., & Veenstra-VanderWeele, J. (2017). OCD candidate gene SLC1A1/EAAT3 impacts basal ganglia-mediated activity and stereotypic behavior. *Proceedings of the National Academy of Sciences, 114*(22), 5719–5724. https://doi.org/10.1073/pnas.1701736114

Chapter 8

Trauma- and stressor-related disorders

Just the facts

In this chapter, you'll learn:

◆ possible causes of trauma and stressor-related disorders

◆ signs and symptoms of trauma and stressor-related disorders

◆ assessment and interventions for patients with trauma and stressor-related disorders.

A look at trauma- and stressor-related disorders

Trauma- and stressor-related disorders can develop after an individual experiences a traumatic or stressful event. A traumatic event or trauma is defined as an exposure to actual or threatened death, serious injury, or sexual violence in one or more ways: from directly experiencing or witnessing the event, or learning the event happened to a close family member, or experiencing repeated exposure to adverse events (American Psychiatric Association [APA], 2013; Jones-Wilkins et al., 2017). A stressor-related disorder is defined as an abnormal response to prolonged anxiety resulting in a decline in mental health or causing new or worsening health problems. Experiencing a traumatic or stressful event at any time throughout an individual's lifespan may lead to trauma- and stressor-related disorders such as posttraumatic stress disorder (PTSD), reactive attachment disorder (RAD), disinhibited social engagement disorder (DSED), and adjustment disorders (AJDs) (APA, 2013; Boyd, 2018).

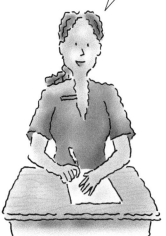

A patient with PTSD may become hypervigilant and easily startled.

Posttraumatic stress disorder

PTSD is considered a trauma- and stressor-related disorder. There is a close relationship between anxiety disorders and PTSD. However, there are marked differences that place PTSD in a different diagnostic category (APA, 2013). PTSD can occur after someone experiences or witnesses a serious traumatic event, such as wartime combat, a natural disaster, rape, murder, childhood sexual abuse, or torture.

The disorder is characterized by symptoms that are grouped into four categories: intrusive memories, avoidance, negative changes in thinking and mood, and hyperarousal. These symptoms can be different from person to person and may vary over time (Iyadurai et al., 2019). Intrusive memories are sensory-perceptual impressions of the event that occur involuntarily after a patient experiences a traumatic event that has resulted in PTSD. These impressions may take the form of visual images known as flashbacks or nightmares; may include sounds, smells, tastes, and bodily sensations; and may be associated with negative emotions (Iyadurai et al., 2019). The patient may demonstrate avoidance as their way of attempting to cope with the traumatic event. To avoid stimuli that trigger memories of the traumatic event, the patient with PTSD may become hypervigilant, easily aroused, and easily startled. When patients have changes in negative thinking and mood, they may express feelings of hopelessness and have difficulty maintaining close relationships. Clinical manifestations related to trouble sleeping, concentrating, and being easily startled fall within the hyperarousal category (APA, 2013; Kaczkurkin et al., 2016). In addition, the patient may experience survivor's guilt and a sense of being permanently damaged. Impairments caused by PTSD can be mild to severe, affecting nearly every aspect of the person's life.

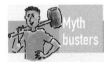

Posttraumatic stress disorder by the numbers

Experiencing or witnessing trauma is relatively common; 60% of men and 50% of women experience at least one traumatic event in their lives. Women are more likely to experience sexual violence, whereas men are more likely to experience accidents, physical violence, or witness death or serious injury. In the United States, 7% to 8% of the population has experienced PTSD in their lifetime. Approximately 8 million adults suffer from PTSD annually (The National Center for PTSD, 2019).

Up to 16% of patients with PTSD have a psychiatric comorbidity such as depressive disorders, anxiety disorders, and substance misuse disorders (Sareen, 2019).

Causes

A traumatic event (or events, such as in chronic childhood sexual abuse) can lead to PTSD. Not all individuals experiencing a traumatic event will have PTSD. However, some individuals may be biochemically predisposed to the disorder. Serotonin, a neurotransmitter found in the brain, has been known to have a role in the development and continued symptoms of PTSD (Schuch et al., 2016).

Posttraumatic stress disorder: Not just for war veterans

When some people hear the term PTSD, the image of a male war veteran pops into mind. However, the typical victim is more likely to be female.

Myth: Most PTSD victims are war veterans.

Reality: In the United States, 4% of men develop PTSD in their lifetime compared to 10% of women (The National Center for PTSD, 2019).

Other neurotransmitters, such as glutamate, neuropeptide Y, gamma-aminobutyric acid (GABA), and endogenous opioids, have shown to be altered in those with PTSD (Gore, 2018). In addition, gluco-corticoids can also induce PTSD-like symptoms due to activation of norepinephrine (Liu et al., 2019). MRI scans have shown abnormalities in the subcortical regions including the amygdala, hippocampus, and thalamus in clients with PTSD (Zhong et al., 2015). Although preexisting psychopathology may predispose a person to this disorder, PTSD can develop in anyone—especially if the stressor is extreme. Genetic factors may also play a role.

Risk factors

Risk factors for PTSD include:

- inadequate social support
- avoidant coping
- high anxiety levels; prior diagnosis of acute stress disorder
- low self-worth
- initial severity of reaction to the traumatic event
- history of psychiatric disorders (personal or in the family) (Mor & Dardeck, 2018).

Signs and symptoms

Common signs and symptoms of PTSD may include:

- anger
- poor impulse control
- chronic anxiety and tension
- avoidance of people, places, and things associated with the traumatic experience
- avoidance of talking about the event
- flashbacks, nightmares
- recklessness or self-destructive behaviors
- emotional detachment or numbness
- depersonalization (loss of personal identity)
- difficulty concentrating
- difficulty falling or staying asleep
- hypervigilance, hyperarousal, and exaggerated startle reflex
- inability to recall details of the traumatic event
- labile affect (rapid, easily changing affective expression)
- social withdrawal
- decreased self-esteem
- loss of sustained beliefs about people or society
- hopelessness
- sense of being permanently damaged
- relationship problems
- survivor's guilt.

Diagnosis

Diagnosing a patient with PTSD is based on a comprehensive clinical interview where numerous screening tools are used. The diagnosis is confirmed if the patient exhibits clinical manifestations that last longer than 30 days and cause a significant disruption in daily life (Iyadurai et al., 2019).

Treatment

Recovery takes time, support systems, and a collaborative approach. The major components of treatment involve psychotherapy and pharmacotherapy (Boyd, 2018).

Treatment is individualized and may differ between individuals based on preexisting conditions and current clinical presentation. Non-pharmacologic treatment options include prolonged exposure (PE), de-sensitization (systematic desensitization, eye movement desensitization and reprocessing [EMDR]), relaxation techniques, cognitive processing therapy (CPT), and psychotherapy (see table on therapies below).

Individual psychotherapy gives the patient a chance to talk through the traumatic experience with a nonthreatening person and thus gain perspective about the experience. Promoting feelings of loss, grief, and anxiety may aid in resolving the emotional numbness associated with PTSD. Group therapy helps the patient realize that they are not alone. A skilled group therapist can assist group members in confronting stressful feelings in a supportive environment. CPT and PE are the most commonly used nonpharmacologic treatments for PTSD for the newly diagnosed patient (Stein, 2019). Therapies can be used alone or in conjunction with others.

Therapies	Purpose
PE	Exposes the patient to the trauma in a safe way. Patients face and learn to control fears.
EMDR	The patient reviews and visualizes traumatic events with guidance under deep relaxation while focusing on the clinician's finger movements.
Relaxation techniques	Meditation, yoga, deep breathing can help reduce physiologic symptoms of PTSD.
CPT	Helps the patient understand the condition and its impact on daily life. Focus is on how the traumatic experience changed thoughts and beliefs.
Psychotherapy	Talk therapy helps patients understand their thoughts and feelings associated with the traumatic event.

Boyd, M. (2018). *Psychiatric nursing: Contemporary practice* (6th ed.). Wolters Kluwer; Scotland-Coogan, D., & Davis, E. (2016). Relaxation techniques for trauma. *Journal of Evidence Informed Social Work, 13*(5), 434–441. https://doi.org/10.1080/23761407.2016.1166845

Pharmacologic treatment

The major pharmacologic classifications used for patients with PTSD include selective serotonin reuptake inhibitors (SSRIs), benzodiazepines, and selective-norepinephrine reuptake inhibitors (SNRIs). (See *Meds matters: Pharmacologic therapy for posttraumatic stress disorder*, page 194.) Other medications may be prescribed based on the patient's psychiatric and medical comorbidities. Pharmacotherapy and psychotherapy can be used in a variety of combinations to effectively reduce symptoms of PTSD.

Suicide risk

A majority of research studies suggest an increased risk of suicide in patients with PTSD; however, more research is needed to corroborate these findings (Gradus, 2018). A thorough assessment, including a suicide risk assessment, should be performed to ensure the safety of the patient.

Nursing interventions

These nursing interventions may be appropriate for patients with PTSD:
- Work to establish a trusting relationship and build rapport with the patient. Assign the same care providers whenever possible. Promote an attitude of openness and acceptance (Boyd, 2018).
- Encourage the patient to express grief, complete the mourning process, and gain coping skills to relieve anxiety and desensitize the patient to memories of the traumatic event.
- Provide positive feedback to the patient for expressing thoughts and feelings about the traumatic event (Videbeck, 2017).
- Teach relaxation techniques.
- Use crisis intervention techniques as needed.
- Deal constructively with the patient's displays of anger. Encourage the patient to assess angry outbursts by identifying how the anger escalates.
- Help the patient regain control over angry impulses by identifying situations in which the patient lost control and by talking about past and precipitating events.
- Use a direct, nonjudgmental approach in discussing suicide or substance misuse.

Perspectives

- Reassure the patient of the ability to return to a previous level of functioning. Encourage the patient to make future plans.
- Help the individual put his or her behavior into perspective, recognizing isolation and self-destructive behavior as forms of atonement, and accept forgiveness from self and accept forgiveness from self and from others.
- Carefully review the healing process with the patient. Remind the individual not to equate setbacks with treatment failure.

Pharmacologic therapy for posttraumatic stress disorder

This chart highlights Food and Drug Administration (FDA)-approved drugs used to treat PTSD.

Drug	Adverse effects	Contraindications	Nursing considerations
SSRIs			
Sertraline (Zoloft) Paroxetine (Paxil) Fluoxetine (Prozac) Escitalopram (Lexapro) Citalopram (Celexa)	• Sweating • Dry mouth • Drowsiness • Indigestion/nausea • Sexual side effects • Hyponatremia	Do not use: • in pregnant women • or within 14 days of taking a monoamine oxidase inhibitor (MAOI)	• Monitor serum sodium levels. • Monitor for suicidal ideation. • Give in the morning with or without food. • Monitor for weight loss if nausea occurs. • Instruct patient to avoid alcoholic beverages. • Tell patient to report adverse effects, especially rash or itching. • Advise patient that stopping medication abruptly may cause serotonin withdrawal syndrome. • Monitor for serotonin syndrome such as high body temperature, dilated pupils, increased reflexes, tremor, sweating.
Benzodiazepines			
Alprazolam (Xanax) Chlordiazepoxide (Librium) Clonazepam (Klonopin) Clorazepate (Tranxene) Diazepam (Valium) Lorazepam (Ativan) Oxazepam (Serax)	• Ataxia • Confusion • Constipation • Double or blurred vision • Dry mouth • Sedation • Skin reactions (rash, urticaria, photosensitivity) • Vertigo • Weight change	• Do not use in patients with: – Acute alcohol intoxication – Acute angle-closure glaucoma or untreated open-angle glaucoma – Coma – Depression or psychosis without anxiety – Pregnancy or breast-feeding – Shock – Within 14 days of taking an MAOI	• Monitor closely after giving each dose because of a possible disinhibitory effect (excitement) rather than calming effect. • Administer cautiously in the elderly and in patients with epilepsy, myasthenia gravis, impaired hepatic or renal function, history of substance abuse, or other central nervous system (CNS) depressant use. • Assess for unexplained bleeding. • Monitor liver function and blood counts. • Instruct patient to avoid alcohol, antidepressants, and anticonvulsants. • Caution patient not to drive or operate hazardous machinery until drowsiness subsides. • Stress the importance of avoiding abrupt drug withdrawal.

Pharmacologic therapy for posttraumatic stress disorder *(continued)*

Drug	Adverse effects	Contraindications	Nursing considerations
SNRIs			
Duloxetine (Cymbalta) Venlafaxine (Effexor)	• Gastrointestinal (GI; nausea, diarrhea, decreased appetite, dry mouth, constipation) • Insomnia, sedation, dizziness • Sexual dysfunction • Increase in blood pressure (2 mm Hg) • Urinary retention • Rare reactions: seizures, induction of hypomania, activation of suicidal ideations and behavior	• Uncontrolled narrow angle-closure glaucoma • Substantial alcohol use • If patient is taking thioridazine or an MAOI • Proven allergy to duloxetine	• Give in the morning with or without food. • Monitor for weight loss if nausea occurs. • Instruct patient to avoid alcoholic beverages. • Monitor blood pressure. • Tell patient to report adverse effects, especially rash or itching. • Advise patient that stopping medication abruptly may cause serotonin withdrawal syndrome.
Other PTSD agents			
Alpha1 adrenergic blocker: Prazosin (Minipress) Beta adrenergic blocker: Propranolol (Inderal)	• Syncope, especially with the first dose • Drowsiness • Headache – Bradycardia – Dizziness – Emotional lability – Heart block – Hypotension – Impotence/decreased libido	• Use cautiously in patients with: – hypotension or orthostatic hypotension – heart disease – renal disease – glaucoma • Avoid using in patients with: – asthma – bradycardia – sick sinus syndrome or atrioventricular (AV) block – concomitant use of reserpine, MAOIs, digoxin, calcium channel blockers, theophylline, norepinephrine, or dopamine	• Tell patients not to abruptly stop the medication. • Take the first dose at bedtime to reduce the risk of falling. • Monitor blood pressure. • Tell patients not to drive or operate heavy machinery until effect of drug is known. • Instruct patients to limit alcohol. • Tell patient to take the drug at the same time every day. • Monitor blood pressure. • Assess apical heart rate for one full minute. • Tell patient to avoid alcohol. • Tell patient to inform the health care provider if shortness of breath, sudden weight gain (>2 lb/week), or lightheadedness occurs. • Assess for signs of depression. • If patient is diabetic, monitor glucose levels as this drug may mask hypoglycemia.

Medications

- Administer prescribed medications, as ordered.
- Teach the patient about prescribed medications and adverse effects. Advise the patient not to discontinue medication without first consulting the health care provider.
- Evaluate the patient's response to the prescribed drug regimen.
- Be aware that although benzodiazepines are fast acting, they may lose their effectiveness with prolonged use.

Referrals

- Refer the patient to clergy and community resources as appropriate.
- Refer the individual to group therapy with other victims for peer support.
- Encourage patient to contact community or online resources for support.

Acute stress disorder

Acute stress disorder has symptoms consistent with psychological disturbances similar to those of PTSD. Symptoms start as early as 2 days after the trauma is witnessed or experienced. Acute stress disorder has a maximum duration of 1 month, and if symptoms last longer than a month, the diagnosis is changed to PTSD (Santana et al., 2017).

Unlike PTSD, acute stress disorder resolves within 4 weeks. Acute stress disorder may begin as early as 2 days after the trauma. Duration of symptoms is 3 days to 1 month.

The American Institute of Stress (2019) estimates that between 5% and 20% of individuals experiencing a traumatic event develop acute stress disorder; of those 50% develop PTSD. Risk factors for acute stress disorder are similar to those of PTSD (e.g., history of a psychiatric disorder, female gender, trauma severity, and avoidant coping) (Bryant, 2019a).

Progression

Prognosis depends on such factors as severity and duration of the trauma and the patient's level of functioning. With immediate psychological care and much social support, recovery may be more rapid. If untreated, acute stress disorder may progress to PTSD, which can lead to substance misuse or major depression.

Causes

Exposure to trauma is the major precipitant of acute stress disorder. The trauma may involve serious physical or emotional injury or

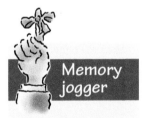

Memory jogger

The word "acute" is the key to remembering the difference between acute stress disorder and PTSD. Both cause similar symptoms but differ in their timing: Acute stress disorder happens shortly after the trauma and PTSD takes a bit longer to emerge (delayed).

threats to one's life. It is not clear what specific factors cause acute stress disorder. Several theories posit causes that focus on fear at the time of the traumatic event, cognitive processes (unrealistic appraisals of the event), and dissociation (Bryant, 2019a).

Signs and symptoms

Signs, symptoms, and clinical features of acute stress disorder, which are similar to those of PTSD, include intrusive memories, avoidance, negative changes in thinking and mood, and hyperarousal (Iyadurai et al., 2019).

A hallmark of acute stress disorder is dissociation—a defense mechanism in which the patient separates anxiety-provoking thoughts and emotions from the rest of the psyche. The world may seem dreamlike or unreal to the patient, or the patient may feel like he or she is observing himself or herself from a distance or that a body part has somehow changed. Dissociation may be accompanied by poor memory of the traumatic event or even complete amnesia of it.

Diagnosis

Physical examination helps rule out organic causes of signs and symptoms. The patient is diagnosed with acute stress disorder based on clinical manifestations of less than 30 days and recent history of trauma or traumatic event.

Treatment

Treatment of acute stress disorder is aimed at reducing symptoms and preventing progression to PTSD (Bryant, 2019b). Treatment of acute stress disorder may include social supports, psychotherapy, cognitive-behavioral therapy (CBT), and pharmacotherapy.

The first line of treatment for a patient diagnosed with acute stress disorder is CPT. CPT may involve trauma education, cognitive restructuring of the traumatic event to help the patient see it from a different perspective, and gradual reexposure with less avoidance (Jones et al., 2017). Supportive counseling or short-term psychotherapy helps the patient examine the trauma in a supportive environment, strengthen previously helpful coping mechanisms, and learn new coping strategies.

Medications may be used if nonpharmacologic methods aren't effective. The health care provider may prescribe short-term use of benzodiazepines and the beta adrenergic blocker propranolol (Inderal). SSRIs and SNRIs are generally not effective for patients with acute stress disorder.

Nursing interventions

These nursing interventions may be appropriate for patients with acute stress disorder:

- Encourage the patient to discuss the stressful event and identify it as traumatic. This validates that the situation was indeed beyond the patient's personal control.
- Urge the patient to talk about the feelings of anxiety and feelings about the trauma. This helps the patient cope with the reality of the event.
- Encourage the patient to identify any feelings of survivor guilt, inadequacy, or blame. Expressing these feelings helps the patient understand that survival may have been due to chance and not related to any personal action or inaction.
- Teach relaxation techniques, such as progressive muscle relaxation.
- Administer medications, as prescribed.
- If the patient is taking a medication, stress the importance of complying with prescribed therapy. Teach the patient about adverse drug reactions and what needs to be reported to the prescriber.

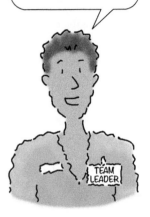

With survivor's guilt, your patient may feel better if they understand that their survival was due to chance alone.

Reactive attachment disorder overview

RAD occurs in children 6 months to 2 years of age. These children do not establish attachments with their direct caregivers, and their basic needs for comfort, affection, and nurturing are not met (Vega et al., 2019). Children with RAD are at greater risk of developing behavioral, social, and substance misuse disorders.

Causes

The common causes of RAD include:

- Early neglect
- Childhood abuse
- Abrupt separation from caregivers
- Absence of responsible caregivers

Risk factors

Children who:

- live in a facility or other institution
- frequently change foster homes or caregivers
- have caregivers with mental health or substance use disorders
- have a prolonged separation from caregiver

Signs and symptoms

- Unexplained withdrawal, fear, or irritability
- Sad appearance
- Not seeking comfort or showing no response when comfort is given
- Failure to smile
- Not engaging in social interaction
- Failure to ask for support or assistance
- Failure to reach out when picked up
- No interest in playing peekaboo or other interactive games
- Aggression
- Manipulation of caregivers

Diagnosis

RAD is diagnosed based on clinical manifestation and if the child has been exposed to a pattern of extremes of insufficient care (Bosmans et al., 2019).

Treatment

Treatment of RAD is aimed at providing a safe and secure environment. In addition, family therapy treatments such as trust-based relational intervention (TBRI) therapy can be effective. TBRI focuses on developing positive interactions between the child and caregiver (Losinski et al., 2016; Vega et al., 2019). Cognitive and dialectical behavioral therapy, a type of cognitive therapy, has also been effective in treating children with RAD. Dialectical behavioral therapy focuses on changing negative thinking patterns into positive thinking patterns. Parental training classes may also be beneficial.

Meds or no meds?

Currently, there are no recommended pharmacologic treatments for RAD except managing symptoms.

Nursing interventions

These nursing interventions may be appropriate for a patient with RAD:
- Establish a trusting relationship with the child and caregiver.
- Educate caregivers about RAD and need for safe, stable, and structured environment.

- Teach bonding or attachment activities such as piggy backs, games such as twister, or dancing.
- Teach caregivers about providing proper nutrition.
- Assess nonverbal cues of unspoken needs.
- Assess for self-destructive behaviors.
- Encourage use of community and online resources for support.

Disinhibited social engagement disorder

Overview

DSED is a pattern of behavior in which a child actively approaches and interacts with unfamiliar adults (APA, 2013). DSED affects children in their first 2 years of life because of insufficient caregiving; is characterized by functional impairments, inattention, and hyperactivity; and is similar to RAD. One of the main differences between DSED and RAD is that the child with DSED has no fear of going to strangers and the child with RAD is withdrawn (Guyon-Harris et al., 2019).

Causes

The causes of DSED include:
- Early neglect
- Childhood abuse
- Abrupt separation from caregivers
- Absence of responsible caregivers.

Risk factors

Children who:
- Live in a facility or other institution
- Frequently change foster homes or caregivers
- Have caregivers with mental health or substance use disorders
- Have a prolonged separation from caregiver.

Signs and symptoms

- No fear of strangers
- Impulsive and hyperactive behaviors
- Excessive self-disclosure
- Overfriendly and intrusive
- Developmental delays (social and motor skills)
- Unusually comfortable talking to, touching, and leaving a location with a stranger (Kennedy et al., 2017).

Diagnosis

To diagnose DSED, it must be established that the unusual social behavior is reactive to exposure to extremes of insufficient care, such as social neglect and deprivation, frequent changes in primary caregivers, and growing up in an environment that limited the ability for attachment to foster (Giltaij et al., 2017).

Treatment

Treatment is focused on family therapies, such as TBRI, that is centered on developing positive interactions between the child and caregiver (Losinski et al., 2016). Cognitive and dialectical behavioral therapy has also been effective in treating children with DSED. Expressive therapies such as play and art therapy may be beneficial.

Pharmacologic treatment

Currently, there is no recommended pharmacologic treatment for DSED except managing symptoms.

Nursing interventions

These nursing interventions may be appropriate for a patient with DSED:
- Educate caregivers about DSED
- Demonstrate consistency in delineating social boundaries
- Teach self-control strategies
- Encourage use of community and online resources for support (Scheper et al., 2019).

Adjustment disorders

Overview

AJD is a disorder that appears in response to some identifiable stressful event such as separation, job loss, or diagnosis of a disease. AJD is characterized by emotional and behavioral symptoms in response to the stressful event occurring within 3 months from the beginning of the stressor, causing marked distress (Yaseen, 2017). The individual with AJD has a difficult time coping with the stressor.

Causes

Causes of AJD include:
- Involuntary job loss
- Divorce
- Family conflicts
- Affairs
- Domestic abuse
- Diagnosis of disease
- Academic failure.

Risk factors

- Loss (such as loss of a loved one, employment, residence)
- Lack of appropriate coping skills
- Repeated and significant life changes
- Being a victim of violence and/or neglect.

Signs and symptoms

The signs and symptoms of AJD include:
- Marked impairment in different functional areas of patients' lives such as family, friendships, school/work
- Guilt
- Depression
- Anxiety
- Anger
- Physical complaints such as abdominal pain, trembling, or twitching
- Social withdrawal
- Difficulty in thinking of the future.

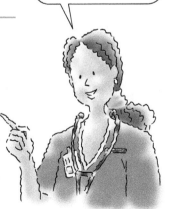

Behavioral, cognitive, physical, and psychological symptoms may occur in patients with AJD.

Diagnosis

Diagnosis is based on an identified stressor, clinical manifestations, and timing of the symptoms: within 3 months of the stressful event and subsiding within 6 months following resolution of the stressor or its consequences (Rachyla et al., 2018).

Treatment

CBT is the preferred method of treatment. However, there are few evidence-based interventions for AJD. The lack of specific treatment guidelines for this disorder often results in the worsening of clinical symptoms because patients do not receive appropriate help (Rachyla et al., 2018). Some research shows humor promotes positive emotions and can be an efficient tool for dealing with negative or stressful life situations. Humor also has positive effects on other aspects of our daily lives such as social or physical functioning (Tagalidou et al., 2019).

Pharmacologic treatment

There is no definitive pharmacologic treatment for AJD except to treat symptoms on an individual case-by-case basis.

Nursing interventions

These nursing interventions may be appropriate for a patient with AJD:
- Establish a trusting relationship with the patient
- Provide emotional support
- Assess coping mechanisms, encourage use of past successful coping strategies, assist the patient with developing new coping strategies
- Monitor for suicidal behavior or self-inflicted injuries
- Teach stress reduction methods such as relaxation techniques.

Quick quiz

1. Flashbacks of an unpleasant, terrifying, or painful experience are associated with which trauma- and stressor-related disorder?
    A. PTSD
    B. RAD
    C. AJD
    D. DSED

Answer: A. Flashbacks are characteristic of PTSD. They aren't major components of RAD, AJD, or DSED.

2. Which medication will the nurse prepare to teach a patient with acute stress disorder?
    A. Sertraline (Zoloft)
    B. Fluoxetine (Prozac)
    C. Prazosin (Minipress)
    D. Propranolol (Inderal)

Answer: D. Propranolol (Inderal) may be prescribed if nonpharmacologic therapies are ineffective. Short-term benzodiazepines may also be prescribed.

3. Which statement reflects the purpose of CPT?
   A. Talk therapy that helps the patients understand their thoughts and feelings associated with the traumatic event.
   B. Exposes the patient to the trauma in a safe way. Patients face and learn to control fears.
   C. The patient reviews and visualizes traumatic events with guidance under deep relaxation while focusing on the clinician's finger movements.
   D. Helps the patient understand the condition and its impact on daily life. Focus is on how the traumatic experience changed thoughts and beliefs.

Answer: D. CPT helps the patient understand the condition and its impact on daily life. Focus is on how the traumatic experience changed thoughts and beliefs. A is psychotherapy; B is PE; C is EMDR.

4. EMDR has been effective in treating which trauma/stress-related disorder?
   A. PTSD
   B. Panic disorder
   C. AJD
   D. DSED

Answer: A. EMDR is an effective treatment for PTSD. In EMDR, the patient reviews and visualizes traumatic events with guidance under deep relaxation while focusing on the clinician's finger movements.

Scoring

☆☆☆ If you answered all four items correctly, terrific! You're doing a great job!

☆☆ If you answered three correctly, you have a basic knowledge of trauma- and stress-related disorders.

☆ If you answered fewer than three items correctly, stop those negative thoughts—and then reexpose yourself to the chapter for further study.

Selected references

American Psychiatric Association. (2013). *Diagnostic and statistical manual of mental disorders* (5th ed.). Author.

American Institute of Stress. (2019). Acute stress disorder. Retrieved from https://www.stress.org/acute-stress-disorder

Bosmans, G., Spilt, J., Vervoort, E., & Verschueren, K. (2019). Inhibited symptoms of reactive attachment disorder: Links with working models of significant others and the self. *Attachment & Human Development, 21*(2), 190–204. https://doi.org/10.1080/14616734.2018.1499213

Boyd, M. (2018). *Psychiatric nursing: Contemporary practice* (6th ed.). Wolters Kluwer.

Bryant, R. (2019a). Acute stress disorder in adults: Epidemiology, pathogenesis, clinical manifestations, course, and diagnosis. *UpToDate.* https://www.uptodate.com/contents/acute-stress-disorder-in-adults-epidemiology-pathogenesis-clinical-manifestations-course-and-diagnosis

Bryant, R. (2019b). Treatment of acute stress disorder in adults. *UpToDate.* https://www.uptodate.com/contents/treatment-of-acute-stress-disorder-in-adults

Giltaij, H., Sterkenburg, P., & Schuengel, C. (2017). Convergence between observations and interviews in clinical diagnosis of reactive attachment disorder and disinhibited social engagement disorder. *Clinical Child Psychology and Psychiatry, 22*(4), 603–619. https://doi.org/10.1177/1359104517709049

Gore, A. (2018, November 14). What is the pathophysiology of the brain in post-traumatic stress disorder (PTSD). *Medscape.* https://www.medscape.com/answers/288154-95784/what-is-the-pathophysiology-of-the-brain-in-post-traumatic-stress-disorder-ptsd

Gradus, J. (2018). Posttraumatic stress disorder and death from suicide. *Current Psychiatric Reports, 20*(11), 98. https://doi.org/10.1007/s11920-018-0965-0

Guyon-Harris, K., Humphreys, K., Miron, D., Gleason, M., Nelson, C., Fox, N., & Zeanah, C. (2019). Disinhibited social engagement disorder in early childhood predicts reduced competence in early adolescence. *Journal of Abnormal Child Psychology, 47*(10), 1735–1745. https://doi.org/10.1007/s10802-019-00547-0

Iyadurai, L., Visser, R., Lau-Zhu, A., Porcheret, K., Horsch, A., Holmes, E., & James, E. (2019). Intrusive memories of trauma: A target for research bridging cognitive science and its clinical application. *Clinical Psychology Review, 69,* 67–82. https://doi.org/10.1016/j.cpr.2018.08.005

Jones Wilkins, M., Owen, T., & Kilpatrick, B. (2017). Trauma and stress related disorders: Relevance to DSM-5 and life care planning. *Journal of Life Care Planning, 15*(2), 39–47. International Association of Rehabilitation Professionals. www.rehabpro.org

Kaczkurkin, A., Anaani, A., Alpert, E., & Foa, E. (2016). The impact of treatment condition and the lagged effects of PTSD symptom severity and alcohol use on changes in alcohol craving. *Behaviour Research and Therapy, 79,* 7–14. https://doi.org/10.1016/j.brat.2016.02.001

Kennedy, M., Kreppner, J., Knights, N., Kumsta, R., Maughan, B., Golm, D., & Sonuga-Barke, E. (2017). Adult disinhibited social engagement in adoptees exposed to extreme institutional deprivation: Examination of its clinical status and functional impact. *The British Journal of Psychiatry, 211*(5), 289–295. https://doi.org/10.1192/bjp.bp.117.200618

Liu, X., Zhu, R., Hao, B., Shi, Y., Wang, X., Xue, L., & Zhao, H. (2019). Norepinephrine induces PTSD-like memory impairments via regulation of the β-adrenoceptor-cAMP/PKA and CaMK II/PKC systems in the basolateral amygdala. *Frontiers in Behavioral Neuroscience, 13,* 43. https://doi.org/10.3389/fnbeh.2019.00043

Losinski, M., Katsiyannis, A., Wite, S., & Wiseman, N. (2016). Addressing the complex needs of students with attachment disorders. *Intervention in School & Clinic, 51*(3), 184. https://doi.org/10.1177/1053451215585800

Mor, N., & Dardeck, K. L. (2018). Quantitative forecasting of risk for PTSD using eco-
logical factors: A deep learning application. *Journal of Social, Behavioral, and
Health Sciences, 12*, 61–73. https://doi.org/10.5590/JSBHS.2018.12.1.04

National Center for PTSD. (2019). PTSD and death from suicide. *PTSD Research Quarterly, 28*(4), 1–8. https://www.ptsd.va.gov/publications/rq_docs/V28N4.pdf

Rachyla, I., Perez-Ara, M., Moles, M., Campos, D., Mira, A., Botella, C., & Quero, S.
(2018). An internet-based intervention for adjustment disorder (TAO): Study
protocol for a randomized controlled trial. *BMC Psychiatry, 18*(1), 161.
https://doi.org/10.1186/s12888-018-1751-6

Santana, M., Zatti, C., Spader, M., Malgarim, B., Salle, E., Piltcher, R., Cereser, K., Bastos,
A., & Freitas, L. H. (2017). Acute stress disorder and defense mechanisms:
A study of physical trauma patients admitted to an emergency hospital. *Trends
in Psychiatry and Psychotherapy, 39*(4), 247–256. https://doi.org/10.1590/
2237-6089-2016-0071

Sareen, J. (2019). Posttraumatic stress disorder in adults: Epidemiology, pathophysiology, clinical manifestations, course, assessment, and diagnosis. *UpToDate.*
https://www.uptodate.com/contents/posttraumatic-stress-disorder-in-adults-
epidemiology-pathophysiology-clinical-manifestations-course-assessment-
and-diagnosis

Scheper, F., Groot, C., de Vries, A., Doreleijers, T., Jansen, L., & Schuengel, C. (2019).
Course of disinhibited social engagement behavior in clinically referred
home-reared preschool children. *Journal of Child Psychology and Psychiatry,
60*(5), 555–565. https://doi.org/10.1111/jcpp.12994

Schuch, L., Yip, A., Nouri, K., Gregersen, M., Cason, B., Kukreja, J., Wozniak, C., Brzez-
inski, M. (2016). Serotonin syndrome following an uncomplicated orthope-
dic surgery in a patient with posttraumatic stress disorder. *Military Medicine,
181*(9), e1185–e1188. https://doi.org/10.7205/MILMED-D-15-00461

Scotland-Coogan, D., & Davis, E. (2016). Relaxation techniques for trauma. *Journal of
Evidence Informed Social Work, 13*(5), 434–441. https://doi.org/10.1080/23761
407.2016.1166845

Stein, B. (2019). Approach to treating posttraumatic stress disorder in adults. *UpToDate.*
https://www.uptodate.com/contents/approach-to-treating-posttraumatic-
stress-disorder-in-adults

Tagalidou, N., Distlberger, E., Loderer, V., & Laireiter, A. (2019). Efficacy and feasibility
of a humor training for people suffering from depression, anxiety, and adjustment disorder: A randomized controlled trial. *BMC Psychiatry, 19*, 93. https://
doi.org/10.1186/s12888-019-2075-x

Vega, H., Cole, K., & Hill, K. (2019). Interventions for children with reactive attachment
disorder. *Nursing, 49*(6), 50–55. https://doi.org/10.1097/01.NURSE.
0000554615.92598.b2

Videbeck, S. (2017). *Psychiatric-mental health nursing* (7th ed.). Wolters Kluwer.

Yaseen, Y. A. (2017). Adjustment disorder: Prevalence, sociodemographic risk factors,
and its subtypes in outpatient psychiatric clinic. *Asian Journal of Psychiatry, 28*,
82–85. https://doi.org/10.1016/1.ajp.2017.03.012

Zhong, Y., Zhang, R., Li, K., Qi, R., Zhang, Z., Huang, Q., & Lu, G. (2015). Altered cortical and subcortical local coherence in PTSD: Evidence from resting-state fMRI.
Acta Radiologica, 56(6), 746–753. https://doi.org/10.1177/0284185114537927

Chapter 9

Dissociative disorders

Just the facts

In this chapter, you will learn:

◆ general characteristics of dissociative disorders

◆ diagnostic tools used to evaluate dissociative disorders

◆ signs, and symptoms of dissociative disorders

◆ assessment and interventions for patients with dissociative disorders.

A look at dissociative disorders

Dissociative disorders are marked by disruption of the fundamental aspects of waking consciousness—memory, identity, consciousness, and the general experience and perception of oneself and one's surroundings. Dissociation is used as an unconscious defense mechanism to separate anxiety-provoking feelings and thoughts from the conscious mind (American Psychiatric Association [APA], 2013).

Dissociation is a common occurrence that ranges from normal to pathologic. Normal types of dissociation include daydreams, highway hypnosis (also known as "white line fever," a trancelike feeling that can occur when driving), and getting "lost" in a book, movie, or program to the point that someone fails to notice the time or surroundings. Pathologic dissociation occurs in dissociative disorders (APA, 2013).

This chapter discusses depersonalization/derealization disorder (DDD), dissociative amnesia (which includes dissociative fugue), and dissociative identity disorder (DID).

> One type of dissociation is highway hypnosis, a trancelike feeling that occurs when driving.

Too awful to remember

Usually, dissociative disorders result from overwhelming stress caused by a traumatic event that has been experienced or witnessed or by intolerable psychological conflict. The disorder occurs as the mind isolates the unacceptable information and feelings.

Dissociation is not fully understood. Dissociative disorders (especially dissociative amnesia) have been associated with "forgotten" childhood traumas and repressed memories. Some experts believe dissociation is a common defense mechanism used by a child who has experienced abuse or trauma (Spiegel, 2019a). Dissociative disorders are extremely rare, occurring in less than 1% of the population (Foote, 2018). Symptoms may arise suddenly or gradually. Many dissociative episodes are transient; however, if they persist, such episodes may cause functional impairments (APA, 2013).

> Dissociation is thought to be a defense mechanism.

Causes

There are several theories that attempt to explain dissociative disorders via psychological, biological, and learning theories.

Psychological theories

According to psychological theories, dissociative disorders are a response to severe trauma or abuse. To cope with the trauma or abuse, the patient tries to repress the unpleasant experience from awareness. If repression fails, dissociation occurs as a defense mechanism: The patient separates the experience from the conscious mind because it's too traumatic to integrate it. (See *Delving into dissociation*.)

Biological theories

Biological theories are most closely linked with DDD. Researchers point out that this disorder shares a key symptom—a sense of loss of one's own reality—with certain neurologic disorders (such as epilepsy and tumors), several psychiatric disorders, and the effects of certain drugs (most notably, barbiturates, benzodiazepines, hallucinogens, and marijuana) (Spiegel, 2019b).

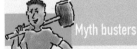

Myth busters

Delving into dissociation

Dissociation is a mysterious and often misunderstood phenomenon.
Myth: A person who experiences dissociation or derealization after a traumatic event can consciously control the dissociation.
Reality: Dissociation and derealization occur because the traumatic event has overwhelmed the person's ability to cope using any other method. The dissociations are beyond conscious control.
Myth: People in dissociative fugue states behave in a confused manner.
Reality: Most people in dissociative fugue states behave in a normal manner.

Learning theory

According to learning theory, dissociative disorders represent a learned response of avoiding stress and anxiety, and with opportunity and practice, a person can become highly skilled at dissociating. This learned behavior of forcing the memory from awareness is common in people with a history of abuse (Spiegel, 2019b).

Evaluation

Because a dissociative disorder can mimic a physical illness or another psychiatric disorder, the patient should undergo a complete physical examination.

Trials of trauma

A mental health professional should obtain a careful personal history from the patient and family members. The interview should include questions about childhood and/or adult trauma, abuse, and any of the below experiences:

- blackouts or "lost" time
- fugues—travel away from home with no memory of what happened on these trips
- unexplained possessions that may have been purchased during a fugue
- relationship changes
- fluctuations in skills and knowledge
- unclear or spotty recollection of one's own history
- occurrence of spontaneous trancelike state, or age regression.

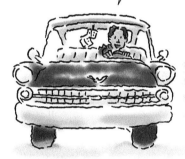

A person who experiences dissociative amnesia with dissociative fugue may find themselves far from home with no memory of how they got there.

Diagnostic toolbox

Patients with dissociative disorders may be evaluated with any of these diagnostic tools.

- Dissociative Experiences Scale II (DES-II). This brief self-report scale measures the frequency of dissociative experiences. The patient quantifies their experiences for each item (Bernstein & Putnam, 1986; Carlson & Putnam, 1993). If the patient scores high, further evaluation is necessary.
- Dissociative Disorders Interview Schedule. This highly structured interview is used to diagnose trauma-related disorders. The patient answers questions that the examiner must ask in a precisely designated order. The interview takes 30 to 45 minutes (Ross et al., 1989).
- Structured Clinical Interview for Dissociative Disorders (SCID-D). This semi-structured interview assesses the nature and severity of five dissociative symptoms—amnesia, depersonalization, derealization, identity confusion, and identity alteration. It also enables

the clinician to diagnose a dissociative disorder based on the *Diagnostic and Statistical Manual of Mental Disorders*, 5th Edition (*DSM-5*) criteria.

- Cambridge Depersonalization Scale. This self-report scale requires that the patient rate the frequency and duration of 29 types of depersonalization and derealization experiences. A high score of 70 or above indicates that the patient's experiences are not better explained by various mood, anxiety, or neurologic disorders (Sierra & Berrios, 2000).
- Multidimensional Inventory of Dissociation. This self-report scale consists of 218 items that are ranked on a scale of "never" to "always." It can take up to 90 minutes to complete and the results can be categorized according to potential diagnoses (Dell, 2006).
- Diagnostic Drawing Series. This test is used by art therapists to aid in diagnosis of dissociative disorders. The patient is instructed to draw a tree and a picture of their feelings (Cohen, 1983).

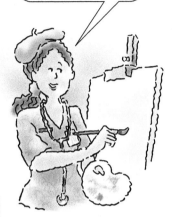

An art therapist may use the Diagnostic Drawing Series to help diagnose a dissociative disorder.

Depersonalization/derealization disorder

DDD is marked by a persistent or recurrent feeling that one is detached from one's own mental processes or body, or by feelings of detachment from other persons, objects, or their surroundings. The patient seldom loses touch with reality completely. However, depersonalization episodes may cause severe distress and impair functioning (APA, 2013).

Shrinking away?

During episodes of depersonalization, self-awareness (or a portion of it) is altered or lost temporarily. The sense of depersonalization may be restricted to a single body part, such as a limb, or it may encompass the whole self. The patient may feel as if a body part or the entire body has shrunk or grown. Awareness of others is temporarily altered as well. Another person, object, or their surroundings may seem veiled, flat, seemingly artificial, or lifeless. Other persons or objects may seem larger, smaller, closer, or farther away than they really are (APA, 2013).

Watching the world go by

The patient may perceive the change in consciousness as a barrier between himself or herself and the outside world. The patient may feel as if he or she is passively watching from the outside or as if the external world is unreal or distorted (APA, 2013).

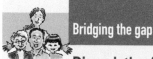

Bridging the gap

Dissociation/derealization and cultural considerations

If your patient has symptoms of a dissociative disorder, make sure to find out about cultural and religious practices before drawing conclusions about their mental state.

Possession trances
Meditative and trancelike practices are a part of some religions and cultures. Some of these practices may resemble a dissociative disorder (particularly DDD).

If a patient's cultural or religious practices include elements of spiritual possession and/or dissociation, then a dissociative disorder is not applicable (APA, 2013).

Not so unusual

Although DDD is rare, the experience of depersonalization or derealization is not rare. It occurs in many average people for brief periods of time and should not be confused with a psychiatric disorder. In fact, 50% of people have had a brief experience of depersonalization or derealization in their lives. However, only about 2% of people meet the criteria for clinical diagnosis of DDD (Spiegel, 2019b).

For example, many people occasionally report feeling "spaced out" or as if they are in a dream or looking at themselves from the outside. When intoxicated, some people feel they are out of control of their actions. Situational depersonalization or derealization can also follow life-threatening danger, such as an accident, assault, serious illness, or injury. It can occur as a symptom in other psychiatric disorders, in medical conditions like seizures, as a side effect of medication, or as part of certain religious practices (APA, 2013). Situational depersonalization or derealization is brief and has no lasting effect. However, DDD is considered a chronic illness (APA)." (See *Dissociation/derealization and cultural considerations*.)

Prevalence and onset

The prevalence of DDD is believed to be about 2% and affects males and females equally (Morrison, 2014; Spiegel, 2019b). Onset of DDD usually occurs by the early 20s and is considered a chronic illness (Morrison). Onset can be sudden or gradual, usually in childhood or adolescence. It rarely occurs after age 40 (APA, 2013).

The disorder often progresses and becomes chronic, with exacerbations and remissions. Exacerbations can be caused by stress and overstimulation (APA, 2013).

Causes

As a separate disorder, DDD has not been studied widely and its exact cause is unknown. It typically occurs in people who have experienced severe stress or complex trauma early in life, such as combat, violent crime, accidents, or natural disasters (APA, 2013). It can also be induced by illicit drug use, in particular, marijuana, ketamine, and hallucinogens (Spiegel, 2019b).

Other factors linked to its development include:

- immature defense mechanisms
- sensory deprivation
- neurophysiologic factors, such as epilepsy or a concussion
- history of physical or mental abuse or neglect
- history of substance abuse

Signs and symptoms

A patient with DDD may report feeling emotionally numb and detached from their entire being and body, as if they were a robot or were watching themselves from a distance or living in a dream. The patient may report that they feel as if "in a fog" and that their vision and/or hearing is distorted (APA, 2013). However, it is important to note that although a patient may feel and experience these sensations, they maintain a sense of what is real. For example, they may report that they feel as if they were a robot, but they know that they are not one (Morrison, 2014).

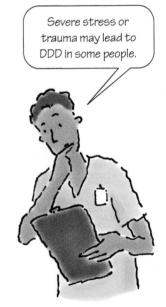

Severe stress or trauma may lead to DDD in some people.

Rumination and disconsolation

Other signs and symptoms may include:

- obsessive rumination
- depression
- anxiety
- fear of going insane
- disturbed sense of time
- slow recall
- physical concerns, such as dizziness
- impaired social and occupational functioning.

Diagnosis

The health care provider must rule out physical disorders, substance abuse, and other dissociative disorders. Psychological tests and special interviews may aid diagnosis. Standard tests include the DES-II and the Dissociative Disorders Interview Schedule, both of which can demonstrate the presence of dissociation. The Cambridge Depersonalization Scale is the most specific scale in the diagnosis of DDD (Sierra & Berrios, 2000).

Treatment

Even without treatment, many patients recover completely. Treatment is warranted, however, if the disorder is persistent, recurrent, or distressing.

Treatment measures include supportive psychotherapy and psychoeducation that give the patient information about the disorder, reduce associated guilt and stigma, and provide hope for the future. Cognitive-behavioral therapy (CBT) or dialectical behavior therapy (DBT) has been shown to be helpful (National Association on Mental Illness [NAMI], 2020). Mindfulness (Zerubavel & Messman-Moore, 2015) and eye movement desensitization and reprocessing (EMDR) (Shapiro, 2018) are also tools trained therapists are using to treat dissociative disorders.

Psychotherapy

If DDD is linked to a traumatic event, psychotherapy focuses on helping the patient recognize the event and the anxiety it has evoked. Then, the therapist teaches the patient to use reality-based coping strategies instead of detaching from the situation.

Pharmacologic therapy

In addition to psychotherapy, paroxetine and naloxone have been found to have some effect in controlling depersonalization symptoms, particularly when they co-occur with posttraumatic stress disorder (PTSD) or borderline personality disorder (Sutar & Sahu, 2019).

Nursing interventions

Nursing interventions that are appropriate for a patient with DDD include:

- Establish and maintain a therapeutic, nonjudgmental relationship.
- Encourage the patient to recognize that depersonalization is a defense mechanism used to deal with anxiety caused by a traumatic event.

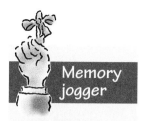

Memory jogger

ABCDES of depersonalization

Altered perceptions of self

Belief that one is observing oneself from outside the body

Characteristics of the body are perceived as altered

Detachment from the environment

Errors in the perceived sense of time

Sense of unreality

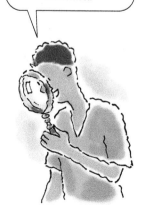

For treatment to succeed, all stressors linked to onset of the disorder must be identified.

- Encourage the patient to recognize and confront anxiety-producing experiences with appropriate behavioral techniques.
- Assist the patient in establishing supportive relationships.

Dissociative amnesia

The key feature of dissociative amnesia is an inability to recall important personal information that cannot be explained by ordinary forgetfulness. Commonly, the patient forgets basic autobiographical information, such as their name, people spoken to recently, and what was said, thought, experienced, or felt recently. It usually comes on suddenly but may be delayed for hours, days, or longer following a traumatic event. It may resolve quickly but sometimes becomes chronic (APA, 2013).

In most cases, an acute memory loss is triggered by a severe psychological stress. Recovery is usually complete and recurrence is rare, although the patient may be unable to recall certain life events. (See *Myths about memory lapses*.)

When dissociative amnesia is accompanied by sudden, unexpected travel away from one's home or workplace as well as the inability to recall one's past and confusion about one's personal identity (or assumption of a new identity), the term *dissociative amnesia with dissociative fugue* is used. The travel during a fugue may range from brief trips lasting hours or days to complex wandering for weeks or months. In some cases, the person travels thousands of miles (APA, 2013). (See *Memory jogger* for dissociative fugue.)

During the fugue state, the patient may appear normal and attract no attention. However, confusion about identity—or the return to original identity—may make the patient aware of the memory loss. At that time, distress can ensue.

A rough landing

Although the patient may be asymptomatic during a fugue, they may experience various symptoms when it ends—depression, discomfort, grief, shame, intense conflict, or even suicidal ideation or aggressive impulses. Failure to remember the events that took place during the fugue may cause confusion, or even terror.

Types of dissociative amnesia

Dissociative amnesia occurs in three main types (APA, 2018):

1. In *localized amnesia*, the most common type, the patient cannot remember a specific event or period of time. For example,

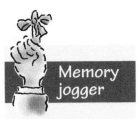

Memory jogger

The word **TRAIL** is your clue to ineffective coping in patients with dissociative amnesia with dissociative fugue.

TRavels or runs away to escape severe distress

Amnesia and anxiety are experienced

Identity changes are experienced

Low self-esteem may ensue when the memory returns

a patient may not be able to recall the moments when they were in the midst of a tornado.

2. In *selective amnesia*, the patient can recall some, but not all, of the events during a circumscribed time period. For instance, a soldier may be able to recall only some parts of a violent combat experience.

3. In *generalized amnesia*, the rarest type, the patient experiences prolonged loss of identity and life history.

Time warp

Most patients with dissociative amnesia are aware that they have "lost" some time. But a few have "amnesia for amnesia"—they realize they have lost time only after seeing evidence that they have done things they do not recall. Some patients are distressed over their amnesia; others are not distressed at all (APA, 2013).

Unlike other types of amnesia, dissociative amnesia does not result from an organic disorder (such as a stroke or dementia) (APA, 2013).

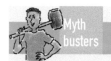

Myths about memory lapses

Myth: Memory lapses are a sign of psychosis.
Reality: Occasional, brief memory lapses are common—and normal—experiences. If these lapses recur often and cause impairment, they may reflect an injury or an underlying psychiatric or physical disorder.

Prevalence and onset

The prevalence of dissociative amnesia is believed to be about 1.8%, about twice as high for women than for men (Spiegel, 2019a). Most common in adolescents and young women, the disorder is also seen in young men after combat.

Unfilled memory voids

The prognosis depends mainly on life circumstances, particular stressors and conflicts associated with the amnesia, and the patient's overall psychological adjustment. (See *Patient safety and family strain.*) Although most patients recover, some never break through the barriers to reconstruct their missing past, and those patients usually remain impaired in both their relationships and vocations. Patients who experience amnesia with dissociative fugue are particularly at risk for poorer outcomes (APA, 2013; Spiegel, 2019a).

Causes

Dissociative amnesia is thought to result from severe stress associated with a traumatic experience, major life event, or severe internal conflict (APA, 2013).

Patient safety and family strain

During an episode of dissociative amnesia or fugue, the patient may pose a safety risk to themselves because of impaired memory and reduced awareness of their surroundings. Not only is the patient at high risk for falls and other injuries, but, if obviously confused, the patient is easy prey for con artists and criminals. Self-care may suffer as well.

Family strain

If the patient experiences frequent amnesia or fugue episodes, the family may feel helpless to cope with the patient's behavior. Family therapy is recommended to help family members recognize symptoms of recurrence.

Factors that may contribute to development of this disorder include:
- history of a traumatic event or repeated trauma
- history of physical, emotional, or sexual abuse, particularly in childhood
- mild traumatic brain injury.

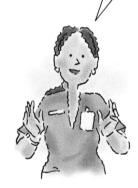

I am reluctant to show her as a nurse spinning around - we need our nurses to be competent and stable.

Signs and symptoms

During an amnesic episode, the patient may seem perplexed and disoriented, wandering aimlessly, especially if experiencing a fugue. The patient is unable to remember the event that precipitated the episode and usually does not even recognize the inability to recall information. The patient may have mild to severe social impairment.

Once the amnesic episode ends, the patient usually is not aware that there has been a memory disturbance. However, the patient may gradually recall some memories and may experience distress or symptoms of PTSD, which may lead to self-destructive or suicidal behaviors (APA, 2013).

Diagnosis

As with all psychiatric illnesses, the patient should undergo a thorough physical examination to rule out an organic cause for the symptoms. Blood and urine tests may be done to rule out drug use and other conditions. Electroencephalography (EEG) can exclude a seizure disorder and an MRI can detect structural abnormalities.

Diagnostic Toolbox

The patient should also undergo a psychiatric examination. Psychological tests help characterize the nature of the patient's dissociative experiences. These tests include the Diagnostic Drawing Series, DES, and Dissociative Disorders Interview Schedule (Bernstein & Putnam, 1986; Cohen, 1983; Ross et al., 1989).

The diagnosis of dissociative amnesia is confirmed if the patient meets the criteria in the *DSM-5* (APA, 2013). If dissociative amnesia occurs as a symptom of another psychiatric disorder, it is not diagnosed separately (APA).

Treatment

Sometimes, the amnesia resolves by itself, often suddenly with total recollection of memories (Morrison, 2014). If not, psychotherapy is used to help the patient recognize the traumatic event that triggered the amnesia and the anxiety it has produced. A supportive, trusting therapeutic relationship is essential to achieving this goal. An accepting environment may in itself enable the patient to gradually recover missing memories. The psychotherapist subsequently attempts to teach the patient reality-based coping strategies.

Recovery and clarification

Filling in the memory gaps can be useful in restoring the continuity of the patient's identity and sense of self. Once these gaps have been filled, treatment helps the patient clarify the trauma or conflicts and resolve the problems associated with the amnesic episode (Spiegel, 2019a).

Mission: Memory retrieval

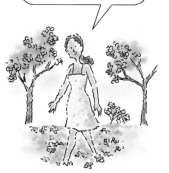

It's all coming back to me … I feel like my old self again.

When the need to recover memories is urgent, the patient may be questioned under hypnosis or in a drug-induced semi-hypnotic state, which may help the patient to relax enough to recall forgotten information. However, such memory retrieval techniques must be used cautiously because the circumstances that triggered the memory loss are likely to be highly distressing to the patient (van der Hart, 2019). This process should only be conducted by a trained therapist or health care provider.

Also, the validity of "recovered" memories is controversial, and external corroboration is required to validate their accuracy. (See *First do no harm*, page 218.)

First do no harm

Dissociative amnesia usually arises as a reaction to a trauma too overwhelming for the patient to integrate into waking consciousness. In other words, the patient has experienced something they want to forget.

Although you may encourage the patient to express feelings, do not try to elicit forgotten memories.

Only a mental health professional with special training and education in addressing unconscious memories should attempt to do this. The techniques used to elicit memories, such as hypnosis, guided imagery, and free association, carry certain risks and could prove harmful to the patient.

Pharmacologic therapy

Drugs used during treatment for dissociative amnesia may include short-acting barbiturates or benzodiazepines for anxiety (Spiegel, 2019a).

Nursing interventions

These nursing interventions are appropriate for a patient with dissociative amnesia:

- Establish a therapeutic, nonjudgmental relationship.
- Encourage the patient to verbalize feelings of distress.
- Help the patient to recognize that memory loss is a defense mechanism used to cope with anxiety and trauma.
- Help the patient deal with anxiety-producing experiences.
- Teach and assist the patient in using reality-based coping strategies when under stress rather than strategies that distort reality.
- If the patient is resolving a dissociative fugue state, monitor for signs of overt aggression toward self or others.

Dissociative identity disorder

DID is marked by two or more distinct identities or subpersonalities (or alters) that recurrently take control of the patient's consciousness and behavior. Each identity may exhibit unique behavior patterns, memories, and social relationships (APA, 2013). Patients with DID may exhibit symptoms frequently associated with other psychiatric illnesses including mood, personality, and somatic disorders and thus be misdiagnosed (Brand et al., 2016).

Differences are key

In some cases, the primary personality (identity) is radically different from the subpersonalities.

This personality may be strongly religious, or behave aggressively, or lack sexual inhibitions. They may have a different gender, sexual orientation, religion, or race than the primary personality—and may even differ in hand dominance, vocal qualities, intelligence level, language, and EEG readings (APA, 2013).

The primary personality may be unaware of the subpersonalities and may wonder about lost time and unexplained events. Some of the subpersonalities may interact with one another outside of the primary personality, creating their own inner world (Spiegel, 2019c).

About face!

The transition from one personality to another often is triggered by stress or a meaningful social or environmental cue. Although usually sudden (seconds to minutes), the transition can take hours or days. The switch from one personality to another may be accompanied by trancelike behavior, a change in posture, and/or rolling or blinking of the eyes (APA, 2013).

Prevalence and onset

It is estimated that up to 1% of adults have DID (Foote, 2018). Men are affected at a slightly higher rate (1.6%) than women (1.4%) (APA, 2013). However, there is growing research that shows that DID is underdiagnosed and, if not specifically addressed in treatment, goes unresolved (Brand et al., 2016).

It can get very complicated

DID may lead to severe social and occupational impairment, depending on the nature of the subpersonalities and their interrelationships. Often, one or more of the subpersonalities has an overlapping psychiatric disorder, such as generalized anxiety disorder, borderline personality disorder, or mood disorder. Suicide attempts, self-mutilation, externally directed violence, and psychoactive drug dependence may occur (APA, 2013).

Causes

No known single cause for DID exists, but many experts believe the disorder results primarily from trauma, extreme stress, or severe physical and sexual abuse—especially in childhood. Symptoms may become apparent at any age.

Survival through splitting

Some psychiatrists believe victims of severe trauma and abuse develop DID as a survival mechanism. A child exposed to overwhelming trauma may evolve multiple personalities to dissociate himself or herself from the traumatic situation. The dissociated contents then become linked with one of many possible influences that shape personality organization (APA, 2013).

Besides emotional, physical, or sexual abuse, factors that may contribute to DID include:

- genetic predisposition
- lack of nurturing experiences to assist in recovering from abuse
- removal of the original stressor
- combat or a traumatic event
- prison conditions (APA, 2013).

Signs and symptoms

Signs and symptoms of DID may include:

- lack of recall about personal past history that exceeds normal forgetfulness
- inability to recall how to perform past skills, such as how to read or use a computer
- confrontation with evidence of activity they do not recall or "awakening" during an activity they do not remember initiating
- hallucinations, particularly auditory and visual
- posttraumatic symptoms, such as flashbacks, nightmares, and an exaggerated startle response
- recurrent depression
- sexual dysfunction and difficulty forming intimate relationships
- sleep disorders
- eating disorders
- somatic pain disorders
- substance abuse
- guilt and shame
- self-mutilation
- suicidal tendencies or other self-harming behaviors, such as excessive risk taking; unprotected sex with multiple partners; self-neglect; or excessive drinking, smoking, or eating (APA, 2013).

Baffling vacillations

The patient's history may include unsuccessful psychiatric treatment, periods of amnesia, and disturbances in time perception. Family members and friends may describe incidents that the patient cannot recall as well as pronounced changes in the patient's facial presentation, voice, and behavior (Brand et al., 2016).

Diagnosis

Many patients with DID spend months or even years being examined before being diagnosed correctly. Common misdiagnoses include psychotic disorders, PTSD, substance abuse disorder, borderline personality disorder, and bipolar disorder (Brand et al., 2016). Standard tests for DID include the Minnesota Multiphasic Personality Inventory, Diagnostic Drawing Series, Dissociative Disorders Interview Schedule, and the SCID-D (Brand et al.).

Treatment

Treatment of DID is a long-term complex process that may take years to complete. The goal of therapy is to integrate all the patient's personalities and to help with understanding that the different presenting affects can be expressed within a single personality (APA, 2013; Brand et al., 2016).

Can't they all just get along?

Experts recommend a tristaged treatment approach. After first stabilizing the patient and decreasing the degree of dissociation, the therapist tries to identify the personality that remembers the trauma and enhance cooperation and co-consciousness among the subpersonalities, and ultimately merge them into one personality (Brand et al., 2013).

Unifying the parts

Although the therapist may address the different personalities separately, an increased connectedness is the measure of success (Brand et al., 2016). Whether disagreeable or congenial, all of the patient's personalities must be treated with equal respect and empathetic concern (Brand et al). (See *Promoting recovery from dissociative identity disorder*.)

Advice from the experts

Promoting recovery from dissociative identity disorder

Integrating the subpersonalities is the goal of therapy for a patient with DID. Certain actions by the therapist and caregivers can promote connectedness among the subpersonalities. It is important to remember:

- *Do not* encourage the patient to create additional subpersonalities.
- *Do not* suggest that the patient adopt names for unnamed subpersonalities.
- *Do not* encourage subpersonalities to function more autonomously.
- *Do not* encourage the patient to ignore certain subpersonalities.
- *Do not* exclude unlikable subpersonalities from therapy.

Respecting boundaries

Clearly delineating boundaries is also important in treating patients with DID. Many grew up in environments without clear boundaries or where personal boundaries were not always respected.

Family focus

Family and couples therapy may be helpful in reinforcing coping mechanisms for caregivers of a patient with DID (NAMI, 2020).

Hypnosis

Some therapists may use hypnosis for the purpose of:
- obtaining additional history
- identifying previously unrecognized identities
- inducing abreactions (Spiegel, 2019c). (See *Memory jogger* for ABREACTIONS.)

Tiffs over trances

The role of hypnosis in DID treatment is controversial. Patients and therapists may become overconfident in the accuracy of information arrived at during a hypnotic trance and traumatic experiences may be reexperienced (van der Hart, 2019). To reduce the risk that the patient will alter details of what is recalled during hypnosis, the therapist must minimize the use of leading questions.

Informed consent should be obtained before the use of hypnosis, and its benefits, risks, and limitations should be discussed (Hutchinson, 2015). The therapist should inform the patient that anything recalled while in a trance may not be admissible as evidence in legal actions (United States Department of Justice, 2020).

Pharmacologic interventions

Drugs used to treat DID include antidepressants, anxiolytics, mood stabilizers, and anticonvulsants. Psychopharmacology is used for management of the associated symptoms of depression, anxiety, and drug abuse, but these drugs do not treat the dissociation itself (Spiegel, 2019c).

Nursing interventions

These nursing interventions are appropriate for a patient with DID:
- Establish a trusting relationship with each subpersonality. If the patient has a history of abuse, be aware that it may cause difficulty trusting others.
- Promote interventions that help the patient identify each subpersonality, with the goal of integration.
- Encourage the patient to identify emotions that occur under stress.

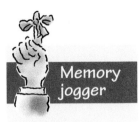

Memory jogger

ABREACTION refers to the purging of distressing memories or feelings. This term will help you remember key interventions for patients with DID.

Abuse is identified

Blend or integrate all the personalities into one personality

Recall the trauma in detail and process it

Encourage the patient to maintain a safe environment

Anxiety needs to be decreased

Conflict resolution is taught

Talk about the patient's feelings, especially guilt and shame

Inform the patient about the use of hypnosis to help mobilize memories

Orient the patient to surroundings as necessary

New coping strategies are developed

- Recognize even small gains that the patient makes.
- Teach the patient effective defense mechanisms and coping skills, including use of available social support systems.

Encourage patience

- Teach the importance of continuing with psychotherapy. Prepare the patient to expect prolonged therapy, with alternating successes and failures, and the possibility that one or more of the subpersonalities may resist treatment.
- Monitor the patient for violence directed at self or others.
- Monitor the patient for suicidal ideation and behavior as patients with DID are at high risk for suicidal behavior—over 70% have attempted suicide and multiple attempts are common (APA, 2013). Implement precautions as needed.

Quick quiz

1. Which events does the nurse identify that are possible causes of dissociative amnesia? *Select all that apply.*
    A. Being in a car accident
    B. Experiencing sexual assault
    C. Having a mild traumatic brain injury
    D. Witnessing a violent criminal act
    E. Living through a natural disaster

Answers: A, B, C, D, E. Experiencing or witnessing a traumatic event such as a car accident, sexual assault, violent crime, or natural disaster is a possible cause of dissociative amnesia. Having a mild traumatic brain injury has also been associated with development of dissociative amnesia.

2. Which assessment finding does the nurse anticipate in a patient with depersonalization disorder?
    A. Forgetting one's whereabouts
    B. Reports of feeling in a dreamlike state
    C. Identifying two or more distinct personalities
    D. Claiming to be an important historical figure

Answer: B. Depersonalization disorder is characterized by a sense of being in a dreamlike state or being a detached observer. Forgetting one's whereabouts is associated with dissociative amnesia. Identifying two or more distinct personalities is associated with DID. Claiming to be an important historical figure is reflective of a grandiose delusion.

3. The nurse is caring for a patient who reports having six different personalities. The nurse associates this assessment finding with
which disorder?
    A. Dissociative fugue
    B. Depersonalization disorder
    C. Dissociative amnesia
    D. DID

Answer: D. DID is the condition of identifying two or more distinct
personality states within the same person.

4. Which risk factor does the nurse identify that may contribute to
DID? *Select all that apply.*
    A. History of seizures.
    B. Emotional, physical, or sexual abuse.
    C. Genetic predisposition.
    D. Extreme stress and trauma.
    E. Cardiac structural anomalies.

Answers: B, C, D. A history of seizures and cardiac structural anomalies have not been linked to the development of DID. Abuse, genetic
predisposition, and extreme stress and trauma are all risk factors that
may contribute to DID.

5. Signs and symptoms of dissociative amnesia with dissociated
fugue are most pronounced:
    A. weeks before the fugue episode.
    B. during the fugue episode.
    C. after the fugue episode.
    D. moments before the onset of the fugue episode.

Answer: C. After a fugue, the patient may experience depression,
grief, shame, intense conflict, confusion, terror, or suicidal or
aggressive impulses. In contrast, a fugue in progress is rarely recognized. There are no short- or long-term warning signs of an impending fugue episode.

Scoring

☆☆☆ If you answered all five items correctly, unreal! You've integrated all
of the important aspects into your conscious mind.

☆☆ If you answered three or four items correctly, fantastic! It's all coming together for you nicely.

☆ If you answered fewer than three items correctly, don't despair! Just
thumb through the chapter again and try to fill in those memory
gaps.

Selected references

American Psychiatric Association. (2013). *Diagnostic and statistical manual of mental disorders* (5th ed.). Author.

American Psychiatric Association. (2018). *What are dissociative disorders?* https://www.psychiatry.org/patients-families/dissociative-disorders/what-are-dissociative-disorders

Bernstein, C., & Putnam, F. W. (1986). Development, reliability and validity of a dissociative scale. *Journal of Nervous and Mental Disease, 174,* 727–735.

Brand, B. L., McNary, S. W., Myrick, A. C., Classen, C. C., Lanius, R., Loewenstein, R. J., Pain, C., & Putnam, F. W. (2013). A longitudinal naturalistic study of patients with dissociative disorders treated by community clinicians. *Psychological Trauma: Theory, Research, Practice, and Policy, 5*(4), 301–308.

Brand, B. L., Sar, V., Stavropoulos, P., Krüger, C., Korzekwa, M., Martínez-Taboas, A., & Middleton, W. (2016). Separating fact from fiction: An empirical examination of six myths about dissociative identity disorder. *Harvard Review of Psychiatry, 24*(4), 257–270. http://doi.org/10.1097/HRP.0000000000000100

Carlson, E. B., & Putnam, F. W. (1993). An update on the dissociative experience scale. *Dissociation, 6*(1), 16–27.

Cohen, B. M. (1983). Diagnostic drawing series. In S. L. Brooke (Ed.), *Tools of the trade: A therapist's guide to art therapy assessments* (2nd ed., pp. 56–65). Charles C. Thomas.

Dell, P. (2006). The multidimensional inventory of dissociation (MID): A comprehensive measure of pathological dissociation. *Journal of Trauma & Dissociation, 7*(2), 77–106.

Foote, B. (2018). Dissociative identity disorder: Epidemiology, pathogenesis, clinical manifestations, course, assessment, and diagnosis. *UpToDate.* https://www.uptodate.com/contents/dissociative-identity-disorder-epidemiology-pathogenesis-clinical-manifestations-course-assessment-and-diagnosis

Foote, B., & Van Orden, K. (2018). Adapting dialectical behavior therapy for the treatment of dissociative identity disorder. *American Journal of Psychotherapy, 70*(4), 343–364. https://doi.org/10.1176/appi.psychotherapy.2016.70.4.343

Hutchinson, K. (2015). *Psychiatric-mental health nursing* (5th ed., pp. 253–257). Nursing Knowledge Center.

Morrison, J. (2014). *DSM-5 made easy: The clinician's guide to diagnosis.* The Guildford Press.

National Association on Mental Illness. (2020). *Dissociative disorders.* https://www.nami.org/Learn-More/Mental-Health-Conditions/Dissociative-Disorders/Treatment

Ross, C., Heber, S., Norton, G. R., Anderson, D., Anderson, G., & Barchet, P. (1989). The Dissociative Disorders Interview Schedule: A structured interview. *Dissociation, 2*(3), 69–189. https://www.empty-memories.nl/dis_89/Ross_structuredinterview.pdf

Shapiro, F. (2018). *Eye movement desensitization and reprocessing therapy: Basic principles, protocols and procedures* (3rd ed.). The Guildford Press.

Sierra, M. B., & Berrios, G. E. (2000). The Cambridge Depersonalization Scale: A new instrument for the measurement of depersonalization. *Psychiatry Research, 93*, 153–164.

Spiegel, D. (2019a). Dissociative amnesia. *Merck Manual Professional Version.* https://www.merckmanuals.com/professional/psychiatric-disorders/dissociative-disorders/dissociative-amnesia

Spiegel, D. (2019b). Depersonalization/derealization disorder. *Merck Manual Professional Version.* https://www.merckmanuals.com/professional/psychiatric-disorders/dissociative-disorders/depersonalization-derealization-disorder

Spiegel, D. (2019c). Dissociative identity disorder. *Merck Manual Professional Version.* https://www.merckmanuals.com/professional/psychiatric-disorders/dissociative-disorders/dissociative-identity-disorder

Sutar, R., & Sahu, S. (2019). Pharmacotherapy for dissociative disorders: A systematic review. *Psychiatry Research, 281*, 112529. https://doi.org/10.1016/j.psychres.2019.112529

United States Department of Justice. (2020). *Admissibility at trial.* https://www.justice.gov/jm/criminal-resource-manual-288-admissibility-trial

van der Hart, O. (2019). The value of hypnosis in the resolution of dissociation: Clinical lessons from World War I on the integration of traumatic memories. *Quaderni di Psicoterapia Cognitiva, 44*, 12–49. http://ojs.francoangeli.it/_ojs/index.php/qpcoa/article/view/8148/414

Zerubavel, N., & Messman-Moore, T. L. (2015). Staying present: Incorporating mindfulness into therapy for dissociation. *Mindfulness, 6*(2), 303–314. https://doi.org/10.1007/s12671-013-0261-3

Chapter 10

Somatic symptom and related disorders

Just the facts

In this chapter, you will learn:

♦ how stress can manifest in physical symptoms

♦ signs and symptoms of somatic symptom and related disorders

♦ nursing assessment and interventions for individuals with somatic symptom and related disorders.

A look at somatic symptom and related disorders

Somatic symptom and related disorders are a group of psychiatric conditions in which the individual has persistent somatic (physical) concerns associated with significant distress and impairment. This category is characterized by distressing somatic symptoms combined with abnormal thoughts, feelings, and behaviors in response to the somatic symptoms. The patient may have a diagnosed medical disorder or be experiencing symptoms that have not yet been medically explained. Because symptoms are physical in nature, somatic disorders are seen more frequently in medical primary care offices or consultation-liaison practices than in mental health settings. It is important to note that in this diagnostic category, these somatic symptoms cannot be attributed to substance misuse or another mental disorder. Instead, the symptoms are linked to psychological factors. Distress and preoccupation with the symptoms can lead to occupational, academic, social, and other impairments (American Psychiatric Association [APA], 2013).

This chapter discusses somatic symptom disorder, illness anxiety disorder, conversion disorder, factitious disorder (FD), and psychological factors affecting other medical conditions.

They're not faking it

Individuals with somatic disorders don't feign ("fake") their symptoms. Because they don't produce the symptoms intentionally or feel

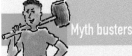
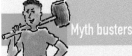

The scoop on somatic symptom and related disorder

Many people misunderstand the nature of somatic symptom and related disorders. To separate yourself from the masses, read on.

Myth: A patient with somatic symptom or a related disorder experience symptoms that are "only in their head."

Reality: Patients with somatic symptom or a related disorder experience symptoms that are very real to them. These symptoms cause a tangible degree of distress or impairment.

a sense of control over them, they may have trouble accepting that the symptoms have a psychological origin.

Converting stress into symptoms

Somatization is an informal term used to describe the presentation of patients who have medically unexplained symptoms that cause a level of distress or impairment (Levenson, 2020c). Individuals with somatic symptom and related disorders internalize anxiety, stress, and frustration. Instead of confronting these feelings directly, it is thought that they express them unconsciously through physical symptoms. (See *The scoop on somatic symptom disorder.*)

Not all in the head

It is important to remember that the patients experiencing symptoms of somatic symptom disorder or a related disorder are not told "it is all in your head." Failure to recognize somatization and manage it appropriately can lead to frustrating, costly, and potentially unnecessary tests and treatments, as well as more distress for the individual.

Some individuals will travel to numerous health care providers in search of a diagnosis and treatment, only to obtain minimal or no relief.

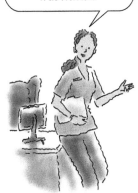

Individuals with somatic symptom and related disorders internalize anxiety, stress, and frustration.

Coexisting disorders

Other disorders such as depression or anxiety may coexist with somatic symptom or related disorders. Comorbidities often result in more severe disability and treatment resistance.

Some of the common combinations include the following:

- Individuals with somatic symptom disorder may also experience panic disorder.
- Somatic disorders that include persistent pain may exist alongside depression, increasing the risk for suicide.

Cultural and ethnic factors

Cultural norms and expectations can influence how people express physical discomfort; in certain cultures, it is normal for people to express pain outwardly, whereas in other cultures, suppression of emotions associated with pain is considered normal (Boyd, 2018). The relationships that exist between somatic symptoms and depression are very similar around the world and even between varied cultures within the same country (APA, 2013).

Causes

Although the pathogenesis of these disorders is not fully understood, researchers have identified several factors that appear to affect vulnerability to these disorders. Risk factors include (Levenson, 2020c):

- Female gender
- Fewer years of education
- Lower socioeconomic status
- Personal history of chronic childhood illnesses
- Family history of chronic illnesses
- Existing general medical or psychiatric conditions.

Developmental factors, a history of physical and sexual abuse, difficulties with self-expression, and cognitive and perceptual disorders accompanied by behavioral abnormalities have been identified as factors accompanying somatic symptom and related disorders (Levenson, 2020c). It is thought that an individual with one of these disorders experiences overwhelming stress without adequate coping skills to deal with the predisposing factors. Which individuals cope adequately or develop somatic disorders is thought to be influenced by personality factors, genetic determinants, and environmental factors such as availability or lack of social support.

Individuals who have predisposing factors and do not develop symptoms, or who develop symptoms but quickly recover and return to normal functioning, are referred to as being *resilient* (Smith et al., 2018).

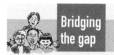
Bridging the gap

How culture influences treatment choices

An individual's cultural or ethnic background may influence their treatment preferences and choices. Some cultures may be unsupportive of alternative therapies, whereas those from other cultures may often use alternative techniques. Some patients who use complementary or alternative therapies are hesitant to disclose this if they fear that their health care provider would not support their choice of intervention.

Family stress

Among children and adolescents, family stress is thought to be a common cause of somatic disorders. For instance, a child may unconsciously reflect or imitate a parent's behavior—especially if the parent reaped considerable secondary gain (such as attention) from the symptoms. (See *Primary and secondary gain*.)

Learned responses

Behavioral theorists view psychosomatic symptoms as responses the patient has consciously learned and subsequently maintains because they bring some type of reward. The symptoms, for instance, may allow the patient to:
- gain concern or sympathy
- avoid unpleasant tasks
- explain or justify failures.

Heightened body sensations

Somatic symptom and related disorders may be linked to a heightened awareness of normal body sensations. Paired with a cognitive bias, this heightened awareness may predispose the patient to interpret any physical symptom as a sign of physical illness.

An individual who is worried about physical disease may focus attention on common variations in bodily sensations (hunger, pressure, stiffness, etc.) to the point that these sensations become disturbing and unpleasant. The patient thinks the sensations confirm the suspected presence of physical disease. The perception of such altered sensations exacerbates an individual's concerns, further increasing their anxiety and amplifying the sensations.

Increased autonomic arousal

Some patients with somatoform disorders may have heightened autonomic arousal. Such arousal may be associated with the effects of body chemicals that cause norepinephrine release, resulting in symptoms as tachycardia or gastric hypermotility. Heightened autonomic arousal also may contribute to pain and muscle tension associated with muscular hyperactivity, as in muscle tension headache.

Perceived need to be sick

Individuals with somatic disorders may seek the "sick" role because it provides relief from stressful interpersonal expectations and, in some cultures, offers attention and caring.

Primary and secondary gain

Primary gain refers to relief of the unconscious psychological conflict, wish, or need that is causing the physical symptom. As the individual's anxiety increases and threatens to emerge into consciousness, they unconsciously "convert" this to physical symptoms. This relieves the pressure to deal with the source of anxiety directly.

Secondary gain, in contrast, refers to the benefit, resources, or advantages that come from having the symptom—such as avoiding difficult situations, work, or getting emotional support or sympathy that the individual might not otherwise receive.

Somatic symptom disorder

Somatic symptom disorder is characterized by multiple and often vague physical concerns that are distressing to the patient and interfere with the patient's daily functioning. Excessive thoughts, feelings, and behaviors related to the somatic symptoms may preoccupy the patient. Typically, the symptoms are recurrent.

Concerns may involve any body system and often persist for years. They may begin or get worse after a job loss, death of a close relative or friend, or the occurrence of some other type of significant loss. Stress tends to intensify the symptoms.

An ongoing search for the cause

Patients with somatic symptom disorder may have impairments in occupational, social, and other functioning and may become extremely dependent in their relationships. Patients may seek medical care from multiple health care providers, which can lead to multiple treatment plans that overlap or leave gaps in care. Even when presented with contrary medical evidence, patients with somatic symptom disorder may still think the worst about their health and be convinced that a medical disorder is at the root of their symptoms (APA, 2013).

Commonly, the patient undergoes repeated medical evaluations, which (unlike the symptoms themselves) can be potentially damaging and debilitating. When the patient grows dissatisfied with the medical care he or she is receiving, the patient may seek another provider and may continue to ask for more tests and treatments. These patients may even undergo unnecessary surgery. However, unlike the individual with illness anxiety disorder, the patient with somatic symptom disorder isn't preoccupied with the belief in a specific disease that has caused their symptoms.

Prevalence and onset

Somatic symptom disorder affects an estimated 5% to 7% of the general population (Kurlansik & Maffei, 2016). It's 10 times more common in females (Kurlansik & Maffei, 2016; Yates et al, 2019). Symptoms begin before age 30, often in adolescence or early adulthood. Somatic symptom disorder is a chronic condition of fluctuating course. Evidence shows that some patients experience chronic symptoms of varying degrees over a period of time, yet 50% to 75% of patients demonstrate functional improvement (Kurlansik & Maffei, 2016). A strong patient-provider relationship is needed to achieve better patient outcomes, with the provider being supportive, yet firm in not testing or medicating without absolute cause (Kurlansik & Maffei, 2016).

Ever-present illness

Symptoms may be most obvious during early adulthood, but few patients are entirely asymptomatic or go more than 1 or 2 years without seeking medical attention.

Somatic symptom disorder often coexists with other psychiatric conditions, including major depression and anxiety. These patients are at an increased risk for substance misuse involving prescription medications, as well as drug interactions from prescriptions written by multiple providers.

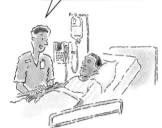

This is your third admission to the hospital this year, isn't it?

Causes

Somatic symptom disorder has no specific cause, but genetic, environmental, and psychological factors may contribute to its development (Levenson, 2020c).

Signs and symptoms

Signs and symptoms may involve any body system but commonly involve the gastrointestinal (GI), neurologic, cardiopulmonary, or reproductive systems. Nonspecific symptoms such as fatigue, dizziness, and syncope are often reported, as are pain symptoms (Levenson, 2020c). It is not uncommon for patients to report multiple symptoms at the same time. (See *Common assessment findings in somatic symptom disorder.*)

An important clue to this disorder is a history of multiple medical evaluations by different providers at different health care facilities (sometimes simultaneously)—without significant findings.

It is important to remember that in somatic symptom disorder, patients do not have voluntary control over their symptoms (Halter, 2018). The individual may report concerns and previous medical evaluations in an exaggerated fashion. The patient may have a complicated medical history in which many physical diagnoses have been considered. They may also seem quite knowledgeable about tests, procedures, and medical terminology.

Diagnosis

Diagnosis of somatic symptom disorder can be challenging. Because of the nature of this condition, health care providers must rule out

Common assessment findings in somatic symptom disorder

Signs and symptoms of somatic symptom disorder may mimic actual disorders and are just as real to the individual as the physical disorders that can cause them. They often involve a few key body systems (Levenson, 2020c).

Cardiopulmonary symptoms
- Chest pain
- Dizziness
- Palpitations
- Shortness of breath (without exertion)

GI signs and symptoms
- Abdominal pain (excluding menstruation)
- Diarrhea
- Flatulence
- Intolerance to foods
- Nausea and vomiting (excluding motion sickness)

Pain
- In extremities
- In the back
- During urination

Pseudoneurologic signs and symptoms
- Amnesia
- Blindness
- Difficulty walking, paralysis, or weakness
- Double or blurred vision
- Dysphagia
- Dysuria or urinary retention
- Fainting or loss of consciousness

- Loss of voice or hearing
- Seizures

Reproductive or sexual signs and symptoms
- Burning sensation in sexual organs or rectum (except during intercourse)
- Dyspareunia or lack of pleasure during sex
- Impotence
- Sexual indifference
- Excessive menstrual bleeding or irregular menses

physical origins for the symptoms. The patient should undergo a physical examination and appropriate diagnostic testing to rule out physical conditions that may produce their reported symptoms. There is no specific diagnostic test that reveals the disorder; however, the Patient Health Questionnaire-15 and the Somatic Symptom Scale-8 screening tools can be helpful in substantiating a diagnosis.

A psychological evaluation should be done to rule out related psychiatric disorders, such as major depressive disorder, schizophrenia, or illness anxiety disorder.

Ultimately, the diagnosis is confirmed if the patient meets the criteria in the *Diagnostic and Statistical Manual of Mental Disorders*, 5th Edition (*DSM-5*), which center on persistent physical symptoms that interrupt daily life and function (APA, 2013). The manner in which the diagnosis is explained by the health care provider is very important to avoid more distress and embarrassment.

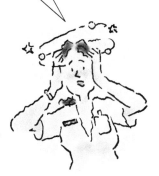

What a complicated medical history! It's typical for a patient with somatic symptom disorder.

Treatment

Somatic symptom disorder is challenging to manage (Boyd, 2018). The patient may not acknowledge any psychological aspect of the symptoms or be willing to consider psychiatric treatment.

The goal is control

The goal of treatment is to help the patient learn to control and cope with symptoms rather than eliminate them completely (Levenson, 2020d). Telling the patient that symptoms are imaginary won't help. It is very important to develop a relationship and trusting therapeutic rapport with the patient and to validate feelings while also presenting factual information and supportive care. For example, as the nurse, you may say, "You do not have a serious illness, but I will continue to provide care to help ease your symptoms."

A single gatekeeper and consistent team

Management also focuses on preventing unnecessary medical and surgical interventions and turning the patient's attention away from the symptoms. Ideally, an individual with a somatic disorder should develop a long-term relationship with a single, trusted primary health care provider. This helps guard against unnecessary tests, treatments, and surgeries. It is best when the primary health care provider works in conjunction with a consistent, supportive team to provide interprofessional care. The key to success is communication between the provider, team, and patient as this helps to create consistency and decreases the opportunity for unnecessary medical intervention (Halter, 2018). The interprofessional team should work together to support healthy and adaptive behaviors and encourage the patient to move beyond the somatization and work toward effective management of life.

Pharmacologic treatment

There is unclear evidence regarding the use of medications in the treatment of somatic symptom disorder. If the patient has a coexisting depressive or anxiety disorder, antidepressant drugs, such as selective serotonin reuptake inhibitors (SSRIs), may ease preoccupation with symptoms. Short-term antianxiety medication may also be used, although only in extreme circumstances and with careful monitoring due to the potential for misuse of these types of drugs. The goal of pharmaceutical treatment by the health care provider is to only treat what is absolutely necessary and to taper and discontinue any unnecessary medication (Levenson, 2020d).

Nursing interventions

These nursing interventions may be appropriate for a patient with somatic symptom disorder.

- Acknowledge the individual's symptoms and support efforts to function and cope despite distress. Don't tell the patient that the symptoms are imaginary—but do inform them of diagnostic test results and their implications.

- Encourage the patient to keep a symptom journal. This validates what the patient is feeling. Have the patient bring the journal with them to the next appointment and look for symptomatic patterns. This is helpful in educating the patient and also increases feelings of control over their symptoms (Boyd, 2018).

Strength in positive statements

- Emphasize the patient's strengths. For example, say "It's good that you can still work even though you're in pain. That is an admirable accomplishment."
- Help the patient make the connection of the link between stressful events and the onset of physical symptoms.
- Keep in mind that your goal, as the nurse, is to help the individual find ways to manage symptoms, not eliminate them.
- Because these patients seek medical care frequently, they often associate health care providers as their support network versus looking to develop healthy relationships with family and friends. Work to establish a trusting therapeutic rapport while fostering their independence by helping the patient strengthen social relationships (Boyd, 2018).

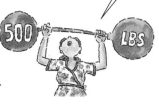

Emphasize the individual's strengths and point out accomplishments.

Attitude assessment

Assess your own feelings and attitudes periodically. If you think you've developed a nontherapeutic attitude, acknowledge your feelings honestly. Be sure that your body language does not display frustration or anger toward the patient. It is important to remember that the patient really does believe that what he or she is feeling is real even though there is no physical basis for the symptoms. Caring for these patients can be challenging for the nurse. Care conferences (team or unit-based meetings) are an important way to keep focused on providing the best possible care for the patient as part of the interprofessional team.

Patient's role

The patient must be encouraged to take an active role in treatment and be willing to take responsibility for moving forward with the treatment plan (such as by keeping a diary of symptoms and activities). Also, he or she should be encouraged to attend physical therapy or get regular exercise because self-initiated physical activity fosters responsibility and a sense of control. Periodic conferences should be scheduled with the patient (and the family, if the patient agrees) to provide a forum for communication and education. Patients with this disorder often find comfort in having a regularly scheduled appointment with their health care provider, as this may decrease the number of "urgent" visits related to somatic symptomology.

Therapeutic approaches

Cognitive-behavioral therapy (CBT) is one of many therapeutic approaches that can be used in patients with somatic symptom disorder (Lieftink et al., 2018; Newby et al., 2018). The goal is better adaptation and coping mechanisms (Henningsen, 2018).

Family therapy
Family therapy may be recommended for children or adolescents with somatic disorders. If the caregivers seem to use the child to divert attention from other difficulties, or use the child's symptoms as means to obtain attention for themselves, remain alert. This type of disorder is called *factitious disorder imposed on another* (see *Facts about factitious disorders* later in this chapter) and is a serious mental illness and a form of child abuse; nurses are accountable to report cases of suspected abuse to authorities.

Illness anxiety disorder

Illness anxiety disorder is marked by the persistent conviction that one has or is likely to get a serious disease, despite medical evidence and reassurance to the contrary. There is a very high level of anxiety about health status even if significant symptoms are not present. This individual focuses on the fear of having or developing a serious physical illness as opposed to the individual with somatic symptom disorder who focuses on the symptoms. For example, an individual with illness anxiety disorder who is fearful of developing breast cancer may often check breasts for lumps (often multiple times daily, as opposed to the normal once-monthly self-examination). This same individual may request or insist upon frequent diagnostic testing (e.g., blood tests, mammograms) when no clinical signs or risk factors exist that require this volume of testing.

Illness anxiety disorder may lead to physical illness

A long history of previously unfounded health concerns may contribute to the health care provider overlooking a serious organic disease. The individual is also at risk for complications from multiple evaluations, tests, and invasive procedures.

Prevalence and onset
The prevalence of illness anxiety disorder is estimated at up to 13% within the general population (Scarella et al., 2019). Illness anxiety disorder affects as many men as women (Levenson, 2020a). Onset of

illness anxiety disorder is unknown, but appears to be more common in individuals between the ages of 35 and 64 (Levenson, 2020a).

Illness anxiety disorder is considered a chronic and relapsing condition (APA, 2013). Flare-ups often follow stressful events and the specific feared illness may vary. It is relevant to note that some cases of illness anxiety disorder are transient and are associated with more medical comorbidity versus psychological morbidity (APA, 2013). In other words, for some people, the disorder is less severe and does not last for a long period of time.

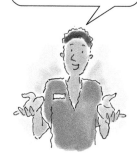

A patient with illness anxiety disorder often worries about developing a specific medical disorder.

Causes

The exact cause of illness anxiety disorder isn't known. There are numerous potential causative factors discussed.

Just like parents

Psychological factors are thought to play a role in the development of this disorder. For instance, children may report physical symptoms that resemble those of other family members.

Needing care

In adults, illness anxiety disorder may reflect a wish to be taken care of by someone else. The condition enables the patient to take on a dependent sick role while another person (or persons) tends to their needs.

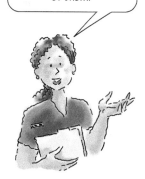

An adult patient with illness anxiety disorder may wish for someone to take care of them.

Contributing factors

Factors that may contribute to illness anxiety disorder include (Levenson, 2020a):

- family member or friend with a serious illness
- reading about a celebrity's illness
- a history of serious illness.

In older adults, illness anxiety disorder may be associated with depression, grief, or loneliness. (Refer to *Advice from the experts* on page 238.)

Signs and symptoms

Signs and symptoms of illness anxiety disorder range from specific to general concerns. Usually, the patient reports multiple concerns over a minimum of 6 months; the focus of illness may vary over that period of time (APA, 2013). The individual may have excessive contact with health care providers (termed as the "care-seeking type") or totally avoid contact with such (termed as "care-avoidant type") (APA, 2013).

Assessing older adults for illness anxiety or somatic symptom disorders

Older adults may perceive themselves to be in poor health (or at risk for poor health) even if they have no significant physical impairments. Their tendency to present with somatic concerns can pose a challenge to assessment and management.

As a first step, the individual should undergo a comprehensive medical evaluation (and laboratory tests, as needed) to check for a physical basis for concerns. Cognitive and psychiatric examinations may be warranted, too.

Essential assessment data

When assessing an older adult, always gather a complete history. Be sure to assess:
- past level of functioning
- extent of current ability
- presence of any cognitive deficits
- signs of emotional distress.

Also assess the patient's psychosocial status, including:
- living situation
- social supports
- role within the family
- key support persons outside the family.

To verify the individual's information, obtain a collaborative history from family members, if possible.

Family stress and abuse

Be aware that the family may respond to the patient's somatic symptoms by giving the patient more time and attention. In some cases, however, family members become angry and frustrated as conflicts arise and escalate. The individual may even suffer neglect and abuse. If you suspect this is happening, make sure to report this to the proper authorities.

Multiple sources and details

Patients with illness anxiety disorder often focus on something specific at any given time, although the focus may change from visit to visit. Examples of focus include (Levenson, 2020a):
- A particular diagnosis (e.g., cancer)
- A specific bodily function (e.g., bowel movements)
- A normal variation in the function of a body part (e.g., the heart)
- Vague somatic sensations (e.g., "tired lungs")

Typically, the individual describes the symptom's location, quality, and duration in specific detail. Yet, these symptoms rarely follow a recognizable pattern of organic dysfunction and usually aren't associated with abnormal physical findings.

Don't confuse me with the facts

Examination and reassurance by a health care provider don't relieve the patient's concerns. Instead, the patient may report that the provider has failed to find the real cause of the disorder.

Diagnosis

Just like somatic symptom disorder, diagnosis of illness anxiety disorder is challenging. Patient symptoms change frequently and are often associated with normal bodily functioning (such as the patient's report of abdominal pain, which is diagnosed to come from flatulence). A complete history, with an emphasis on current psychological stressors, is helpful. Tests to rule out underlying organic disease may be used, although invasive procedures should be minimized. Typically, test results are inconsistent with the reported concerns and physical findings.

Let's make it official

Although history and physical findings may suggest illness anxiety disorder, the diagnosis is official only if the patient meets the criteria in the *DSM-5* as determined by the health care provider. There is a persistent preoccupation over a period of at least 6 months of having or acquiring a serious disease without symptoms being present (APA, 2013).

Breaking the not-so-awful news

After the medical evaluation is complete, the individual should be told by the health care provider that he or she doesn't have a serious disease, and that continued follow-up will be designed to manage symptoms. Linking the diagnosis to psychological stressors also can be therapeutic. Although providing this diagnosis may not make symptoms disappear, it may ease some of the anxiety.

Treatment

The goal of treatment is to help the individual improve coping. Appropriate teaching and a supportive therapeutic relationship with a single competent, trusted health care professional are crucial.

Follow-up care

Regular outpatient follow-up care can help the patient deal with symptoms.

Psychotherapy

Most patients with illness anxiety disorder don't acknowledge any psychological influence on their symptoms and resist psychiatric treatment. However, a patient who's willing to try psychotherapy may be treated individually, in a group, or as part of a family.

The first line of treatment for illness anxiety disorder is CBT (Levenson, 2020b). Mindfulness-based cognitive therapy, acceptance and commitment therapy, or psychoeducation can also be considered if CBT is ineffective (Levenson, 2020b).

Pharmacologic therapy

Although no drug is specifically approved for illness anxiety disorder, certain medications may be prescribed to help patients manage symptoms such as SSRIs or serotonin-norepinephrine reuptake inhibitors (SNRIs) (Levenson, 2020b).

Medication can be especially helpful for patients with overlapping psychiatric conditions, such as depression or other anxiety disorders.

Nursing interventions

Because there is a close relationship between somatic symptom disorder and illness anxiety disorder, the nursing care often overlaps. In addition to the nursing interventions discussed on page 235 for somatic symptom disorder, these nursing interventions may also be appropriate for a patient with illness anxiety disorder:

- Provide teaching about illness anxiety disorder in a nonjudgmental, therapeutic manner.
- Help the individual expand coping skills.
- Assess the patient's level of knowledge about the effects of emotions and stress on physiologic functioning.
- Encourage the patient to express feelings to deter emotional repression, which can have physical consequences.

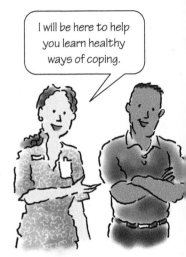

I will be here to help you learn healthy ways of coping.

Relaxation techniques

If your patient has symptoms related to stress or anxiety, relaxation techniques may help. Simple relaxation techniques include deep breathing, in which the patient takes a series of slow, deep breaths and releases each breath slowly. Encourage the patient to be deliberately mindful of the mechanics of breathing, which diverts attention from other physical symptoms that the patient may be focused upon.

To teach your patient how to perform deep breathing, first instruct them to sit in a comfortable position with their eyes closed. Next, tell the patient to focus on a peaceful sound or image, and then breathe in through their nose to a count of 4. Have the patient hold their breath for a count of 2. Then instruct them to breathe out through their mouth for a count of 6. The patient should repeat this cycle for 30 seconds to 5 minutes.

Change the subject

- Respond to the individual's symptoms objectively to reduce secondary gain that the patient may get from talking about them.
- Create a supportive relationship that helps the patient feel cared for and understood.
- Keep in mind that the patient with illness anxiety disorder experiences real distress. Don't deny their symptoms or challenge behavior. Instead, help the patient find new ways to deal with stress other than focusing on physical symptoms.

Remain objective

Recognize that the patient may never be symptom-free. Stay objective and professional with the patient and do not demonstrate frustration or anger. Such behavior can drive the patient away to yet another unnecessary medical evaluation.

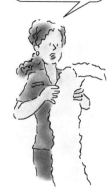

Yikes! This patient's history is long!

Conversion disorder

Conversion disorder, also referred to as *functional neurologic symptom disorder*, is marked by the loss of, or change in, voluntary motor or sensory functioning (e.g., sudden blindness or paralysis) that suggests a physical illness but has no demonstrable physiologic basis. The symptom likely has a psychological basis, although it may not be readily identifiable.

The conversion symptom itself isn't life-threatening and usually has a short duration. However, it's clinically significant and distressing enough to disrupt social, occupational, or other important areas of functioning.

Involuntary response

The symptom isn't under the individual's voluntary control. The patient with conversion disorder doesn't feign or intentionally produce the symptoms, although they may have the unconscious motives of primary or secondary gain. (See *Facts about factitious disorders*, page 242.)

Complications and consequences

Conversion symptoms can severely impede the individual's normal activities. In fact, the severity of the symptoms are comparable to what people who have the actual condition experience (APA, 2013).

Facts about factitious disorders

FDs are conditions in which a patient deliberately produces or exaggerates symptoms of a physical or psychiatric illness to assume the role of a sick person. These disorders aren't a form of malingering (pretending illness for a clear benefit, such as financial gain). Instead, the patient has a deep-seated need to be seen as ill or injured.

Patients may simply report symptoms or use other methods such as contaminating urine samples with blood, or taking hallucinogens, to create symptoms.

There are two types of FD. The first type is *factitious disorder imposed on self*. (This diagnosis was previously referred to as *Munchausen syndrome*.) In this form of the disorder, the individual falsifies physical or psychological symptoms or induces illness on themselves. The second type is *factitious disorder imposed on another*. (This diagnosis was previously referred to as *Munchausen syndrome by proxy*.) In this form of the disorder, an individual falsifies symptoms or induces illness upon another person (a victim). The key element of both is deception.

Factitious disorder imposed on self

In FD imposed on self, the individual convincingly presents with intentionally feigned physical symptoms. These symptoms may be:
- fabricated (e.g., acute abdominal pain without underlying disease)
- self-inflicted (e.g., deliberately infecting an open wound)
- an exacerbation or exaggeration of a preexisting disorder (e.g., taking penicillin despite a known allergy to it)
- a combination of the characteristics above.

Some patients with this type of FD go so far as to convince health care providers of their disorder, which can lead to repeated major surgeries.

History lessons

The patient with an FD may have a history of:
- multiple admissions to various hospitals, typically across a wide geographic area
- extensive knowledge of medical terminology
- pathologic fabrication
- shifting concerns, signs, and symptoms
- poor interpersonal relationships
- refusal of psychiatric examination
- psychoactive substance or analgesic use
- eagerness to undergo unnecessary procedures, even if high risk or painful in nature
- evidence of previous treatments, such as surgery
- discharge against medical advice to avoid detection.

Factitious disorder imposed on another

In this type, the same patterns of behavior or symptomatology may be present but in the caregiver versus the patient. The illness is being imposed on another (the victim) by the person with the disorder.

The individual (typically, a parent) intentionally produces or causes a physical illness or condition in another person (most often a child) through such actions as:
- falsifying the child's medical history
- tampering with laboratory tests to make the child appear sick
- injecting toxic substances into the child
- tampering with treatments (for instance, intravenous or ventilator settings)
- biting or mutilating the child.

This diagnosis is assigned to the caregiver, not the victim. The victim may be assigned a diagnosis of abuse, if assessed as such (APA, 2013).

Prevalence

This disorder is not usually diagnosed in primary care but rather in the secondary care environment. It is seen in up to 20% of patients in neurologic and psychiatric settings (Feinstein, 2018). Conversion disorder was once thought to affect more females than males; however, current evidence shows that certain symptoms are more prevalent in males, and others are more prevalent in females (Stone & Sharpe, 2019). Very few studies are available to establish a known age of onset, although it is extremely rare to find a documented case of conversion disorder in patients under 10 years old.

Causes

Conversion disorder is not fully understood, yet is thought to have biological and psychosocial factors that influence the course of the disorder (Stone & Sharpe, 2019).

Biological factors
There may be a connection between neurobiological changes in the brains of those with conversion disorder. Neuroimaging of patients with conversion disorder has shown some evidence of altered brain structure (compared to brain structure of individuals without conversion disorder). Findings include reduced thalamic volume and increased cortical thickness, although these have not been correlated by research as foundational to the development of the disorder (Stone & Sharpe, 2019).

Psychosocial factors
A history of trauma, interpersonal conflicts, and stressors has been connected to conversion disorder, as has a history of childhood sexual abuse. However, these factors are present in many physical and psychiatric conditions, so their association with conversion order is not unique (Stone & Sharpe, 2019). Having a history of preexisting psychiatric diagnoses such as depression, anxiety, or personality disorder increases risk factors for conversion disorder, especially when the patient then experiences a neurologic physical concern (Stone & Sharpe, 2019). It is also thought that conversion disorder may be a response to a life stressor that is relieved by the physical symptomology, but would otherwise be present if the disorder resolved (Stone & Sharpe, 2019).

Signs and symptoms

The patient's history may reveal the sudden onset of a single, debilitating sign or symptom that prevents normal function of the affected body part, such as weakness, paralysis, or sensation loss.

Other common conversion symptoms include:
- pseudoseizures (seizure-like attacks that are thought to be psychogenically produced)

- loss or impairment of a sense, such as vision (blindness or double vision), hearing (deafness), or touch
- aphonia (inability to use the voice) or slurring of speech
- dysphagia (difficulty swallowing)
- impaired balance or coordination
- weakness or paralysis
- urinary retention.

The patient may report that the symptom began after a traumatic event.

La belle indifférence

Some individuals with conversion disorder may not show concern over the symptoms or their functional limitations (van Meerkerk-Aanen et al., 2017). Called *la belle indifférence* (French for "the beautiful indifference"), this apathy is associated with conversion disorder but should not be used as an isolated indicator of the disorder (APA, 2013).

Things just don't add up

Conversion symptoms rarely conform fully to the known anatomic and physiologic mechanisms underlying a true physical disorder. Here are three examples:

1. Tendon reflexes may be normal in a "paralyzed" body part.
2. Reported loss of function fails to follow anatomic patterns of innervation.
3. Normal pupillary responses and evoked potentials are present in an individual who reports blindness.

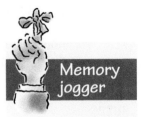

Memory jogger

The word **convert** is your clue to what happens in conversion disorder. Convert means to change from one form or function to another. It is hypothesized that patients with conversion disorder may unknowingly convert stress into physical symptoms.

Diagnosis

The diagnosis of conversion disorder is considered only after extensive physical examination and laboratory tests fail to reveal a physical disorder that explains the symptoms. Nonetheless, early consideration of the disorder may avoid tests that increase patient costs and risks, and that may reinforce the patient's symptoms.

Process of elimination

Depending on the individual's symptoms, he or she may undergo a neurologic evaluation to rule out physical illnesses that affect sensory function (e.g., blindness) or voluntary motor function (such as paralysis or the inability to walk or stand). Diseases with a vague early symptomology (such as multiple sclerosis or systemic lupus erythematosus) must also be ruled out.

Laboratory tests can identify such conditions that would negate a diagnosis of conversion disorder, such as:

- hypoglycemia or hyperglycemia
- electrolyte disturbances
- renal failure
- systemic infection
- toxins
- effects of prescribed, over-the-counter, or illicit drugs.

Scans, X-rays, and punctures

Diagnostic studies may be ordered to rule out medical conditions, such as:

- computed tomography or magnetic resonance imaging scans to exclude a space-occupying lesion in the brain or spinal cord
- chest X-ray to rule out neoplasms
- lumbar puncture for spinal fluid analysis, which can rule out infection and other causes of neurologic symptoms
- electroencephalogram to help distinguish pseudoseizures from true seizures.

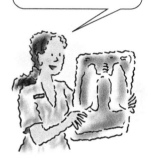

A chest X-ray may be ordered to rule out neoplasms in an individual with possible conversion disorder.

Inconsistency's the key

In conversion disorder, physical and diagnostic findings are inconsistent with the patient's reports and symptoms. The diagnosis is confirmed if the individual fulfills the diagnostic criteria listed in the *DSM-5* regarding having symptoms of altered motor or sensory function that is not explained by a medical or psychiatric condition (APA, 2013). The diagnosis can be further specified as acute or persistent and with or without a psychological stressor.

Treatment

A trusting, therapeutic relationship between the health care provider and patient is essential. In many cases, receiving education that the symptom doesn't indicate a serious underlying disorder can be reassuring (Stone & Sharpe, 2019). Therefore, education is the first line of treatment.

The second line of treatment, specifically for patients with motor conversion symptoms, is physical therapy (Stone & Sharpe, 2019). CBT should also be considered to help the patient reframe distorted thoughts (Stone & Sharpe, 2019).

Third-line treatment, used for patients who do not respond to first- or second-line treatment, can include pharmacotherapy (such as antidepressants), hypnosis, inpatient therapy, group therapy, and/or family therapy (Stone & Sharpe, 2019).

Nursing interventions

These nursing interventions may be appropriate for a patient with conversion disorder.

- Establish a supportive relationship that communicates acceptance of the individual but keeps the focus away from the symptoms. Doing this helps the patient learn to recognize and express underlying anxiety versus the symptomatic manifestation.
- Don't force the individual to talk, but convey a caring attitude that encourages them to share feelings.
- Encourage the patient to seek psychiatric care if they are not already receiving it.

Identify emotional links

- Help the individual identify any emotional conflicts that preceded symptom onset to help clarify the link between the conflict and the symptom.
- Do not imply that the symptoms are all in the patient's head.
- Help the individual increase coping ability, which can reduce anxiety and enhance self-esteem.
- Use measures to maintain the integrity of the affected body system or part. For instance, regularly exercise a "paralyzed" limb to prevent muscle wasting and contractures. Frequently change the position of a patient who is bedridden to prevent pressure injuries.

Ditch the insistence

- Don't insist that the individual use the affected body part or body system. This may frustrate the patient, which can impede a therapeutic relationship.
- Ensure adequate nutrition even if the individual reports GI distress.
- Promote social interaction to decrease the individual's self-involvement.

Call for a casting change

- Identify constructive coping mechanisms to encourage the individual to use practical coping skills.
- Include the family in the patient's care, if the patient agrees. Family therapy can help them understand if they are contributing to the patient's perceived stress; they are also essential in providing support and helping the patient regain normal function.

Prognosis

Although prognosis for individuals with conversion disorder has historically been poor, there are factors that are associated with a more favorable outcome. These include (Stone & Sharpe, 2019):

- Early diagnosis and intervention
- Good response to initial treatment plan
- Favorable therapeutic relationship with the health care provider.

Quick quiz

1. How does the nurse document the manifestation of physical symptoms caused by psychological distress?
    A. Somatization.
    B. Pain disorder.
    C. Conversion disorder.
    D. Psychosomatic disorder.

Answer: A. Somatization occurs when a psychological state causes or contributes to the development of physical symptoms.

2. The nurse is caring for a patient who has been diagnosed with somatic symptom disorder. What teaching about this condition will the nurse provide?
    A. "Your symptoms are all inside your head."
    B. "Regular visits with a counselor can be helpful."
    C. "Certain medications will cure this type of condition."
    D. "There is no chance you will recover from this disorder."

Answer: B. Counseling can be beneficial for patients with somatic symptom disorder. This gives patients an opportunity to explore the root cause of symptoms and learn to manage themselves more effectively. Symptoms associated with somatic symptom disorder are not inside a patient's head; they truly experience distress related to their symptoms. Medications can be used to treat symptoms, but they do not cure somatic symptom disorder. Evidence shows that many patients with this disorder do improve with adherence to therapy and treatment.

3. The nurse is caring for a patient whose therapist has the patient physically say the word "stop" when a negative thought enters the patient's mind. How will the nurse document this technique associated with cognitive-behavioral therapy (CBT)?
    A. Thought stopping.
    B. Aversion therapy.
    C. Implosion therapy.
    D. Response prevention.

Answer: A. CBT uses techniques such as thought stopping and thought reframing to assist with changes in thoughts and behaviors.

4. The nurse is caring for a patient who frequently misinterprets bodily sensations or symptoms. Which disorder does the nurse anticipate?
    A. Malingering.
    B. Somatization.
    C. Conversion disorder.
    D. Illness anxiety disorder.

Answer: D. A patient with illness anxiety disorder misinterprets the severity and significance of bodily sensations or symptoms as indications of illness.

Scoring

☆☆☆   If you answered all four items correctly, kudos! You've obviously converted all the information in this chapter to your brain!

☆☆   If you answered three items correctly, nice job! There's very little missing about your understanding of somatoform disorders.

☆   If you answered two or fewer items correctly, don't convert your disappointment into symptoms. Just flood yourself with the concepts in this chapter, and then give it another try.

Selected references

American Psychiatric Association. (2013). *Diagnostic and statistical manual of mental disorders* (5th ed.). Author.

Boyd, M. (2018). *Psychiatric nursing: Contemporary practice* (6th ed.). Lippincott Williams & Wilkins.

Feinstein, A. (2018). Conversion disorder. *Behavioral Neurology and Psychiatry, 24*(3), 861–872. http://doi.org/10.1212/CON.0000000000000601

Gierk, B., Kohlmann, S., Kroenke, K., Spangenberg, L., Zenger, M., Brähler, E., & Löwe, B. (2014). The Somatic Symptom Scale-8 (SSS-8): A brief measure of somatic symptom burden. *JAMA Internal Medicine, 174*(3), 400.

Halter, M. (2018). *Varicolis' foundation of psychiatric mental health nursing: A clinical approach* (8th ed.). Elsevier.

Henningsen, P. (2018). Somatic symptom disorder and illness anxiety disorder. In J. Levenson (Ed.), *Textbook of psychosomatic medicine and consultation-liaison psychiatry* (p. 305). American Psychiatric Association Publishing.

Kroenke, K., Spitzer, R., & Williams, J. (2002). The PHQ-15: Validity of a new measure for evaluating the severity of somatic symptoms. *Psychosomatic Medicine, 64*(2), 266.

Kurlansik, S. L., & Maffei, M. S. (2016). Somatic symptom disorder. *American Family Physician, 93*(1), 49–54.

Levenson, J. (2020a). Illness anxiety disorder: Epidemiology, clinical presentation, assessment and diagnosis. *UpToDate.* https://www.uptodate.com/contents/illness-anxiety-disorder-epidemiology-clinical-presentation-assessment-and-diagnosis

Levenson, J. (2020b). Illness anxiety disorder: Treatment and prognosis. *UpToDate.* https://www.uptodate.com/contents/illness-anxiety-disorder-treatment-and-prognosis

Levenson, J. (2020c). Somatic symptom disorder: Epidemiology and clinical presentation. *UpToDate.* https://www.uptodate.com/contents/somatic-symptom-disorder-epidemiology-and-clinical-presentation/print

Levenson, J. (2020d). Somatic symptom disorder: Treatment. *UpToDate.* https://www.uptodate.com/contents/somatic-symptom-disorder-treatment

Lieftink, S. E., Diener, M. J., van Broeckhuysen, S. A. M., & Geenen, R. (2018). Predictors of response to psychological treatment in somatoform disorder and somatic symptom disorder: A meta-analysis. *Journal of Psychosomatic Research, 109*, 116.

Newby, J. M., Smith, J., Uppal, S., Mason, E., Mahoney, A. E., & Andrews, G. (2018). Internet-based cognitive behavioral therapy versus psychoeducation control for illness anxiety disorder and somatic symptom disorder: A randomized controlled trial. *Journal of Consulting and Clinical Psychology, 86*(1), 89.

Scarella, T., Boland, R., & Barsky, A. (2019). Illness anxiety disorder: Psychopathology, epidemiology, clinical characteristics, and treatment. *Psychosomatic Medicine, 81*(5), 398–407.

Smith, B., Shatté, A., Perlman, A., Siers, M., & Lynch, W. D. (2018). Improvements in resilience, stress, and somatic symptoms following online resilience training: A dose–response effect. *Journal of Occupational and Environmental Medicine, 69*(1), 1–5.

Stone, J., & Sharpe, M. (2019). Conversion disorder in adults: Epidemiology, pathogenesis, and prognosis. *UpToDate.* https://www.uptodate.com/contents/conversion-disorder-in-adults-epidemiology-pathogenesis-and-prognosis

van Meerkerk-Aanen, P., de Vroege, L., Khasho, D., Foruz, A., van Asseldonk, J. T., & van der Feltz-Cornelis, C. M. (2017). La belle indifférence revisited: A case report on progressive supranuclear palsy misdiagnosed as conversion disorder. *Neuropsychiatric Disease and Treatment, 13*, 2057–2067.

Yates, W. R., Shortridge, A. B., & Forrest, J. S. (2019). Somatic symptom disorders. https://emedicine.medscape.com/article/294908-overview

Chapter 11

Feeding and eating disorders

Just the facts

In this chapter, you'll learn:

◆ major features of the most common feeding and eating disorders

◆ proposed causes of feeding and eating disorders

◆ assessment findings and nursing interventions for patients with feeding and eating disorders

◆ recommended treatments for patients with feeding and eating disorders.

A look at eating disorders

Eating disorders are serious and sometimes fatal psychological and medical illnesses associated with persistent and severe disturbances in a person's eating behaviors and related thoughts and emotions. Eating disorders impact a person's physical and emotional health, productivity, and relationships with others. An individual with an eating disorder is preoccupied with thoughts of food, weight, and body shape to the extent that it disrupts daily life. Serious and life-threatening consequences occur if the condition is left untreated.

Several different feeding and eating disorders have been identified and classified by the American Psychiatric Association (APA, 2013) based on presentation of symptoms. Although some individuals only present with partial symptoms of a feeding or eating disorder, called subthreshold or subclinical or partial syndromes, these individuals still require treatment.

About 30 million individuals in the United States will suffer from a clinically significant eating disorder at some time in their lives (Hudson, 2018). Subthreshold eating disorders may be as high as 11% of the population (National Institute of Mental Health, 2017). Eating disorders can occur in all ages (7 to 70 years), affect both genders, and can be found in all ethnic groups and backgrounds. (See *Getting past stereotypes*.) The symptoms most frequently appear in adolescence or young adulthood and generally begin between the ages of 13 and 17. Eating disorders are the third leading type of

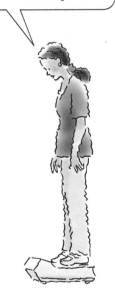

People with feeding and eating disorders are preoccupied with food, and/or weight, and/or body size.

chronic illness in children and adolescents (Frank & Shott, 2016), and females have a significantly higher incidence of these diseases.

Illness inventory

This chapter discusses the three most common psychiatric feeding and eating disorders:

- anorexia nervosa (AN)
- bulimia nervosa (BN)
- binge-eating disorder (BED).

Eating disorders occur on a spectrum of severity from mild to severe. All three of the most common eating disorders involve disordered eating patterns. In some individuals, the specific type of eating disorder may change over time. For example, a person with a diagnosis of AN may begin to binge and purge when weight is restored. There can be significant overlap of symptoms of all three of these eating disorders (Mehler & Andersen, 2017).

These disorders may be physically and psychologically debilitating. Extreme cases can lead to death from physical complications or suicide. Eating disorders have the highest rate of mortality than any other psychiatric disorder.

As with other disorders, early recognition and treatment leads to a better outcome. Long-standing illness and comorbid psychiatric problems, such as substance use disorders, depression and anxiety disorders, obsessive-compulsive disorder (OCD), or personality disorders, complicate treatment and tend to have a poorer prognosis.

Causes

Currently, the causes of eating disorders involve a complex interaction of genetics, biological and psychodynamics factors, and social and family influences.

Genetic and biological theories

Eating disorders have a 50% to 70% genetic contribution (Mehler & Andersen, 2017). Eating disorders tend to run in families. There is a higher rate of eating disorders in monozygotic twins than in dizygotic twins.

Some behaviors associated with eating disorders are linked to specific chromosomal abnormalities. Gene mutations that affect hormone functioning and neurotransmitter regulation (especially serotonin, norepinephrine, and dopamine) are implicated in these diseases. Neuroanatomic brain changes are also seen with these disorders.

Risk factors

Risk factors or factors that may increase susceptibility for feeding and eating disorders (Boyd, 2018; Hudson, 2018) include:

- ○ gender: being female
- ○ age: being an adolescent or young adult
- family history:
  - ○ having a parent or sibling with an eating disorder
  - ○ family history of mood disorders or substance use disorders
  - ○ parental overconcern with the child's weight
- psychosocial history:
  - ○ concurrent depressive disorder, anxiety disorder, mood disorder, OCD, or a personality disorder
  - ○ history of childhood depression or anxiety disorder
  - ○ personality traits of high anxiety, perfectionism, low self-esteem, and high achievement orientation
  - ○ conflicts over identity, sexual identify, role development, and body image
  - ○ history of trauma, physical and sexual abuse, and severe neglect
- situational:
  - ○ transitioning in life such as moving, beginning college, or other life changes
- social:
  - ○ being an athlete, actor, dancer, model, or in a profession in which weight and appearance are emphasized
  - ○ interpersonal conflicts, especially bullying (about weight) in children and adolescents

In addition to these risk factors, adolescent girls with type 1 diabetes are twice as likely to have disordered eating behavior than their nondiabetic counterparts and may omit insulin as a weight reduction strategy (Davenport, 2019).

Social influences

Society sets unrealistic expectations for appearance, equating thinness with being successful, powerful, and popular. These expectations are conveyed through omnipresent images of thin, beautiful people on television and in films, magazines, and social media.

General signs of a feeding and eating disorder

Common indicators of a feeding and eating disorder (Hudson, 2018) include the following:

- Dramatic or frequent fluctuations in weight
- Eating differently than the rest of the family, avoiding eating with others, or secretive eating

- Dieting, extreme food restrictions, or rigid eating rituals
- Preoccupation with food, body shape, and weight
- Expressing excessive body dissatisfaction
- Secretive exercise
- Feelings of guilt after eating
- Frequent weighing of self.

Anorexia nervosa

AN is a syndrome in which the affected person relentlessly pursues thinness, sometimes to the point of fatal emaciation, as the person becomes preoccupied with food and body image. Despite the extreme thinness, these individuals perceive themselves as being overweight because they have distorted body image. This syndrome is also characterized by an extreme self-induced starvation and excessive weight loss that result in medical abnormalities. Generally, a person is deemed to have AN when body weight is significantly below expectations for the person's age, height, development, and health. (See *Name games*.)

Disorder subtypes

Two AN subtypes are recognized by the APA (2013):
- Restricting—dieting and fasting
- Binge/purge—episodes of eating large amounts of food followed by behaviors (self-induced vomiting) that prevent weight gain

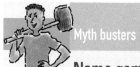

Myth busters

Name games

Many people confuse the medical diagnosis of AN with the symptom of anorexia.

Myth: AN is the clinical term for anorexia.

Reality: The two conditions are not the same thing. *Anorexia* refers to loss of appetite. A common symptom of gastrointestinal (GI) and endocrine disorders, anorexia may also accompany anxiety, chronic pain, poor oral hygiene, increased body temperature caused by fever or hot weather, and aging-related changes in taste or smell. Some drugs may also cause anorexia.

AN, on the other hand, is an eating disorder marked by a distorted body image, an extreme fear of gaining weight, and a restricted nutritional intake to maintain a minimally normal body weight. Persons with AN perceive themselves as overweight even when extremely underweight.

Complications

Serious medical complications can result from malnutrition, dehydration, and electrolyte imbalances caused by the prolonged starvation, vomiting, and laxative and diuretic misuse associated with this disorder. AN tends to have the highest mortality risk (Mehler, 2019), with about 10% to 20% from both physiologic complications and suicide (Bernstein, 2019a).

Prolonged starvation seen in severe cases of AN also brings additional psychological and neurologic consequences (such as acute cognitive dysfunction) that tends to resolve when weight is restored.

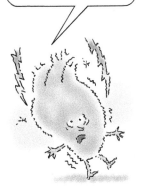

If malnutrition leads to edema or hypokalemia, ventricular arrhythmias may occur.

Disheartening complications

Cardiovascular complications of AN can be life-threatening. They include:

- bradycardia
- hypotension and orthostatic hypotension
- reduced cardiac output
- cardiac palpitations and arrhythmias (associated with hypokalemia)
  - may result in sudden death
  - electrocardiograph (ECG) changes, such as nonspecific ST intervals, T-wave changes, and prolonged PR intervals and Q-T intervals
- decreased left ventricular muscle mass and chamber size
- congestive heart failure—increased risk during refeeding process.

Other complications and lab abnormalities

Endocrine and metabolic

- amenorrhea (cessation of menstrual periods) may occur with loss of 25% of normal body weight
- estrogen deficiency can cause reproductive problems and delayed psychosexual development
- hypothermia, cold intolerance
- increased growth hormone, cortisol, cholesterol, and liver function studies
- abnormal blood glucose levels.

Gastrointestinal

- bloating, nausea, constipation, and abdominal pain
- esophageal erosion, ulcers, tears, and bleeding as well as tooth and gum erosion and dental caries with excessive vomiting.

Hemolytic

- bone marrow suppression:
  - ↓ White blood cells (WBCs) = ↑ susceptibility to infection

- ○ ↓ Red blood cells (RBCs) lead to anemia, low energy levels, and weakness
- ○ ↓ platelets lead to ↑ bleeding and bruising
- ○ ↓ hemoglobin and hematocrit.

Fluid and electrolyte imbalances

- dehydration with poor skin turgor and dry mucosa
- hypokalemia, hypomagnesemia, hyponatremia, hypophosphatemia, metabolic alkalosis (with vomiting), metabolic acidosis (reduced sodium bicarbonate related to laxative misuse)
- peripheral edema (with refeeding)
- renal dysfunction (↑ creatinine, blood urea nitrogen, diluted urine).

Multiple vitamin and mineral insufficiencies

- osteoporosis from ↓ calcium levels
- ↓ thiamine disrupts cell physiology.

Dermatologic

- dry flaking skin, brittle nails, hair loss
- development of *lanugo* (downylike hair that develops due to loss of subcutaneous fat).

Neurologic

- vertigo and fainting
- development of rigidity of thinking, decreased concentration, and confusion
- clinical depression and high levels of anxiety and irritability.

Refeeding process

- The refeeding process used to treat the severely malnourished persons diagnosed with AN requires careful monitoring to prevent life-threatening complications (Mehler & Andersen, 2017) associated with serious metabolic and neurologic complications.

Prevalence and onset

Statistics on the onset and prevalence of AN are variable. It is estimated that AN has a lifetime prevalence rate of 0.3% to 1%, with some studies indicating a rate as high as 4% for females (Bernstein, 2019a; Wolfe et al., 2016). Approximately 90% of those diagnosed with AN are adolescent and young adult women. Males and older and younger individuals of both genders can also struggle with this illness. The age of onset is generally between 13 and 18 years of age (Bernstein, 2019a).

Causes

No one knows exactly what causes AN. Experts suspect it results from an interplay of genetic, biological, behavioral, environmental, family, and psychosocial factors.

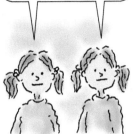

We're identical twins, so if one of us gets AN, the other has an increased risk.

Genetic causes

The genetic contribution to this disease is as high as 50% to 80% (Bernstein, 2019a). AN is more common among sisters and mothers of those with the disorder when compared to the general population. Identical twins have a higher risk for AN than fraternal twins. Genetic abnormalities on chromosome 12 have been linked to AN (Duncan et al., 2017).

Biological causes

Neuroendocrine theories identify hypothalamic dysfunction as a contributing factor to AN. Neurochemical theories suggest that below normal levels of several neurotransmitters such as serotonin and norepinephrine are associated with this disorder.

Brain abnormalities are seen in computed tomography (CT) and positron emission tomography (PET) scans in individuals who have AN during starvation. However, the association of these abnormalities with AN is not clear. Decreased activity in the parietal and occipital lobes with increased activity in the frontal cortex is associated with those diagnosed with AN. Alterations in areas of the brain (insula and the orbitofrontal cortex) that are involved in normal biological food-reward circuitry and anxiety symptoms have also been identified in this population (Frank & Shott, 2016).

Behavioral and environmental factors

Because AN is more common in Western and industrialized countries, some experts blame the disorder on societal standards of ideal

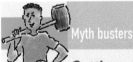

Myth busters

Getting past stereotypes

If you have preconceived notions about who gets AN, you may mistake this disorder for another condition.

Myth: Only young women get AN.

Reality: Although young females are more commonly diagnosed with AN, the disorder is increasingly showing up in children, males of all ages, and older women.

body shape and the constant pressure to be thin. Many people first learn about feeding and eating disorders from friends and the media. Some theorists believe feeding and eating disorders may represent *learned behaviors* in response to strong social pressures to be thin.

Stress may also play a role. As with other psychiatric disorders, stressful events may increase the risk of AN in those with a genetic predisposition.

Psychological factors

Experts have observed low self-esteem, perfectionism, and a sense of powerlessness in those with a diagnosis of AN. It is believed that the disorder may be an attempt to defend against feelings of inadequacy.

> Restricting calories gives the patient with AN a sense of power and control.

Power and perfection

It is hypothesized that individuals with AN feel powerless and unable to control their life or environment. The individual strives to regain a personal sense of power and control through caloric restriction. The individual may come to believe that achieving the "perfect" body leads to achieving the "perfect" life.

A shield against sexuality

Some psychiatrists see refusal to eat as a subconscious effort to protect oneself from dealing with issues surrounding sexuality.

Family dynamics

Families with adolescents diagnosed with *AN* tend to report interpersonal boundary problems in which there may be *separation and autonomy* developmental issues (Cerniglia et al., 2017). Other family factors that may play a role in the disorder include:

* A family system in which one parent is dominant and the other parent is passive
* A family system that places a high value on achievement
* A family system that has trouble resolving conflict and expressing anger

Families often report feeling powerless in the face of some of the mystifying behaviors associated with eating disorders. It is unclear if some of the problematic behaviors observed in the family system contribute to the development of the eating disorder or result from the acute frustration of seeing a loved one struggling with an eating disorder.

Signs and symptoms

The key features of AN are:
- self-imposed starvation, despite the patient's obvious emaciation
- significant weight loss with no organic reason
- a morbid fear of being "fat" with frantic efforts to be thin.

Physical findings

Physical findings that suggest AN include:
- emaciated appearance
- skeletal muscle atrophy
- loss of fatty tissue
- breast tissue atrophy
- lanugo (a covering of soft, fine hair) on the face and body
- dryness or loss of scalp hair
- hypotension
- bradycardia and/or irregular heart rhythm
- fatigue
- sleep difficulties
- cold intolerance
- constipation
- bowel distention
- loss of libido
- amenorrhea.

Psychosocial findings

Common psychosocial findings of AN include:
- preoccupation with body size
- distorted body image
- extreme fear of weight gain
- lack of insight: inability to comprehend the severity of the situation
- descriptions of self as "fat"—"fat phobia"
- dissatisfaction with a particular aspect of the appearance
- low self-esteem
- social isolation/withdrawal
- perfectionism
- paradoxical obsession with food such as preparing elaborate meals for others
- feelings of despair, hopelessness, and worthlessness
- suicidal thoughts
- self-harm behaviors such as cutting

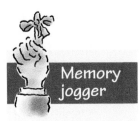

Memory jogger

The word **HUNGER** is your guidepost to the major features of AN.

Has an obsession with food and weight

Underweight or emaciated

Nutritional needs go unmet

Gross distortion of body image

Exercises, vomits, or uses laxatives and diuretics to lose weight

Refuses to eat

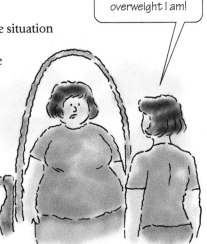

Look at how overweight I am!

Behavioral findings

Behavioral signs of AN include:

- wearing of oversized clothing in an effort to disguise body size
- ritualistic eating patterns
- behaviors to prevent weight gain
- layering of clothing or wearing of unseasonably warm clothing to compensate for cold intolerance and loss of adipose tissue
- restless activity and vigor (despite undernourishment)
- excessive exercising with no apparent fatigue
- high academic or athletic performance

Comorbid conditions

Approximately half of those diagnosed with AN will present with symptoms for at least one major psychiatric disorder (Westmoreland et al., 2017). These include anxiety disorders, depressive disorders, substance use disorders, and personality disorders. OCD or traits and rigidity of thinking are frequently seen with those with a diagnosis of AN.

Suicide and self-harm behaviors like cutting are increased with this disorder.

Diagnosis

Although AN should be suspected in any young person with weight loss, health care providers often miss the diagnosis because the patient is secretive about symptoms.

The SCOFF questionnaire is an example of a standardized, validated screening tool available to primary care providers to assess for eating disorders (Bernstein, 2019a). Two "yes" answers suggest a possible eating disorder and the need for a more in-depth assessment.

- **Sick:** Do you make yourself sick or vomit after a meal because you feel uncomfortably full?
- **Control:** Do you fear loss of control over how much you eat?
- **One stone:** Have you gained 14 lb (equivalent to one stone in Great Britain) in a 3-month period?
- **Fat:** Do you believe you are fat even when others tell you that you are too thin?
- **Food:** Does food dominate your life?

A complete physical examination with laboratory tests should be done.

Laboratory findings

Laboratory tests help rule out endocrine, metabolic, and central nervous system abnormalities; cancer; malabsorption syndrome; and other disorders that cause physical wasting (such as human immunodeficiency virus [HIV]).

Deviations from the norm

In a patient who has lost more than 30% of their normal weight, findings may include:

- below normal hemoglobin, platelet count, WBC count, erythrocyte sedimentation rate, creatinine, blood, urea, nitrogen, uric acid, cholesterol, total protein, albumin, chloride, calcium, fasting blood glucose, luteinizing and follicle-stimulating hormone, and triiodothyronine levels
- prolonged bleeding time
- above-normal amylase
- dilute urine.

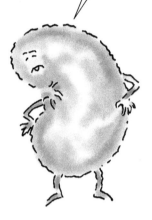

AN may impair the kidney's ability to concentrate urine.

Exclusion of other medical or psychiatric disorders: Differential diagnosis

AN must be differentiated from other medical conditions or psychiatric disorders.

Medical conditions include:
- GI disease
- hyperthyroidism
- occult malignancies
- HIV.

Psychiatric disorders include:
- substance use disorders (especially with stimulants, such as cocaine and amphetamines)
- anxiety disorders (especially social phobia)
- OCD
- mood disorders (such as major depression and bipolar disorder)
- personality disorders (especially histrionic, borderline, and narcissistic personality disorders)
- schizophrenia.

The diagnosis of AN is based on the patient's presentation of symptoms.

Treatment

Although statistics vary, most people who meet the criteria for this diagnosis will not seek help voluntarily. This is related to *lack of insight* and *stigma and shame* associated with this disorder.

The priority treatment for AN aims to promote weight gain, correct malnutrition, and normalize eating habits. It is important to resolve the underlying psychological, physical, interpersonal, and social issues that perpetuate the disease for long-term recovery. The most effective strategy has been psychotherapy coupled with weight restoration to within 10% of normal. An interdisciplinary team of medical and mental health clinicians and dietitians who have experience in treating AN enhances outcomes.

As appropriate, treatment measures may include:
- refeeding consisting of a reasonable diet, with or without liquid supplements
- vitamin and mineral supplements
- activity curtailment as needed (such as for arrhythmias or other physical reasons)
- group, family, or individual psychotherapy
- behavior modification, with privileges based on weight gain.

Hospitalization

Some patients with AN can be treated successfully as outpatients. However, the patient who exhibits any of the following signs or symptoms requires hospitalization in a medical or psychiatric unit:
- rapid weight loss equal to 15% or more of normal body mass or a body mass index (BMI) less than 16
- persistent bradycardia (heart rate of 50 beats/minute or less)
- systolic blood pressure of 90 mm Hg or lower
- hypothermia (a core body temperature of 97°F [36.1°C] or less)
- medical complications
- persistent sabotage or disruption of outpatient treatment
- denial of the disorder and the need for treatment
- risk for suicide
- nonsuicidal, self-injurious behaviors (such as cutting).

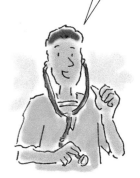

Hospitalization is warranted if the patient's systolic blood pressure drops to 90 mm Hg or lower.

Two years??

When hospitalization is required, it may be as brief as 2 weeks or as long as 2 years or more. Many clinical centers now have inpatient and outpatient programs specifically for managing eating disorders. Generally, about a third of patients with an eating disorder fully recover, a third retain subthreshold symptoms, and a third maintain a chronic eating disorder (Franco et al., 2017).

Psychotherapy

All forms of psychotherapy, from psychoanalysis to hypnotherapy, have been tried in the treatment of AN—with varying success. To be effective, psychotherapy must address the underlying problems of low self-esteem, guilt, anxiety, depression, and the disordered perceptions and thinking processes. Psychotherapy is aimed at helping the person develop more constructive, nonfood-related coping skills.

Common evidence-based therapies used for the treatment of AN include:
- Enhanced cognitive-behavioral therapy (CBT-E) is a type of CBT specifically designed to challenge the cognitive distortions associated with eating disorders. It helps the patient think differently about weight and body image.

- Interpersonal psychotherapy (ITP) is a therapy aimed at improving interpersonal relationships, which has been shown to effectively decrease AN symptoms.
- Maudsley/family-based therapy (FBT) and other types of family therapy. Family therapy involves therapy for the family as a whole or in part and offers the most effective treatment for adolescents.

Pharmacotherapy

No definitive medications have shown solid evidence of improvement in the symptoms of AN. Antidepressants can be used to treat comorbid conditions such as depressive and anxiety disorders. There is some evidence that suggests low doses of antipsychotics such as olanzapine (Zyprexa) will reduce ruminative thinking about food and excessive levels of anxiety about weight gain. In general, medication is initiated after weight is restored.

Nursing interventions

All nursing interventions start with the development of a therapeutic nurse-patient relationship. This is especially true for individuals with eating disorders. It was found that the motivation for patients to adhere to treatment was likely to increase when the nursing approach was person-centered and when nurses' attitudes were characterized by presence, genuine commitment, and motivation (Salzmann-Erikson & Dahlén, 2017).

Specific nursing interventions that facilitate recovery for patients with AN include:

- Regular monitoring of vital signs, nutritional status, and fluid intake and output during hospitalization
- Regular assessment of skin turgor and mucous membranes
- Determination of, with the patient and health care team, a target weight and support of the person's efforts to achieve that goal
- Some programs use a behavior modification approach to support weight gain. Unit privileges (such as participation in activities) are taken away if the person does not gain weight. The nurse can explain and support the plan to facilitate treatment adherence.
- Monitor the patient for passive or active suicidal potential and potential for self-harm behaviors. Weight gain can increase these urges in the early stages of treatment.

It is important to recognize that the patient's great fear of weight gain may interfere with achievement of treatment goals. Lack of treatment adherence can be frustrating to the nurse and to significant others. Empathy, respect, and the ability to be nonjudgmental are essential components of a supportive nurse-patient relationship that lead to better outcomes.

Person to person

- Maintain one-on-one supervision of the patient during meals and for 1 to 3 hours afterward to ensure that the patient is complying with the dietary treatment program and not vomiting as a way to maintain a low weight after eating. Remember that for a hospitalized patient with AN, food is considered a medication.
- The person is usually given a limited time to complete a meal (such as 30 minutes).
- Food choices must be done in conjunction with a dietitian to prevent reinforcing dysfunctional eating patterns.
- Allow the person to exercise control when possible over nonfood-related activities in the therapeutic environment.

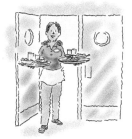

Food is considered a medication for a patient hospitalized with AN.

Liquidation strategy

- Be aware that during an acute anorexic episode, nutritionally complete liquids are sometimes more acceptable because they don't require the patient to select foods (something patients with AN commonly find difficult).
- If tube feedings or other special feeding measures become necessary, explain these measures to the patient and be ready to discuss patient's fears or reluctance. However, limit the discussion about the food itself.

Pound by pound

- Weigh the patient daily (after voiding and before breakfast) on the same scale, at the same time, and in the same clothing. Before weighing the patient, monitor closely. Patients may add hidden objects in clothing or drink large amounts of fluids to falsely increase weight.
- Keep in mind that a patient's weight should increase from morning to night.
- Anticipate a weight gain of about 1 to 3 lb/week.

Defusing fat fears

- If edema or bloating occurs after resuming normal eating behavior, reassure the patient that this is temporary. Otherwise, they may fear that they are getting fat and may stop complying with the treatment plan.
- Encourage the patient to recognize and assert feelings freely. If the patients understand that they can be assertive, they may gradually learn that expressing their true feelings will not result in losing control or love.
- Explain how improved nutrition can reverse the effects of starvation and prevent complications.
- Advise family members to avoid discussing food with the patient.

Preservation tactics

- Remember that patients with AN use exercise, preoccupation with food, ritualism, and even manipulation as mechanisms to preserve the only control they think they have in their life.
- If a patient requires hospitalization, maintain contact with the patient's outpatient treatment teams to promote a smooth return to the outpatient setting.
- Patients and families may benefit from therapy that assists the family and significant others to develop strategies for improved communication and to search for ways to be comfortably supportive to the patient.
- Families frequently feel much guilt about a loved one's illness. It is important not to assign blame to the person or the family. Patients and families are not responsible for causing an illness; all are responsible for participating in treatment and recovery.
- There are a variety of support groups available to patients and families to help with recovery. Two online examples such as the National Association of Anorexia Nervosa and Related Eating Disorders, Inc. (www.anred.org) and the National Eating Disorders Association (http://www.nationaleatingdisorders.org) provide education and support to those seeking information about eating disorders.
- Unfortunately, social media can also interfere with recovery efforts. Websites and blogs, perpetuate the myth that excessive thinness and disordered eating can be a legitimate lifestyle choice. These websites describe, endorse, and motivate users to continue their efforts with disordered eating behaviors. It is important to monitor patient's internet activities, especially adolescents, to support use of appropriate resources.

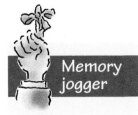

Memory jogger

Give your patient and family **CUES** *to eating disorders by covering these topics during teaching:*

Causes of eating disorders

Understanding how to overcome power struggles and issues of separation and autonomy

Effects of the eating disorder on physical and mental health

Symptoms of eating disorders and signs of relapse

Bulimia nervosa

BN is marked by episodes of binge eating. Binge eating is defined as eating a large amount of food in a short period of time. During the binge-eating episode, the patient feels a loss of control over the eating behavior. The binge-eating episode is usually followed by "purging" or use of problematic behaviors to eliminate the calories consumed. Feelings of guilt, humiliation, depression, and self-condemnation usually accompany the binge-purge episodes. Binge episodes may occur up to several times a day. Another important feature of BN is an extreme concern with body shape and weight. (See *Erroneous beliefs about eating disorders*.)

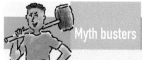

Erroneous beliefs about eating disorders

What you don't know about eating disorders could prevent you from assessing the condition accurately.

Myth: All patients with eating disorders are either very thin or very overweight.
Reality: A patient with BN may have a weight within a normal range.
Myth: Open conflict and verbal fighting are common among families of adolescents with eating disorders.
Reality: Conflict *avoidance*, not open conflict, is typical in these families.

Eating to excess

Although males are diagnosed with BN, it is young women of normal or nearly normal weight who typically develop the condition after a history of extended dieting. As dieting continues, the individual may experience a growing impulse to eat restricted foods. Eventually (usually after an anxiety-producing situation), the individual eats to excess, temporarily relieving this impulse. Fearing that the binge eating will lead to excessive weight gain, compensatory mechanisms such as induced vomiting and diuretic or laxative use (or both) are usually implemented to prevent weight gain.

Catalogue of complications

Physiologic complications of BN are usually caused by the consequences of the binge-eating behavior and the problematic compensatory behaviors to purge. This includes excessive vomiting and excessive use of diuretics and laxatives. Mortality rates for BN are lower than AN but are still present (Hilty, 2019).

The following are important potential complications:

Gastrointestinal
- bloating, nausea, and abdominal pain; irritation of GI tract due to self-induced vomiting
  - esophageal erosion, ulcers, tears, and bleeding
  - tooth and gum erosion and dental caries
- gastroesophageal reflux disease (GERD)
- laxative overuse may cause chronic irregular bowel movements and constipation

Deadly imbalances
- dehydration

- electrolyte imbalances including hypokalemia, hypomagnesemia, hyponatremia, hypophosphatemia, metabolic alkalosis (with vomiting), metabolic acidosis (reduced sodium bicarbonate related to laxative use)

Cardiac

- edema and electrocardiogram (EKG) changes
- increased risk of arrhythmias and sudden death from electrolyte imbalances
- toxicity from ingestion of substances such as ipecac to induce vomiting associated with severe cardiac disease

Prevalence and onset

BN is more common than AN and has a better prognosis. The disorder usually begins in late adolescence or young adults. As in AN, BN also affects both females and males but with a 10:1 female to male ratio. Some believe that the actual number of males affected may be as high as 20% (Hilty, 2019). Approximately 1% to 3% of the population meets the diagnostic criteria for BN—but up to 5% to 15% may have some symptoms of the disorder (Wolfe et al., 2016). These numbers may be a gross underestimation because many sufferers are able to hide their symptoms.

The prognosis for BN is variable with 50% to 70% recovery rates. Unfortunately, some studies show that about half of those patients may relapse. Unlike AN, there is an increased probability of recovery from BN even after 10 years (Hilty, 2019).

Comorbid conditions

Most patients with a diagnosis of BN will present symptoms for at least one major mental illness. Depressive disorder, anxiety disorder, and OCD are the most common comorbid conditions. One-third of these individuals will have a substance use disorder. There is a higher risk of suicide and self-harm behaviors associated with this disorder when compared to the general population

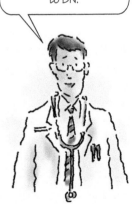

Researchers have proposed genetic links at chromosomes 1, 3, and 10p related to BN.

Causes

The exact cause of BN is unknown. As with AN, experts suspect it results from an interplay of genetic, biological, behavioral, environmental, family, and psychosocial factors.

Genetic and biological factors

There is an increased incidence of BN in first-degree relatives of individuals with the disorder. Researchers have noted genetic links at chromosomes 1, 3, and 10p related to BN (Hilty, 2019). This provides strong evidence that genes play a determining role in susceptibility to the disorder.

Some studies suggest that altered serotonin and norepinephrine levels and multiple hormone levels in the brain play a role in the development of BN. An increase in endorphins (feel-good hormones) in the brain during binge-eating episodes may reinforce BN and BEDs (Hilty, 2019).

Other factors

Other factors associated with the development of BN are related to social and psychological influences. Modern society's overemphasis on appearance and thinness is integral in the development of BN. Additional factors include:

- prior history of AN
- family system dysfunctions
  ○ poor conflict resolution issues
  ○ families described as being noncohesive with lack of nurturance
- trauma: neglect and physical and sexual abuse
- family history of substance use disorders, eating disorders, and other psychiatric illnesses
- maladaptive learned behavior
- struggle for self-control or self-identity.

Signs and symptoms

The history of an individual with BN typically includes episodic binge eating within a period of 2 hours, occurring up to several times a day. During bingeing episodes, the individual continues to eat until interrupted by abdominal pain, sleep, or another person's presence. Most patients with BN prefer foods that are sweet, soft, and high in calories and carbohydrates. There is a perceived loss of control of eating during these episodes. Compensatory behaviors are used to prevent weight gain. These can include:

- self-induced vomiting
- use of laxatives and diuretics
- use of appetite suppressants
- use of drugs to stimulate metabolism (such as thyroid medication)
- excessive exercise
- periods of extreme fasting
- failure to use insulin properly for those with type 1 diabetes.

Physical findings

Physical findings that suggest BN include:
- weight/body shape may be thin, within the normal weight range or slightly overweight with frequent weight fluctuations
- persistent sore throat and heartburn (from vomited stomach acids)
- calluses or scarring on the back of the hands and knuckles (from forcing the hand down the throat to induce vomiting)
- salivary gland swelling, hoarseness, throat lacerations, and dental erosion (from repetitive vomiting)
- tooth staining or discoloration
- dizziness and light-headedness
- severe GI reflux symptoms, abdominal and epigastric pain (from acute gastric dilation)
- amenorrhea and menstrual irregularities.

Psychosocial findings

Individuals with a diagnosis of BN express great dissatisfaction with body shape and weight.

Stay alert for these psychosocial features:
- perfectionism
- distorted body image
- preoccupation and overconcern with weight and appearance
- self-image based upon weight and appearance
- exaggerated sense of guilt
- feelings of alienation
- recurrent anxiety
- an image as the "perfect" student, parent, or career professional (a child may be distinguished for participating in competitive activities, such as ballet or gymnastics)
- poor impulse control
- chronic depression
- low tolerance for frustration
- self-consciousness
- difficulty expressing such feelings as anger
- impaired social or occupational adjustment
- history of childhood trauma (especially sexual abuse)
- history of unsatisfactory interpersonal relationships
- parental obesity
- family dysfunction.

Behavioral findings

Behavioral signs of BN include:
- evidence of binge-eating episodes
- disappearance of large amounts of food over short periods

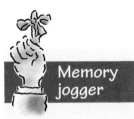

Memory jogger

Although not all individuals with bulimia engage in purging, the term **RIDS BODY** can help you remember the clinical features of bulimia.

Recurrent binge-eating episodes

Intense exercise

Diuretic, laxative, and enema use

Self-induced vomiting

Body image distortion

Ordinary eating alternating with episodes of binge-purge cycles

Depression and anxiety disorders may be present

Yo-yo effect of tension relief and pleasure experienced with bingeing; guilt and depression following purging

- presence of containers and wrappers
- evidence of purging
- frequent trips to the bathroom after meals
- sounds and smells of vomiting
- presence of packages of diuretics and laxatives
- peculiar eating habits or rituals
- excessive, rigid exercise regimen despite poor weather, fatigue, illness, or injury
- a complex schedule (to make time for binge-and-purge sessions)
- withdrawal from friends and usual activities
- hyperactivity
- frequent weighing
- other behaviors suggesting that weight loss, dieting, and control of food are becoming primary concerns.

Diagnosis

The individual should undergo a medical evaluation to rule out other causes of symptoms, such as an upper GI disorder that can cause repeated vomiting. The individual should also undergo a neuropsychological evaluation to identify BN and other comorbid psychiatric disorders. When individuals are honest about the length and extent of their behavior, this can help ascertain the seriousness and the severity of their BN disorder.

Lab tests

Laboratory tests can determine the presence and severity of complications. For example:

- serum electrolyte studies (see *Complications*) may reveal above-normal bicarbonate levels and decreased potassium and sodium levels
- blood glucose testing may detect hypoglycemia
- baseline ECG to rule out cardiac arrhythmias from electrolyte disturbances
- complete blood count to rule out anemias
- amylase levels—excessive amounts indicate excessive vomiting.
  The diagnosis of BN is based on the patient's presentation of symptoms.

Treatment

Like other eating disorders, most people do not seek treatment due to stigma and shame and denial of the seriousness of the illness. Health care providers may miss the diagnosis because the person may be of normal weight and not "look" sick. Early recognition and treatment of BN is crucial because patients treated early are more likely to recover more fully than those who delay treatment. Treatment is most effective when it addresses the issues that cause the behavior, not the behavior itself. Usually, treatment involves individual, group, and family therapy; nutritional counseling; and, in many cases, medications.

> The sooner a person gets treatment for bulimia, the greater the chance of a full recovery.

Spotlight on structure

At all levels of care, treatment requires a high degree of structure and a behavioral treatment plan based on the person's weight and eating behaviors. The focus of treatment is on eliminating the binge-purge cycle, treating physical complications, and changing core dysfunctional thoughts and attitudes that perpetuate the dysfunctional eating pattern. A multidisciplinary approach is recommended.

Psychotherapy

Psychotherapy focuses on breaking the binge-purge cycle and helping patients regain control over their eating behavior. Treatment may take place in an inpatient or outpatient setting. It usually includes behavior modification therapy, possibly in highly structured psychoeducational group meetings.

The same therapies for AN show effectiveness for treating BN. These include:

- CBT-E
- ITP
- Maudsley/FBT and other types of family therapy

Nutritional counseling and education support the development of healthy eating patterns and well-balanced exercise regimes.

The use of psychotropic medications may be recommended as a supplement to therapy. Fluoxetine (Prozac), a selective serotonin reuptake inhibitor (SSRI), is the only Food and Drug Administration (FDA)-approved medication for BN. Other antidepressants, especially those that increase serotonin levels in the brain, are sometimes prescribed. The risk of side effects, including the increased risk of suicide for antidepressants, must be considered when antidepressants are prescribed. The use of antidepressants may also treat comorbid depressive and anxiety disorders and obsessive-compulsive traits.

Anonymous help

Patients may benefit from participation in a self-help group such as Overeaters Anonymous or other support groups. Cautious use of *appropriate* online resources for education and support can be useful adjuncts to formal therapy.

Hospitalization

If binge eating and purging have caused serious physical harm, hospitalization may be necessary to provide around-the-clock observation of all eating and elimination (urinating, bowel movements, and vomiting). As symptoms abate and the eating behaviors and weight stabilize, patients gradually resume control over their eating.

Nursing interventions

The following nursing interventions are recommended for a patient with BN:

- Facilitating the development of a therapeutic nurse-patient relationship is the first nursing intervention. The nurse needs to empathize with feelings of low self-esteem, worthlessness, sadness, and anxiety. An accepting, nonjudgmental approach, along with a comprehensive understanding of the subjective experience of the patient, is essential.
- Establish a contract with the patient that specifies the amount and types of food that must be eaten at each meal.
- Discourage fasting or restrictive food intake because this may trigger a binge episode.
- Supervise the patient during mealtimes and for a specified period afterward (usually 1 to 2 hours) to prevent purging.
- Set a time limit for each meal. Provide a pleasant, relaxed eating environment.
- Teach the patient to keep a journal to document time of eating, food eaten, mood, life events, and binge urges and behaviors.
  - The purpose of a food journal is to identify triggers for binge episode (hunger from inadequate intake, emotional distress, automatic conditioning response) (Mehler & Andersen, 2017).
- Reinforce the need to maintain a healthy weight.
- Encourage patients to recognize and verbalize their feelings and mood states.
- Identify the patient's elimination patterns.
- Encourage the patient to talk about stressful issues, such as achievement, independence, socialization, sexuality, family problems, and control.

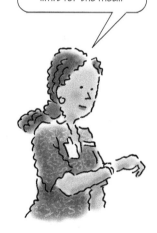

When supervising a patient with BN at mealtimes, set a time limit for the meal.

Misuse aversion

- Explain the medical complications associated with excessive vomiting and the risks of laxative, emetic, and diuretic use.
- Provide assertiveness training to help patients gain control over their behavior and achieve a realistic and positive self-image.
- Assess the patient's passive and active suicide potential and risk for self-harm.

The long haul

- Offer support and encouragement to help the patient stay in treatment. Treatment may need to continue for years to prevent relapse.

  Refer the patient and family to appropriate websites. The *National Association of Anorexia Nervosa and Related Eating Disorders*, Inc. (www .anred.org) and the *National Eating Disorders Association* (http://www .nationaleatingdisorders.org) provide additional education and support regarding eating disorders.

Binge-eating disorder

BED involves a regular occurrence of rapidly eating large amounts of food, usually in secret. Binge eating is associated with feeling out of control about food intake. These episodes are followed by guilt, shame, and acute emotional distress. The individual usually does not engage in compensatory behaviors, which may result in excessive weight gain. BED can occur in those with normal weight, those that are moderately overweight, or those that are obese.

Complications

Individuals with BED often have the same health risks as those with clinical obesity, including:
- high blood pressure
- high cholesterol levels
- heart disease
- noninsulin-dependent diabetes mellitus
- gallbladder disease
- musculoskeletal problems
- obstructive sleep apnea.

Prevalence and onset

BED is the most common eating disorder in the United States. At some point in their lives, up to 3.5% of females and 2% of males will experience BED (Bernstein, 2019b; Wolfe et al., 2016). BED affects women slightly more than men, with the average onset occurring in young adulthood, slightly later than for other eating disorders. Long-term favorable outcomes are slightly better than for other eating disorders. Individuals with BED also frequently have comorbid conditions such as anxiety disorders, mood disorders, and/or substance use disorders. The risk for suicide and self-harm behaviors is higher when compared to those without this disorder (Bernstein, 2019b).

Causes

BED has also been shown to run in families and is believed to have both genetic and environmental influences. Hereditary factors as causation for BED are estimated to be from 41% to 57% (Bernstein, 2019b). As with the other eating disorders, brain chemistry changes are seen in those with BED. Stressful life events increase the risk of developing BED.

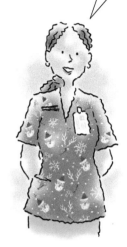

Up to 10% of the U.S. population may suffer from an eating disorder at some point in their life.

Signs and symptoms

The key feature of BED is bingeing without compensatory behaviors and acute distress over the bingeing behavior. Other findings include:

Physical findings
- insomnia
- normal weight, slightly above-normal weight, or obesity (BMI > 30).

Psychosocial findings
- constant thoughts of food
- eating in private
- feeling disgusted, guilty, and/or worthless after eating
- feeling powerless to stop eating
- interpersonal isolation and loneliness
- depression, anxiety, and substance use disorders are common comorbidities.

Behavioral findings
- feeling out of control when eating
- eating even when uncomfortably full
- emotional eating—eating to escape stress or for comfort.

Diagnosis

The patient should undergo a medical evaluation to rule out other causes of bingeing or excessive weight gain. Assessing for complications associated with obesity and completing a neuropsychological evaluation to identify BED and other comorbid psychiatric disorders are also essential.

Treatment

Treatment of this disorder has two components. The first component is to find strategies to interrupt the binge-eating episodes. The second component is to find strategies to facilitate weight loss if appropriate.

For patients with BED, psychotherapy, including cognitive-based therapy and behavioral therapy and family therapy, has been shown to be the most effective in helping patients identify triggers and strategies to interrupt or stop binges. Because binge episodes are frequently triggered by stressful events, general relaxation techniques like mindfulness meditation are useful adjuncts to formal therapy.

Pharmacologic therapy includes the following:

- Antidepressants to lessen bingeing episodes and reduce depression
  - SSRIs such as fluoxetine (Prozac)
  - Selective serotonin/norepinephrine reuptake inhibitors (SNRIs) such as venlafaxine (Effexor)
- Lisdexamfetamine (Vyvanse) is a stimulant that is FDA approved to treat moderate-to-severe BED in adults. It lessens binge eating in this population.

Other classifications of drugs sometimes used include glucagon-like agonists to improve glycemic control to control weight, anorexiants to decrease food consumption, lipase inhibitors to inhibit nutrient absorption, and anticonvulsants to decrease the compulsive behavior.

Treatment also should involve nutritional counseling to facilitate healthy weight management. Behavioral- based weight loss programs can be useful.

Nursing interventions

The following nursing interventions are recommended for a patient with BED:

Person to person

- Establish a therapeutic nurse-patient relationship.
- Promote an accepting, nonjudgmental atmosphere. Control your reactions to the patient's behavior and feelings.

Setting goals

- Help patients to formulate daily goals and develop a plan to reach the goals.
- Help patients to establish a target weight and support efforts to achieve this goal.

Maintaining control

- Allow the patient to maintain control over the types and amounts of food they eat.
- Teach patients how to keep a food journal, including the types of foods they eat, eating frequency, and feelings associated with eating. Help patient identify triggers to binges.
- Maintain a routine weighing session to help patients assess goal achievement.
- Help patients to learn other coping strategies (other than eating) for dealing with emotions.

Support

- Offer support and encouragement to help the patient stay in treatment.
- Refer patients and families to support groups like Overeaters Anonymous.
- Refer patients and their families to appropriate websites, such as National Association of Anorexia Nervosa and Related Eating Disorders, Inc. (www.anred.org) and *National Eating Disorders Association* (http://www.nationaleatingdisorders.org) to provide additional education and support.

Quick quiz

1. Which is the most serious concern for a patient diagnosed with AN?
   - A. Risk of mortality.
   - B. Coexisting depression.
   - C. Poor family relationships.
   - D. Social isolation.

Answer: A. AN has a mortality rate of 10% to 20%.

2. In caring for a patient with BED, the nurse would perform which action?
   - A. Monitor BMI.
   - B. Prescribe an antidepressant.
   - C. Provide mental health counseling.
   - D. Confirm the binge-eating diagnosis.

Answer: A. The patient's BMI indicates the efficacy of treatment. Options B, C, and D are outside the scope of a registered prepared nurse.

3.   The nurse is caring for a patient with BN who presents with binge-purge cycles. Which patient characteristic does the nurse anticipate would trigger purge behavior?
   A.   Sensations of fullness or bloating.
   B.   Guilt, humiliation, and self-condemnation.
   C.   Fear of being discovered as a binge eater.
   D.   Feelings of nausea.

Answer: B. Guilt, humiliation, and self-condemnation usually trigger the desire to purge. Physical sensations, such as fullness, bloating, or nausea, aren't triggers to purging nor is the fear of being discovered.

4.   Which medication teaching will the nurse include in the teaching plan for a patient who has BN disorder?
   A.   Clozapine (Clozaril)
   B.   Risperidone (Risperdal)
   C.   Ziprasidone (Geodon)
   D.   Fluoxetine (Prozac)

Answer: D. SSRIs such as Prozac are commonly used to treat BN. Clozaril, Risperdal, and Geodon are medications used in treating schizophrenia and are not associated with the treatment of eating disorders.

Scoring

☆☆☆   If you answered all four items correctly, savor the moment! You've done well on this chapter.

☆☆   If you answered two or three items correctly, swell! You've just gained important knowledge.

☆   If you answered just one item correctly, review the chapter again.

Selected references

American Psychiatric Association. (2013). *Diagnostic and statistical manual of mental disorders* 5th ed.). Author.

Bernstein, B. E. (2019a). Anorexia nervosa. *Medscape.* https://emedicine.medscape.com/article/912187-overview

Bernstein, B. E. (2019b). Binge eating disorder (BED). *Medscape.* https://emedicine.medscape.com/article/2221362-overview#a1

Boyd, M. (2018). *Psychiatric nursing: Contemporary practice* (6th ed.). Wolters Kluwer.

Cerniglia, L., Cimino, S., Tafà, M., Marzilli, E., Ballarotto, G., & Bracaglia, F. (2017). Family profiles in eating disorders: Family functioning and psychopathology. *Psychology Research and Behavior Management, 2017*(10), 305–312. https://doi.org/10.2147/PRBM.S145463

Davenport, L. (2019). Emotional support key to unlocking eating disorders in T2D. *Medscape*. https://www.medscape.com/viewarticle/910463

Duncan, L., Yilmaz, Z., Gaspar, H., Walters, R., Goldstein, J., Anttila, V., Bulik-Sullivan, B., Ripke, S.; Eating Disorders Working Group of the Psychiatric Genomics Consortium, Thornton, L., Hinney, A., Daly, M., Sullivan, P. F., Zeggini, E., Breen, G., & Bulik, C. M. (2017). Significant locus and metabolic genetic correlations revealed in genome-wide association study of anorexia nervosa. *American Journal of Psychiatry, 174*(9), 850–858. https://doi.org/10.1176/appi.ajp.2017.16121402

Franco, K., Sieke, E., Dickstein, L., & Falcone, T. (2017). Eating disorders. *Cleveland Clinic Center for Continuing Education.* http://www.clevelandclinicmeded.com/medicalpubs/diseasemanagement/psychiatry-psychology/eating-disorders/

Frank, G. K., & Shott, M. E. (2016). The role of psychotropic medications in the management of anorexia nervosa: Rationale, evidence and future prospects. *CNS Drugs, 30*(5), https://doi.org/10.1007/s40263-016-0335-6

Hilty, D. M. (2019). Bulimia nervosa. *Medscape.* https://emedicine.medscape.com/article/286485-overview

Hudson, L. (2018). Warning signs of eating disorders and proven treatment to help. *Michigan Health.* https://healthblog.uofmhealth.org/health-management/common-signs-of-eating-disorders-and-proven-treatments-to-help

Mehler, P. (2019). Anorexia nervosa in adults: Evaluation for medical complications and criteria for hospitalization to manage these complications. *UpToDate.* https://www.uptodate.com/contents/anorexia-nervosa-in-adults-evaluation-for-medical-complications-and-criteria-for-hospitalization-to-manage-these-complications

Mehler, P., & Andersen, A. (2017). *Eating disorders: A guide to medical care and complications* (3rd ed.). Johns Hopkins University Press.

National Institute of Mental Health. (2017). *Eating disorders.* https://www.nimh.nih.gov/health/statistics/eating-disorders.shtml

Salzmann-Erikson, M., & Dahlén, J. (2017). Nurses' establishment of health promoting relationships: A descriptive synthesis of anorexia nervosa research. *Journal of Child and Family Studies, 26*(1), 1–13. https://doi.org/10.1007/s10826-016-0534-2

Westmoreland, P., Krantz, M., & Mehler, P. (2016). Medical complications of anorexia nervosa and bulimia. *American Journal of Medicine, 129*(1), 30–37. https://doi.org/1016/j.amjmed.2015.06.031

Wolfe, B., Dunne, J., & Kells, M. (2016). Nursing care considerations for the hospitalized patient with an eating disorder. *Nursing Clinics, 51*(2), 213–235. https://doi.org/10.1016/j.cnur.2016.01.006

Chapter 12

Elimination disorders

Just the facts

In this chapter, you'll learn about:

♦ encopresis, a stool elimination disorder

♦ enuresis, a urine elimination disorder

♦ diagnosis, treatment, and nursing interventions for patients with encopresis or enuresis.

A look at elimination disorders

Before reviewing elimination disorders, it is important to understand developmentally appropriate elimination, including both bowel and bladder continence. Achieving bowel and bladder continence, through toilet training, is considered a developmental milestone according to the American Academy of Pediatrics (Wolraich, 2016). However, children's progress, success, and timeline in achieving this expectation may vary based on both physiologic and psychosocial factors. Physiologic factors that could impact both bowel and bladder continence include anatomic abnormalities and issues with normal urine flow through the kidneys and bladder, recurrent urinary tract infections (UTIs), and poor or low-fiber diets (Gaither et al., 2018; Korczak et al., 2017; Shaikh et al., 2016). Psychosocial factors that may predispose children to bowel and/or bladder dysfunction include stressful or traumatic life events, particularly sexual or physical abuse, difficult temperament and emotional or behavioral problems, and academic impairment (Join-son et al., 2019b; Martins et al., 2016; Philips et al., 2015).

The American Academy of Pediatrics recommends the process of toilet training begin when the child is developmentally ready or shows signs of readiness, such as the ability to ambulate to the toilet, stability when sitting on the toilet, the ability to remain dry for several hours, receptive and expressive language skills, ability to imitate behaviors, expression of interest in toilet training, and the desire for independence (Kaerts et al., 2012). Typically, parents or guardians can begin to consider toilet training at 12 months of age, with most children completing toilet training by 36 months of age (Greer et al., 2016). Nonetheless, children who may struggle with achieving bowel and bladder incontinence, or who alternatively may succeed and then "lose" their ability, may present with an elimination disorder, including encopresis or enuresis.

Typically, encopresis and enuresis are thought of as childhood disorders, as many children's symptoms will resolve with appropriate treatment. Some adults may continue to experience symptoms of encopresis and enuresis, although this is more common in individuals with intellectual or neurodevelopmental disorders. Although the disorders are fairly common in children and adolescents, it is still critical to assess for not only medical or physiologic causes to the symptoms, but also psychosocial precipitating factors, including history of abuse and/or trauma. These disorders may be voluntary or involuntary and can coexist or may occur separately.

Parents or guardians of children diagnosed with an elimination disorder may experience significant stress in managing these symptoms. Additionally, parental factors may influence symptoms and the risk for disorder development, including maternal history of anxiety and highly controlling parenting styles (Kessel et al., 2017). Further, without the provision of adequate patient education, some parents or guardians may not understand that symptoms comprise a psychiatric disorder, subsequently may believe symptoms are intentional or behavioral, and may implement punitive interventions or punishment when their child is incontinent of bowel or bladder. When parents or guardians punish children for their symptoms of elimination disorders, children are less likely to have an improvement in symptoms.

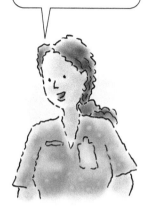

"Encopresis is one type of elimination disorder that involves inappropriate passage and elimination of stool."

Encopresis

Encopresis is one type of elimination disorder that involves inappropriate passage and elimination of stool. According to the *Diagnostic and Statistical Manual of Mental Disorders*, 5th Edition (*DSM-5*), diagnostic criteria encompass repeated passages of stool in inappropriate places, whether involuntarily or intentionally (American Psychiatric Association [APA], 2013). The child must be at least 4 years old and have inappropriate stooling events monthly over a 3-month period (APA, 2013). This disorder can occur with constipation and overflow incontinence, where there is evidence of constipation based on history or physical examination, and without constipation and overflow incontinence, where there is no evidence of constipation based on history or physical examination.

Characteristics of the disorder will vary on the basis of a presentation with or without constipation. Children who present with encopresis with constipation and overflow incontinence often have poorly formed stool that leaks either infrequently or continuously. Constipation can occur due to an organic cause (structural issues, poor diet), but can also occur due to psychosocial factors, such as anxiety or pain with bowel movements, that ultimately result in the child retaining stool. The stool can then become impacted and hard in texture, resulting in "overflow," or the leaking of poorly formed stool around the impaction. Typically, these children may present with high degrees of anxiety, and often this underlying anxiety requires treatment. Those with constipation and overflow incontinence are often thought to present with involuntary symptoms.

Alternatively, those who present without constipation and overflow incontinence are more likely to present with intentional symptoms. Stool is likely to be of typical consistency, and episodes occur intermittently rather than continuously. These children may present with comorbid oppositional defiant disorder or conduct disorder, and these underlying disorders must be treated and addressed. This subtype of encopresis is much less common than those who present with constipation.

Primary encopresis occurs when an individual has never established bowel incontinence, whereas secondary encopresis occurs when symptoms develop after an established period of bowel continence. The disorder is more common in biological males than females (Olaru et al., 2016), and rates will vary based on developmental age, with 1.5% of children between the ages of 5 and 8 years meeting diagnostic criteria for encopresis (Rijlaarsdam et al., 2015).

Causes

The cause of encopresis will vary based on the presence or absence of constipation and overflow incontinence. For individuals with encopresis with constipation and overflow incontinence, it is critical to understand the pathophysiology of constipation. Poor or slow intestinal motility can lead to constipation, as can dehydration and a low-fiber diet. Immune dysfunction and inflammation, in addition to alterations in microflora, may also lead to constipation and subsequent symptoms of encopresis (Drossman, 2016). Anatomic abnormalities that may reduce rectal sensitivity may also lead to constipation; those who lack sensitivity to stool may require a large volume of stool to trigger a sensation that a bowel movement is imminent and may also be predisposed to constipation (Vuletic, 2017). A history of painful bowel movements or anxiety surrounding bowel incontinence may also lead to constipation, as the child may retain stool.

For those with encopresis without constipation and overflow incontinence, causative factors and pathophysiology are not as well understood. Issues with discipline, behavioral issues, and mental health disorders such as oppositional defiant disorder and conduct disorder may lead to intentional defecation in inappropriate places.

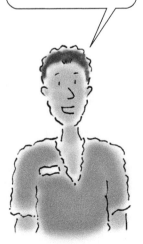

"A history of painful bowel movements or anxiety surrounding bowel incontinence may also lead to constipation, as the child may retain stool."

Finally, in both encopresis with and without constipation and overflow incontinence, it is critical to assess for the potential that significant trauma or abuse is a causative agent. This is particularly true for children with secondary encopresis, who had previously been successful with bowel continence. It has been documented that the prevalence of stressful life events, including childhood physical and sexual abuse, is higher in those with encopresis compared to their healthy peers (Philips et al., 2015). It is recommended that trauma is included within differential diagnoses in children who present with encopresis, and further evaluation is certainly warranted (Adams et al., 2018).

Risk factors

Risk factors for encopresis are usually similar to the causative agents:
- Constipation
- Painful passage of stool
- Dehydration
- Anxiety
- Oppositional defiant disorder or conduct disorder
- History of physical or sexual abuse
- High levels of parental anxiety.

Signs and symptoms

Common signs and symptoms of encopresis include:
- Passage of feces in inappropriate places (e.g., a closet, into clothing)
- May be voluntary or involuntary
  - Symptoms, subsequently, may or may not include symptoms of constipation (abdominal pain or distension, continuous leakage of stool, hesitation or refusal to use the toilet).

Additionally, children may present with comorbid mental health symptoms, such as anxiety, and/or mental health disorders such as oppositional or defiant behavior.

Diagnosis

Diagnosing a patient with encopresis is based on a comprehensive history. The diagnosis is confirmed if the patient meets the criteria for the disorder defined in the *DSM-5*.

Physical examination findings will be helpful in distinguishing if the disorder is occurring with or without constipation and overflow incontinence. Assess for potential causes of constipation and for the presence of hypothyroidism. An abdominal examination is needed, assessing for abdominal distension and pain, in addition to the quality and quantity of bowel sounds. A neurologic examination may be warranted. Finally, a rectal examination may confirm hard stool in the rectal vault and can assess rectal tone. Imaging studies may be beneficial, for example, an X-ray of the kidneys, ureters, and bladder or plain radiographs of the abdomen, to assess for the presence of excessive stool in the colon or for fecal impaction (Allen & Lawrence, 2019; Xinias & Mavroudi, 2015).

Treatment

Effective treatment requires a collaboration between health care providers, parents, and the child. Patient and parent education is paramount, and it is critical that parents or guardians understand that soiling represents a physiologic or psychological symptom; thus, punishment or scolding is not encouraged. Behavioral interventions are also recommended to address pain and stool withholding. The child should be encouraged to sit on the toilet in regular, scheduled intervals, typically after a meal, for up to 10 minutes approximately three times a day. This procedure should occur at a consistent time per day and should be followed even in times of transition, such as vacations, weekends, or special occasions. It may be helpful for parents or guardians to provide children with a foot stool or rest for support—this position can assist in raising the knees above hip level and can subsequently relax the pelvic floor and promote defecation. It is also helpful for parents or guardians to monitor bowel movements via a diary or log. Monitoring should include number of bowel movements and characteristics of such, the use of medications, episodes of fecal incontinence, periods of abdominal pain, and dietary characteristics.

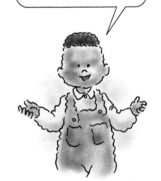

"Today is a big day for me. I'm wearing training pants and my parents took me to the bathroom and helped me sit on the toilet seat!"

Another behavioral intervention that may be beneficial is a reward system or token economy. Children can be rewarded for their effort (sitting on the toilet, attempting to have a bowel movement), rather than for their success. Rewards should be developmentally appropriate and inexpensive.

Dietary interventions such as increases in fiber and fluid intake, the avoidance or elimination of cow's milk, and probiotic supplementation may also be a worthwhile and prudent trial. Monitoring of symptoms should occur when dietary interventions are implemented.

Psychotherapy may be helpful for children who have an underlying or comorbid psychiatric disorder, such as anxiety, oppositional defiant disorder, or conduct disorder. Psychotherapy can be individualized and occur between a child and a therapist, or can be family-based through which parents and guardians are involved in the therapeutic intervention.

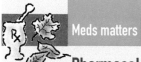

Pharmacologic therapy for encopresis

This chart highlights medications used to treat encopresis.

Drug class	Adverse effects	Contraindications	Nursing considerations
Osmotic laxative • Polyethylene glycol (Miralax, Glycolax, Restoralax) • Magnesium hydroxide (milk of magnesia) • Lactulose	• Bloating • Diarrhea • Dehydration • Electrolyte abnormalities	• Hypersensitivity to medication formulation • Known or suspected bowel obstruction	• Monitor for diarrhea or loose stool • Encourage adequate fluid intake and hydration status • Monitor for signs and symptoms of electrolyte abnormalities
Lubricant laxative • Mineral oil	• Abdominal cramps • Nausea • Diarrhea • Oily rectal leakage	• Children less than 6 years • Pregnancy • Use longer than 1 week • Difficulty swallowing	• Monitor for diarrhea or loose stool • Encourage adequate fluid intake and hydration status • Monitor for signs and symptoms of electrolyte abnormalities
Stimulant laxative • Senna • Bisacodyl	• Abdominal cramps • Diarrhea • Nausea • Vomiting • Electrolyte disturbances	• No documented contraindications	• Monitor for diarrhea or loose stool • Encourage adequate fluid intake and hydration status • Monitor for signs and symptoms of electrolyte abnormalities
Stool softeners • Docusate (Colace)	• Diarrhea • Nausea • Vomiting	• Use for longer than 7 days • Concomitant use with mineral oil	• Monitor for diarrhea or loose stool • Encourage adequate fluid intake and hydration status • Monitor for signs and symptoms of electrolyte abnormalities
Other pharmacologic agents • Linaclotide (Linzess) • Lubiprostone (Amitiza)	• Diarrhea • Nausea • Headache • Abdominal pain • Flatulence • Dehydration	• Pediatric patients younger than 6 years of age (for linaclotide) • Known or suspected gastrointestinal obstruction	• Monitor for diarrhea or loose stool • Encourage adequate fluid intake and hydration status • Monitor for signs and symptoms of electrolyte abnormalities

Pharmacologic treatment

There are no current Food and Drug Administration (FDA)-approved medications to treat encopresis. Pharmacologic treatment for encopresis primarily seeks to resolve constipation and overflow incontinence. This can be accomplished via oral medications or medications that are administered via a rectal route, such as suppositories or enemas. These include laxatives, stool softeners, and other, newer pharmacologic agents such as linaclotide (Linzess) or lubiprostone (Amitiza). As with nonpharmacologic interventions, underlying or comorbid psychiatric disorders should also be addressed as indicated.

Nursing interventions

These nursing interventions may be appropriate for patients with encopresis.

- Provide parent or guardian education on the importance of scheduled, routine periods where the child should sit on the toilet and attempt to have a bowel movement. It is helpful if this occurs shortly after a meal.
- Monitor fluid intake and hydration status. Dehydration not only can lead to constipation, but can also be a side effect of treatment.
- Encourage adequate dietary fiber intake.
- Parents or guardians and children should be educated on stress management techniques.
- Parents or guardians may have to coordinate with others (school nurses, teachers, daycare attendants, coaches) to ensure that bowel retraining expectations are upheld, even while the child is not at home or in the presence of a parent or guardian.

Enuresis

Like encopresis, enuresis is frequently considered a childhood disorder; however, it is critical to note that older adults may be impacted by new-onset enuresis. Enuresis involves inappropriate elimination of urine, and symptoms include repeated voiding of urine in inappropriate places. According to the *DSM-5*, diagnostic criteria include repeated voiding of urine in bed or clothes, which can be intentional or involuntary (APA, 2013). The child must be at least 5 years old, with episodes of inappropriate urination occurring at least twice per week over a period of 3 months. Enuresis can be nocturnal, diurnal, or a combination. Nocturnal enuresis describes voiding that only occurs at night. Diurnal enuresis describes voiding during the day. A combination enuresis pattern occurs during the day and night.

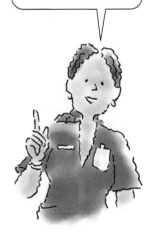

"Enuresis can be nocturnal, diurnal, or a combination."

Occasionally, symptoms begin concurrently with UTIs, but can persist after infection has resolved.

Nocturnal enuresis is the most common subtype of enuresis. Typically, voiding occurs in the first third of sleep, during rapid eye movement (REM) sleep, and may accompany a dream in which the child reports they dreamt they were voiding.

Although diurnal enuresis is less common, there are still key distinguishable characteristics. Typically, children with diurnal enuresis will delay voiding until incontinence eventually occurs and often report anxiety or intense focus on play or activities as a reason for voiding avoidance. Like encopresis, diurnal enuresis can be associated with high rates of oppositional behavior, including oppositional defiant disorder.

Recently, nocturnal enuresis has been found to be as high as over 9%, and it is more common in males than females (Sarici et al., 2016). Diurnal incontinence, however, is more common in females. The *DSM-5* also notes that rates decrease with age, with prevalence of enuresis as high as 10% in 5-year-old children and is reduced to 1% in those older than 15 years (APA, 2013).

Similar to encopresis, primary enuresis occurs when a child fails to gain urinary continence as developmentally appropriate, whereas secondary enuresis occurs when symptoms develop after an established period of continence was achieved.

Causes

There are a variety of causative or predictive factors for the development of enuresis, which include both physiologic or biological variables and psychosocial variables. In adults, sleep disorders such as obstructive sleep apnea may accompany nocturnal enuresis (Koo et al., 2016). In children, as well, sleep disorders or issues may accompany nocturnal enuresis, including bedtime resistance, sleep duration disorder, night awakening, sleep anxiety, sleep-disordered breathing, and daytime sleepiness (Ma et al., 2018). Family history is another strong risk factor, as there is a known genetic association in regard to enuresis. The *DSM-5* notes that heritability has been established, and another recent study found that a history of maternal enuresis was associated with a fourfold increase in risk for enuresis in offspring (APA, 2013; Joinson et al., 2019a).

Psychosocial factors have also been found to contribute to the development of enuresis. Various studies have supported increased stress, whether familial or individual, as a contributing factor toward the development of enuresis as well as behavioral and emotional symptoms (Joinson et al., 2016, 2019a; Vasconcelos et al., 2017).

Impaired global functioning, depression, anxiety, and attention-deficit hyperactivity disorder (ADHD) may also precede enuresis (Kessel et al., 2017). Children who are refugees are also at risk for enuresis (Jurković et al., 2019), although this could be mediated through stress.

Risk factors

Like encopresis, risk factors for enuresis frequently mirror causative or precipitating agents.

Risk factors for enuresis include:
- History of UTIs, particularly recurrent UTIs
- Psychiatric disorders, including depression, anxiety, and ADHD
- Developmental delays, including autism spectrum disorder
- Sleep disorders, particularly REM sleep disorders
- Positive family history of enuresis.

Signs and symptoms

Common signs and symptoms of enuresis include:
- "Bedwetting," often at night
- Avoidance of urination throughout the day, either due to anxiety or intense focus on play or activities.

Diagnosis

Diagnosing a patient with enuresis is based on a comprehensive history. The diagnosis is confirmed if the patient meets the criteria for the disorder defined within the *DSM-5*.

Physical examination is required to determine if the incontinence is related to an underlying medical condition. An abdominal examination and genitourinary examination should be conducted. Palpation of the bladder and percussion of the kidneys may also be helpful to determine physiologic abnormalities. Laboratory studies that may be beneficial include urinalysis and culture to assess for current UTI.

> "Physical examination is required to determine if the incontinence is related to an underlying medical condition."

Treatment

Effective treatment includes collaboration between health care providers, patients, and families. Behavioral interventions or modifications are frequently used with success for both nocturnal and diurnal enuresis.

Diurnal enuresis

For diurnal enuresis, it is critical to address any underlying comorbidities, including oppositional defiant disorder, ADHD, or mood disorders, with specific interventions for the comorbid disorder. Behavioral rehearsal is recommended as a nonpharmacologic intervention to treat diurnal enuresis (Thurber, 2017). This consists of assisting the child in "practicing" appropriate voiding. The child should be instructed and observed as they repeatedly attempt to void in the toilet, and positive reinforcement should be provided thereafter. Overcorrecting interventions may also be helpful, and parents should work to ensure that children are involved in the "cleaning-up" aspect of inappropriate voiding, including laundering clothes, cleaning the urine, as developmentally appropriate (Thurber, 2017).

Nocturnal enuresis

Interventions may differ for nocturnal enuresis. Conditioning therapy with a bell-pad alarm remains a first-line intervention for children struggling with nocturnal enuresis (Raj, 2016; Thurber, 2017). Essentially, this apparatus uses an electrical current to connect a bell with a pad. The child sleeps on the pad, and when voiding occurs, the moisture stimulates an electrical current that runs from the pad to the bell, resulting in the bell "alarming." This typically will awaken the child. Similar systems have been developed to place electrodes or sensors near the child's urinary meatus, which will alarm when urination occurs. Over time, conditioning occurs so that the child awakens on their own prior to voiding and can appropriately void with success. Other techniques include planned, scheduled awakenings throughout the night (approximately every 5 hours) that allow the child to void appropriately. Fluids should certainly be reduced or restricted in the hours prior to bedtime. Additionally, overnight diapers or pull-ups should be avoided. Use of such interventions will desensitize the child to the voiding sensation, as they are absorbent and the child will not feel "wet." Such an intervention, while perhaps convenient to the child and family, can actually result in prolonged symptoms and difficulty responding to treatment in the future.

Finally, as mentioned earlier in the chapter, encopresis and enuresis can co-occur. Children should be assessed for the presence of constipation, and appropriate interventions should be implemented as needed.

> "Two medications are commonly used in the treatment of nocturnal enuresis: desmopressin (DDAVP), a vasopressin analog, and imipramine (Tofranil), a tricyclic antidepressant."

Pharmacologic treatment

Two medications are commonly used in the treatment of nocturnal enuresis: desmopressin (DDAVP), a vasopressin analog, and imipramine (Tofranil), a tricyclic antidepressant. Desmopressin is a vasopressin, or antidiuretic hormone, analog. Antidiuretic hormone functions through the hypothalamic-pituitary

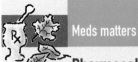

Pharmacologic therapy for enuresis

This chart highlights FDA-approved drugs used to treat enuresis.

Drug	Adverse effects	Contraindications	Nursing considerations
Vasopressin analog			
Desmopressin (DDAVP)	• Hyponatremia • Dry mouth • Hypertension • Headache • Dizziness	• Known hypersensitivity to desmopressin • Hyponatremia or history of hyponatremia • Renal impairment (creatinine clearance < 50 mL/minute)	• Monitor for hyponatremia • Can offer oral mouth spray to combat dry mouth • Should closely monitor blood pressure
Tricyclic antidepressant			
Imipramine (Tofranil)	• Cardiac arrhythmia (prolonged QTc interval) • Sedation, fatigue, dizziness, weakness • Anxiety, nervousness, restlessness • Sexual dysfunction, sweating • Dry mouth, constipation, blurred vision, urinary retention • Heartburn • Headache • Weight gain • Hypotension • Seizures	• Hypersensitivity to imipramine • Recovery period after myocardial infarction • Use of monoamine oxidase inhibitors within 14 days	• Antidepressants are associated with an FDA Black Box Warning for increased risk of suicidal thinking in children, adolescents, and young adults with major depressive disorder. Nurses must assess for the presence of mood symptoms and implement safety planning as needed • Monitor closely for symptoms of cardiac arrhythmia, including heart palpitations, dizziness, syncope • Must monitor for orthostatic hypotension and provide patient education to stand from a seated or reclined position slowly and carefully • Can utilize eye drops for blurred vision and mouth spray for dry mouth

axis to increase water reabsorption from nephron tubules. In increasing water reabsorption, urinary volume and frequency are reduced, which can improve symptoms of enuresis.

Imipramine is a tricyclic antidepressant that is used for nocturnal enuresis. This medication not only decreases the amount of time in REM sleep, but also stimulates vasopressin, or antidiuretic hormone, secretion. Imipramine is used after behavioral interventions and/or desmopressin fails.

Occasionally, anticholinergic medications, such as oxybutynin (Ditropan), are utilized. Anticholinergic medications have not been found effective in treating nocturnal enuresis alone, but may be beneficial for those who have nocturnal and diurnal enuresis in reducing daytime incontinence (Raj, 2016).

Nursing interventions

These nursing interventions may be appropriate for patients with enuresis:

- Nurses should encourage behavioral modifications, as outlined earlier, to both parents or guardians and children. This includes the bell-pad alarm and overcorrection techniques, such as encouraging the child to launder his/her own clothes or to assist with cleaning up urination.
- Nurses should encourage that fluid intake is restricted or minimized in the hours prior to bed.
- Parents or guardians and children should be educated on stress management techniques.
- Parents or guardians may have to coordinate with others (school nurses, teachers, daycare attendants, coaches) to ensure that voiding expectations are upheld, even while the child is not at home or in the presence of a parent or guardian.
- Children with nocturnal enuresis may wish to spend the night at a friend's house, at an overnight camp, etc. Parents or guardians may have to coordinate with other adults to ensure symptoms are appropriately managed. This includes minimizing fluid intake in the hours prior to bedtime and potentially planning for scheduled nighttime awakenings when voiding could occur.

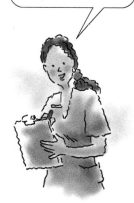

"Nurses should encourage that fluid intake is restricted or minimized in the hours prior to bed."

Quick quiz

1. How will the nurse document encopresis the started after a child had already developed bowel continence?
- A. Primary encopresis.
- B. Constipation.
- C. Secondary encopresis.
- D. Inconsistent encopresis.

Answer: C. Secondary encopresis occurs after a child has already demonstrated bowel continence.

2. What assessment data will the nurse anticipate in a child diagnosed with encopresis with constipation and overflow incontinence? Select all that apply.
    A. Leaking of stool
    B. Normal stool consistency
    C. Anxiety
    D. Intermittent symptoms
    E. Comorbid mental health disorder

Answer: A, C. Children who present with encopresis with constipation and overflow incontinence often have poorly formed stool that leaks either infrequently or continuously. The stool is often hard in texture and can lead to impaction, allowing stool to leak around the impaction. Passing stool can be painful and is associated with high anxiety in the child.

3. Which parental action for a child with nocturnal enuresis requires additional nursing education?
    A. Placing a moisture alarm on the bed.
    B. Putting a pull-up on the child before bed.
    C. Restricting fluids after dinner.
    D. Waking the child at night to void.

Answer: B. Parents should avoid the use of diapers or pull-ups for a child with nocturnal diuresis as they are designed to keep the child from feeling wet. This can desensitize the child to voiding sensation as they do not feel wet when they void. This action requires additional nursing education.

4. What behavior will the nurse anticipate with a child who has diurnal enuresis? Select all that apply.
    A. Periods of diarrhea
    B. Incontinence during the day
    C. Delay of voiding
    D. Intense focus during playtime
    E. Frequent nightmares

Answers: B, C, D. Although diurnal enuresis is less common, there are still key distinguishable characteristics. Typically, children **with diurnal enuresis** will delay voiding until incontinence eventually occurs and often report anxiety or intense focus on play or activities as a reason for voiding avoidance.

Scoring

⭐⭐⭐ If you answered all four items correctly, superb! Your knowledge of elimination is "moving!"

⭐⭐ If you answered three items correctly, well done! You're obviously moving forward with elimination disorders.

⭐ If you answered fewer than three items correctly, don't despair! You have plenty of time to move through the material in this *Incredibly Easy* resource!

Selected references

Adams, J. A., Farst, K. J., & Kellogg, N. D. (2018). Interpretation of medical findings in suspected child sexual abuse: An update for 2018. *Journal of Pediatric and Adolescent Gynecology, 31*(3), 225–231.

Allen, P., & Lawrence, V. N. (2019). Pediatric Functional Constipation. In *StatPearls* [Internet]. StatPearls Publishing.

American Psychiatric Association. (2013). *Diagnostic and statistical manual of mental disorders* (5th ed.). Author.

Drossman, D. A. (2016). Functional gastrointestinal disorders: History, pathophysiology, clinical features, and Rome IV. *Gastroenterology, 150*(6), 1262–1279.

Gaither, T. W., Cooper, C. S., Kornberg, Z., Baskin, L. S., & Copp, H. L. (2018). Risk factors for the development of bladder and bowel dysfunction. *Pediatrics, 141*(1), e20172797.

Greer, B. D., Neidert, P. L., & Dozier, C. L. (2016). A component analysis of toilet-training procedures recommended for young children. *Journal of Applied Behavior Analysis, 49*(1), 69–84.

Joinson, C., Grzeda, M. T., von Gontard, A., & Heron, J. (2019a). A prospective cohort study of biopsychosocial factors associated with childhood urinary incontinence. *European Child & Adolescent Psychiatry, 28*(1), 123–130.

Joinson, C., Grzeda, M. T., von Gontard, A., & Heron, J. (2019b). Psychosocial risks for constipation and soiling in primary school children. *European Child & Adolescent Psychiatry, 28*(2), 203–210.

Joinson, C., Sullivan, S., von Gontard, A., & Heron, J. (2016). Stressful events in early childhood and developmental trajectories of bedwetting at school age. *Journal of Pediatric Psychology, 41*(9), 1002–1010.

Jurković, M., Tomašković, I., Tomašković, M., Smital Zore, B., Pavić, I., & Roić, A. C. (2019). Refugee status as a possible risk factor for childhood enuresis. *International Journal of Environmental Research and Public Health, 16*(7), 1293.

Kaerts, N., Van Hal, G., Vermandel, A., & Wyndaele, J. J. (2012). Readiness signs used to define the proper moment to start toilet training: A review of the literature. *Neurourology and Urodynamics, 31*(4), 437–440.

Kessel, E. M., Allmann, A. E., Goldstein, B. L., Finsaas, M., Dougherty, L. R., Bufferd, S. J., Carlson, G. A., & Klein, D. N. (2017). Predictors and outcomes of childhood primary enuresis. *Journal of the American Academy of Child & Adolescent Psychiatry, 56*(3), 250–257.

Koo, P., McCool, F. D., Hale, L., Stone, K., & Eaton, C. B. (2016). Association of obstructive sleep apnea risk factors with nocturnal enuresis in postmenopausal women. *Menopause, 23*(2), 175.

Korczak, R., Kamil, A., Fleige, L., Donovan, S. M., & Slavin, J. L. (2017). Dietary fiber and digestive health in children. *Nutrition Reviews, 75*(4), 241–259.

Ma, J., Li, S., Jiang, F., Jin, X., Zhang, Y., Yan, C., Tian, Y., Shen, X., & Li, F. (2018). Relationship between sleep patterns, sleep problems, and childhood enuresis. *Sleep Medicine, 50*, 14–20.

Martins, G., Minuk, J., Varghese, A., Dave, S., Williams, K., & Farhat, W. A. (2016). Non biological determinants of paediatric bladder bowel dysfunction: A pilot study. *Journal of Pediatric Urology, 12*(2), 109.e1–e6.

Olaru, C., Diaconescu, S., Trandafir, L., Gimiga, N., Olaru, R. A., Stefanescu, G., Ciubotariu, G., Burlea, M., & Iorga, M. (2016). Chronic functional constipation and encopresis in children in relationship with the psychosocial environment. *Gastroenterology Research and Practice, 2016*, 7828576.

Philips, E. M., Peeters, B., Teeuw, A. H., Leenders, A. G., Boluyt, N., Brillesljiper-Kater, S. N., & Benninga, M. A. (2015). Stressful life events in children with functional defecation disorders. *Journal of Pediatric Gastroenterology and Nutrition, 61*(4), 384–392.

Raj, V. M. S. (2016). Review in enuresis. *ARC Journal of Pediatrics, 2*(1), 9–16.

Rijlaarsdam, J., Stevens, G. W., van der Ende, J., Hofman, A., Jaddoe, V. W., Verhulst, F. C., & Tiemeier, H. (2015). Prevalence of DSM-IV disorders in a population-based sample of 5-to 8-year-old children: The impact of impairment criteria. *European Child & Adolescent Psychiatry, 24*(11), 1339–1348.

Rostion, C. G., Galaz, M. I., Contador, M., Aldunate, M., Benavides, S., & Harz, C. (2016). Helpfulness of rectoanal endosonography in diagnosis of sexual abuse in a child. *Journal of Pediatric Surgery, 51*(7), 1151–1161.

Sarici, H., Telli, O., Ozgur, B. C., Demirbas, A., Ozgur, S., & Karagoz, M. A. (2016). Prevalence of nocturnal enuresis and its influence on quality of life in school-aged children. *Journal of Pediatric Urology, 12*(3), 159.e1–e6.

Shaikh, N., Hoberman, A., Keren, R., Gotman, N., Docimo, S. G., Mathews, R., Bhatnagar, S., Ivanova, A., Mattoo, T. K., Moxey-Mims, M., Carpenter, M. A., Pohl, H. G., & Greenfield, S. (2016). Recurrent urinary tract infections in children with bladder and bowel dysfunction. *Pediatrics, 137*(1), e20191071.

Thurber, S. (2017). Childhood enuresis: Current diagnostic formulations, salient findings, and effective treatment modalities. *Archives of Psychiatric Nursing, 31*(3), 319–323.

Vasconcelos, M. M., East, P., Blanco, E., Lukacz, E. S., Caballero, G., Lozoff, B., & Gahagan, S. (2017). Early behavioral risks of childhood and adolescent daytime urinary incontinence and nocturnal enuresis. *Journal of Developmental and Behavioral Pediatrics, 38*(9), 736–742.

Vuletic, B. (2017). Encopresis in children: An overview of recent findings. *Serbian Journal of Experimental and Clinical Research, 18*(2), 157–161.

Wolraich, M. (2016). *Guide to toilet training* (2nd ed.). American Academy of Pediatrics.

Xinias, I., & Mavroudi, A. (2015). Constipation in Childhood. An update on evaluation and management. *Hippokratia, 19*(1), 11.

Chapter 13

Sleep-wake disorders

Just the facts

In this chapter, you'll learn:

♦ sleep stages and circadian rhythms

♦ types of sleep disorders and their causesis

♦ assessment findings in patients with sleep disorders

♦ special procedures used to diagnose sleep disorders

♦ treatments and nursing interventions for patients with sleep disorders.

A look at sleep disorders

Sleep is a natural state of rest during which muscle movement and awareness of surroundings diminish. Sleep is essential to restore energy, to maintain physical and mental well-being, and allows us to function optimally (Garside et al., 2018). Unlike other states resembling sleep (such as coma), sleep is easily interrupted—or prevented—by both external and internal stimuli. External stimuli include light, noise, or an uncomfortable sleep environment. Internal factors, such as stress and anxiety, can impair an individual's ability to achieve quality of sleep (Watson et al., 2015).

It has been estimated that 35.2% of adults in the United States experience chronic sleeping problems (Centers for Disease Control and Prevention [CDC], 2018b). Nearly one-third of patients seen in primary care settings report occasional sleep difficulties (CDC, 2018b). Quality sleep is recognized as a priority in national health as indicated in the goals in Healthy People 2020. This chapter discusses major sleep disorders—breathing-related sleep disorders, circadian rhythm sleep disorders, narcolepsy, hypersomnolence, and insomnia.

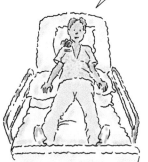

All of this research on sleep disorders is making me sleepy.

Causes

Sleep disorders may be acute or chronic, occurring primary or secondary to a medical or mental health disorder, substance misuse, or environmental factors. Various medical conditions can cause sleep disorders including chronic pain, neurodegenerative disorders such as Parkinson disease and Huntington disease, viral encephalitis, thyroid disease, and hormonal imbalances (Potter et al., 2016).

Mental health disorders, including depression, anxiety, and schizophrenia, are the most common causes of chronic insomnia. High levels of stress also may contribute to sleep disorders (Cox & Olatunji, 2016).

Substances that can disrupt sleep include alcohol, caffeine, and prescription medications—most notably, antihistamines, corticosteroids, and central nervous system (CNS) stimulants (Potter et al., 2016).

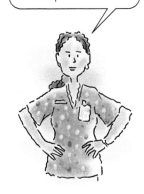

High levels of stress may contribute to sleep disorders.

Impact of sleep disorders

Sleep disorders can lead to sleep deprivation, which can seriously interfere with a person's overall functioning, including impairment in one's family life, occupation, driving ability, and social activities. Medical costs related to sleep disorders amount to at least $63 billion annually—with indirect costs incurred from such factors as lost productivity (CDC, 2018b; Hafner et al., 2017; Potter et al., 2016).

Chronic sleep deprivation can cause or contribute to accidents, social and marital disruption, and cause or worsen psychiatric disturbances. It is also an independent risk factor for cardiovascular and gastrointestinal (GI) disorders (Hafner et al., 2017; Potter et al., 2016).

Driving while drowsy

Sleepy drivers and sleepy heavy equipment operators are the cause of many accidents. Experts believe that sleepy drivers on the road pose an even greater safety threat than intoxicated drivers. It has been estimated that up to 21% of fatal car crashes are caused by drowsy driving (CDC, 2018a; Garbarino et al., 2017).

Someone who isn't well rested in the workplace is unable to perform at their best. Poor work performance can lead to workplace errors or accidents, resulting in corrective action and even job dismissal.

Dangerous deprivation

Sleep-deprived health care professionals are more likely to use poor judgment and make potentially life-threatening mistakes. Sleep-deprived factory workers may cause injury to themselves or others as well as contribute to the manufacture of defective products (CDC, 2018a). Multiple major environmental incidents have been linked to lack of sleep, including the near-nuclear disaster of Three Mile Island in 1979, the nuclear meltdown at Chernobyl in 1986, and the oil spill of Exxon Valdez in 1989.

Fuel for family feuds

Research supports that someone who doesn't sleep well is more likely to feel tense, unhappy, lonely, and more socially disconnected (Chu et al., 2019). These feelings can compromise healthy interpersonal relationships.

Sleep disturbances can also have a direct impact on other family members' sleep patterns. For example, snoring may awaken the patient's partner, or prevent the partner from falling asleep in the first place.

Sleep stages

Sleep occurs in five stages. With each stage, sleep becomes deeper and brain waves grow progressively larger and slower, as shown by electroencephalography (EEG). Using an EEG to identify disruptions of these stages, through evaluation of the waves, can provide information about potential sleep disorders. (See *Sleep stages and brain waves*, page 297.) Throughout sleep, a person cycles through the different stages over and over again, with the first cycle lasting approximately 100 to 120 minutes. Most people will go through five to seven cycles per night (Potter et al., 2016).

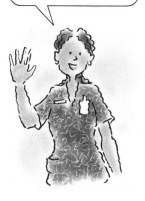

> Sleep occurs in five stages, growing progressively deeper with each stage.

Stage 1

The lightest stage of sleep, stage 1, occurs as a person falls asleep. The muscles relax and theta waves are produced that are fast and irregular. During this stage, the patient can be easily awakened by sounds, light, and other stimuli. Individuals can also experience muscle spasms or feelings of falling in this stage. Stage 1 accounts for approximately 5% of an adult's total sleep time and generally lasts around 10 to 15 minutes.

Stage 2

During stage 2, a relatively light stage of sleep but considered the first stage of non–rapid eye movement (NREM) sleep, theta waves continue but become interspersed with sleep spindles (sudden increases in wave frequency—increased waves per second) and K complexes (sudden increases in wave amplitude—increased height of waves). It is hypothesized that K complexes and sleep spindles protect the brain from awakening. Stage 2 comprises approximately 50% of total sleep time. In this stage, the heart rate slows, body temperature decreases, and the muscles relax more as the body prepares for deep sleep.

Stages 3 and 4

Stages 3 and 4 are the deepest stages of sleep. Delta waves—large, slow waves of high amplitude and low frequency—appear on the EEG. Stages 3 and 4 differ only in the percentage of delta waves seen. During stage 3, delta waves account for less than 50% of brain waves, whereas during stage 4, they account for more than 50%. Stages 3 and 4 are where sleep walking and sleep talking, also known as parasomnias, occur.

Conserve as you sleep

Arousing a sleeper from stage 3 or 4 is harder than during any other stage. Because these stages are marked by decreased body temperature and metabolism, researchers believe they function to conserve energy. They account for 10% to 20% of total sleep time. As night fades into morning, stages 3 and 4 get progressively shorter. During the last few cycles of the sleep period, no delta wave sleep occurs at all.

Stage 5

Stage 5 is a deep sleep called REM sleep. During this stage, the sleeper shows darting eye movements; muscle twitching; and short, rapid brain waves resembling those seen during the waking state. (See *Sleep stages and brain waves*, page 297.)

REM sleep usually begins about 90 minutes after sleep onset. Over the course of the night, REM periods lengthen. Overall, REM sleep accounts for 20% to 25% of total sleep time.

To sleep, perchance to dream

Most storylike dreams take place during REM sleep. People awakened from REM sleep commonly report vivid dreams. In contrast, people awakened during stages 1 through 4 rarely report vivid dreams.

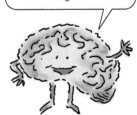

REM is my friend! Scientists think REM sleep may stimulate brain growth.

Functions of REM and NREM sleep

Scientists believe REM and NREM sleep serve different biological functions, although they don't know exactly what these functions are. REM sleep may stimulate brain growth or consolidate memory. A person deprived of REM sleep tends to have longer REM cycles during the next sleep episode. These longer REM cycles are more intense, with more eye movements per minute.

Make-up sleep

Similarly, people deprived of NREM sleep have longer NREM sleep during the next sleep period—and the "make-up" NREM sleep produces different EEG patterns than normal NREM sleep.

Sleep stages and brain waves

Each sleep stage generates distinctive brain waves, as measured by EEG.

Stage 1: Theta waves

During stage 1, which occurs as a person falls asleep, fast, irregular, low-amplitude brain waves called *theta waves* appear on the EEG.

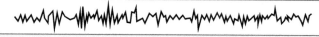

Stage 2: Theta waves with sleep spindles and K complexes

During stage 2, theta waves are interspersed with wave phenomena called *sleep spindles* and *K complexes*.

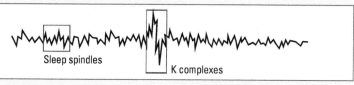

Stage 3 and 4: Delta waves

During stages 3 and 4, the EEG shows large, slow, high-amplitude waves called *delta waves*.

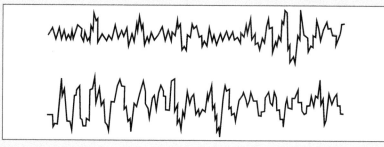

Stage 5: REM sleep

During stage 5, called *rapid eye movement (REM) sleep*, short, rapid brain waves appear.

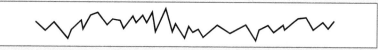

Neurologic regulation of sleep stages

The various sleep stages are influenced by different parts of the brain. REM sleep is controlled by the pons (a part of the brainstem) and adjacent portions of the midbrain. Chemical stimulation of the pons may induce long periods of REM sleep, whereas damage to the pons may reduce or prevent REM sleep.

Paralysis and the pons

During REM sleep, neurons in the pons and midbrain that control muscle tone show various levels of activity: Some are active, whereas others aren't. Reflecting this variable activity, certain body muscles remain inactive during REM sleep—especially those of the back, neck, arms, and legs. As a result, the sleeper is effectively paralyzed and can't act out dreams. However, if these regulatory neurons malfunction, the sleeper may be more active during dreams, thrashing about or becoming violent.

Baths and the basal forebrain

The basal forebrain, located in front of the hypothalamus, controls NREM sleep. Damage to this region of the brain may cause difficulty falling or staying asleep. Some neurons in the basal forebrain are activated by heat, which may explain the sleep-promoting benefits of taking a warm bath in the evening.

Factors that affect sleep

Factors that affect sleep quality and quantity include the patient's age, lifestyle, sleep environment, and medication use.

Age

Amounts and patterns of sleep differ at each major stage of the life cycle. Both REM and NREM sleep periods decrease with age.

Newborns and toddlers
Newborns sleep the most, averaging 17 to 18 hours a day; newborns do not have distinctive sleep stages until about 4 months old. Sleep is differentiated into "active," "quiet," and "indeterminate." Active sleep most resembles REM sleep, which allows for frequent awakening to feed; active sleep accounts for the majority of total infant sleep time.

Go to sleep-y, little baby
At first, a newborn sleeps in episodes of 3 to 4 hours. Gradually, by about age 3 or 4 months, the infant begins to sleep more at night and sleep stages begin to resemble adult sleep. A 6-month-old typically sleeps 12 hours a night and naps 1 to 2 hours each day. Sleep in children plays an important role in growth and brain development.

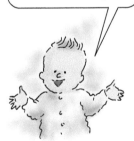

Newborns need their sleep! On average, they sleep 17 to 18 hours a day.

Toddlers sleep about 11 or 12 hours a night, with a 1- to 2-hour nap after lunch. Nap requirements vary depending on the individual child, with some children taking naps up to age 5.

By age 5, children typically sleep 10 to 12 hours a day, with REM sleep accounting for about 20% of the total.

Tweens and teens

Preadolescents need approximately 10 hours of sleep. Adolescent requirements aren't well defined. Many teenagers get too little sleep because of their busy schedules, overuse of personal electronics, and academic pressures. Growth spurts can result in an increased need for sleep (Hale et al., 2018).

Young adults

A typical young adult needs about 8 hours of sleep, although the requirement varies widely. Some young adults need as little as 6 or 7 hours, whereas others may need 9 or 10 hours to function optimally. Lifestyle choices make this group vulnerable to sleep disturbances (Dickinson et al., 2018).

Middle-aged adults

In middle-aged adults, sleep requirements may remain unchanged from those of a young adult. Typical sleep disturbances during middle age may stem from hormonal changes in women, breathing-related disorders, and insomnia.

Older adults

Sleep problems are common among older adults (Suzuki et al., 2017). Besides taking longer to fall asleep, they spend less time in deep NREM sleep, so their sleep is more easily interrupted or fragmented. (See *Sleep requirements of older adults*.)

Bathroom breaks

Early awakening is also common in older adults and may result from an earlier rise in body temperature. Finally, many older adults have trouble falling back to sleep after awakening to urinate.

Environment

Sleep environment can greatly affect sleep quality. Environmental influences on sleep include excessive noise, bright lights or sunlight, excessive activity, an uncomfortable bed, and an uncomfortable room temperature. When these influences are prominent, sleep can be difficult even for someone who is sleepy.

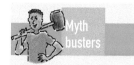

Sleep requirements of older adults

Another misconception about elderly adults bites the dust.

Myth: Older adults need less sleep than younger adults.

Reality: Sleep requirements increase in older adults because they tend to get decreased amounts of deep restorative sleep and suffer frequent sleep interruptions.

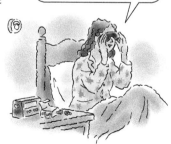

Darkness, silence, a comfortable bed, and a comfortable room temperature promote sleep.

Removing such stimuli produces an environment that's more conducive to sleeping.

Lifestyle

Travel, shift work, stress, and anxiety can greatly influence sleep. A person who travels through different time zones may suffer jet lag, which is worse when traveling west to east. A "jet-setter" typically tries to sleep when he or she isn't tired (traveling west to east) and tries to stay awake when it's daylight (traveling east to west).

Night shift blues

Over 20% of night shift workers experience problems with sleep due to disruption of the body's natural rhythms (Kerkhof, 2018).

Medications and substances

Medications of any kind have the potential to alter sleep patterns. Prescription drugs may cause somnolence (drowsiness) at inappropriate times and some may cause insomnia. Use of illicit drugs may also disturb established sleep patterns (Potter et al., 2016).

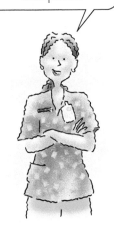

Although alcohol initially may increase the amount of slow-wave sleep, it later causes sleep disruptions.

Alcohol

Alcohol's effect on sleep varies with the amount, time, and frequency of consumption. In individuals who do not consume alcohol on a regular basis, alcohol may have a sedative effect. Alcohol increases the amount of slow-wave sleep for the first 4 hours after sleep onset. After alcohol's effects wear off, sleep may be disrupted, with an increased amount of REM sleep and anxiety-causing dreams.

Individuals with alcoholism may have trouble falling and staying asleep because of REM sleep disturbances caused by chronic heavy alcohol use.

Withdrawal woes

During alcohol withdrawal, sleep deprivation is common. When sleep occurs, it's usually fragmented and accompanied by nightmares and anxiety-causing dreams.

Approach to assessment

The most important symptoms of sleep disturbances are insomnia at night (the most common symptom) and sleepiness during waking hours. A thorough medical and psychological history should be obtained from a patient who reports sleep problems. The family may also need to be questioned because the patient may be unaware of his or her sleep behavior.

Sometimes, a physical examination is also warranted. Because sleep disorders are commonly linked to mood disorders, psychological tests may be administered as well.

Breathing-related sleep disorders

Breathing-related sleep disorders are marked by abnormal breathing during sleep that causes the sleeper to awaken at inappropriate times. Obstructive sleep apnea (OSA) is the most common breathing-related sleep disorder and occurs in up to 22% of adults (Senaratna et al., 2017). Other disorders in this category include central sleep apnea syndrome and central alveolar hypoventilation syndrome (Javaheri et al., 2017).

Breathing blockade

In OSA, the upper airway becomes blocked during sleep, impeding airflow. Reduced airway muscle tone and the pull of gravity in the supine position further limit airway size during sleep. As tissue collapse worsens, the airway may become completely obstructed. (See *Airway obstruction during sleep apnea*, page 302.)

With either partial or complete airway obstruction, the patient struggles to breathe. Blockage of airflow lasts a minimum of 10 seconds up to 1 minute and arouses the patient from sleep as the brain responds to decreased blood oxygen levels. (However, arousal is commonly partial and the patient may not recognize this brief disruption in sleep.)

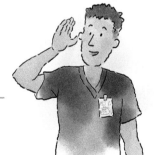

I hear a symphony … of snoring. That patient needs to be checked for sleep apnea.

Snoring, then silence

This pattern causes disturbed and fragmented sleep, with periods of loud snoring or gasping when the airway is partly open alternating with silence when the airway is blocked. (It should be noted that not everyone who snores has OSA.)

Airway obstruction during sleep apnea

In a patient with OSA, the airway is blocked by increased tissue of the soft palate or tongue, increased amounts of fat around the pharynx, or a small or receding jaw that leaves too little room for the tongue.

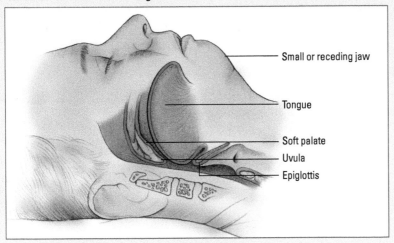

— Small or receding jaw

— Tongue

— Soft palate
— Uvula
— Epiglottis

With arousal, the muscle tone of the tongue and airway tissues increases, causing the patient to awaken just enough to tighten the upper airway muscles and open the trachea. However, when falling back to sleep, the tongue and soft tissue relax again—and the cycle begins anew. This cycle may repeat up to a hundred times in an hour, significantly impairing the individual's ability to reach all stages of sleep (Rotariu et al., 2016).

Complications

Repetitive cycles of snoring, airway collapse, and arousal may lead to increased risk for diabetes and cardiovascular problems such as hypertension, arrhythmias, myocardial infarction, or stroke. In some high-risk patients, sleep apnea may lead to sudden death from respiratory arrest during sleep (Yu et al., 2017).

Drowsy, irritable, and indifferent

Frequent awakenings leave the patient sleepy during the day and can cause irritability or mental health disorders including anxiety and depression. The patient may experience morning headaches, impaired mental functioning, and a reduced sex drive. People with severe, untreated sleep apnea have two or three times the risk of motor vehicle accidents.

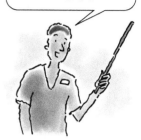

Sleep apnea is common, affecting 22% of men and 17% of women.

Prevalence

OSA affects an average of 22% of men and 17% of women. Incidence increases with age—especially after age 50. It's most common in overweight, middle-aged men but can affect females and males of any age. In women, menopause is a significant precipitating factor (Franklin & Lindberg, 2015; Rotariu et al., 2016).

Causes

Many patients with OSA are overweight with a short, thick neck and fat infiltration around the pharynx that increases the risk of airway blockage. Some have an unusually large soft palate, including large tonsils and tongue.

Apnea and anatomy

In people who aren't overweight, OSA typically results from a small upper airway, an oval-shaped airway, and a long upper airway. Other structural causes of OSA include malformations of the oropharynx or jaw and tumors and other growths that narrow the airway. Among elderly adults, loss of muscle tone may contribute to the condition (Chen et al., 2016).

Rotational forces

People with rotating work schedules may be at higher risk for OSA. The use of alcohol or sedatives may increase the frequency and length of apneic episodes.

Signs and symptoms

Patients with OSA may report chronic daytime sleepiness. Some also report snoring, which may be pronounced enough to disturb the sleep of other household members. In fact, the patient may not be aware of heavy snoring and nocturnal arousals, so the nurse may need to question family members about these symptoms (Miller & Berger, 2016).

Other symptoms in a patient with OSA include:

- awakening feeling unrested
- frequent headaches
- general feeling of tiredness and fatigue
- frequent daytime naps (which usually aren't effective in restoring energy)
- irritability
- difficulty paying attention
- learning or memory problems
- depression
- excessive urination at night
- impotence
- heartburn or acid indigestion (suggesting esophageal reflux).

Body reconnaissance

During the physical examination, stay alert for:

- obesity
- hypertension
- jaw malformation
- signs and symptoms of tumors or other tissue abnormalities
- reduced chest excursion (from obesity)
- indications of cardiovascular and cerebrovascular conditions.

Diagnosis

Polysomnography, a sleep study performed in a sleep laboratory, is the gold standard for diagnosing OSA.

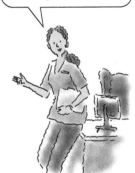

Polysomnography is a sleep study used to evaluate patients for sleep disorders.

Treatment

Treatments for OSA include lifestyle changes, continuous positive airway pressure (CPAP) therapy, and dental devices that modify tongue or jaw position.

Lifestyle changes

Lifestyle changes—especially weight loss—are the simplest treatments for OSA. Weight loss reduces the amount of excess tissue in and around the airway. Decreasing the body mass index to 30 or less significantly reduces the frequency of obstructive sleep episodes. However, even small weight reductions can improve the patient's condition.

Supine is not sublime

Sleeping on the side rather than in a supine (back-lying) position may reduce apneic episodes. Avoiding alcohol and sleeping medications can decrease the number and duration of these episodes.

Continuous positive airway pressure

CPAP therapy during sleep is the most common and effective treatment for OSA. Positive pressure helps to maintain an open airway, preventing its collapse. The desired level of pressure varies with the type and pressure setting of CPAP device used. The patient can wear either a full facial mask or a nasal mask. Proper mask fit is essential for CPAP functioning and comfort.

Dental devices

Oral appliances worn during sleep may help to relieve airway obstruction by moving the jaw forward, which creates a larger airway opening. However, they may be uncomfortable for some patients and may cause excessive salivation.

Surgery

Surgical procedures used to correct OSA include:
*   tonsil and adenoid removal to increase the size of the pharynx
*   removal of any growths or nasal polyps obstructing the airway
*   correction of jaw abnormalities
*   uvulopalatopharyngoplasty—surgical revision of the uvula, tonsils, soft palate, and soft tissues of the oropharynx.

Nursing interventions

These nursing interventions may be appropriate for a patient with OSA:
*   Remember the patient is likely to be tired and irritable. Be helpful and supportive.
*   If the patient reports associated symptoms, such as esophageal reflux, nocturia, or impotence, refer for appropriate treatment.
*   Assist the patient in a weight loss program, if indicated.
*   Advise the patient to stop smoking, if indicated.
*   Encourage the patient to avoid alcohol and illicit drug use.
*   Help family members deal with issues related to the patient's snoring.

Polysomnography: It knows when you're asleep

Polysomnography is an overnight sleep study performed in a special laboratory or a sleep center that measures various physiologic functions related to sleep and wakefulness. Sensor leads and other detectors are placed on the patient to gather the following information:

• Brain wave activity, recorded by EEG. The EEG reveals the stage of sleep that the patient is in during any given period.

• Eye movements, recorded by electrooculography (EOG). The EOG determines when the patient is experiencing REM sleep. Along with the EEG, it also helps determine how long it takes the patient to fall asleep, total sleep time, time spent in each sleep stage, and the number of arousals from sleep.

• Muscle movements, measured by electromyography (EMG). The EMG recording helps document wakeful periods, arousal, or spastic movements.

• Respiratory effort, which determines chest and abdominal excursion during breathing. Velcro bands are placed around the patient's chest and around the abdomen and connected to a transducer. The force of chest and abdominal expansion on the bands stretches the transducer and alters the signal to a recorder.

• Oxygen saturation, recorded by a pulse oximeter probe placed on the finger, earlobe, or other appropriate site, to determine oxygen levels during an apneic episode.

• Electrocardiography (ECG), which can reveal whether low oxygen saturation during apneic episodes leads to arrhythmias. The ECG also alerts the technician to any emergency condition.

• Airflow, recorded by a thermistor secured to the patient's nose. The thermistor detects the amount of air moving into and out of the airways, thus revealing apneic or hypopneic (inadequate breathing) episodes.

• Blood pressure, to detect dangerous blood pressure elevations (sometimes caused by apneic episodes).

Optional monitoring includes core body temperature, penile tumescence, and the pressure and pH at various esophageal levels. Information gathered from all the leads and sensors is fed into a computer and transformed into a series of waveform tracings.

Smile for the camera

The patient may be videotaped so the technician can determine whether any abnormal waveforms were caused by an actual arousal, a period of wakefulness, or normal movement in bed. Sound recordings may be made to evaluate snoring.

Sleep latency testing

The day after polysomnography, the patient may undergo multiple sleep latency testing (MSLT) to evaluate excessive daytime sleepiness or narcolepsy. MSLT records sleep patterns (including napping) throughout the day.

MSLT usually involves five testing periods spaced about 2 hours apart. For each testing period, the patient is taken to a "sleeping" room, where electrodes are attached to the face and scalp to record eye movements, muscle tone, and brain waves.

Then the lights are turned off and the patient is asked to sleep for 15 to 20 minutes, during which recordings are taken. The technician awakens the patient after the testing period. Even if the patient can't sleep during the test, the information can be useful. All told, MSLT takes about 8 hours.

Circadian rhythm sleep disorder

In circadian rhythm sleep disorder, the patient's internal sleep-wake pattern is out of sync with the demands of work schedule, travel requirements, or social activities. The result is insomnia and daytime sleepiness.

Tick tock, it's the body clock

The human body has an internal "clock" that follows a 24-hour cycle of wakefulness and sleepiness. This clock runs on circadian rhythms, which are linked to nature's cycle of light and darkness.

Critical organs, such as the heart, liver, and kidneys, have their own "clocks" that work in a coordinated fashion with the body's master clock located in a specific area of the brain. Researchers know, for example, that certain cardiac events, such as heart attacks and sudden cardiac death, occur more often during specific times of the circadian cycle.

Lark versus owl

The body's clock keeps us alert during daylight hours and makes us sleepy when night falls. All of our physiologic functions are geared toward being active during the day and resting at night. The desire to sleep is strongest between 12 and 6 a.m.

Nonetheless, individual patterns of alertness vary, explaining why some people are relatively more alert during the day ("larks"), whereas others are more alert at night ("night owls") and others fall somewhere in between these two tendencies.

Mighty melatonin

The body's internal clock is influenced by melatonin, a hormone that causes sleepiness. Melatonin is secreted by the pineal gland, a structure located in the roof of the brain's third ventricle. Influenced by light, the pineal gland slows melatonin production during daylight hours to promote alertness and increases production when darkness falls, causing sleepiness.

With age, the body produces less melatonin. Not surprisingly, many elderly adults suffer from sleep disorders. Some pharmacologic therapies try to increase the level of melatonin or enhance its effectiveness to try and readjust the internal clock.

Circadian lullaby

Circadian refers to the biological rhythms with a cycle of about 24 hours. (*Circadian* comes from the Latin "circa" meaning around or about, and "diem" meaning a day.) The circadian rhythm functions as the body's internal "clock," regulating the 24-hour sleep-wake cycle and other body functions, such as body temperature, hormones, and heart rate. (See *Tick tock, it's the body clock.*)

The body's internal clock can reset itself to help a person adjust to disturbances such as seasonal changes, transitions to or from daylight savings time, or the start of a new workweek. However, it can't always overcome longer lasting disruptions resulting from shift work or jet lag (air travel across time zones).

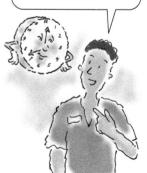

The body's internal clock governs the sleep-wake cycles and many other body functions.

Weirded-out rhythms

Disruption of circadian rhythms may cause sleep difficulties, fatigue, poor concentration, impaired cognitive abilities (such as poor judgment and decision making), and even GI disorders (Stranks & Crowe, 2016).

Types of circadian rhythm sleep-wake disorders

The main types of circadian rhythm sleep-wake disorders include the delayed sleep phase disorder, advanced sleep phase disorder, irregular sleep-wake, non–24-hour sleep-wake disorder, shift work type, and jet lag (American Psychiatric Association [APA], 2013).

Delayed sleep-wake phase disorder

In delayed sleep-wake phase disorder, the patient sleeps according to a delayed clock time, relative to the light-dark cycle and social, economic, and family demands. Typically, individuals have trouble falling asleep until the early hours of the morning and the patient ends up sleeping through much of the day. This disorder often begins in childhood and is relatively common among adolescents. These patients may consider themselves "night owls."

Advanced sleep-wake phase disorder

With advanced sleep-wake phase disorder, the patient wakes up earlier than is desired or socially acceptable. The patient will often force himself or herself to stay awake later than they would prefer but continues to wake up early. This disruption in their natural circadian rhythm results in sleep deprivation and daytime sleepiness. These patients may consider themselves "early birds or larks."

Non–24-hour sleep-wake disorder

In the non–24-hour sleep-wake pattern disorder, the patient will experience a sleep-wake cycle that does not correlate with a typical 24-hour environment. For these patients, sleep is characterized by a daily drift toward later sleep and wake times (APA, 2013). This disorder occurs frequently in blind individuals who are unable to regulate their circadian rhythm through environmental cues.

Shift work

In the shift work sleep disorder, night shift work or frequently changing work schedules cause insomnia during the major sleep period or excessive sleepiness during the major awake period. The patient typically suffers chronic sleep disruption.

Asleep on the job

Few, if any, night workers regularly get restful restorative day sleep. An estimated 10% to 20% of night workers report falling asleep on the job, usually during the second half of the shift. Twenty percent of

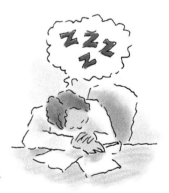

the U.S. workforce is engaged in shift work, placing them at risk for circadian rhythm disorders (Kerkhof, 2018).

Prevalence

The prevalence of circadian rhythm sleep disorders is unclear. However, there are estimates associated with night shift workers that range from 5% to 10%. Prevalence is also indicated to increase with age (APA, 2013).

Causes

Circadian rhythm sleep disorders result from either intrinsic or extrinsic factors. Intrinsic factors are those where the individual's circadian rhythm significantly deviates from societal norms. Extrinsic factors occur when the individual's circadian rhythm is in sync with light and dark cycles but lifestyle factors such as jet lag or shift work impact sleep.

Signs and symptoms

Assessment findings vary with the type of circadian rhythm sleep disorder.

Symptoms in delayed sleep phase type

Patients with delayed sleep phase may report:
- inability to fall asleep before 2 a.m. to 6 a.m.
- difficulty awakening in the morning
- feeling of being sleep deprived
- significant social or work impairment
- need for multiple means to awaken before natural awakening time (several alarm clocks, other persons, telephone wake-up calls, or a combination of these).

Symptoms in shift work type

Patients with shift work type commonly report:
- sleepiness while performing their jobs, especially if working nights
- insufficient daytime sleep because of family or social demands or environmental disturbances
- significant social or work impairment.

Diagnosis

The patient's history may suggest a circadian rhythm sleep disorder. A sleep diary or wrist-worn motion/sleep detector may be used to assist in determining a diagnosis. The diagnosis is confirmed through comparison of the history with current diagnostic criteria (APA, 2013).

Treatment

Various treatments have been used for circadian rhythm disorders.

Chronotherapy

Chronotherapy involves manipulating the patient's sleep schedule by progressively delaying or advancing bedtime by between 15 minutes each night until the patient can go to sleep and wake up at appropriate times. Chronotherapy is most commonly used to treat delayed sleep-wake phase disorders.

Light therapy

Light therapy is the use of a bright light to manipulate the circadian system. Typically administered with therapeutic light boxes, it's safe and effective when used according to recommendations.

Here comes the sun

For patients with delayed sleep phase–type sleep-wake disorder, some health care providers recommend exposure to bright light on awakening. Sunlight exposure for night shift workers or individuals traveling between time zones can help reset the circadian clock to environmental time.

The value of nursing assessment

Many times, the nurse is the first to identify that a sleep disorder may be an issue for a patient. Over time, patients become used to living in a constant state of feeling "tired." In addition, because lack of sleep isn't often recognized as a problem, patients will minimize feeling tired and chalk it up to lifestyle or life demands. When asked appropriate questions, the data emerge that can show trends in sleeping patterns.

Sleep disorder assessment questions:
1. Do you have difficulty falling asleep?
2. Do you feel well rested when you wake up?
3. Do you take medication to help you fall or stay asleep or stay awake?
4. What is your caffeine intake on a normal day?
5. Do you feel sleepy at "normal" sleep times?
6. When do you prefer to sleep and does this coincide with your work and social schedule?

Chronopharmacotherapy

Chronopharmacotherapy involves the use of drugs to induce sleep or promote wakefulness when desired. Short-acting sedative-hypnotic drugs may be used to promote sleep, especially when associated with jet lag.

Many night shift workers use caffeine to keep themselves awake on the job. However, some become tolerant to caffeine's effects over time and may require prescription medications.

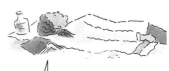

Mellowing out with melatonin

Supplemental melatonin therapy has been studied as a treatment for circadian rhythm sleep disorders. Data are limited regarding effectiveness of melatonin therapy. However, recent research into prolonged use of melatonin has shown some promise especially in children and older adults (Matheson & Hainer, 2017).

Sunlight exposure can help a night shift worker or jet-setter adjust the body clock.

Bypassing jet lag

To prevent jet lag, some experts suggest that travelers attempt to reach their destination by early evening and go to sleep around 10 p.m. local time. To prepare their bodies for the change, they should go to sleep at the new bedtime for a few days before the trip. Properly hydrating, avoiding alcohol and caffeine in-flight may also help minimize jet lag.

Nursing interventions

These nursing interventions may be appropriate for a patient with a circadian rhythm sleep disorder:

- Be sure to include a thorough assessment that includes sleep pattern and wake pattern assessment.
- To promote adherence to sleep interventions, review the required procedures with the patient. Assess understanding of these procedures by having patient repeat instructions back to you.
- If the patient is using chronotherapy, ensure patient understands how to adjust bedtime correctly.
- Teach the patient about purpose, administration, and adverse effects of prescribed drugs such as sedative-hypnotics. Monitor for adverse effects and medication overuse.
- If the patient is taking a herbal supplement such as melatonin, reinforce this product isn't always manufactured under quality-controlled conditions.

Narcolepsy

Narcolepsy is characterized by sudden, uncontrollable attacks of deep sleep lasting up to 20 minutes. These "sleep attacks" come on without warning and may be accompanied by paralysis and hallucinations. Although the brief sleep is refreshing, the urge to sleep soon returns.

Sleep paralysis and hallucinations typically occur during sleep onset (hypnagogic hallucinations) or during the transition from sleep to wakefulness (hypnopompic hallucinations). Mostly visual, these hallucinations are intense, dreamlike images commonly involving the immediate environment.

A confounding cataplexy

Some patients with narcolepsy experience attacks of cataplexy—sudden loss of muscle tone and strength. (In more subtle forms of cataplexy, the patient's head may drop or jaw may slacken.)

Cataplexy is commonly triggered by intense generally positive emotions—for example, the knees may buckle after the patient laughs, gets angry, or feels elated or surprised. Cataplexy typically lasts just a few seconds, and the patient remains alert during the episode. However, in severe cases, the patient falls down and becomes completely paralyzed, usually lasting no more than 2 minutes.

Complications

Narcoleptic sleep attacks may occur at any time of day. All too often, they occur during activities that call for undivided attention, such as driving or work. Narcolepsy can be disabling, impairing work performance and disrupting leisure activities and interpersonal relationships. Coworkers may perceive the patient as lazy; an employer may suspect illegal drug use.

Jeers from their peers

In children, narcolepsy impairs school performance and social relationships and invites ridicule from peers. Teenagers with the disorder are at increased risk for automobile accidents.

Prevalence and onset

Narcolepsy is not rare, as it is estimated to occur in up to 1 out of every 2,000 people. However, it is also believed to be underrecognized and underdiagnosed (Scheer et al., 2019).

Narcolepsy is the second leading cause of daytime sleepiness diagnosed by sleep specialists. (OSA is the most common.) The disorder affects males and females equally. The usual onset is during young adulthood, but has been documented as early as 5 years old, and can be abrupt or progressive in nature (APA, 2013; Ruoff & Rye, 2016).

Causes

The exact cause of narcolepsy is unknown. However, most patients with narcolepsy have a deficit in the neurotransmitter orexin, which helps people stay awake (Scheer et al., 2019). Narcolepsy isn't related to the amount of sleep a person gets.

Signs and symptoms

Assessment findings in narcolepsy include:
- excessive daytime sleepiness, even during active states, such as eating and talking
- cataplexy
- brief episodes of sleep paralysis (inability to move or speak when falling asleep or waking up)
- dreamlike hallucinations at sleep onset or when awakening from sleep
- disturbed nighttime sleep, such as tossing and turning, leg jerks, nightmares, frequent awakenings, and abnormal REM sleep.

Diagnosis

A history of excessive daytime sleepiness, uncontrollable sleep, and observed cataplexy strongly suggest narcolepsy. However, other possible causes of excessive daytime sleepiness—heart disease, brain tumors, anemia, and depression, to name a few—must be ruled out.

Napping on demand

Overnight polysomnography and an MSLT may be performed. After these naps, the time required to fall asleep (sleep latency) is averaged. In narcolepsy, sleep latency is less than 8 minutes. Diagnosis is confirmed by using the diagnostic criteria in the *Diagnostic and Statistical Manual of Mental Disorders*, 5th edition (*DSM-5*) and can be further classified as mild, moderate, or severe (APA, 2013).

Modafinil: Narcolepsy treatment

A CNS stimulant that promotes wakefulness and alertness, modafinil (Provigil) is used to prevent excessive daytime sleepiness in patients with narcolepsy. When taken as directed, it should not interfere with nighttime sleep.

Modafinil is considered safe, effective, and generally well tolerated. It's less likely than traditional stimulants (such as amphetamines and methylphenidate) to cause jitteriness, anxiety, excessive motor activity, or a rebound effect. The medication may cause mild psychological dependence.

How it works

Modafinil is a central alpha-1 adrenergic agonist that induces wakefulness partly through its action in the brain's hypothalamus. It acts selectively through the brain's sleep-wake center, stimulating the patient only when stimulation is required and avoiding the highs and lows caused by other stimulants.

How it's given

The standard dosage is 200 mg/day, given as a single dose in the morning. Adverse effects are mild and may include headache, anxiety, nervousness, palpitations, insomnia, and nausea.

Nursing considerations

- Teach the patient about the drug, including the dosage, purpose, administration, and adverse effects.
- Monitor the patient for adverse effects.
- Instruct the patient not to drive or operate other complex machinery until understanding how the drug affects their ability to function.
- Advise patient to avoid alcohol while using this drug.
- Tell patient to call the health care provider if the following develop: skin rash, hives, or an allergic reaction.
- Know that patients with severe hepatic impairment should receive one-half of the standard dosage.
- Be aware that older adult patients may need a decreased dosage.
- Don't give this drug to patients who have a history of cardiovascular disease or are taking oral contraceptives, cyclosporine, theophylline, diazepam, phenytoin, warfarin, or propranolol.

Treatment

Although no cure exists for narcolepsy, symptoms can be controlled with behavioral and pharmacologic interventions. Behavioral interventions include lifestyle adjustments, such as regulating sleep schedules and taking scheduled daytime naps.

A stimulating strategy

Symptomatic treatment is focused on excessive somnolence and cataplexy. CNS stimulants may be prescribed (such as methylphenidate [Concerta] or modafinil [Provigil]) to decrease daytime sleepiness and antidepressants (such as imipramine [Tofranil] or fluoxetine [Prozac]) to reduce cataplectic attacks. (See *Modafinil: Narcolepsy treatment.*)

Nursing interventions

These interventions may be appropriate for a patient with narcolepsy:

- Review recommended lifestyle changes.
- Help the patient plan and maintain a regular sleep schedule.
- Discuss the need for ample sleep opportunity with the patient.
- Teach about the purpose, administration, and adverse effects of prescribed drugs.
- Monitor for adverse effects.

Hypersomnolence disorder

Hypersomnia is a condition of excessive sleepiness and excessive difficulty waking from daytime naps and nighttime sleep periods occurring nearly every day. During long periods of drowsiness, the patient may exhibit automatic behavior, acting in a semicontrolled fashion. There may be trouble meeting work and family obligations, and driving can be negatively affected. The diagnosis of hypersomnolence disorder is reserved for those patients who have no other direct cause of daytime sleepiness such as OSA or narcolepsy (Becker et al., 2017; Billiard & Sonka, 2016).

Signs and symptoms

The primary symptom associated with hypersomnolence disorder is feeling tired to the point where the feeling interferes with the activities of daily living. Patients may report extended sleep periods at night or the desire to nap frequently during the day. In some cases, behavior upon awakening can resemble "drunkenness" in the manifestation of confusion, disorientation, poor motor coordination, and slowness on awakening (Billiard & Sonka, 2016).

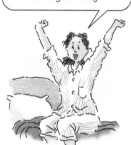

Even after 12 hours of sleep, a patient with hypersomnia may feel drowsy during the day.

Prevalence

The prevalence of hypersomnolence disorder in the general population isn't known.

"Hypersomnolence fully manifests in most cases in late adolescence or early adulthood, with a mean age at onset of 17 to 24 years. Individuals with hypersomnolence disorders are diagnosed, on average, 10 to 15 years AFTER the appearance of the first symptoms" (APA, 2013, p. 370).

Causes

Based on the underlying cause of the disorder, experts have identified two possible risk and prognostic factors.

Environmental

Alcohol use and psychological stress can lead to increased hypersomnolence on a temporary basis. In addition, viral infections such as HIV, pneumonia, mononucleosis, and Guillain-Barré syndrome can also lead to hypersomnolence (APA, 2013). Even after the infectious process resolves, these patients continue to need significantly more sleep and feel very tired upon awakening.

Genetic and physiologic

There may be a genetic modality associated with hypersomnolence, with some studies suggesting an autosomal dominant inheritance pattern (APA, 2013).

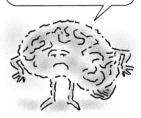

A viral infection with neurologic symptoms has been linked to some cases of hypersomnia.

Signs and symptoms

In patients with hypersomnolence disorder, assessment findings typically include:

- excessive sleepiness on a daily basis
- daytime napping without feeling refreshed
- long nighttime sleeping (8 to 12 hours)
- difficulty awakening in the morning.

Many patients also report irritability, depression, memory loss, headache, poor concentration, impaired work or school performance, fainting episodes, and dizziness on standing (from orthostatic hypotension). A few report hypnagogic hallucinations and sleep paralysis.

Diagnosis

Physical examination, a complete blood cell count, and thyroid-stimulating hormone tests may rule out other possible causes of excessive sleepiness or prolonged nocturnal sleep, including:

- OSA
- circadian rhythm sleep-wake disorders
- narcolepsy
- thyroid abnormalities
- chronic pain
- CNS disorders, damage, or malfunction
- viral infection

- bipolar depression, atypical depression, or dysthymia
- medication withdrawal
- adverse drug effects.

Out like a light

Polysomnography typically reveals short sleep latency, long sleep duration, and a normal sleep pattern.

Diagnosis is confirmed by using the diagnostic criteria in the *DSM-5* and can be further classified as acute, subacute, or persistent. The level of severity can also be determined as mild, moderate, or severe (APA, 2013).

Treatment

Treatment focuses on relieving symptoms and may include behavioral approaches, sleep hygiene techniques, and pharmacologic interventions.

Awake and wired

Drugs used to treat hypersomnolence disorder include antidepressants and stimulants (such as modafinil [Provigil], methylphenidate [Ritalin, Concerta], and dextroamphetamine [Adderall]). Stimulants are the most effective agents; however, they often provide only partial relief. Typically, the patient is maintained on daily stimulants, with the dosage titrated so the patient can stay alert during the day with minimal side effects (Becker et al., 2017; Billiard & Sonka, 2016). Medications in the stimulant category are considered controlled substances, and misuse of these medications can occur and should be a consideration during the patient assessment.

Java jolt therapy

Self-medicating with caffeine is probably the most commonly tried treatment. The stimulating effects of caffeine temporarily improve psychomotor performance and increase alertness.

- Teach patient about prescribed drugs; include purpose, administration, and adverse effects.
- Caution the patient about driving or using dangerous machinery when drowsy. Help develop an alternate plan, such as taking public transportation or carpooling.
- Inform the patient that excessive caffeine may cause anxiety, irritability, jitteriness, and tolerance.
- Provide information on the causative ties between excessive caffeine intake and angina.

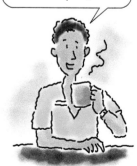

Many patients with hypersomnia rely on caffeine to keep them perky.

Insomnia disorder

The most common sleep disorder, insomnia, encompasses many types of sleep problems—difficulty falling asleep, sleeping too lightly, frequent awakenings during the night, inability to fall back to sleep once awakened, and waking up in the early morning and being unable to fall back to sleep.

Obsessing over insomnia

Insomnia can be episodic, persistent, or recurrent. With persistent insomnia, the person may become preoccupied with getting enough sleep. The more the patient tries to sleep, the greater the sense of frustration and distress—and the more elusive sleep becomes.

Consequences

Insomnia commonly leads to daytime drowsiness, poor concentration, memory impairments, difficulty coping with minor problems, irritability, and reduced ability to enjoy family and social relationships.

You snooze, you lose

People with insomnia are more than twice as likely as the general population to have a fatigue-related motor vehicle accident. Those who sleep less than 5 hours per night may have a higher death rate, too.

Prevalence

Insomnia disorder occurring over 1 month is found in approximately 6% to 10% of the population. Prevalence increases with age and is greater in women. Insomnia can present as its own disorder or, commonly, is observed as a comorbid condition with another medical or mental health disorder (APA, 2013).

Causes

Episodic insomnia often stems from a specific event—a physical stressor (such as illness), a significant life change or emotional stressor (such as divorce), or an environmental disturbance that makes sleep difficult (such as noise, unwanted light, or an uncomfortable room temperature).

You booze, you may not snooze

Persistent insomnia may result from either a single factor or multiple factors. Everyday stress and anxiety, caffeine consumption, and alcohol use are the most common culprits.

Risk factors for developing persistent insomnia include:
- history of being a light sleeper
- tendency toward easy arousal at night
- inability to fall asleep or stay asleep after an initial stressful situation is resolved
- repression of feelings resulting in physical symptoms, rather than expressing them outright or dealing with them constructively.

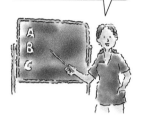

Alcohol, caffeine, and anxiety are the main culprits in persistent insomnia.

Signs and symptoms

A patient with insomnia disorder may report or exhibit:
- difficulty falling asleep
- difficulty staying asleep
- waking up too early in the morning
- inability to fall back to sleep once awakened
- nonrestorative sleep
- daytime fatigue and lack of energy
- haggard appearance
- irritability
- short attention span
- poor concentration
- excessive anxiety over his or her health
- interpersonal, social, or occupational problems stemming from anxiety over sleeplessness
- inappropriate use of sedative-hypnotic drugs, alcohol, or caffeine.

(See *Key questions to ask when assessing for insomnia*, page 320.)

Diagnosis

Insomnia disorder may be diagnosed from the patient history and physical findings. Polysomnography can rule out other sleep disorders such as OSA. Polysomnography usually shows increased stage 1 sleep and decreased slow-wave sleep.

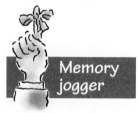

Memory jogger

Typical findings in patients with **INSOMNIA**

Intermittent wakefulness

Not able to fall asleep easily

Stressed by the inability to fall asleep

Overly concerned with the consequences of not sleeping

May medicate with inappropriate drugs

Needs frequent daytime naps

Irritable

Attention and concentration problems

Key questions to ask when assessing for insomnia

When assessing a patient who reports insomnia, ask the following questions:
• When did the problem begin?
• Do you have a medical or mental health disorder that might affect your ability to sleep?
• What's your sleep environment like? Is it dark? Quiet? Bright? Noisy? Does it have a comfortable room temperature?
• Do you use your bedroom for things other than sleep or sexual activity (such as watching television, eating, or working)?
• What time do you usually go to bed?
• What time do you usually get up in the morning on weekdays? On weekends?
• Do you drink alcohol or smoke? Are you taking prescribed medications? Nonprescription preparations? Illicit drugs?
• What's your typical work schedule?
• How do you feel in the day after a poor night's sleep?

Family inquiries
If possible, ask the patient's partner or other family members if the patient snores or has unusual limb movements when sleeping.

Sleep scribblings

To aid diagnosis, the health care provider may ask the patient to keep a sleep diary for 1 to 2 weeks. (See *Dear sleep diary*, pages 322 and 323.) In the acute care setting, sleep-wake logs are a commonly utilized technique.

Diagnosis of insomnia disorder is confirmed by using the diagnostic criteria in the *DSM-5* and can be further classified as episodic, persistent, or recurrent (APA, 2013).

Treatment

Treatment for insomnia disorder may involve relaxation techniques, improved sleep hygiene, behavioral interventions, cognitive behavioral therapy for insomnia, alternative and complementary measures, or pharmacologic options.

Nipping it in the bud

With episodic insomnia, the need for treatment is based on the severity of daytime symptoms and duration of the episode. A patient who suffers brief episodes of insomnia should be monitored for prolonged negative effects because untreated episodic insomnia can lead to a chronic condition.

Relaxation techniques

Because patients with insomnia display high levels of physiologic and cognitive arousal (both at night and during the day), relaxation-based interventions may provide relief. Techniques that help deactivate the arousal system include progressive muscle relaxation, abdominal or deep breathing, biofeedback, and imagery training (Baron et al., 2017).

Sleep hygiene

For some patients, insomnia responds well to lifestyle changes, referred to as *sleep hygiene* (Baron et al., 2017; Chung et al., 2018). Such changes include going to bed at the same time every night, optimizing sleeping conditions, and avoiding naps during the day. (See *Getting hygienic about sleep*, page 324.)

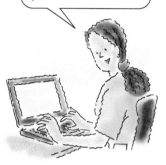

Recording bedtimes, awakening times, and other sleep-related information can help the healthcare provider diagnose a patient with insomnia.

Behavioral interventions

Behavioral interventions aim to change maladaptive sleep habits, reduce autonomic arousal, and alter dysfunctional beliefs and attitudes. A wide range of behavioral techniques may be used to treat persistent insomnia (Baron et al., 2017). Stimulus control is a behavioral intervention that connects behavior associated with sleep hygiene to sleep behavior. For example, with behavioral intervention, patients are instructed to go to bed only when sleepy and make the behavioral choice to get out of bed when realizing that sleep is not naturally occurring after a brief period of time (Baron et al., 2017).

Stimulus control is based on the theory that insomnia represents a learned response to bedtime and bedroom cues.

Bedroom behavior

Give your patient these instructions:
- Go to bed only when sleepy and having difficulty staying awake. (See *Getting hygienic about sleep*, page 324.)
- Use the bed and bedroom only for sleep (or sex).
- If you can't fall asleep or stay asleep, get out of bed and go to another room. Return to bed only when you feel sleepy.
- Awaken and get out of bed at the same time every morning regardless of how much sleep you got.
- Avoid naps.

Dear sleep diary

A sleep diary, like the one shown here, can aid the diagnosis and treatment of insomnia disorder. The diary provides a night-by-night account of the patient's sleep schedule and perception of sleep. The sleep diary serves as a baseline for monitoring treatment efficacy. In the diary, the patient records information such as:

- bedtime of the previous night
- total sleep time
- time elapsed before sleep onset
- number and duration of awakenings
- morning awakening time
- total time awake
- use of sleep medications
- subjective rating of sleep quality and daytime symptoms.

Sample sleep diary

Name _Willa Selby_

		Mon 5/12	Tues 5/13
	Date	Mon 5/12	Tues 5/13
Complete in AM	**Bedtime (previous night)**	11:00 pm	10:45 pm
	Awakening time	7:30 am	7:45 am
	Estimated time to sleep onset (previous night)	45 minutes	1 hour
	Estimated number of awakenings and total time awake (previous night)	6 times/total of 3 hours	5 times/total of 4 hours
	Estimated amount of sleep obtained (previous night)	4 1/2 hours	5 hours
Complete in PM	**Naps (time and duration)**	4:00 pm for 30 minutes	4:30 pm for 30 minutes
	Alcoholic drinks (number and time)	2 drinks at 8:00 pm	1 drink at 9:00 pm
	Stresses experienced today	Car wouldn't start, argued with boss	none
	Rate how you felt today 1—Very tired/sleepy 2—Somewhat tired/sleepy 3—Fairly alert 4—Wide awake	1	2
	Irritability 1—Not at all 5—Very	5 (very)	3
	Medications	Benadryl	Benadryl

Encourage the patient to complete the diary each morning using estimates rather than exact times to make the process less disruptive to sleep.

	Wed 5/14	Thu 5/15	Fri 5/16
	11:00 pm		
	7:30 am		
	30 minutes		
	6 times/total of 3 hours		
	4 1/2 hours		
	4:00 pm for 45 minutes		
	2 drinks at 8:00 pm		
	argued with a friend		
	1		
	4		
	Benadryl		

Getting hygienic about sleep

For most patients with insomnia, lifestyle measures—termed *sleep hygiene*—are recommended as first-line treatment. When teaching your patient about sleep hygiene, cover the following dos and don'ts.

Sleep-promoting measures
- Use the bed only for sleep and sex—not for reading, watching television, or working.
- Establish a regular bedtime and a regular time for getting up in the morning. Stick to these times even on weekends and on vacations.
- Exercise in the evening. Energy levels bottom out a few hours after exercise, promoting sleep at that time.
- Take a hot bath 90 minutes to 2 hours before bedtime. This alters core body temperature and can help you fall asleep more easily.
- During the 30 minutes before bedtime, do something quiet and relaxing, such as reading, meditating, or taking a leisurely walk.
- Keep the bedroom quiet, dark, relatively cool, and well ventilated.
- Eat dinner 4 to 5 hours before bedtime. At bedtime, a light snack (low in sugar and calories) may promote sleep.
- Spend 30 minutes in the sun each day. (However, be sure to take precautions against overexposure.)

- If you don't fall asleep after 15 or 20 minutes, get up and go into another room. Read or perform a quiet activity, using dim lighting, until you feel sleepy.
- If your bed partner distracts you, consider moving to another bedroom or the sofa for a few nights.

What not to do
- Don't use the bedroom for work, reading, or watching television.
- Avoid large meals immediately before bedtime.
- Don't look at the clock. Obsessing over time makes it harder to sleep.
- Avoid naps, especially in the evening.
- Don't drink a large amount of fluid after dinner, or the need to urinate may disturb your sleep.
- Avoid exercising close to bedtime because this may make you more alert.
- Avoid alcohol and caffeine in the evening.
- Don't take a bath just before bedtime because this could increase your alertness.
- Don't engage in highly stimulating activities before bed, such as watching a frightening movie or playing competitive computer games.
- Don't smoke because nicotine's effects may contribute to sleep loss.
- Don't toss and turn in bed. Instead, get up and read or listen to relaxing music. However, don't watch television because it emits too bright of a light.

Paradoxical intention

In paradoxical intention, the patient does the opposite of what is wanted, sometimes taking it to an extreme. For instance, instead of going through activities that promote sleep, the patient prepares to stay awake and might be doing something energetic. If worry is a factor in insomnia, it may intensify.

Biofeedback

In biofeedback, the patient is connected to a device that measures brain waves and other body functions. Then the patient is given feedback to help learn to recognize certain states of tension or sleep stages—and either avoid or repeat these states voluntarily.

Sleep restriction

Sleep restriction creates a mild state of sleep deprivation, which may promote more rapid sleep onset and more "efficient" sleep. The patient limits the amount of time spent in bed based on calculations of their actual time spent sleeping. As sleep efficiency improves, the patient incrementally increases their time in bed with the goal of increasing the total amount of time spent asleep.

Bedtime amendments

To maintain a consistent sleep-wake pattern, the patient usually alters bedtime rather than rising time. However, time in bed shouldn't be reduced to less than 5 hours a day. Naps aren't allowed (except in older adults).

Cognitive therapy

Cognitive therapy helps the patient identify dysfunctional beliefs and attitudes about sleep (such as "I'll never fall asleep") and replace them with positive ones. Changing beliefs and attitudes can decrease the anticipatory anxiety that interferes with sleep. Cognitive therapy also focuses on actions intended to change behavior.

Alternative and complementary therapies

Alternative and complementary therapies that may be used to treat insomnia include acupressure, acupuncture, aromatherapy, massage, biofeedback, chiropractic, homeopathy, light and dark therapy, meditation, reflexology, visualization, and yoga.

Supplements to sleep by

Some patients use herbal preparations (such as St. John's wort and chamomile), nutritional substances, and other nonprescription preparations to treat insomnia. However, few of these products have been demonstrated to be safe and effective. There is also a lack of standardized dosing or purity control among nutritional supplements. Therefore, potency and actual dosage can vary based on the manufacturer.

Dietary supplements sometimes recommended for insomnia relief include vitamins B_6, B_{12}, and D. Some practitioners also recommend calcium and magnesium. Tryptophan may relieve insomnia in some patients, but the patient must be monitored for adverse effects.

Melatonin is a hormone that is released from the pineal gland and can help regulate sleep-wake cycles. Melatonin is also found in

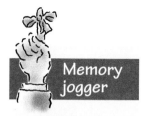

Memory jogger

Help your patient **DISCOVER** ways to overcome sleep disorders.

Define what may be causing the problem.

Identify changes in the patient's sleep pattern.

State an understanding of "good" sleep.

C Calculate how many hours of sleep is needed.

Offer assistance on ways to promote sleep.

Venting feelings about sleep problems can be therapeutic.

Educate the patient about how sleep patterns change throughout life.

Review the negative effects of stress on sleep.

a number of plants including St. John's wort and in fruits such as grapes and cherries. It is believed to bind to melatonin receptors in the body, leading to their activation (agonist). Activation of these receptors is then believed to help restore the sleep-wake cycle. Few side effects have been found, primarily drowsiness and a worsening of orthostatic hypertension.

Valerian is a perennial flowering plant native to Europe commonly used in the treatment of anxiety and insomnia. It is believed to have a pharmacologic mechanism similar to benzodiazepines, in which an effect is exerted on an inhibitory neurotransmitter (gamma-aminobutyric acid [GABA]). Evidence is mixed as to whether or not this can be an effective treatment for sleep disorders. It can result in stomach upset and nausea. Additional side effects are a sense of asthenia (lack of energy) and allergic reactions.

Pharmacologic options

If insomnia persists despite other measures, the prescribing health provider may recommend medication therapy (Sateia et al., 2017). The most commonly prescribed drugs are short-acting sedative-hypnotics (primarily benzodiazepines), antidepressants, and antihistamines. (See *Pharmacologic therapy for sleep disorders*.)

Sleep aids

Sedative-hypnotics—usually temazepam (Restoril) and zolpidem (Ambien)—are commonly prescribed for short-term management of insomnia. Benzodiazepines such as temazepam (Restoril) help maintain sleep, whereas nonbenzodiazepines such as zolpidem (Ambien) help the patient fall asleep. Recently, zolpidem (Ambien) has developed a controlled release (CR) form labeled Ambien CR that helps the patient also stay asleep longer. Newer sedative-hypnotics such as zaleplon (Sonata) and ramelteon (Rozerem) are also used according to the symptoms the patient describes that interrupt the sleep-wake cycle (Sateia et al., 2017).

Both prescription and nonprescription antihistamines can be used for short-term management of insomnia, particularly with adolescents and the elderly. The most common over-the-counter agents are doxylamine (Unisom) and diphenhydramine (Benadryl). Adverse effects include daytime sedation, cognitive impairment, and anticholinergic effects (e.g., dry mouth, constipation, or urinary retention). Tolerance or reliance may also occur.

Sedating antidepressants may be given in low dosages—especially if the patient has related psychiatric disorders or a history of substance abuse. These medications can also be effective in the treatment of chronic pain. However, some antidepressants can exacerbate other disorders, such as mania or restless leg syndrome, so the patient should be monitored closely (Sateia et al., 2017).

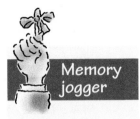

Memory jogger

Cover these basic **TEACHING** points to help your patient get better sleep.

Take prescribed sleep medications appropriately.

Eliminate caffeine, alcohol, and nicotine at least 4 hours before bedtime.

Attend to adequate sleep hygiene.

Consider the effects of foods and fluids on sleep.

Have a consistent bedtime routine.

Initiate relaxation strategies before bedtime.

Nightmares and dreams that disrupt sleep must be addressed.

Get family support, as needed.

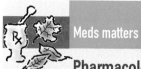

Pharmacologic therapy for sleep disorders

Several different medications are used to treat sleep disorders. A patient with insomnia may receive a benzo-diazepine, a nonbenzodiazepine hypnotic, an antidepressant, or a medication that influences melatonin. All of these therapies can lead to drowsiness and should not be taken in combination with other sedating medication or alcohol (Sateia et al., 2017).

Drug	Adverse effects	Contraindications	Nursing interventions
Antihistamines			
Diphenhydramine hydro-chloride (Benadryl)	Drowsiness Dry mouth Possible increase in heart rate	Should not be used in acute asthma Use of monoamine oxidase inhibitors	Avoid alcohol and other sedating agents. Be cautious when operating heavy machinery after taking medication. Recommend hard candies to aid in alleviating dry mouth if experienced.
Benzodiazepines			
Temazepam (Restoril)	Dizziness Drowsiness	Pregnancy and breast-feeding	Teach the patient about drug action, dosage, and adverse effects.
Triazolam (Halcion)	Lethargy Orthostatic hypotension	Triazolam should not be taken at the same time as ketoconazole, itraconazole, or ne-fazodone therapy	Caution the patient not to drink alco-hol, drive a motor vehicle, or operate machinery while under the influence of this drug. Advise the patient to change position slowly to avoid dizziness. Inform the patient of potential for physical and psychological dependence.
Nonbenzodiazepines			
Eszopiclone (Lunesta) Zaleplon (Sonata) Zolpidem (Ambien)	Amnesia Dizziness Fugue states (sleepwalking and performing other ac-tivities such as driv-ing while appearing asleep)	Pregnancy and breast-feeding Hepatic impairment	Teach the patient about drug action, dosage, and adverse effects. Avoid alcohol and other sedating agents. Be cautious when operating heavy machinery after taking medication.
Melatonin receptor agonists			
Ramelteon (Rozerem)	Dizziness Fatigue Headache Nausea	Angioedema Hepatic impairment Should not be taken at the same time as fluvoxamine	Teach the patient about drug action, dosage, and adverse effects. Avoid alcohol and other sedating agents. Be cautious when operating heavy machinery after taking medication.

(continued)

Pharmacologic therapy for sleep disorders *(continued)*

Drug	Adverse effects	Contraindications	Nursing interventions
Antidepressants			
Amitriptyline (Elavil) Doxepin (Silenor)	Blood dyscrasias Ataxia Blurred vision Dry mouth Increased heart rate Palpitation Priapism	Certain cardiovascular disorders, particularly those associated with prolonged QT interval	Monitor for a compromised immune system. Assess for changes in mood and potential suicidal ideation. Avoid alcohol and other sedating agents. Be cautious when operating heavy machinery after taking medication. Can increase liver function test results.

Nursing interventions

These nursing interventions may be appropriate for a patient with insomnia disorder:

- Provide teaching about prescribed medications, including drug purpose, administration, and adverse effects. Inform the patient that taking these drugs for more than a few weeks may lead to tolerance and withdrawal, making it even more difficult to sleep when the medication is stopped.
- Monitor the patient for adverse drug effects.
- Instruct the patient in good sleep hygiene, such as maintaining a regular bedtime and awakening times; avoiding naps; and eliminating caffeine, alcohol, and nicotine.
- Encourage the practice of relaxation routines, such as progressive muscle relaxation or meditation.
- Caution about the possible dangers of using unproven therapies.
- Advise the patient to move the alarm clock away from the bed if it's distracting.

Quick quiz

1. What actions characterize REM sleep?
   A. Light sleep
   B. Paralysis of the voluntary muscles
   C. Restricted eye movements
   D. Nonvivid dreams

Answer: B. During REM sleep, many muscles are effectively paralyzed so the sleeper won't act out dreams. Eye movements are rapid.

2. What regulates NREM sleep?
    A. Pons
    B. Hypothalamus
    C. Basal forebrain
    D. Amygdala

Answer: C. The basal forebrain controls NREM sleep. The pons and midbrain control REM sleep.

3. Which assessment data is a hallmark sign of OSA?
    A. Snoring
    B. Sneezing
    C. Early morning awakening
    D. Bursts of energy

Answer: A. Snoring is a hallmark of OSA. Sneezing, bursts of energy, and early morning awakening aren't common in this disorder.

4. Which treatment is not used as a primary treatment for circadian rhythm sleep disorders?
    A. Chronotherapy
    B. Short-acting sedative-hypnotics
    C. Relaxation techniques
    D. Light therapy

Answer: C. Relaxation techniques aren't used as primary treatments for circadian rhythm sleep disorders.

5. What data will the nurse teach the patient to include in a sleep diary?
    A. Usual bedtime
    B. Foods consumed before bedtime
    C. Daily weights
    D. Fluid consumption

Answer: A. In a sleep diary, the patient records sleep-related items, such as usual bedtime and awakening times, time elapsed before sleep onset, number of nightly awakenings, and total time spent in sleep. Food and fluid consumption and daily weights aren't relevant.

Scoring

✩✩✩   If you answered all five items correctly, stupendous! Your study of snoozing and snoring has succeeded beyond our wildest dreams!

✩✩   If you answered four items correctly, remarkable. Your solid grasp of sleep disorders should make for a sweet slumber tonight.

✩   If you answered fewer than three items correctly, consider this your wake-up call. Read the chapter again—but try not to doze off this time.

Selected references

American Psychiatric Association. (2013). *Diagnostic and statistical manual of mental disorders* (5th ed.). American Psychiatric Publishing.

Baron, K. G., Perlis, M. L., Nowakowski, S., Smith, M. T., Jungquist, C. R., & Orff, H. J. (2017). Cognitive behavioral therapy for insomnia. In H. Attarian (Ed.), *Clinical handbook of insomnia* (pp. 75–96). Springer.

Becker, L. A., Murray, C. F., Hoque, R., & Trotti, L. M. (2017). Medications for daytime sleepiness in individuals with idiopathic hypersomnia. *Cochrane Database of Systematic Reviews*, (7), CD012714.

Billiard, M., & Sonka, K. (2016). Idiopathic hypersomnia. *Sleep Medicine Reviews*, 29, 23–33.

Centers for Disease Control and Prevention. (2018a). Drowsy driving asleep at the wheel. *CDC Features*. https://www.cdc.gov/features/dsdrowsydriving/index.html

Centers for Disease Control and Prevention. (2018b). Sleep and sleep disorders. *Data and statistics*. https://www.cdc.gov/sleep/index.html

Chen, H., Aarab, G., de Ruiter, M. H., de Lange, J., Lobbezoo, F., & van der Stelt, P. F. (2016). Three-dimensional imaging of the upper airway anatomy in obstructive sleep apnea: A systematic review. *Sleep Medicine*, 21, 19–27.

Chu, C., Hom, M. A., Gallyer, A. J., Hammock, E. A., & Joiner, T. E. (2019). Insomnia predicts increased perceived burdensomeness and decreased desire for emotional support following an in-laboratory social exclusion paradigm. *Journal of Affective Disorders*, 243, 432–440. https://doi.org/10.1016/j.jad.2018.09.069

Chung, K. F., Lee, C. T., Yeung, W. F., Chan, M. S., Chung, E. W. Y., & Lin, W. L. (2018). Sleep hygiene education as a treatment of insomnia: A systematic review and meta-analysis. *Family Practice*, 35(4), 365–375.

Cox, R. C., & Olatunji, B. O. (2016). A systematic review of sleep disturbance in anxiety and related disorders. *Journal of Anxiety Disorders*, 37, 104–129.

Dickinson, D. L., Wolkow, A. P., Rajaratnam, S. M., & Drummond, S. P. (2018). Personal sleep debt and daytime sleepiness mediate the relationship between sleep and mental health outcomes in young adults. *Depression and Anxiety*, 35(8), 775–783.

Franklin, K. A., & Lindberg, E. (2015). Obstructive sleep apnea is a common disorder in the population—A review on the epidemiology of sleep apnea. *Journal of Thoracic Disease*, 7(8), 1311.

Garbarino, S., Magnavita, N., Guglielmi, O., Maestri, M., Dini, G., Bersi, F. M., Toletone, A., Chiorri, C., & Durando, P. (2017). Insomnia is associated with road accidents. Further evidence from a study on truck drivers. *PLoS One*, 12(10), e0187256. https://doi.org/10.1371/journal.pone.0187256

Garside, J., Stephenson, J., Curtis, H., Morrell, M., Dearnley, C., & Astin, F. (2018). Are noise reduction interventions effective in adult ward settings? A systematic review and meta analysis. *Applied Nursing Research*, 44, 6–17.

Hafner, M., Stepanek, M., Taylor, J., Troxel, W. M., & van Stolk, C. (2017). Why sleep matters—The economic costs of insufficient sleep: A cross-country comparative analysis. *RAND Health Quarterly*, 6(4), 11.

Hale, L., Kirschen, G. W., LeBourgeois, M. K., Gradisar, M., Garrison, M. M., Montgomery-Downs, H., Kirschen, H., McHale, S. M., Chang, A. M., &

Buxton, O. M. (2018). Youth screen media habits and sleep: Sleep-friendly screen behavior recommendations for clinicians, educators, and parents. *Child and Adolescent Psychiatric Clinics, 27*(2), 229–245.

Javaheri, S., Barbe, F., Campos-Rodriguez, F., Dempsey, J. A., Khayat, R., Javaheri, S., Malhotra, A., Martinez-Garcia, M. A., Mehra, R., Pack, A. I., Polotsky, V. Y., Redline, S., & Somers, V. K. (2017). Sleep apnea: Types, mechanisms, and clinical cardiovascular consequences. *Journal of the American College of Cardiology, 69*(7), 841–858.

Kerkhof, G. A. (2018). Shift work and sleep disorder comorbidity tend to go hand in hand. *Chronobiology International, 35*(2), 219–228.

Matheson, E., & Hainer, B. L. (2017). Insomnia: Pharmacologic therapy. *American Family Physician, 96*(1), 29–35

Miller, J. N., & Berger, A. M. (2016). Screening and assessment for obstructive sleep apnea in primary care. *Sleep Medicine Reviews, 29*, 41–51.

Potter, G. D., Skene, D. J., Arendt, J., Cade, J. E., Grant, P. J., & Hardie, L. J. (2016). Circadian rhythm and sleep disruption: Causes, metabolic consequences, and countermeasures. *Endocrine Reviews, 37*(6), 584–608.

Rotariu, C., Cristea, C., Arotaritei, D., Bozomitu, R. G., & Pasarica, A. (2016). *Continuous respiratory monitoring device for detection of sleep apnea episodes.* Presented at the 2016 IEEE 22nd International Symposium for Design and Technology in Electronic Packaging (SIITME) (pp. 106–109). IEEE.

Ruoff, C., & Rye, D. (2016). The ICSD-3 and DSM-5 guidelines for diagnosing narcolepsy: Clinical relevance and practicality. *Current Medical Research and Opinion, 32*(10), 1611–1622.

Sateia, M. J., Buysse, D. J., Krystal, A. D., Neubauer, D. N., & Heald, J. L. (2017). Clinical practice guideline for the pharmacologic treatment of chronic insomnia in adults: An American Academy of Sleep Medicine clinical practice guideline. *Journal of Clinical Sleep Medicine, 13*(2), 307–349.

Scheer, D., Schwartz, S. W., Parr, M., Zgibor, J., Sanchez-Anguiano, A., & Rajaram, L. (2019). Prevalence and incidence of narcolepsy in a US health care claims database, 2008–2010. *Sleep, 42*, zsz091.

Senaratna, C. V., Perret, J. L., Lodge, C. J., Lowe, A. J., Campbell, B. E., Matheson, M. C., Hamilton, G. S., & Dharmage, S. C. (2017). Prevalence of obstructive sleep apnea in the general population: A systematic review. *Sleep Medicine Reviews, 34*, 70–81.

Stranks, E. K., & Crowe, S. F. (2016). The cognitive effects of obstructive sleep apnea: An updated meta-analysis. *Archives of Clinical Neuropsychology, 31*(2), 186–193.

Suzuki, K., Miyamoto, M., & Hirata, K. (2017). Sleep disorders in the elderly: Diagnosis and management. *Journal of General and Family Medicine, 18*(2), 61–71.

Watson, N. F., Badr, M. S., Belenky, G., Bliwise, D. L., Buxton, O. M., Buysse, D., Dinges, D. F., Gangwisch, J., Grandner, M. A., Kushida, C., Malhotra, R. K., Martin, J. L., Patel, S. R., Quan, S. F., & Tasali, E. (2015). Recommended amount of sleep for a healthy adult: A joint consensus statement of the American Academy of Sleep Medicine and Sleep Research Society. *Journal of Clinical Sleep Medicine, 11*(6), 591–592.

Yu, J., Zhou, Z., McEvoy, R. D., Anderson, C. S., Rodgers, A., Perkovic, V., & Neal, B. (2017). Association of positive airway pressure with cardiovascular events and death in adults with sleep apnea: A systematic review and meta-analysis. *JAMA, 318*(2), 156–166.

Selected Internet-Based Resources

American Academy of Sleep Medicine—http://www.aasmnet.org/practiceguidelines.aspx

American Sleep Apnea Association—http://sleepapnea.org/

American Sleep Association—http://www.sleepassociation.org/index.php

National Sleep Foundation—http://www.sleepfoundation.org/

Sleep.com—http://www.sleep.com/

Willis-Ekbom Disease Foundation—http://www.rls.org/Selected references

Chapter 14

Paraphilic disorders and sexual dysfunctions

Just the facts

In this chapter, you'll learn about the following:

◆ stages of sexual development

◆ phases of the sexual response cycle

◆ categories and definitions of sexual dysfunctions and paraphilic disorders and their causes

◆ assessment findings in patients with sexual dysfunctions or paraphilic disorders

◆ treatments and nursing interventions for patients with sexual dysfunctions or paraphilic disorders.

A look at sex

In its simplest and most straightforward definition, sex, or sexual intercourse, describes the means behind biological reproduction across species. In humans, sex is often much more nuanced than a reproductive act alone and includes biological or endocrine responses, psychological or social factors, and an aspect of one's internalized gender or sexual identity. Gender identify is the way the person feels inside, and how they experience gender. This may or may not correlate with their recorded sex at birth, whereas sexual identify is an "inherent or immutable enduring emotional, romantic, or sexual attraction to other people" (Human Rights Campaign, 2020). Nonetheless, sex is known to motivate human behavior, and how an individual understands or experiences sex or their sexuality may vary based on psychological variants, social or cultural norms and expectations, and past sexual experiences, including trauma or abuse. In many cultures, sex remains a taboo subject and is something that is not often talked about, even in health care settings. For all nurses and health care workers, particularly those working in psychiatric or mental health, it is critical to understand that sexuality is a key component of one's identity. To provide holistic, culturally competent, and patient-centered care, an understanding of patients' sexuality and how it may influence their clinical presentation is paramount.

A look at sexual dysfunctions and paraphilic disorders

Sexuality is expressed in an individual's attitude, behaviors, appearance, and relationships. Influenced by ongoing biophysical and psychosocial factors, sexuality starts to take shape during early childhood and is solidified or reshaped throughout the life span.

A sexual dysfunction can cause distress and anxiety for individuals, can create strife in intimate relationships, and can impair overall functioning. An international study that examined sexual dysfunction of men and women found rates as high as 55% and 50%, respectively, for certain sexual dysfunction (McCabe et al., 2016). These conditions not only can lead to sexual dissatisfaction, but may also be associated with low self-esteem and issues with body image (van den Brink et al., 2018), depression and other mental health issues (Chokka & Hankey, 2018), and sleep disorders (Seehuus & Pigeon, 2018). Additionally, it is well documented that psychiatric disorders and associated medications can cause sexual dysfunction (Montejo et al., 2018), as can other chronic physical health problems, such as heart disease (Ibrahim et al., 2018), neurologic deficits (Purwata et al., 2019), and endocrine dysfunction (Zamorano-Leon et al., 2018). Sexual dysfunction are considered psychiatric disorders per the *Diagnostic and Statistical Manual of Mental Disorders*, 5th Edition (*DSM-5*) (American Psychiatric Association [APA], 2013) and thus are commonly identified and treated in psychiatric settings.

Paraphilic disorders are acts or sexual stimuli that are outside of what society consider as normal but are required by some individuals to experience desire, arousal, or orgasm (Halter, 2018, p 383). Many people who meet criteria for paraphilic disorders do not openly act on their desires (Sorrentino, 2016); however, others do and may be found guilty of a sexual offense.

Sexual disorders in the *DSM-5*

Conditions described in the *DSM-5* (APA, 2013) include paraphilic disorders and sexual dysfunctions.

- Paraphilic disorders described in the *DSM-5* (APA 2013) include voyeuristic disorder, enhibitionistic disorder, frotteuristic disorder, sexual masochism disorder, sexual sadism disorder, pedophilic disorder, fetishistic disorder, and transvestic disorder.
- Sexual dysfunctions described in the *DSM-5* (APA, 2013) include delayed ejaculation, erectile disorder (ED), female orgasmic

disorder, female sexual interest/arousal disorder, genito-pelvic pain/penetration disorder, male hypoactive sexual desire disorder, premature ejaculation (PE), and substance/medication-induced sexual dsyfunction.

Defining "abnormal" sexual behavior

The definition of "abnormal" sexual behavior depends largely on cultural and historical context. Accepted norms of sexual behavior and attitudes vary greatly within and among different cultures. In most Western cultures, the work that defines what is "abnormal," or what can be considered a mental illness, is the *DSM*. Published by the APA, the text is periodically revised and was most recently released in its 5th edition (*DSM-5*) in 2013.

Historically, it was often believed that the only "normal" sexual behavior was intercourse between heterosexual partners for procreation. Masturbation and homosexuality were viewed as aberrant. A much broader range of attitudes toward sexuality exists today, which allows for and promotes individual expression of sexuality that is not shamed or stigmatized. Homosexuality is now regarded as a normal variant of sexuality in most cultures (Kite & Bryant-Lees, 2016), and masturbation is accepted as a normal sexual activity (Mosher, 2017).

Stages of sexual development

Beginning in infancy, individuals progress through various phases of sexual and psychosexual development. Characteristic physical attributes and feelings related to sex develop during each phase.

Infancy to age 5

Age of discovery

Genital play as early as infancy is considered part of normal development. Subsequently, between ages 1 and 3 years, children start to observe body differences and show an interest in bathroom habits (see Chapter 12 for a brief overview of toilet training). Curious and explorative, young children, often between the ages of 3 and 5 years, commonly ask "where babies come from" and what their sex organs are for. They're accepting and straightforward about sex and may comment on the differences between genders. Children this age may develop an interest in the genitalia of the opposite sex, and their curiosity may lead to genital or sexual exploration with other children (e.g., playing "doctor" or looking at others' genitals). Typically, this is seen as an expected developmental variant.

Important definitions!

Review these important definitions associated with biological sex, gender role expression, gender identity, and sexual orientation or preference.

Biological sex or assigned sex

Biological sex describes the physical, genetic, and hormonal characteristics of being male or female at birth.

Gender role expression

Gender role is the outward expression of one's gender and may be congruent or incongruent with sociocultural norms and expectations. Labels attached to gender role include masculine or feminine, traditional or conforming, and gender-neutral. Learned by the individual, gender role is influenced by culture, religion, schools, peers, and social messages.

Gender identity

"One's innermost concept of self as male, female, a blend of both or neither – how individuals perceive themselves and what they call themselves. One's gender identity can be the same or different from their sex assigned at birth" (Human Rights Campaign, 2020)

Sexual orientation or preference

Sexual orientation or preference is an "inherent or immutable enduring emotional, romantic, or sexual attraction to other people" (Human Rights Campaign, 2020)

* Heterosexuality is marked by an inherent or immutable enduring emotional, romantic, or sexual attraction to people of the opposite gender.
* Homrosexuality is marked by an inherent or immutable enduring emotional, romantic, or sexual attraction to people of the same gender.
* Bisexuality is "used to describe a person who experiences emotional, romantic and/or sexual attractions to, or engages in romantic or sexual relationships with, more than one sex or gender" (APA, 2020).
* Asexuality is characterized by "having little interest in having sex, even though most individual who identify as asexual desire emotionally intimate relationships" (The Trevor Project, 2020)

A topic apart

Toward the end of this stage, children pick up cues from others that sex is a "different" or taboo topic. They may become shy, ask fewer questions about sex, and show a desire for privacy about their bodies.

Ages 5 to 10

Children aged 5 to 10 years may think in terms of "good" and "bad" parts of their bodies. Children this age are often same gender oriented and seek friendships with individuals of the same gender. Masturbation and sexual exploration remain common during these ages.

Ages 10 to 14

Puberty usually begins at about age 11 years for girls and age 12 years for boys. Young adolescents may be confused, embarrassed, or self-conscious about their bodily changes and may be uncomfortable with, or unaware of, their social roles.

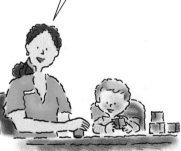

Children as young as 3 years will be curious about where babies come from and note differences in sex organs between genders.

Sexual responsiveness develops during this stage, as can the ability to reproduce. In response to peer pressure and other influences, some young adolescents become sexually active.

Ages 14 and older (adolescence)

From age 14 years onward, children develop more adult characteristics. This may be apparent physically (voice changes, distribution of pubic hair, complete development of secondary sex characteristics), emotionally (more easily able to identify a broad range of emotions, engaging in abstract thought), and socially (may pursue intimate relationships with others). Adolescents this age can be easily influenced by peer pressure and media messages. Adolescents want to be in control of themselves and should work to form their identities and self-concepts.

Sexual activity in adolescence—changing trends

Trends in sexuality and sexual behavior have shifted among adolescents. In 2017, 85.4% of U.S. high school students surveyed identified as heterosexual. Alternatively, 2.4% identified as lesbian or gay, 8.0% identified as bisexual, and 4.2% were unsure of or questioning their sexual identity (Rasberry et al., 2018). Across the United States, 52.2% of surveyed students reported having sexual contact at some point, with 45.3% of students having sexual contact with only the opposite sex, 1.6% having sexual contact with only the same sex, and 5.3% having sexual contact with both sexes (Rasberry et al.). Interestingly, not all students who had sexual contact with only the opposite sex identified as heterosexual; 4.0% identified as gay, lesbian, or bisexual. Further, social media and new communication trends have allowed for the possibility that adolescents can engage in alternative, nonphysical forms of sexual behavior. One study found that 17% of children and adolescents aged between 12 and 18 years sent and received sexual text messages (or "sexts"), whereas 24% of these children and adolescents only received sexts. Both sending and receiving sexts were associated with increased rates of sexual intercourse (Rice et al., 2018).

Adults

By adulthood, sex and sexuality are a part of a person's life. More than 75% of adults are sexually active (Liu et al., 2015). Adults hold views on sexuality that have been influenced by society and its standards of normal behavior, culture, their own personal drives and desires, and familial or social expectations.

Nursing interventions for patients with sexual dysfunctions

You can use the general interventions below when caring for a patient with any type of sexual dysfunction.

Ensure a therapeutic relationship

• Arrange to spend uninterrupted time with the patient. Encourage the patient to express feelings, and accept what the patient says.
• Explain all treatments and procedures, and answer the patient's questions to allay the patient's fear and help the patient regain a sense of control.
• Never say anything that would make the patient feel ashamed. It's the patient's needs and feelings—not your opinions—that matter.
• Realize that treating the patient with empathy doesn't threaten your sexuality.

Assessment

• Perform a thorough patient assessment. A complete assessment is essential in developing a plan of care. The initial assessment includes age, physical health, sexual functioning, current and past medical and mental health alterations, substance use, and factors affecting sexual functioning, such as relationships, diet, rest, stress, and personal hygiene.
• Assess medications, prescribed and over-the-counter, taken regularly and prn.
• Assess personal and intimate relationships and support systems.
• Assess cultural and religious values.
• Assess sexual knowledge, values, and needs.
• Assess body image and self-esteem.
• Assess for lifestyle disruptions or factors affecting emotions and mood.

Promote self-knowledge

• Initiate a discussion about how the need for self-esteem, respect, love, and intimacy influences a person's sexual expression. This helps the patient understand their condition.
• Encourage the patient to ask questions about sexual functioning.
• Encourage the patient to identify feelings—such as pleasure, reduced anxiety, increased control, or

shame—associated with the individual's sexual behavior and fantasies.
• Encourage the patient to express sexual preferences as well as feelings about these preferences.

Promote participation in care

• Encourage the patient to make decisions about their care, to enhance their self-esteem, and increase their sense of mastery over the current situation.

Improve coping skills

• Encourage the patient to use support systems to assist with coping, thereby helping to restore psychological equilibrium and prevent crises.
• Help the patient look at their current situation and evaluate various coping behaviors to encourage a realistic view of the crisis.
• Request feedback from the patient about health coping mechanisms that seem to work. This encourages the patient to evaluate the effect of these behaviors.
• Praise the patient for making decisions and performing activities to reinforce coping behaviors.

Provide referrals

• Refer the patient for professional psychological counseling. If maladaptive behavior has high crisis potential, formal counseling can help ease your frustration, increase your objectivity, and foster a collaborative approach to patient care. As appropriate, refer the patient to a physician, nurse, psychologist, social worker, or counselor trained in sex therapy.

Other actions

• Be aware that whenever possible, a primary nurse should be assigned to the patient to ensure continuity of care and promote a therapeutic relationship.
• If the patient poses a threat to themselves and others, institute safety precautions, according to agency protocol.

Human sexual response cycle

The sexual response cycle refers to the progressive mental, physical, and emotional changes that occur during sexual stimulation. Although the sexual response is highly individualized, nearly everyone experiences certain basic physiologic changes.

The sex scientists

Different researchers have proposed various models of the sexual response cycle, describing three, four, or five distinct phases. For example, Helen Singer Kaplan's model (1979) encompasses three stages—desire, excitement, and orgasm. Masters and Johnson (1966) describe four phases—excitement (arousal), plateau, orgasm, and resolution. Using instruments that monitor changes in heart rate and muscle tension, Masters and Johnson identified the physiologic changes that take place during each phase.

Currently, experts conceptualize a three-cycle sexual response that includes excitement, orgasmic, and resolution phases (Sadock et al., 2015); however, it is also important to examine desire. Notably, the sexual response can occur in completion even in the absence of desire.

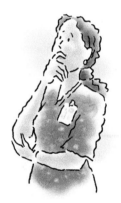

Desire phase

The desire phase is marked by a strong urge for sexual stimulation and satisfaction, either by oneself or with another person. Cultural and societal values affect the range of stimulation that provokes sexual desire.

Potential sexual partners may communicate desire either verbally or through behavior and body language (e.g., flirting). Such communication may be subtle and easily misread (see *Flirting across cultures*) and underscores the importance of obtaining consent prior to engaging in sexual behavior.

Bridging the gap

Flirting across cultures

In different cultures, behaviors meant to communicate sexual desire may vary greatly. Some cultures disapprove of individuals expressing overt communication of their sexual desire—but expect such communication from other individuals.

Culturally defined behaviors can also influence perceptions of what is—and what isn't—flirting. In some cultures, people tend to stand relatively close to each other and make frequent physical contact. Others might misinterpret this behavior as flirting.

In other cultures, people tend to stand farther away and make less physical contact. An individual who isn't aware of these social customs might misconstrue them as a lack of romantic interest—even when such interest is present.

Desire is mental, not physical. Without further mental or physical stimulation, the desire phase may not progress to sexual excitement.

Nice—but not always needed

As mentioned, desire doesn't have to be present for sex to occur. For example, a couple trying to conceive a child may have intercourse, even on days when they lack sexual desire. Also, a person can respond to another's sexual advances, even if they aren't initially experiencing desire.

Excitement or arousal phase

The excitement or arousal phase prepares both partners for intercourse. Muscle tension increases, the heart rate quickens, the skin becomes flushed or blotchy (called *sexual flush*), and the nipples grow hard or erect.

Congested, lubricated, and swollen

Vasocongestion begins during this phase, causing the clitoris, vagina, and labia minora to swell. The vaginal walls start to produce a lubricating fluid, the uterus and breasts enlarge, and the pubococcygeus muscle surrounding the vaginal opening tightens.

The penis becomes erect, the testes become elevated and swollen, the scrotal sac tightens, and the bulbourethral glands (Cowper's glands) secrete a lubricating fluid.

Plateau

With continued stimulation (especially stroking and rubbing of the erogenous zones or sexual intercourse) during full arousal, the plateau stage may be reached. Actually, a person may achieve, lose, and regain a plateau several times without orgasm occurring.

During the plateau stage, the heart and respiratory rates and blood pressure rise further, sexual flush deepens, and muscle tension increases. A sense of impending orgasm occurs. At this point, the clitoris withdraws, vaginal lubrication increases, the labia continue to swell, and the areolae enlarge. The lower vagina narrows and tightens.

In the male genitalia, the ridge of the glans penis becomes more prominent, the Cowper's glands secrete pre-ejaculatory fluid, and the testes rise closer to the body.

Orgasm phase

The orgasm phase is the peak of sexual excitement. Physiologic changes include involuntary muscle contractions, elevated heart rate and blood pressure, rapid oxygen intake, sphincter muscle contraction, and sudden, forceful release of sexual tension.

Describing the indescribable

Orgasm is the shortest phase of the sexual response cycle, typically lasting just a few seconds. Orgasm usually climaxes with the ejaculation of semen. For women, orgasm involves rhythmic muscle contractions of the uterus. Typically, and unless sexual dysfunction is present or the sexual intercourse is not consensual, orgasm is pleasurable for both sexes.

Resolution phase

During the resolution phase, the body returns to its normal, unexcited state. The heart and respiratory rates slow, blood pressure decreases, and muscle tone slackens. Swollen and erect body parts return to normal, and skin flushing disappears. Some of these changes occur rapidly, whereas others take longer. This phase is marked by a general sense of well-being and enhanced intimacy.

Refractory period

For a biological male, the resolution phase includes a refractory period during which the individual can't reach orgasm—although the individual may be able to maintain a partial or full erection. This period lasts a few minutes to several days, depending on such factors as age and frequency of sexual activity. Many biological females, in contrast, can return rapidly to the orgasmic phase with minimal stimulation.

Paraphilic disorders

Paraphilic disorders are complex psychosexual disorders marked by repetitive sexual urges, fantasies, or behaviors that center on:
- inanimate and nonhuman objects
- suffering or humiliation
- children or other nonconsenting persons.

Characteristics of paraphilic disorders

Paraphilic disorders involve an attraction to nonsanctioned sources of sexual satisfaction. The source may be a behavior, as with exhibitionistic disorder or sexual sadism disorder, or a forbidden object of attraction, as with pedophilic disorder or fetishistic disorder.

Paraphilic disorders commonly involve sexual arousal and orgasm, usually achieved through masturbation and fantasy. (See *Puncturing some paraphilic disorder myths*, page 342.) In most people with these disorders, the paraphilic urge, fantasy, or behavior is always present, although its frequency and intensity may remit and recur. Usually, a paraphilic disorder is chronic and lifelong, although it may diminish with age.

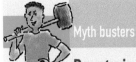

Puncturing some paraphilic disorder myths

Like other sexual topics, paraphilic disorders aren't well understood by the public—and even by some health care professionals. Here are some examples.

Myth: Exhibitionistic disorder is the act of masturbating in front of peers or family members.
Reality: Exhibitionistic disorder is an intense sexual urge to expose one's genitals to an unsuspecting person. Masturbation may occur during an exhibitionist act.

Myth: Pedophilic disorder is defined as exhibitionism in front of a prepubescent child.
Reality: Pedophilic disorder is defined as having sexually arousing fantasies, sexual urges, or behaviors involving sexual activity with a prepubescent child.

Like other mental disorders, paraphilic disorders may worsen during times of increased psychological stress, when other psychiatric disorders are present, or when opportunities to engage in the paraphilia become more available.

Pinning down prevalence

Reliable statistics on the prevalence of paraphilic disorders are difficult to discern. These disorders are rarely diagnosed in clinical settings—most likely because people with paraphilic disorders are secretive about them and may be ashamed. Although some experts believe paraphilic disorders are relatively rare, large commercial markets in paraphilic pornography and paraphernalia, in addition to some preliminary evidence, suggest otherwise. A recent study surveyed over 1,000 individuals and found that one-third of individuals had experience with at least one paraphilic category (Joyal & Carpentier, 2017), calling into question the current definition of what society, and the *DSM-5*, deems normal sexual behavior versus paraphilic sexual behavior.

In clinics specializing in paraphilic disorder treatment, the most commonly seen disorders include pedophilic disorder, voyeuristic disorder, and exhibitionistic disorder. Sexual masochism disorder and sexual sadism disorder are much less common.

The majority of those with paraphilic disorders are males. Those with sexual masochism disorder are the exception, with female-to-male ratio estimated at 20:1.

Criminal compulsions

Some paraphilic disorders are crimes in many jurisdictions. Those that involve or harm another person, particularly pedophilic disorder, exhibitionistic disorder, voyeuristic disorder, and frotteuristic disorder, are commonly considered criminal acts, leading to arrest and possible incarceration.

Individuals with exhibitionistic disorder, pedophilic disorder, and voyeuristic disorder comprise the majority of those apprehended for sex offenses. Sex offenses against children, as in pedophilic disorder, constitute a significant portion of reported criminal sex acts.

Specific paraphilic disorders

The *DSM-5* recognizes eight paraphilic disorders. This chapter discusses three of them in detail. For information on the other disorders, see *DSM-5*(2013).

Exhibitionistic disorder

One of the most common paraphilic disorders, exhibitionistic disorder is marked by sexual fantasies, urges, or behaviors involving unexpected exposure of an individual's genitals to strangers—primarily passersby of the opposite sex in public places. The behavior is usually limited to genital exposure, with no harmful advances or assaults made toward the victim. The individual with exhibitionistic disorder is considered more of a nuisance than an actual danger.

Exhibitionistic disorder has three characteristic features:
- It's typically (but not always) performed by men for unknown women.
- It occurs in a place where sexual intercourse is near impossible, such as a crowded shopping mall.
- It's meant to be shocking; otherwise, it loses its power to produce sexual arousal in the individual with exhibitionistic disorder.

Exhibitionistic disorder is the most prominent sexual offense leading to arrest, accounting for approximately one-third of sexual crimes.

Post-40 fade-out

Exhibitionistic disorder usually begins during adolescence and continues into adulthood. Although it may be a lifelong problem if untreated, it commonly becomes less severe by about age 40 years.

Fetishistic disorder

Fetishistic disorder is characterized by sexual fantasies, urges, or behaviors that involve the use of a fetish—a nonhuman object or a nonsexual part of the body—to produce or enhance sexual arousal.

Fetishistic disorder may involve a partner. Sometimes, focusing on certain parts of the body, such as the feet, hair, or ears, can become a fetish. In some cases, the person can achieve sexual gratification *only* when using the fetish. Usually, fetishes begin during adolescence and persist into adulthood.

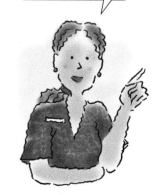

Exhibitionistic disorder usually begins during adolescence and becomes less severe by age 40 years.

Forms of fetishism

Fetishistic disorder commonly presents in two different ways: with arousal occurring via a body part or with arousal occurring via a nonliving object. When arousal occurs via a body part, the individual may engage in sexual activity that focuses on an atypical or not usually sexualized body part, such as the feet, hair, or ears. The latter presentation occurs when an individual seeks sexual arousal from a nonliving object, which can supplement or replace a human partner. This object can include shoes, boots, or particularly fabric, such as velvet or silk. The individual sometimes achieves orgasm when alone and fondling the object.

Pedophilic disorder

Pedophilic disorder is marked by sexual fantasies, urges, or activity involving a child, usually age 13 years or younger. (In adolescents with pedophilic disorder, typically, the child is 5 years younger than the adolescent.) The individual with pedophilic disorder is erotically aroused by children and seeks sexual gratification with them. This urge is their preferred or exclusive sexual activity, although some individuals with pedophilic disorders are also attracted to adults. It should be noted that engaging in sexual contact with a child or person younger than 18 years of age is considered a criminal offense and can result in prison time for convicted perpetrators.

Activity agenda

During sexual activity with a child, the individual with pedophilic disorder may:
- undress the child
- encourage the child to watch the individual masturbate
- touch or fondle the child's genitals
- forcefully perform sexual acts on the child.

Risk factors for victims

Prepubertal children are the most common victims of those with pedophilic disorder. Attraction to girls is almost twice as common as attraction to boys. The individual with pedophilic disorder may sexually abuse their own children or those of a friend or relative.

Behavior profile

Many individuals with pedophilic disorders never come to the attention of authorities. Relatively few engage in other, nonsexual violent behavior. It is also the case that most abusers offend against children that they know or have an established relationship with. In fact, many children have a previous relationship with the perpetrator, and this may impact their willingness to or the likelihood that abuse is reported and treatment is sought (Bottoms et al., 2016).

Typically, the individual with pedophilic disorder behaves seductively, showering the child with money, gifts, drugs, or alcohol, and may be quite attentive to the child's needs to gain loyalty and prevent the child from reporting the encounters (Katz & Barnetz, 2016). The individual with pedophilic disorder will frequently tell the child to keep their activities a secret and will spend an inordinate amount of time doing things with the child. It is also important to note that, in the current era, there has been an increase in online offenses against children, such as Internet child pornography (Ly et al., 2018). Nurses or health care providers who suspect that any child is being sexually abused are mandated reporters, whether the abuse is occurring via direct contact or via Internet or social media.

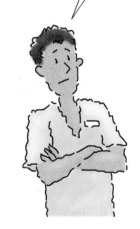

Caution should be taken when an adult is giving a young person excessive gifts of money, other items of value, drugs and/or alcohol, and the like.

Causes of paraphilic disorders

The specific cause of paraphilic disorders is unknown, but experts have proposed behavioral, psychoanalytical, and biological theories to explain these disorders. Behavioral models suggest that a child who was the victim or observer of inappropriate sexual behaviors learns to imitate such behavior and later gains reinforcement for it (Levenson et al., 2018). Biological models, on the other hand, focus on the relationship between hormones, behavior, and the central nervous system (CNS)—especially the role of aggression and male sexual hormones (Holoyda & Kellaher, 2016). It is thought that, in those with paraphilic disorders, levels of circulating testosterone are increased, which can increase sexual drive and impulsivity.

Contributing factors to paraphilic disorders

Based on common patient history findings, some experts have identified factors that may contribute to paraphilic disorders. For example, many individuals with paraphilic disorders come from dysfunctional families marked by isolation and sexual, emotional, or physical abuse (Bijleveld et al., 2016). Some have concurrent mental disorders, such as psychoactive substance use disorders or personality disorders (Frías et al., 2017).

Other factors that may contribute to paraphilic disorders include:
- closed head injury
- CNS tumors
- history of emotional or sexual trauma
- lack of knowledge about sex
- neuroendocrine disorders
- psychosocial stressors.

Signs and symptoms of paraphilic disorders

The patient's history reveals the particular pattern of abnormal sexual fantasies, urges, or behaviors associated with one of the recognized paraphilic disorders.

General assessment findings may include:

- anxiety
- depression
- development of a hobby or an occupation change that makes the paraphilia more accessible
- disturbance in body image
- guilt or shame
- ineffective coping
- multiple paraphilias at the same time
- purchase of books, videos, or magazines related to the paraphilia or frequent visits to paraphilia-related websites
- recurrent fantasies involving a paraphilia
- sexual dysfunction
- social isolation
- troubled social or sexual relationships.

Diagnosis of paraphilic disorders

Diagnosing a patient with a paraphilic disorder is based on a comprehensive history that includes sexual history, fantasies, urges, behaviors, and the duration of symptoms.

Treatment of paraphilic disorders

Those with paraphilic disorders seldom seek help because of their guilt, shame, fear of social ostracism, and/or legal problems. Those who encounter the health care system sometimes do so only at the behest of their family or when forced to by legal authorities. Treatment is mandatory if the patient's sexual behavior is deemed harmful to others or is of a criminal nature. Otherwise, those with certain disorders, such as fetishistic disorder or transvestic disorder, may forego treatment and continue to engage in the paraphilic behavior without significant negative consequences to self or others.

Depending on the specific paraphilic disorder, nonpharmacologic treatment may involve a combination of psychotherapy, cognitive therapy, behavioral therapy, or sex therapy. Pharmacologic interventions can also be effective, such as selective serotonin reuptake inhibitors (SSRIs), which can reduce sex drive and libido as an adverse effect; gonadotropin-releasing hormone analogs, which reduce circulating levels of free testosterone; and medroxyprogesterone acetate (MPA) or cyproterone acetate (CTA), which are synthetic analogs of progesterone that can reduce circulating levels of testosterone (Holoyda & Kellaher, 2016). Surgical interventions are rarely used (Sorrentino et al., 2018).

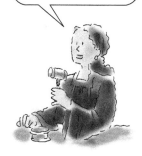

> Some individuals with paraphilic disorder may enter the health care system only because they're forced to by legal authorities.

Improving social skills for those with paraphilic disorders
Some patients with paraphilic disorders have deficient social skills, which are required to obtain sexual satisfaction with consenting adults. Thus, social skills training is an essential part of treatment (Thibaut et al., 2016).

Treatment programs for those with paraphilic disorders who were convicted of a sexual offense
Treatment for those with paraphilic disorders who were convicted of a sexual offense include:
- a specialized sex offender program
- group therapy
- a 12-step sexual addiction or compulsion recovery program
- a rational thinking group
- a structured sexual disorder process group
- educational sessions focusing on the offender's psychological factors, victim impact, and human sexuality
- therapeutically structured recreational activities, adventure-based programming, arts and crafts, team sports, and experimental games
- resident and parent participation in treatment reviews
- alcohol and drug awareness programs
- values clarification
- independent living skills
- vocational exploration.

Pharmacologic therapy
Medications, such as hormones, are generally reserved for individuals with severe cases of paraphilia sexual offenders (Turner & Briken, 2018).

Nursing interventions
Paraphilic disorders are often diagnosed as result of illegal sexual activity.

Care focuses on safety and crisis intervention as comorbid diagnosis of anxiety disorders and depression are common.

Sexual dysfunctions

Sexual dysfunctions are characterized by significant disturbances in an individual's ability to respond sexually or to experience sexual pleasure. These dysfunctions often cause marked distress and interpersonal problems, including relationship discord. They can impair intimate relationships by reducing the enjoyment of sex or preventing the physiologic changes of the sexual response cycle.

In some people, lifelong sexual dysfunction is present at the onset of sexual functioning and activity. In others, dysfunction occurs after a period of relatively normal sexual functioning and is termed *acquired*. Additionally, generalized difficulties are not limited to situations, stimulation, or partners, whereas situational dysfunction refers to difficulties that only occur with certain types of situations, stimulation, or partners.

Although prevalence of sexual dysfunction will vary based on the type of disorder, prevalence rates as high as 55% are found in certain populations (McCabe et al., 2016). Therefore, nurses will undoubtedly interact with patients who are experiencing sexual dysfunction and should be able to appropriately assess for and intervene when such symptoms occur.

In this section, unless otherwise noted, references to "male" and "female" refer to individuals identified as male or female at birth (biological sex).

Categorizing sexual dysfunctions

Sexual dysfunctions are a group of disorders characterized by disturbances in the human sexual response cycle. The *DSM-5* includes the following sexual dysfunctions (APA, 2013):

- premature (early) ejaculation
- delayed ejaculation
- ED
- male hypoactive sexual desire disorder
- female sexual interest/arousal disorder
- female orgasmic disorder
- genito-pelvic pain/penetration disorder
- substance/medication-induced sexual dysfunction.

General signs and symptoms of sexual dysfunctions

Each sexual dysfunction has unique symptoms specific to the sexual disorder; however, it is common for the patient with a sexual dysfunction to present with significant distress and anxiety, strife in intimate relationships, and impairment of overall functioning.

A note about diagnosing sexual dysfunctions

Information from a detailed history, general physical examination, laboratory tests, and other diagnostic tests assists the health care provider in identifying the cause of the sexual dysfunction. The health care provider must rule out possible causes of sexual impairment, such as complications of medical or other mental conditions or side effects of medications or misused substances, before diagnosing sexual dysfunction (APA, 2013).

For most sexual dysfunction diagnoses, the signs and symptoms must have been present for greater than 6 months and occur in nearly all or all sexual encounters (APA, 2013).

Treatment

Identifying the cause of sexual dysfunction is essential in determining the optimal treatment plan. In patients with sexual dysfunctions caused by medical or mental health conditions or substance misuse, treatment is aimed at eliminating the underlying cause as much as possible. If this isn't possible, counseling may help the couple deal with their situation realistically and explore alternatives for sexual expression. If possible, medication dosages may be reduced or other effective medication options may be prescribed. Medical conditions, such as diabetes mellitus, can be controlled to minimize sexual dysfunction symptoms. Abstinence from substances that impair sexual functioning will be included in the treatment plan.

In patients with sexual dysfunctions caused by other factors, treatments may consist of psychotherapy, behavioral therapy, counseling, sex therapy, and pharmacologic therapies (described earlier in the text).

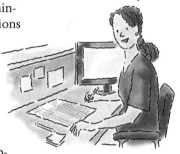

The health care provider will treat sexual dysfunctions caused by medical or other mental health conditions or substance use disorder by eliminating the underlying cause if possible.

Pharmacologic therapy

Specific psychiatric medications can be utilized to combat substance/medication-induced sexual dysfunction. Interestingly, some of these are also antidepressants and include bupropion (Wellbutrin) (Rezaei et al., 2018; Yee et al., 2018) or mirtazapine (Remeron) (Harsh & Clayton, 2018). Other, newer antidepressants, such as vortioxetine (Trintellix) (Salagre et al., 2018), may also result in fewer sexual side effects.

Sensate focus exercises

Many patients with sexual dysfunctions, such as female sexual interest/arousal disorder and male hypoactive sexual desire disorder, may benefit from sensate focus exercises. These exercises minimize the importance of intercourse and orgasm while emphasizing touching and awareness of sensual feelings over the entire body (not just genital sensations).

Sexual dysfunctions

The focus of the sexual dysfunction (excepting paraphilias and gender dysphoria) caused by factors other than medical or mental health conditions or substance misuse is described below:

Premature ejaculation

• An inability to control the ejaculatory reflex during sexual activity. The condition causes an ejaculation to occur prior to or within 1 minute of penetration for nearly all or all sexual encounters (APA, 2013).

• Approximately 4% of men report PE; however, some surveys indicate up to 30% of men having expressed concerns about PE (Snyder & Rosen, 2019). PE is the most common male sexual dysfunction (Boyd, 2018).

• The cause is unknown and research continues relating to genetics, penile hypersensitivity, and negative conditioning (Snyder & Rosen, 2019). Contributing factors may include stress; performance anxiety; feelings of guilt, self-doubt, or inadequacy; or limited sexual experiences.

• Treatment may include behavioral therapy and medications. SSRIs can be therapeutic and are often used to treat PE (Gur et al., 2016). Aside from medication, Masters and Johnson (1966) developed a highly successful intensive treatment program for PE that helps the patient focus on sensations of impending orgasm. The program combines insight therapy, behavioral techniques, and experiential sessions involving both partners. Therapy may include sensate focus exercises (see *Sensate focus exercises*, page 349) and the squeeze technique. (See *Squeeze play for premature ejaculation*, page 354). In addition, the stop-and-start technique helps to delay ejaculation.

Delayed ejaculation

• A delay in ejaculation, infrequent ejaculation, or absence of ejaculation. Men typically report prolonged intercourse to the point of exhaustion or discomfort without successful orgasm or ejaculation. Poor communication in the relationship, poor body image or history of sexual or emotional abuse, psychiatric comorbidity, stress, and medical conditions can also precipitate delayed ejaculation (APA, 2013).

• Treatment may include psychotherapy to address psychogenic factors, lack of knowledge, anxiety, and sexual distress (Abdel-Hamid & Ali, 2017).

Erectile disorder

• ED is the difficulty or inability to obtain or maintain a satisfactory erection during a sexual encounter or a decrease in rigidity of the erected penis.

• It is estimated that between 5% and 20% of men have ED (Boyd, 2018). ED increases with age. Many individuals with ED report low self-esteem and low self-confidence. Psychiatric disorders, such as depression and anxiety, are common.

• Causes of ED may include performance anxiety, relationship stressors, stress, and lack of knowledge.

• Treatment: Sex therapy designed to reduce performance anxiety may effectively cure psychiatrically driven ED. Several Food and Drug Administration (FDA)-approved medications to combat ED, all of which are phosphodiesterase type-5 inhibitors, include sildenafil (Viagra), tadalafil (Cialis), vardenafil (Levitra, Staxyn, or Vivanza), and avanafil (Stendra or Spedra). These medications can cause sustained erection or a precipitous decrease in blood pressure. Other treatments include self-injected vasodilator agents, intraurethral suppositories, and vacuum erection devices. Surgery may be indicated when other measures fail or if penile fibrosis or penile vascular insufficiency is identified (Khera, 2019; Yafi et al., 2016).

Male hypoactive sexual desire disorder

• A recurrent deficient or absent sexual or erotic thoughts, fantasies, or desire for sexual activity

• Prevalence is estimated at 5% to 15%, increases with age, and usually occurs with other sexual disorders (Snyder & Rosen, 2019).

• Nonmedical causes contributing to hypoactive sexual desire disorder include relationship problems, fear of humiliation, fatigue, and other sexual dysfunctions.

• Treatment approaches include formal and informal psychotherapy, including individual and couples therapy.

Female sexual interest/arousal disorder

• An inability to achieve or maintain adequate lubrication and swelling response of sexual excitement, female sexual interest/arousal disorder leads to a reduction in:

  • sexual interest or arousal

Sexual dysfunctions *(continued)*

- sexual excitement or pleasure during sexual encounters
- response to internal or external erotic cues
- genital or nongenital sensations during sexual encounters.
- Prevalence is estimated to be 26% to 43% worldwide and is the most common sexual dysfunction for women (Shifren, 2019).
- Factors contributing to female sexual interest/arousal disorder include relationship stressors, fatigue and stress, age, menopause, inadequate stimulation, psychological factors, and poor body image (Shifren, 2019). Physical indications include lack of vaginal lubrication and absence of signs of genital vasocongestion (Maiorino et al., 2018).
- Treatment includes counseling, couples therapy, sex therapy, lifestyle changes to reduce stress and fatigue, and pharmacotherapy. Flibanserin (Addyi) has been shown to be effective in the treatment of low sexual desire in premenopausal women. Other medications being studied are testosterone combined with sildenafil (Viagra) or buspirone (Buspar), bremelanotide (Vyleesi), BP101, and nasal testosterone (TBS-2) (Both, 2017).

Female orgasmic disorder

- A delayed, infrequent, or absent orgasm following arousal and stimulation, or when orgasmic sensations are markedly reduced. Individuals with this disorder may report difficulty with communicating sexual issues or preferences. Nonetheless, individuals may report high levels of sexual satisfaction despite issues with achieving orgasm (APA, 2013).
- Prevalence is estimated between 15% and 28% in the United States and up to 41% worldwide (McCool et al., 2016).
- Causes include past physical, psychological, or sexual abuse; relationship stressors; lack of knowledge; and guilty feelings about sex.
- Treatment includes psychosocial and behavioral therapies based on causes, situation, and education, such as individual therapy, couples therapy, and partner communication training. Sensate focus exercises, individually or with a partner, are included in the treatment plan. Hormonal therapy, such as phosphodiesterase

type-5 inhibitors, has shown promise in conjunction with psychosocial therapies (Weinberger et al., 2019). For example, flibanserin (Addyi) can be utilized and is generally well tolerated (Joffe et al., 2016).

Genito-pelvic pain/penetration disorder

- Persistent or recurrent difficulties with vaginal penetration during intercourse, or vulvovaginal or pelvic pain during vaginal intercourse or penetration attempts, or fear or anxiety about vulvovaginal or pelvic pain in anticipation of vaginal penetration, or tensing of the pelvic floor muscles during attempted vaginal penetration (APA, 2013). Pain is often described as burning, throbbing, or shooting. Vaginal spasms may occur, resulting in difficult penetration.
- Nonmedical factors contributing to genito-pelvic pain/penetration disorder include fear of pregnancy or losing control; history of frightening, unsatisfying, or painful sexual experiences; or the aftereffects of childbirth (APA, 2013).
- Treatment may include psychotherapy, couples therapy, sensate focus exercises, and progressive use of a plastic dilator or finger to stretch contracted vaginal muscles.

Substance/medication-induced sexual dysfunction

- In medication-induced sexual dysfunction, sexual dysfunction is the result of physiologic effects of such medications as antidepressants, antipsychotics, and antianxiety (benzodiazepines) and cardiovascular (statins, antihypertensives) agents. Substance-induced sexual dysfunction occurs frequently with substances such as alcohol, amphetamines, cocaine, marijuana, nicotine, and opioids (Balon, 2017). Men may present with a loss of sexual interest or desire, inability to achieve or maintain an erection, and difficulty having an orgasm. Women may present with a loss of sexual interest or desire, painful sex, and difficult having an orgasm (National Alliance on Mental Illness, 2019).
- Treatment begins with identifying the cause of the sexual dysfunction. If the cause is medication/substance use, treatment may include changing to other medications, prescribing medications that counteract the side effects of the drug that caused the sexual dysfunction, drug holidays (Balon, 2017), abstinence from substance use, and psychosocial management (Ghadigaonkar & Murthy, 2019).

Sensate focus exercises may be done with a partner. Each partner takes turns giving and then receiving touch and massage. At first, they're instructed to give pleasure without touching the breasts or genitals. The person receiving the pleasure places his or her hand over the giver's to show where the touch should be and what it should feel like. This improves communication and teaches the couple what they *can* achieve rather than what they *can't*.

Later, the ban against genital touching and orgasm is reduced as the couple realizes that mutual pleasure can be derived from simple touching. A sensate focus program may also include masturbation, either alone or together.

Sexual arousal disorder commonly occurs in working mothers with young children. Maybe you're just too exhausted to care about sex.

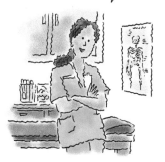

Nursing interventions

In addition to the general interventions listed in *Nursing interventions for patients with sexual dysfunctions*, page 348, these interventions are specific to sexual dysfunction:

- Explain factors that commonly interfere with sexual functioning such as stress, fatigue, prescribed and illicit substances, and medical or mental health conditions.
- Plan time for sexual activity.
- Reinforce education on the use of techniques to facilitate sexual functioning:
  - relaxation techniques to decrease stress and anxiety
  - squeeze play (PE)
  - stop-start technique (PE)
  - sensate focus exercises (PE, female orgasmic disorder, and genito-pelvic pain/penetration disorder)
  - progressive dilation and stretching of vaginal muscles (genito-pelvic pain/penetration disorder)
  - self-injected vasodilators (ED)
  - ureteral suppositories (ED)
  - vacuum erection devices (ED).
- Provide pre- and postoperative care for those men undergoing penile implant surgery (ED).
- Educate on the importance of therapy (individual, couples, and sex therapy) to decrease anxiety and fears related to sexual functioning, increase sexual satisfaction, and enhance communication.
- Encourage communication of sexual needs with sexual partner.
- Educate men about the use of prescribed medications such as phosphodiesterase type-5 inhibitors (ED):
  - Use, purpose, when to take

- ○ Side effects: headache, back pain, muscle pain, gastrointestinal (GI) upset, rash, dizziness, orthostatic hypotension
  - ○ Seek medical help: loss of vision in one or both eyes, blurred vision, priapism (penile erection lasting longer than 4 hours).
- Educate women about the use of a prescribed medication: flibanserin (female sexual interest/arousal disorder):
  - ○ Used only for women who have not undergone menopause.
  - ○ Take at bedtime, avoid grapefruit and alcohol.
  - ○ It may take up to 2 months for improvement in sexual interest/arousal.
  - ○ Side effects: dizziness, dry mouth, insomnia
  - ○ Seek medical help: light-headedness, severe drowsiness.
- Educate on resources for substance use disorder such as smoking cessation support groups and other community resources (substance/medication-induced sexual dysfunction).

Mental health and medications

It is important to remember that sexual problems, including a lack of desire and interest in sex and intimacy and inability or difficulty with performance, can be directly related to the individual's mental health. Any of the mental health disorders can adversely impact how a person feels about sex and their level of interest, particularly if someone is experiencing a mood or anxiety disorder. In addition, a number of illicit substances as well as medications prescribed to treat behavioral disorders are known to cause problems related to sexual interest and performance. (See *Categories of psychotropics that can cause sexual dysfunction*, page 354.) Included among drugs that create problems with performance are alcohol and opioids. In terms of prescribed psychotropic medications, a number of antidepressants, antipsychotics, and anxiolytics can impair erection and ejaculation in males and inhibit or prevent orgasm in women (Montejo et al., 2015). A thorough assessment will ask about the patient's mental health and medications the patient is taking. Most importantly, among the first steps in managing sexual problems is to live as healthy a lifestyle as possible. Simple steps such as watching one's weight; exercising and eating right; and refraining from smoking, drinking to excess, and using drugs can help improve an individual's general health, thus making the road to sexual health a smoother one to travel.

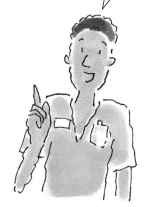

In the stop-and-start technique, the couple starts and stops pelvic thrusting repeatedly to help the man learn to control his ejaculation.

Categories of psychotropics that can cause sexual dysfunction

Antidepressants

Tricyclic antidepressants (TCAs) can cause erectile failure and ejaculation problems in men and anorgasmia and dyspareunia in women. Examples include imipramine (Tofranil), amitriptyline (Elavil), and clomipramine (Anafranil).

SSRIs are the class of antidepressants most commonly associated with sexual dysfunction. They can cause a lack of interest in sex, ED, ejaculatory delay or failure, and anorgasmia. They are also associated with genito-pelvic pain disorder and priapism (sustained erection). Examples include fluoxetine (Prozac), paroxetine (Paxil), and sertraline (Zoloft).

Monoamine oxidase inhibitors (MAOIs) can cause erection difficulties and can delay and inhibit ejaculation and female orgasm. Examples include phenelzine (Nardil), tranylcypromine (Parnate), and isocarboxazid (Marplan).

Antipsychotics

Antipsychotics, both first and second generation, are known to cause a number of problems with sexual functioning, such as decreased sexual desire, diminished or lack of orgasm, a variety of ejaculation disorders, difficulty in achieving an erection, and priapism. Examples of first-generation antipsychotics include haloperidol (Haldol), thioridazine (Mellaril), fluphenazine (Prolixin), and chlorpromazine (Thorazine). Examples of second-generation antipsychotics include olanzapine (Zyprexa), ziprasidone (Geodon), and risperidone (Risperdal).

Anxiolytics

Benzodiazepines can reduce desire because they can cause drowsiness, although in some cases, they can and do increase desire and libido. Examples include diazepam (Valium), chlordiazepoxide (Librium), lorazepam (Ativan), and oxazepam (Serax).

Advice from the experts

Squeeze play for premature ejaculation

The squeeze technique, used to overcome PE, may be practiced either with a partner or alone during masturbation. Advise the patient or his partner to position the fingers correctly around the penis and apply the right amount of pressure. When the patient feels the urge to ejaculate, he or his partner should place a thumb on the frenulum of the penis and place the index and middle fingers above and below the coronal ridge.

Then the patient or partner should squeeze the penis from front to back—more firmly for an erect penis and less firmly for a partially flaccid one. They should apply and release pressure every few minutes during a touching exercise. The goal is to delay ejaculation by keeping the patient at an earlier phase of the sexual response cycle.

The patient should feel pressure but no pain. After several squeezes, he should have a more intense ejaculation than usual.

Anatomic structures and hand position

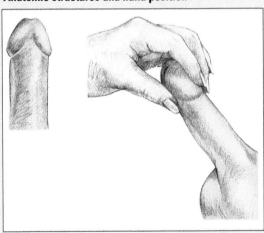

Quick quiz

1. Which phase of the sexual response cycle involves fantasy and expectation?
   A. Desire phase
   B. Excitement phase
   C. Orgasm phase
   D. Resolution phase

Answer: A. The desire phase of the sexual response cycle involves fantasy and expectation.

2. Which factor does the nurse understand may cause or contribute to sexual dysfunction?
   A. Drug use
   B. Dissociative disorders
   C. Supplemental vitamin use
   D. Regimented exercises

Answer: A. Sexual dysfunctions sometimes stem from transient conditions, such as drug or alcohol use.

3. A nurse is caring for a patient with a paraphilic disorder. The nurse understands that a persistent urge to show one's genitalia to a stranger occurs in which disorder?
   A. Fetishistic disorder
   B. Pedophilic disorder
   C. Exhibitionistic disorder
   D. Frotteuristic disorder

Answer: C. An individual with exhibitionistic disorder has sexual fantasies, urges, or behaviors involving exposing the genitals to strangers.

4. Which of the following will the nurse anticipate being part of the treatment plan when caring for a woman with female orgasmic disorder?
   A. Taking soothing bubble bath
   B. Touching the sexual partner
   C. Having sexual intercourse more often
   D. Increasing the degree of sexual arousal

Answer: B. Sensate focus exercises are recommended for female orgasmic disorder. These exercises emphasize touching and awareness of sensual feelings throughout the entire body while minimizing the importance of intercourse and orgasm. The couple takes turns giving and receiving touch.

5. Which disorder involves a person replacing a human partner with a nonliving object?
   A. Fetishistic disorder
   B. Gender dysphoria
   C. Frotteuristic disorder
   D. Female sexual interest/arousal disorder

Answer: A. In one form of fetishistic disorder, a nonliving object completely replaces a human partner. The object may be undergarments, shoes, or a fabric, such as velvet or silk.

6. Which term is used to diagnose a patient who has a sexual attraction to children?
   A. Sexual sadism disorder
   B. Fetishistic disorder
   C. Exhibitionistic disorder
   D. Pedophilic disorder

Answer: D. In pedophilic disorder, the patient has sexual fantasies, urges, or activity involving a child.

Scoring

☆☆☆ If you answered all six items correctly, great work! You know the basics of sexual dysfunction.

☆☆ If you answered four or five items correctly, good job!

☆ If you answered fewer than four items correctly, review what you missed to gain a solid understanding of sexual dysfunction.

Selected references

Abdel-Hamid, I., & Ali, O. (2017). Delayed ejaculation: Pathophysiology, diagnosis, and treatment. *World Journal of Men's Health, 36*(1), 22–40. https://doi.org/10.5534/wjmh.17051

American Psychiatric Association. (2013). *Diagnostic and statistical manual of mental disorders* (5th ed.). American Psychiatric Publishing.

American Psychiatric Association. (2020). *Sexual orientation and gender identity definitions.* https://www.hrc.org/resources/sexual-orientation-and-gender-identity-terminology-and-definitions

Balon, R. (2017). Evaluation and treatment of substance/medication-induced sexual dysfunction. In W. IsHak (Ed.), *The textbook of clinical sexual medicine* (pp. 347–358). Springer.

Bijleveld, C., Hill, J., & Hendriks, J. (2016). Sexual abuse within the family: The intergenerational transmission of victimhood and offending. In H. Kury, S. Redo, & E. Shea (Eds.), *Women and children as victims and offenders: Background, prevention, reintegration* (pp. 905–921). Springer.

Both, S. (2017). Recent developments in psychopharmaceutical approaches to treating female sexual interest and arousal disorder. *Current Sexual Health Reports, 9*(4), 192–199. https://doi.org/10.1007/s11930-017-0124-3

Bottoms, B. L., Peter-Hagene, L. C., Epstein, M. A., Wiley, T. R., Reynolds, C. E., & Rudnicki, A. G. (2016). Abuse characteristics and individual differences related to disclosing childhood sexual, physical, and emotional abuse and witnessed domestic violence. *Journal of Interpersonal Violence, 31*(7), 1308–1339.

Boyd, M. (2017). *Psychiatric nursing:Contemporary practice* (6th ed.). Philadelphia, PA: Lippincott, Wilkins, & Williams.

Chokka, P. R., & Hankey, J. R. (2018). Assessment and management of sexual dysfunction in the context of depression. *Therapeutic Advances in Psychopharmacology, 8*(1), 13–23.

Frías, Á., Gonzβlez, L., Palma, C., & Farriols, N. (2017). Is there a relationship between borderline personality disorder and sexual masochism in women? *Archives of Sexual Behavior, 46*(3), 747–754.

Ghadigaonkar, D., & Murthy, P. (2019). Sexual dysfunction in persons with substance use disorders. *Journal of Psychosexual Health, 1*(2), 117–121. https://doi.org/10.1177/2631831819849365

Gur, S., Kadowitz, P. J., & Sikka, S. C. (2016). Current therapies for premature ejaculation. *Drug Discovery Today, 21*(7), 1147–1154.

Halter, M. (2018). Foundations of psychiatric-mental health nursing (8th ed.). St. Louis, MO: Elsevier.

Harsh, V., & Clayton, A. H. (2018). Sex differences in the treatment of sexual dysfunction. *Current Psychiatry Reports, 20*(3), 18.

Human Rights Campaign. (2020). *Sexual orientation and gender identity definitions.* Retrieved from https://www.hrc.org/resources/sexual-orientation-and-gender-identity-terminology-and-definitions

Holoyda, B. J., & Kellaher, D. C. (2016). The biological treatment of paraphilic disorders: An updated review. *Current Psychiatry Reports, 18*(2), 19.

Ibrahim, A., Ali, M., Kiernan, T. J., & Stack, A. G. (2018). Erectile dysfunction and ischaemic heart disease. *European Cardiology Review, 13*(2), 98.

Joffe, H. V., Chang, C., Sewell, C., Easley, O., Nguyen, C., Dunn, S., Lehrfeld, K., Lee, L. M., Kim, M.-J., Slagle, A. F., & Beitz, J. (2016). FDA approval of flibanserin—Treating hypoactive sexual desire disorder. *New England Journal of Medicine, 374*(2), 101–104.

Joyal, C. C., & Carpentier, J. (2017). The prevalence of paraphilic interests and behaviors in the general population: A provincial survey. *The Journal of Sex Research, 54*(2), 161–171.

Kaplan, H. S. (1979). *Disorders of sexual desire and other new concepts and techniques in sex therapy.* Simon and Schuster.

Katz, C., & Barnetz, Z. (2016). Children's narratives of alleged child sexual abuse offender behaviors and the manipulation process. *Psychology of Violence, 6*(2), 223.

Khera, M. (2019). Treatment of male sexual dysfunction. *UpToDate.* https://www.uptodate.com/contents/treatment-of-male-sexual-dysfunction?search=sexual%20dysfunction%20in%20men%20treatment&source=search_result&selectedTitle=1~150&usage_type=default&display_rank=1

Kite, M. E., & Bryant-Lees, K. B. (2016). Historical and contemporary attitudes toward homosexuality. *Teaching of Psychology, 43*(2), 164–170.

Levenson, J. S., Willis, G. M., & Prescott, D. (2018). Incorporating principles of trauma-informed care into evidence-based sex offending treatment. In E. Jeglic & C. Calkins (Eds.), *New frontiers in offender treatment* (pp. 171–188). Springer.

Liu, G., Hariri, S., Bradley, H., Gottlieb, S. L., Leichliter, J. S., & Markowitz, L. E. (2015). Trends and patterns of sexual behaviors among adolescents and adults aged 14 to 59 years, United States. *Sexually Transmitted Diseases, 42*(1), 20–26.

Ly, T., Dwyer, R. G., & Fedoroff, J. P. (2018). Characteristics and treatment of internet child pornography offenders. *Behavioral Sciences & the Law, 36*(2), 216–234.

Maiorino, M. I., Bellastella, G., & Esposito, K. (2018). Diabetes and sexual disorders. In E. Bonora & R. A. DeFronzo (Eds.), *Diabetes complications, comorbidities and related disorders* (pp. 473–494). Springer.

Masters, W. H., & Johnson, V. E. (1966). *Human sexual response*. Little Brown.

McCabe, M. P., Sharlip, I. D., Lewis, R., Atalla, E., Balon, R., Fisher, A. D., Laumann, E., Lee, S. W., & Segraves, R. T. (2016). Incidence and prevalence of sexual dysfunction in women and men: A consensus statement from the Fourth International Consultation on Sexual Medicine 2015. *The Journal of Sexual Medicine, 13*(2), 144–152.

McCool, M., Zuelke, A., Theurich, M., Knuettel, H., Ricci, C., & Apfelbacher, C. (2016). Prevalence of female sexual dysfunction among premenopausal women: A systematic review and meta-analysis of observational studies. *Sexual Medicine Reviews, 4*(3), 197–212. https://doi.org/10.1016/j.sxmr.2016.03.002

Montejo, A. L., Montejo, L., & Baldwin, D. S. (2018). The impact of severe mental disorders and psychotropic medications on sexual health and its implications for clinical management. *World Psychiatry, 17*(1), 3–11.

Montejo, A. L., Montejo, L., & Navarro-Cremades, F. (2015). Sexual side-effects of antidepressant and antipsychotic drugs. *Current Opinion in Psychiatry, 28*(6), 418–423.

Mosher, C. M. (2017). Historical perspectives of sex positivity: Contributing to a new paradigm within counseling psychology. *The Counseling Psychologist, 45*(4), 487–503.

National Alliance on Mental Illness. (2019). *Medication-induced sexual dysfunction*. https://www.nami.org/Learn-More/Treatment/Mental-Health-Medications/Medication-Induced-Sexual-Dysfunction

Purwata, T. E., Andaka, D., Nuartha, A. A. B. N., Wiratni, C., & Sumada, K. (2019). Positive correlation between left hemisphere lesion and erectile dysfunction in post-stroke patients. *Open Access Macedonian Journal of Medical Sciences, 7*(3), 363.

Rasberry, C. N., Lowry, R., Johns, M., Robin, L., Dunville, R., Pampati, S., Dittus, P. J., & Balaji, A. (2018). Sexual risk behavior differences among sexual minority high school students—United States, 2015 and 2017. *Morbidity and Mortality Weekly Report, 67*(36), 1007.

Rezaei, O., Fadai, F., Sayadnasiri, M., Palizvan, M. A., Armoon, B., & Noroozi, M. (2018). The effect of bupropion on sexual function in patients with schizophrenia: A randomized clinical trial. *The European Journal of Psychiatry, 32*(1), 11–15.

Rice, E., Craddock, J., Hemler, M., Rusow, J., Plant, A., Montoya, J., & Kordic, T. (2018). Associations between sexting behaviors and sexual behaviors among mobile phone-owning teens in Los Angeles. *Child Development, 89*(1), 110–117.

Sadock, B. J., Sadock, V. A., & Ruiz, P. (2015). *Synopsis of psychiatry: Behavioral sciences/clinical psychiatry* (11th ed.). Wolters Kluwer.

Salagre, E., Grande, I., Solé, B., Sanchez-Moreno, J., & Vieta, E. (2018). Vortioxetine: A new alternative for the treatment of major depressive disorder. *Revista de Psiquiatría y Salud Mental, 11*(1), 48–59.

Seehuus, M., & Pigeon, W. (2018). The sleep and sex survey: Relationships between sexual function and sleep. *Journal of Psychosomatic Research, 112*, 59–65.

Shifren, J. (2019). Overview of sexual dysfunction in women: Epidemiology, risk factors, and evaluation. *UpToDate.* https://www.uptodate.com/contents/overview-of-sexual-dysfunction-in-women-epidemiology-risk-factors-and-evaluation? Search =overview%20of%20sexual%20dysfunction%20in%20women&source=search_ result&selectedTitle=1~150&usage_type=default&display_rank=1

Snyder, P., & Rosen, R. (2019). Overview of male sexual dysfunction. *UpToDate.* https://www.uptodate.com/contents/overview-of-male-sexual-dysfunction?search =overview%20of%20male%20sexual%20dysfunction&source=search_result &selectedTitle=1~150&usage_type=default&display_rank=1

Sorrentino, R. (2016). DSM-5 and paraphilias:What psychiatrists need to know. *Psychiatric Times.* Retrieved from https://www.psychiatrictimes.com/dsm-5/dsm-5-and-paraphilias-what-psychiatrists-need-know

Sorrentino, R., Brown, A., Berard, B., & Peretti, K. (2018). Sex offenders: General information and treatment. *Psychiatric Annals, 48*(2), 120–128.

Thibaut, F., Bradford, J. M., Briken, P., De La Barra, F., Haessler, F., & Cosyns, P.; WFSBP Task Force on Sexual Disorders. (2016). The World Federation of Societies of Biological Psychiatry (WFSBP) guidelines for the treatment of adolescent sexual offenders with paraphilic disorders. *The World Journal of Biological Psychiatry, 17*(1), 2–38.

The Trevor Project. (2020). *Asexual.* Retrieved from https://www.thetrevorproject.org/trr_support_center/asexual/

Turner, D., & Briken, P. (2018). Treatment of paraphilia disorders in sexual offenders or men with a risk of sexual offending with luteninizing hormone-releasing hormone agonists: An updated systematic review. *Journal of Sexual Medicine, 15*(1).

van den Brink, F., Vollmann, M., Sternheim, L. C., Berkhout, L. J., Zomerdijk, R. A., & Woertman, L. (2018). Negative body attitudes and sexual dissatisfaction in men: The mediating role of body self-consciousness during physical intimacy. *Archives of Sexual Behavior, 47*(3), 693–701.

Weinberger, J., Houman, J., Caron, A., & Anger, J. (2019). Female sexual dysfunction: A systematic review of outcomes across modalities. *Sexual Medicine Reviews, 7*(2), 223–250. https://doi.org/10.1016/j.smr.2017.12.004

Yafi, F., Jenkins, L., Albersen, M., Corona, G., Isidori, A., Goldfarb, S., Maggi, M., Nelson, C., Parish, S., Salonia, A., Tan, R., Mulhall, J., & Hellstom, W. (2016). Erectile dysfunction. *Nature Reviews Disease Primers, 2*, 16003. https://doi.org/10.1038/nrdp.2016.3

Yee, A., Loh, H. S., Ong, T. A., Ng, C. G., & Sulaiman, A. H. (2018). Randomized, double-blind, parallel-group, placebo-controlled trial of bupropion as treatment for methadone-emergent sexual dysfunction in men. *American Journal of Men's Health, 12*(5), 1705–1718.

Zamorano-Leon, J. J., Segura, A., Lahera, V., Rodriguez-Pardo, J. M., Prieto, R., Puigvert, A., & Lopez-Farre, A. J. (2018). Relationship between erectile dysfunction, diabetes and dyslipidemia in hypertensive-treated men. *Urology Journal, 15*(6), 370–375.

Chapter 15

Gender dysphoria

Just the facts

In this chapter, you'll learn:

♦ gender-related terminology

♦ how gender dysphoria impacts the life span

♦ assessment findings and nursing interventions for patients with gender dysphoria

♦ recommended treatments for patients with gender dysphoria.

Gender-related terminology

Gender is a social construct. Gender dysphoria can exist when there is a conflict between an individual's assigned biological sex and their gender identity. It is important to understand the current gender-related terminology in order to provide patient-centered care (American Psychiatric Association [APA], 2019).

- Assigned gender: the genitalia that is present at birth. Also called "sex," "biological sex," or "natal sex"
- Gender: a social construct of categorization
- Gender identity: the way a person feels inside and how they experience gender. This may or may not correlate with their recorded sex at birth.
- Gender expression: the way that a person chooses to express gender in public; all external behaviors and socially defined characteristics, such as dress, haircut, clothing, social mannerisms, speech, and behavior
- Gender nonconforming: behaviors not typical of individuals of the same assigned gender in a specific society
- Transgender: an adjective—never a noun—that describes a person who identifies as a gender that does not match their biological sex
- Gender dysphoria: a descriptive term reflecting the conflict that occurs when there is an incongruence between a person's physical or assigned natal sex and the gender with which the person identifies

What is gender dysphoria?

Gender dysphoria is the term used to describe the conflict that occurs when gender incongruence causes psychological distress and impaired functioning. People with gender dysphoria question their assigned gender and may determine that it does not match the gender they were assigned at birth (The Trevor Project, 2020).

Individuals with untreated gender dysphoria are at risk for (Kameg & Nativio, 2018):

- discrimination
- bullying
- barriers to health care
- mood disorders
- substance use disorders
- suicidality
- other psychosocial issues.

The gender conflict manifests in various ways. It can affect self-concept, perceptions of an ideal partner, and external expressions of gender through dress, behavior, and mannerisms.

Who am I?

Gender conflict can motivate an individual to seek hormone therapy and/or gender confirmation (or gender-affirming) surgery. This person may choose to express what they believe is their true self, such as dressing in different clothes or using a new name that fits with their new gender identity. New pronouns may also be designated by the person. Some may ask to be addressed with traditional pronouns such as "he/him" or "she/her," whereas others choose nongender-specific pronouns such as "they/them" or "ze/zi" (The Trevor Project, 2020).

The individual may instead choose to deny their conflict and discomfort and try to conform to societal expectations. This can increase distress in many cases. They may feel stigmatized and discriminated against, leading to depression, anxiety, and dysfunction. It may lead to suicidal ideation or suicide attempts. According to Garcia-Vega et al. (2018), almost half of persons who are transgender reported suicidal ideation and 23.8% had attempted suicide. Even after gender confirmation surgery, individuals were about five times more likely to attempt suicide.

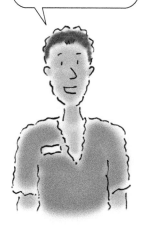

People who are transgender are more likely to attempt suicide.

What gender dysphoria is not...

Gender dysphoria is not a sexual dysfunction. It is not the same as homosexuality, which means a person is sexually attracted to people of the same sex. People who are transgender may identify as straight, gay, lesbian, bisexual, or asexual, and this may change with treatment or with preference.

Incidence and prevalence

It is not known exactly how many individuals experience gender dysphoria, because many people with this disorder never seek help. Gender dysphoria appears to be rare, but the number of individuals diagnosed with this condition is increasing as public awareness grows and stigma decreases.

Demographic details

Gender dysphoria has been known to begin at a very early age (The Trevor Project, 2020). Its prevalence is estimated at 0.56% in the United States, or 560 per 100,000 individuals (Flores et al., 2016; Nolan et al., 2019).

Gender dysphoria is found throughout society. For example, it is estimated that there are 134,000 U.S. Armed Forces veterans with gender dysphoria (Kuzon et al., 2018).

Gender dysphoria can occur with autism spectrum disorder, attention deficit hyperactivity disorder (ADHD), eating disorders, body dysmorphic disorder, substance use disorders, schizophrenia, and obsessive-compulsive disorder. However, it is most commonly found in coexistence with anxiety and depression (Dhejne et al., 2016).

Gender dysphoria across the life span

Gender dysphoria is not limited to one period of life. Gender dysphoria can present across the life span and manifests differently according to stages of life.

Gender dysphoria in childhood

In many cases, gender dysphoria begins to develop in early childhood. One study indicated that children recognized gender dysphoria at a mean age of 8.3 but told their family much later (Olson et al., 2015). A child may not want to wear certain clothing. For example, a girl may not want to wear a dress or a boy may not like wearing pants. Or a boy may prefer to sit when urinating, or a girl may prefer to stand. In many cases this is a temporary preference and does not necessarily persist into adolescence. Only a small percentage of boys and girls treated in gender clinics continue to exhibit gender dysphoria in adulthood.

Children with gender dysphoria may experience bullying at school, loneliness from a sense of being different, and feelings of disgust about their physical appearance, leading to low self-esteem. Diagnosis of gender dysphoria is made by a mental health care provider very carefully in children as this is the time when one's overall sense of identity is developing.

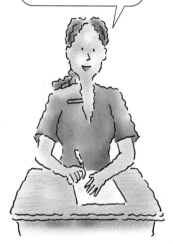

In many cases, gender dysphoria begins to develop in early childhood. *One study indicated that children recognized gender dysphoria at a mean age of 8.3.*

Gender dysphoria in adolescence

In an effort to gain control over unwanted changes of puberty, adolescents may develop anorexia and pathologic weight loss. In a natal female, this may lead to suppression of the menstrual cycle. Some patients may postpone transitioning, while others may wish to move ahead as quickly as possible with hormonal treatment and/or surgical intervention. The issue of competence to make decisions about treatment for gender dysphoria is also important. The mental health care provider works closely with the patient and legal guardian of the child (usually the parent) to make decisions that the child cannot self-make until the age of 18. One of those decisions is about puberty suppression. This can be accomplished with gonadotropin-releasing hormone (GnRH) analogues (synthetic hormones), which can help manage the distress a youth feels when experiencing gender dysphoria at puberty.

Gender dysphoria in adults

Gender dysphoria rarely presents initially in adulthood. It is statistically likely that members of this demographic group have experienced discrimination and social stigma over the years. They face greater risks of poor physical health, victimization, and higher rates of substance abuse and risky sexual behavior compared with adults who live as the sex assigned to them at birth (Johnson et al., 2018).

Causes

The biological mechanisms of gender dysphoria are unclear. There are many theories regarding the cause of gender dysphoria and most suggest a combination of predisposing factors. These factors include:
- Chromosomal abnormalities
- Hormonal imbalances (particularly in utero during brain formation)

- Fetal insensitivity to hormones, known as androgen insensitivity syndrome (AIS), occurs when hormones are not working properly in the womb.
- Congenital adrenal hyperplasia (CAH) occurs when high levels of male hormones are produced in a female fetus. This causes the genitals to become more male in appearance and, in some cases, the baby may be thought to be a natal male when she (a natal female) is born.
- Pathologic defects in early parent-child bonding and child-rearing practices. For example, parents who treat their child as a member of the opposite sex may contribute to gender dysphoria.

Signs, symptoms, and sequelae

Signs and symptoms of gender dysphoria differ among children, adolescents, and adults.

Children

Children may present with the following signs:
- Insisting they are of the opposite assigned gender
- Preferring to play with children of the opposite assigned gender
- Preferring to engage in activities usually associated with the opposite assigned gender
- Wanting to wear clothes typically worn by the opposite assigned gender
- Experiencing severe distress with the physical changes of puberty.

Adolescents and adults

Gender dysphoria is not "just a phase" that an adolescent experiences. Signs of gender dysphoria in adolescents and adults include:
- Feeling sure that one's gender identity is at odds with the assigned gender
- Feeling comfortable only when being in the role of one's truly felt gender identity
- A strong desire to change the outward signs of one's assigned gender, such as body hair removal and voice therapy.

Assessing for gender dysphoria

Adults and adolescents with gender dysphoria believe they were born the wrong sex. They are often interested in eliminating primary and secondary sex characteristics. Some may request hormones, surgery, or other procedures to physically alter their sexual characteristics.

Natal males may describe a lifelong history of feeling feminine and pursuing activities traditionally viewed as feminine. Natal females may exhibit preferences for traditional masculine activities and discomfort with the female role.

Individuals referred for gender dysphoria assessment should have a comprehensive psychological/psychiatric assessment. Remember, gender dysphoria is not a sexual dysfunction. However, it can be associated with mental disorders such as anxiety and depression and requires proper care to manage with a healthy adaptation.

Assessment questions include:

- Is there a clear difference between your natal sex and your gender identity?
- Do you have a strong desire to change the physical characteristics of your assigned gender?
- How are you coping with the consequences of a conflict between your gender identity and assigned gender?
- How much social support do you have, including friends and family?

Signs and symptoms of gender dysphoria

- Anxiety
- Depression
- Attempts to mask or remove the sex organs
- Disturbances in body image (body dysmorphic disorder)
- Dreams of cross-gender identification
- Fear of abandonment by family and friends
- Finding one's genitals "disgusting"
- Maladaptive coping strategies
- Peer ostracism
- Preoccupation with appearance
- Self-hatred
- Self-medication (with alcohol or drugs)
- Insisting they are the opposite assigned gender and hoping they become the opposite assigned gender when they grow up (a sign seen in children)
- Strong attraction to traditional activities of the opposite assigned gender
- Suicide attempts or ideation.

In both natal males and natal females, the crisis related to gender identity is especially acute during puberty. Development of secondary sex characteristics (breasts and pubic hair in the natal female and enlarged penis and testes in the natal male) may trigger intense distress or intensify the internal conflict.

Diagnosis

Patients with gender dysphoria have a marked incongruence between the gender they have been assigned to (usually at birth, referred to as natal gender) and their experienced or expressed gender (APA, 2013). While gender dysphoria presents differently according to age, the underlying component of distress regarding incongruence is a defining characteristic. Diagnosis of gender dysphoria is made according to the diagnostic criteria in the *Diagnostic and Statistical Manual of Mental Disorders*, 5th Edition (*DSM-5*) (APA, 2013).

Testing that may assist with diagnosis includes:
- Karyotyping for sex chromosomes
- Sex hormone assay
- Psychological testing.

Approach to treatment

CARE

Gender-affirming care aims to understand and support the individual's gender experience in a developmental context. An example of an intervention is to provide a message that variations in gender identity and expression are "normal aspects of human diversity and that binary expressions of gender do not always reflect emerging gender identities" (Rafferty, 2018). The Trevor Project (2020) uses the acronym CARE as a reminder:

C: Connect
A: Accept
R: Respond
E: Empower

Holistic, interprofessional, patient-centered care is necessary. A team of health care providers may include plastic surgeons, gynecologists, endocrinologists, urologists, mental health clinicians, nurses, and other providers.

What are the options?

Treatment aims to reduce distress caused by gender dysphoria. Some people may choose to dress and live as a person of their identified gender. For other people, it may mean taking hormones and/or having surgery to alter their physical appearance. Many persons who are transgender choose to permanently alter their body to conform to their gender identity. An evaluation of a person's capacity to make an informed medical decision is a condition for hormonal and surgical treatment.

Therapy

When distress occurs from gender dysphoria, working with a mental health specialist can be helpful. This can include family therapy as well as individual psychotherapy (for children and adults).

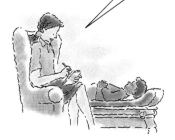

When distress occurs from gender dysphoria, working with a mental health specialist can be helpful.

Group therapy can be very beneficial for adolescents and their parents and also allows for peer support to connect with others experiencing gender dysphoria. Therapy is also important prior to making permanent alterations in body appearance or function. For example, it is suggested that individuals consider whether they may wish to have children in the future. If so, eggs and sperm can be frozen for future use.

An individual may also wish to have speech and language therapy to alter the voice to conform with gender identity. Hair removal therapy is also an option.

Ongoing mental health care may be warranted for individuals who require medications for anxiety and depression, or acute hospitalization for cases of suicidal ideation/plan or self-mutilation.

Social transitions

Sometimes a social transition is made prior to surgery, by living as the gender the person identifies with, at home and in public. This person may also choose to wear clothes and go by a name and desired pronouns that fit. This creates a safe space to explore one's gender and time to thoroughly examine the decision to go forward with surgery, as well as normalizing the experience of gender dysphoria.

Pediatric urologists are starting to see more youth who are transgender and gender nonconforming and have the opportunity to provide supportive and appropriate care for these patients. Referrals often come from mental health providers and, increasingly, from primary care providers.

Pharmacologic therapy

Hormone therapy consists of GnRHs to suppress endogenous hormones. Natal males would receive treatment with antiandrogens and estrogens to become feminized. Natal females receive treatment with androgens to become masculinized. Cross-sex hormonal treatment has been observed to reduce depression, anxiety, and social distress and improve quality of life.

Risk associated with hormone therapy includes (National Health Service, 2016):
- Blood clots
- Gallstones

- Weight gain
- Acne
- Alopecia
- Sleep apnea.

Gender confirmation surgery

For some individuals, gender confirmation surgery may be a desired option. For the natal female who is a transgender male, the surgery may include a bilateral mastectomy, hysterectomy, salpingo-oophorectomy, construction of a penis, scrotoplasty, and a penile implant.

For the natal male who is a transgender female, surgery may include an orchidectomy, penectomy, vaginoplasty, vulvoplasty, clitoroplasty, breast implants, and facial surgery.

Awareness and advocacy

It is important for the nurse to understand the needs of patients experiencing gender dysphoria. Advocacy for the removal of barriers to care for persons with gender dysphoria is needed and is a role nurses are well equipped for (American Nurses Association, 2018). Reducing barriers to health care may improve resilience and increase social support for these patients.

 Quick quiz

1. The nurse is caring for a child who is 9 years old. Which behavior would cause the nurse to suspect gender dysphoria?
    A. A strong desire to be with the parent of the same natal sex
    B. Insistence that he or she is of the opposite natal sex
    C. Preference to play with children of the opposite natal sex
    D. Engaging in games with children of the same natal sex

Answer: B. Gender dysphoria is marked by a repeatedly stated desire to be the opposite natal sex or an insistence that one is the opposite natal sex.

2. The nurse is assessing risk in a client with gender dysphoria. For which condition is the client at higher risk? **Select all that apply.**
    A. Depression
    B. Schizophrenia
    C. Mania
    D. Suicidality
    E. Personality disorder

Answer: A and D. Gender dysphoria places the client at higher risk for depression and suicidality.

3. The nurse is caring for a client with gender dysphoria who is in social transition. What will the nurse anticipate?
    A. The client assumes the natal sex identity while seeking counseling.
    B. The client has undergone gender confirmation surgery.
    C. The client will assume the identity of their preferred gender.
    D. The client will have no changes in outward appearance.

Answer: C. A social transition is often made prior to gender confirmation surgery, by living as the gender the person identifies with, at home and in public.

4. The client states, "I am a natal male." How will the nurse interpret this statement?
    A. The client was born with the assigned gender as a male.
    B. The client's gender identity is male.
    C. The client is transgender.
    D. The client was born with the assigned gender as a female.

Answer: A. Natal male is a term used to describe one's assigned gender at birth.

Scoring

☆☆☆ If you answered all four items correctly, great work! You know the basics of Gender dysphoria .

☆ If you answered fewer than three items correctly, review what you missed to gain a solid understanding of Gender dysphoria.

Selected references

American Psychiatric Association. (2013). *Diagnostic and statistical manual of mental disorders* (5th ed.). American Psychiatric Publishing.

American Psychiatric Association. (2019). *What is gender dysphoria?* https://www.psychiatry.org/patients-families/gender-dysphoria/what-is-gender-dysphoria

Dhejne, C., Van Vlerken, R., Heylens, G., & Arcelus, J. (2016). Mental health and gender dysphoria: A review of the literature. *International Review of Psychiatry, 28*(1), 44–57.

Flores, A., Brown, T. N. T., & Herman, J. L. (2016). *Ethnicity of adults who identify as transgender in the United States.* The Williams Institute.

Garcia-Vega, E., Camero, A., Fernandez, M., & Villaverde, A. (2018). Suicidal ideation and suicide attempts in persons with gender dysphoria. *Psicothema, 30*(3), 283–288.

Johnson, K., Yarns, B. C., Abrams, J. M., Calbridge, L. A., & Sewell, D. D. (2018). Gray and gray session: An interdisciplinary approach to transgender aging. *American Journal of Geriatric Psychiatry, 26,* 719–738.

Kameg, B. N., & Nativio, D. G. (2018). Gender dysphoria in youth: An overview for primary care providers. *Journal of the American Association of Nurse Practitioners, 30*(9), 493–498.

Kuzon, W. M., Jr., Sluiter, E., & Gast, K. M. (2018). Exclusion of medically necessary gender-affirming surgery for America's armed services veterans. *AMA Journal of Ethics, 20*(4), 403–413.

National Health Service. (2016). *Symptoms: Gender dysphoria.* https://www.nhs.uk/conditions/gender-dysphoria/symptoms/

Nolan, I., Kuhner, C. L., & Dy, G. W. (2019). Demographic and temporal trends in transgender identities and gender confirming surgery. *Translational Andrology and Urology, 8*(3), 184–190.

Olson, J., Schrager, S. M., Belzer, M., Simons, L. K., & Clark, L. E. (2015). Baseline physiologic and psychosocial characteristics of transgender youth seeking care for gender dysphoria. *Journal of Adolescent Health, 57*(4), 374–380.

Rafferty, J. (2018). Ensuring comprehensive care and support for transgender and gender-diverse children and adolescents. *Pediatrics, 142*(4), e20182162. www.aappublications.org/news

The Trevor Project. (2020). *Trevor support center: Trans + gender identity.* https://www.thetrevorproject.org/trvr_support_center/trans-gender-identity/

World Professional Association for Transgender Health. (2012). *Standards of care for the health of transsexual, transgender and gender nonconforming people* (7th version). https://www.wpath.org/publications/soc

Selected Internet-Based Resources

American Nurses Association Position Statement. (2018). *The nurse's role in addressing discrimination: Protecting And promoting inclusive strategies in practice settings policy, and advocacy.* http://bit.ly/AddressDiscrimination

Center of Excellence for Transgender Health: Transgender Health Learning Center. http://transhealth.ucsf.edu/trans?page=lib-00-00

The Endocrine Society. *Transgender medicine and research.* https://www.endocrine.org

The Trevor Project. https://www.thetrevorproject.org

World Professional Association for Transgender Health. https://www.wpath.org

Oppositional defiant disorder, conduct disorder, and major depressive disorder in children and adolescents

Just the facts

In this chapter, you'll learn:

◆ theories of growth and development

◆ characteristics of mentally healthy children and adolescents

◆ signs and symptoms of psychiatric disorders in children and adolescents

◆ interventions for children and adolescents with oppositional defiant disorder, conduct disorder, and major depressive disorder

A look at disorders of children and adolescents

Children and adolescents are in a state of rapid change and growth. There are a wide range of behaviors that these individuals experience, many of which are considered normal. Still, an increasing number of children and adolescents experiences emotional and mental distress that is more severe than the expected changes associated with growing up. Some get better over time, while others have serious and persistent problems that affect their daily activities and benefit from professional help.

Alarming statistics show that 48.5% of teens between the ages of 13 and 18 experience a severe mental disorder at some point during their life (National Institute on Mental Health, 2019).

These problems can start early in life and can affect how children achieve their expected developmental, cognitive, and emotional milestones. Undiagnosed and/or untreated mental health concerns can impair the child's or adolescent's ability to function at home, in school, or within community settings and hinder the formation of healthy peer relationships.

It is not always clear whether a child or adolescent has a psychiatric disorder; therefore, assessment by a mental health provider is of high importance. Often, a child or teen may first present with medical problems or demonstrate a range of normal to abnormal emotional behaviors. Further assessment is warranted if the persistent behavior is not age-appropriate, does not conform to the cultural norms, and produces impaired functioning in daily activities.

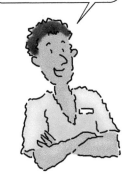

Some psychiatric problems may start in early childhood.

Illness inventory

This chapter discusses more common psychiatric disorders affecting children and teens:

- oppositional defiant disorder (ODD)
- conduct disorder
- major depressive disorder in childhood and adolescence.

Risk factors

Psychiatric disorders occur in children and adolescents of all social classes and backgrounds. Certain factors place children and teens at greater risk, such as:

- low birth weight
- physical health problems
- family history of mental or addictive disorders
- multigenerational poverty
- separation or lack of social support from caregivers
- abuse, neglect, or exposure to violence.

Psychosocial consequences

A child or adolescent with a psychiatric disorder has many challenges to overcome. Despite greater public awareness and understanding of mental disorders, these illnesses still carry a stigma in some settings that can affect the individuals and their families. Children who behave differently may frighten or offend other children and people in the community, placing them at risk to be ostracized.

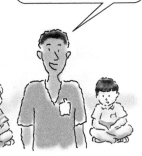

Special classes or special education may be beneficial.

Family discord

Family members may lack adequate knowledge of psychiatric disorders and may feel guilty or embarrassed about having a child who is perceived to be mentally unhealthy or who behaves differently. If the family members do not understand or cannot cope with the child's behavior, they may become frustrated and withdraw, or be overactive in their attempts to control the child's behavior. Ultimately, the caregivers' exasperation may escalate to verbal or physical abuse of the child.

Placement issues

A child whose behavior severely disrupts the family or who can't be integrated into the family unit may require temporary or permanent placement in a structured facility. The placement decision may be influenced by social, financial, religious, and cultural considerations, as well as demographic availability of a facility.

Educational issues

Although most children and adolescents with psychiatric conditions can attend regular schools, those with severe disorders may experience more benefits when enrolled in special classes or special educational facilities. Again, enrollment may be prohibited by financial or geographic considerations.

Childhood development

To understand childhood disruptions and the mental health concerns that can result, nurses must be familiar with the patterns of normal child development. A child typically moves from infancy through childhood to adolescence in an orderly manner. During growth, the personality continually develops from infancy through adulthood.

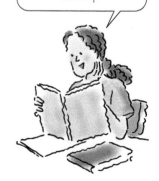

Sigmund Freud, Erik Erikson, and Jean Piaget are important theorists that explained how children develop.

Nature plus nurture

Personality formation is influenced by genetic and environmental factors. Sigmund Freud, Erik Erikson, and Jean Piaget proposed developmental theories to describe the progressive stages of childhood and adolescence. (See *Theories of growth and development,* page 374.)

Nurses who are familiar with theories of growth and development can apply this knowledge to clinical situations and determine a child's expected and actual developmental level by assessing the accomplishment of the tasks defined for each stage.

Recognizing the typical characteristics of mentally healthy young people also helps the nurse compare a child's or adolescent's behavior against the expected norm. (See *Characteristics of mentally healthy young people,* page 375.)

Theories of growth and development

As children grow, they develop intellectually, emotionally, sexually, socially, and spiritually. They learn to think abstractly and logically, to use language, and to explore the world around them. Theorists including Sigmund Freud, Erik Erikson, and Jean Piaget explain how this growth occurs.

Freud: Psychosexual development

Freud theorized that the human mind consists of three major entities—id, ego, and superego. The id seeks instant gratification. The ego orients the person to reality, intercepting impulses from the id. The superego (conscience) develops during childhood—the product of rewards and punishments bestowed on the individual.

According to Freud, children must master each developmental stage before they can move on to the next one.

- **Oral phase (birth to 18 months):** The infant is totally dependent and self-focused and starts to become aware of the self as an individual. Ego development begins.
- **Anal phase (18 months to 3 years):** The child learns to postpone immediate gratification and to manipulate surroundings. Episodes of negativity, rebellion, and conflict may occur. The superego begins to develop.
- **Phallic phase (ages 3 to 6):** The child develops an awareness of anatomic and sexual differences between males and females. The child identifies and adopts the characteristics of the same-sex parent. The skills of cooperation and early socialization occur.
- **Latency period (ages 6 to 12):** As the child identifies with peers, parents become less important. The child's focus is on developing new skills and knowledge and interacting with children of the same gender. Intellectual curiosity increases.
- **Genital (puberty to adult) (age 12 to 20):** The child moves emotionally away from the family and establishes close relationships with peers and the opposite gender. Energy is directed toward work, personal accomplishments, and interpersonal relationships. Adolescent sexual experimentation may begin. Successful resolution of this stage is exhibited by establishing loving and healthy relationships.

Erikson: Psychosocial development

Erikson's theory indicates that major personality changes occur throughout the life cycle. Passage from one stage to another depends on successfully gaining the skills of the preceding stage. Unlike many other theorists, Erikson suggests that new experiences may provide opportunities to cope with deficits in earlier stages.

- **Trust versus mistrust (birth to 18 months):** The infant derives a sense of security from gratification of needs and develops basic trust in the consistent caregiver(s).
- **Autonomy versus shame and doubt (18 months to 3 years):** The child begins to view the self as a person apart from the parents. Children begin to develop a sense of personal control and independence.
- **Initiative versus guilt (ages 3 to 6):** The child starts to behave assertively while exploring and investigating his or her environment. The child develops a beginning sense of purpose.
- **Industry versus inferiority (ages 6 to 12):** Accomplishment occurs and a sense of responsibility develops as the child masters tasks and social skills. A sense of competence develops.
- **Identity versus role confusion (ages 12 to 20):** The adolescent develops a sense of self and personal identity.
- **Intimacy versus isolation (ages 20 to 30):** The ability to establish a commitment to another person occurs. The young adult develops loving, intimate relationships.

Piaget: Cognitive development

Piaget's theory of cognitive development describes successive stages of mental activity that occur during childhood into adolescence. By successfully encountering new experiences, the child adapts and progresses to the next stage.

- **Sensorimotor stage (birth to age 2):** The infant's world focuses on the self. An understanding of the world is experienced through the senses and by motor movements.
- **Preoperational stage (ages 2 to 7):** The child develops language, memory, and imagination. A distinction between the past and the future is made by the child.
- **Concrete operations stage (ages 7 to 12):** The child develops logical thinking and can now use symbols. Abstract concepts such as time, space, categories, numbers, and justice are envisioned.
- **Formal operations stage (ages 12 to adult):** The adolescent begins to think abstractly and systematically and starts to foresee options and possibilities.

Characteristics of mentally healthy young people

When assessing a child for possible psychiatric conditions, the nurse can compare a patient's behavior with what is anticipated for a mentally healthy individual of the same developmental stage. A mentally healthy child or adolescent:

- trusts parents and appropriate caregivers
- views the world as a safe place where needs will be met
- has an age-appropriate sense of reality
- perceives the personal environment realistically
- demonstrates a positive sense of self
- handles age-appropriate stress and frustration effectively
- shows age-appropriate coping skills
- demonstrates mastery of developmental tasks
- communicates or expresses self adequately and appropriately
- has useful and satisfying relationships.

Communicating with children and adolescents

When caring for a child or an adolescent with a psychiatric condition, the nurse's first task is to establish trust. To do this, the nurse must demonstrate empathy and understanding.

Children may be frightened during a first encounter with a health care provider. To establish rapport and build trust, initiate conversation with the child by asking about age-appropriate topics such as toys, hobbies, pets, school, and other subjects that focus on the child's interests.

Communicating with children and adolescents

To further enhance communication with children and adolescents, follow these guidelines:

- Role-model effective ways of communicating.
- Avoid arguments.
- Keep verbal communication brief and use simple language.
- Communicate with kindness, while making expectations clear.
- Ask direct questions when seeking specific information.
- Use body language appropriately.
- Give feedback based on the child's developmental stage.
- Talk about reality by focusing on the "here and now."
- Speak quietly but firmly when reinforcing behavior limits.

Assessment

To fully assess a child or adolescent for a psychiatric condition, the nurse must evaluate the family as well. Begin by collecting biographic data, including the ages of all family members, from the primary caregivers (often the parents or grandparents). Gather information about the family's health, school, housing, economic situation, and religious/spiritual, ethnic, and cultural background.

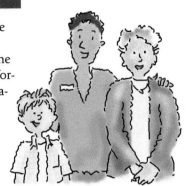

Document an objective description of the primary caregivers, including any communication difficulties, lack of knowledge on growth and development, and family issues and problems.

How do the primary caregivers feel?

Ask the primary caregivers what their concerns are. Ask them how they view the child's behavior, what alleviates or exacerbates the behavior, and how they believe it can be resolved. Evaluate each caregiver's attitude toward the child and the child's present condition. Then obtain the child's developmental history. Find out which, if any, services and agencies are involved in the family's or child's care.

Then begin your interview of the child, including a mental status assessment. (See *Assessing the mental status of a child or adolescent*.)

Diagnosis

A child with signs or symptoms of a psychiatric condition should be first evaluated by a health care provider who specializes in pediatrics and mental health. Based on findings, the provider may recommend further evaluation by a provider who is specialist in child behavioral problems, such as a psychiatrist, psychologist, psychiatric mental health advanced practice nurse, or social worker. When evaluating the child, the provider considers the child's developmental level, social and physical environment, and reports from caregivers and teachers. The purpose of the evaluation is to determine possible causes for the child's behavior and to rule out other possible concerns.

If appropriate, the health care provider makes a diagnosis according to the American Psychiatric Association's *Diagnostic and Statistical Manual of Mental Disorders*, 5th Edition (American Psychiatric Association [APA], 2013).

Oppositional defiant disorder

All children and adolescents at some time will talk back, argue, disobey, and/or defy their caregivers or teachers, especially when they're hungry, tired, ill, or stressed. In fact, for toddlers and young adolescents,

Assessing the mental status of a child or adolescent

When evaluating the mental status of a child or adolescent, be sure to assess:

- physical appearance (age-appropriateness), including hygiene and grooming
- attention level and behavior during the interview
- understanding of his or her role in the interview
- speech or language development
- intellectual functioning
- insight and judgment demonstrated
- demonstrated strengths (e.g., eye contact, appropriate social skills)
- mannerisms, tics, and/or other involuntary movements
- mood and affect
- presence or absence of signs of anxiety, depression, and/or low self-esteem
- ability or inability to listen, follow directions, concentrate, and/or focus
- presence or absence of manipulative, obsessive, impulsive, oppositional, and/or compulsive behaviors
- tolerance for frustration
- difficulty expressing feelings and lack of understanding for other people's feelings
- presence or absence of verbal or physical aggression

- accountability (or lack thereof) for own behavior
- presence or absence of thought disorders, hallucinations, or delusions
- communication problems
- concerns regarding unmet needs for attention, affection, and/or support systems
- perception of emotional closeness to peers and family members
- compliance or noncompliance with family or school rules, society's norms, and laws

Especially for adolescents
- assessment of social skills
- assessment of involvement in, or lack of time for, leisure activities
- academic or employment problems
- discomfort with sexual feelings or inappropriate sexual behaviors
- financial problems
- drug and/or alcohol use and/or disordered eating
- abuse or misuse of technology (e.g., cell phone, Internet)
- legal issues

age-specific oppositional behavior is a normal part of their development. It is important to determine the frequency and tenacity of oppositional behavior in order to ascertain if it is within the normal range of behavior or if it is symptomatic of a psychiatric concern.

Heightened hostility

Hostile, uncooperative behavior in a child may signal ODD, if it is more consistent and severe than that of other children of the same age and developmental level. Another important assessment that may indicate ODD is if the behavior affects the child's social, family, and academic life.

A child with ODD appears exhibits consistently irritable, defiant, noncompliant, antagonistic behavior (Burke & Romano-Verthelyi, 2018). Although this disorder begins in childhood, it is thought to persist into adulthood, causing relational, academic, and occupational difficulties.

No end to the argument

During an argument, children with ODD do not back down, even if they stand to lose privileges. To the child, the struggle overshadows the reality of the situation. If anyone objects to the behavior, the child views it as stimulation to continue the argument. ODD may also be a precursor to conduct disorder (discussed in the following section).

Is oppositional defiant disorder common?

Roughly 1% to 11% (with an average of 3.3%) of school-aged children has ODD (APA, 2013). Onset generally is noted before the age of 8 (APA, 2013).

Prior to adolescence, ODD is more common in males by a 1:4 ratio of males to females. After adolescence, it affects both genders equally (APA, 2013).

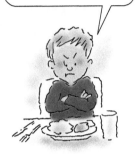

Defiant, disobedient, and hostile—could I have ODD?

Causes

The biological basis of ODD is unknown. However, evidence demonstrates that there is a genetic component that contributes to this disorder (Waldman et al., 2018). Research continues to search for causes related to biological, psychological, and social contributing factors.

Risk factors

Risk factors for development of ODD include:
- acetaminophen use during pregnancy (Ruisch et al., 2018)
- life stressors experienced during pregnancy (Ruisch et al., 2018)
- maternal smoking during pregnancy (Ruisch et al., 2018)
- depression experienced during pregnancy (Ruisch et al., 2018)
- comorbidity with attention deficit hyperactivity disorder (Noordermeer et al., 2017)
- child's natural disposition
- parental difficulties including lack of supervision, harsh discipline, abuse, or neglect
- family conflict or power struggles
- imbalance in brain chemicals (e.g., serotonin)
- limitations or developmental delays in the child's processing of thoughts and feelings.

Signs and symptoms

Signs and symptoms of ODD must occur with more than one authority figure, although they may be more noticeable in one setting versus another. They include (APA, 2013):

- Exhibits a persistent or consistent pattern of angry, irritable, argumentative defiance or vindictiveness, specifically with authority figures
- Disobeys rules directly or indirectly
- Refuses to cooperate with others
- Loses temper frequently
- Is often easily annoyed, angry, and/or resentful
- Makes deliberate attempts to upset or annoy others
- Exhibits spitefulness or vindictiveness
- Blames others for their poor behavior

I'm not going to do that and you can't make me.

Diagnosis

A child with suspected ODD should undergo a complete psychiatric evaluation. The family should be assessed, too, with particular attention given to family interactions, communication patterns, and disciplinary style.

Treatment

Treatment focuses on meeting the child's and family's psychological and psychosocial needs and preventing ODD from progressing to conduct disorder. The child may benefit from individual psychotherapy, with an emphasis on strategies to address anger management.

Teach the caregivers

Caregivers may benefit from educational programs that teach them how to manage the child's behavior, and how to successfully parent. Together, the caregivers and child may undergo family psychotherapy to improve communication, promote adaptive coping skills, and practice positive behaviors.

There are no drug therapies currently approved for treatment of ODD. Other medications may be used to treat symptoms of accompanying anxiety or depression.

Nursing interventions

These nursing interventions are appropriate for a child with ODD:
- Convey a nonjudgmental attitude to help establish a trusting and therapeutic relationship with the child.
- Discuss openly and objectively what consequences will occur when limits are exceeded.

Negate the negativity

- Address negative feelings, especially feelings of anger and resentment. Determine appropriate strategies for handling these feelings.

- Assist in identifying and addressing situations and issues that trigger negative thoughts and feelings.
- Discuss appropriate strategies to use for handling negative emotions (such as shame, blame, and anxiety) and the feelings of "wanting to get even."

Stop the plotting

- Demonstrate how to accept responsibility for personal behavior rather than becoming defensive and plotting revenge.
- Teach methods of controlling temper, and how to express anger appropriately.
- Identify and discuss vindictive behavior, evaluate its effect on others, and devise strategies to eliminate it.

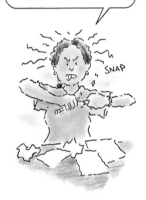

Role model appropriate communication and behaviors

Role-play and reinforce

- Role model appropriate communication and behaviors.
- Teach problem-solving and communication skills. Provide role-playing opportunities to become comfortable and more self-confident when using these new skills.
- Convey acceptance of the child and separate the child's unacceptable behaviors from his or her worth and dignity as a person.
- Reinforce the child's acceptable behavior and positive behavior changes.
- Work with the child and family to address conflict, establish clear expectations, and improve communication skills.

Conduct disorder

Displaying aggressive physical behavior and violating the rights of others are commonly seen in children with conduct disorder. They demonstrate ongoing aggression to people and animals, destroy property, engage in deceit or theft, and seriously violate rules (APA, 2013). Typically, the child has poor relationships with peers and adults and tends to perceive the intentions of other people as hostile and threatening even when this is not the case. Some of the identified personality characteristics of these children include poor self-control and frustration tolerance, frequent outbursts of temper, lack of sensitivity to consequences, and reckless behaviors. The child lacks feelings of remorse or guilt.

Future legal problems

Children with conduct disorder tend to become involved in behaviors that violate the norms of society, which include assault, theft, vandalism, truancy, substance use, running away, and prostitution. Violent behaviors may cause suspension or expulsion from school

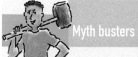

Just a rambunctious child?

All children misbehave now and then, and such behavior is associated with certain stages of normal development. However, misbehavior that is persistent and pronounced, and that interferes with functioning, is **not** normal.

Myth: A child with conduct disorder is just a rambunctious kid involved in normal misbehavior.
Reality: Conduct disorder is a serious mental health problem. A child with

this disorder engages in dangerous behavior, which may lead to involvement with the juvenile justice system or even incarceration.

and the need for placement in foster care, a group home, or a juvenile detention center.

Gender considerations

Conduct disorder affects both genders, but it is more common in males (Mohan & Ray, 2019). Although conduct disorder may occur as early as the preschool years, it is usually diagnosed between middle childhood and early adolescence. (See *Just a rambunctious child?*)

Consequences

A child with conduct disorder is at high risk for:
- school suspension or expulsion
- occupational problems
- risk-taking behaviors (that may result in sexually transmitted diseases, pregnancy)
- rape
- physical injuries and accidents
- substance abuse
- legal problems
- depression with suicidal thoughts, suicide attempts, and suicide itself.

Causes

The cause of conduct disorder isn't fully known, but research indicates that it may be due to genetic and environmental factors. Research shows that a combination of factors such as brain damage, child abuse/neglect, genetic factors, school failure, and/or trauma may contribute to the development of conduct disorder (American Academy of Child and Adolescent Psychiatry, 2018).

Other considerations

Some children diagnosed with conduct disorder also have attention deficit hyperactivity disorder (ADHD), anxiety, or mood disorders. These coexisting conditions may increase the use of drugs and alcohol and involvement in risky behaviors at an early age.

Social risk factors

Various social factors may predispose a child to conduct disorder. All of these factors can lead to lack of attachment to the parents or family unit and eventually to lack of regard for societal rules. They include:

- early caregiver neglect and/or rejection
- separation from caregivers, with no adequate alternative caregiver available
- aggressive behavior leading to unhealthy relationships
- early institutionalization
- family violence
- frequent verbal abuse from parents, teachers, or other authority figures
- a parent with a psychiatric illness, substance abuse, or marital discord
- history of ODD
- large family size, crowding, and poverty.

Other risk factors

Certain physical factors and other conditions also increase the risk of conduct disorder. These include:

- neurologic damage caused by low birth weight or birth complications
- under-arousal of the autonomic nervous system
- lower than average intelligence and learning disabilities
- insensitivity to physical pain and punishment.

Signs and symptoms

Signs and symptoms of conduct disorder include:

- fighting with family members and peers
- speaking to others in a nasty manner
- engaging in cruelty to people or animals
- vandalizing or destroying property
- cheating or cutting classes from school
- running away from home
- using cigarettes, drugs, or alcohol
- stealing or shoplifting
- engaging in precocious sexual activity
- abusing others sexually.

Diagnosis

Understanding the patterns of behavior that a child with conduct disorder uses to violate the rights of others requires an interprofessional team approach, including medical and psychiatric evaluations, caregiver feedback, a school consultant's input, a case manager's plan, and a probation officer's report. A team approach is important because antisocial behaviors go underreported, and earlier intervention has the chance to lead to better outcomes.

What else may be going on?

- Educational assessments must be reviewed to determine if the child also has cognitive deficits, learning disabilities, or problems in intellectual functioning. A neurologic examination may be performed if the child has a history of head trauma, which has been shown to correlate with subsequent use and risky behaviors (Kennedy et al., 2017; Williams et al., 2018).

Treatment

Treatment focuses on coordinating the child's psychological, physiologic, and educational needs. Psychotherapy can help the child learn problem-solving skills, social skills, how to decrease disruptive symptoms, and modify antisocial behavior. Educational strategies focus on encouraging and helping the child to succeed and continue to stay in school. There are no drug therapies currently approved for treatment of conduct disorder. Other medications may be used to treat symptoms of accompanying ADHD or anxiety.

ID them early

Early identification of at-risk children is important because many signs and symptoms of conduct disorder emerge in the earlier life when the child's temperament or personality characteristics emerge and correlate with behavioral problems.

Parental vigilance is needed

Caregivers of an at-risk child should be taught how to set limits and stop the child's aggressive, defensive, and manipulative behavior. They need to learn to create healthy interactions and facilitate the child's self-worth.

Juvenile justice system

Unfortunately, some children with conduct disorder seriously act out and eventually enter the juvenile justice system. Juvenile justice

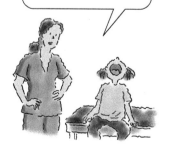

Caregivers must act and not overlook, deny, or make excuses for a child's inappropriate or aggressive behavior.

interventions provide structured rules and a means for monitoring and controlling the child's behavior.

Nursing interventions

These nursing interventions are appropriate for a child (or adolescent) with conduct disorder:

- Establish a trusting, therapeutic relationship with the child. Convey acceptance of the child while setting limits and following through with actions to help him or her to address inappropriate behavior.
- Provide clear behavior guidelines, including consequences for disruptive and manipulative behavior.
- Discuss making acceptable choices, handling anger, and coping with disappointments and frustrations.
- Teach and role-model effective problem-solving skills and have the child demonstrate them in return.
- Partner with caregivers and teachers to identify personal needs and the best strategies for meeting them.
- Teach ways to develop and sustain healthy relationships.

Avert abuse

- Identify abusive communication, such as threats, sarcasm, and disparaging comments.
- Teach options and alternatives and ways of taking responsibility to stop being verbally abusive.
- Teach ways to express difficult and negative feelings appropriately through constructive methods to release stress and frustrations.
- Monitor anger as well as signs of internalization, which may present as signs of depression or suicidal ideation.

Rein in revenge

- Teach ways of taking responsibility for behavior rather than blaming others, becoming defensive, and wanting revenge.
- Teach effective coping skills and social skills.
- Use role-playing to practice ways of handling defensiveness and gaining skill and confidence in managing problematic situations.

Major depressive disorder in children and teens

Everyone feels sad now and then. Mood changes are normal in adults as well as in children and adolescents. Depression is a health problem, which can interfere with the person's ability to function. Persistence of a depressed mood can cause difficulties in eating, sleeping, concentrating, and/or functioning.

Ripple effect

Depression can have widespread effects on a child's adjustment and functioning. A child who is depressed may feel unloved, pessimistic, or hopeless about the future. They may think life isn't worth living. A child with depression is at increased risk for physical illness and psychosocial difficulties that persist long after the depressive episode resolves.

Depression

Major depression (also called *clinical* or *unipolar depression*) is characterized by a depressed mood or a loss of interest in almost all usual activities. There is impaired functioning, a sad or irritable mood, disturbances in sleep and appetite, lethargy, and inability to experience pleasure.

Bipolar possibility

Evidence shows that individuals who initially exhibit depression symptoms may later develop bipolar disorder (Children and Adults with Attention-Deficit/Hyperactivity Disorder [CHADD], 2020). The risk is higher in children and adolescents, as 20% to 40% are thought to develop bipolar disorder later in life (CHADD, 2019). This increased risk underscores the importance of performing a thorough assessment and creating an individualized plan of care as soon as possible.

Two excruciatingly long weeks

Major depressive disorder is characterized by one or more major depressive episodes, defined as episodes of depressed mood lasting at least 2 weeks (APA, 2013). Many patients experience a single episode and recover completely, while others experience recurrences over the life span.

Agonizing episode

In children and adolescents, a major depressive episode can last several months. In addition to feelings of persistent sadness and loss of interest in activities that were previously enjoyable, irritability and difficulty making decisions or concentrating may be noticed. Children and teens with depression may lack energy or motivation and may neglect their appearance and hygiene if not carefully monitored by a caregiver.

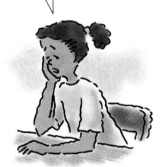

Depression puts children at risk for illnesses and lingering psychosocial problems.

Many miserable kids

In the United States, approximately 3.2% of children aged 3 to 17 years (1.9 million) have been diagnosed with depression

(Ghandour et al., 2018). Early-onset depression can persist, recur, and continue into adulthood. Depression in youth may predict more severe depressive illness in adult life.

Substances and suicide

Teens with depression are at increased risk for substance abuse and suicidal behavior. Suicide attempts peak during the mid-adolescent years. The incidence of death from suicide increases steadily throughout the adolescent years. Suicide is the second leading cause of death for individuals between the ages of 10 and 34 (Centers for Disease Control and Prevention, 2020).

Causes

The multiple causes of depression are not completely understood. Research suggests possible genetic, familial, biochemical, physical, psychological, and social causes. In some patients, the history identifies a specific personal loss or severe stress that likely interacts with a person's predisposition for major depression. Factors such as childhood experiences, stressors, traumatic events, medical illnesses, and exposure to toxic substances can precipitate depression.

Biological tip-offs

The etiology of depression is not fully understood. Genetics, functionality of neurotransmitters, immune responses, and psychosocial factors have all shown some association with this condition (Merck Manual, 2019). Research continues on the use of imaging (such as computed tomography [CT], positron emission tomography [PET], and magnetic resonance imaging [MRI]) to identify structural associations with depression.

Melancholy genes

Studies involving families and twins have demonstrated strong evidence that genetic factors contribute to the risk for depression (Shadrina et al., 2018).

Medical miseries

Depression has been linked to certain medical conditions, such as cardiovascular disease, metabolic syndrome, sleep abnormalities, inflammatory disorders, and the postsurgical period.

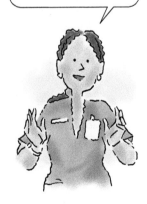

Depression has been linked to certain chromosomal abnormalities.

Risk factors

Common risk factors associated with major depression include (National Council for Behavioral Health, 2019):

- Female gender
- Another psychiatric condition such as anxiety
- Substance use (including cigarettes)

Signs and symptoms

Early diagnosis and treatment of depression is crucial for healthy emotional, social, and behavioral development. Assess the child for such signs and symptoms as:

- experiencing persistent sadness, and or/ an irritable mood
- reporting physical concerns, especially headaches or stomach aches
- persistent crying for no apparent reason
- demonstrating an inability to concentrate or make decisions
- withdrawing from peers and social situations
- being restless, fidgeting, or moving frequently
- lacking interest in daily activities
- having difficulty sleeping or sleeping more than usual
- being fatigued or reporting a lack of energy
- feeling worthlessness, or rejection from others
- experiencing thoughts of death, suicidal ideation, suicide attempts, and other high-risk behaviors
- struggling with normal developmental adjustments
- not growing or developing at an expected rate.

Under the radar

Depression may go unrecognized by the child's family, health care provider, and teachers. Signs and symptoms may be mistaken for the normal mood swings typical of a particular developmental stage. Also, symptoms of depression may be expressed in varying ways depending on the child's developmental stage.

Children and young adolescents may have trouble identifying and describing their emotional states. Instead of expressing how they are feeling, they may act out, which may be interpreted as misbehavior. Often, young people experience irritability associated with depression, which is directly correlated to an increased risk for suicide (Orri et al., 2019).

Depression with a difference

Despite some similarities, childhood depression differs from adult depression in two key ways.

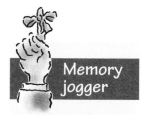

Memory jogger

To help remember the major signs and symptoms of depression in children and adolescents, think of SWAP.

School problems

Withdrawal

Alterations in sleep, appetite, and energy levels

Physical health problems

1. Adolescents experience more changes in weight and/or appetite than adults, which may impact normal and expected growth.
2. Adults frequently experience loss of interest in activities; younger individuals also experience more instances of loss of energy and sleep changes (Bonin, 2020; Rice et al., 2018).

Diagnosis

The diagnosis of depression can be made by the health care provider after gathering information from patient self-reports, family input, interviews, and objective observation.

Tool time

Certain tools may be useful in screening children and adolescents for major depression. Examples of tools include:

1. Children's Depression Inventory 2 (CDI2) for ages 7 to 17
2. Beck Youth Inventory (2nd edition) (BYI-2)—all, or any combination of these tools found within the BYI-2 can be useful:
    o   The Beck Depression Inventory for Youth (BDI-Y)
    o   The Beck Anxiety Inventory for Youth (BAI-Y)
    o   The Beck Anger Inventory for Youth (BANI-Y)
    o   The Beck Disruptive Inventory for Youth (BDBI-Y)
    o   The Beck Self-Concept Inventory for Youth (BSCI-Y)
3. Reynolds Adolescent Depression Scale 2.

A child who screens positive on one of these instruments should undergo a comprehensive diagnostic evaluation by a mental health professional. An interprofessional team approach is crucial. The team should include a medical and psychiatric evaluation, assessment of the patient's psychosocial condition, a school consultant's input, and feedback from caregivers.

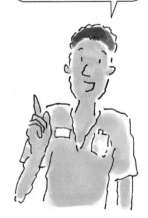

The child may be screened with the Children's Depression Inventory 2 or one of the Beck tools.

Treatment

Treatment of major depression may entail psychotherapy (particularly cognitive behavioral therapy), medication, or a combination. Targeted interventions are most helpful when designed for the specific home and school environments.

Focus on relationships

Cognitive behavioral therapy and interpersonal therapy are evidence-based psychotherapy options that can be used with a child or adolescent with depression. Cognitive-based therapy focused on feelings and thoughts that influence behavior, while interpersonal therapy focuses on working through disturbed relationships that may contribute to depression.

Don't stop too soon

Continuing psychotherapy for several months after symptom remission may help patients and families strengthen the skills they learned during the acute phase of depression. It may also help them cope with depression's aftereffects, address environmental stressors, and understand how the child's thoughts and behaviors could contribute to a relapse.

Pharmacotherapy

Although antidepressant drugs can be effective treatments for adults with depressive disorders, their use in children and adolescents has been controversial. The National Institute of Mental Health recommends the use of antidepressants only when the benefits outweigh the risks. In 2018, the U.S. Food and Drug Administration (FDA) expanded the black box warning on certain agents used to treat children and adolescents who have depression. The revised labeling includes the boxed warning, expanded warning statements about increased risk of suicidality in this population, and accompanying information from pediatric studies (FDA, 2018). (See *Pharmacologic options for treating depression*, page 390.)

Preventing a relapse

After symptom remission, the doctor may recommend that the child continue drug therapy because of the high risk that depression will recur or gradually discontinue the medication under the provider's supervision.

Nursing interventions

These nursing interventions are appropriate for a child or adolescent with major depression:

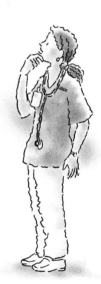

- Structure and maintain a safe, secure environment.
- Sustain a typical routine.
- Monitor for dangerous or self-destructive behavior.
- Address physiologic and psychosocial needs.
- Encourage ways of becoming more social with peers.
- Provide appropriate times to eat, rest, sleep, and play or relax.
- Facilitate development of a support system.

Addressing problems

- Discuss concerns and issues that are upsetting or bothersome.
- Facilitate talking through problems and stressors.
- Teach methods to express strong emotions appropriately.
- Identify techniques to combat self-defeating behaviors, negative verbalizations, and self-statements.

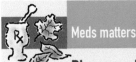

Pharmacologic options for treating depression

A child or adolescent with major depressive disorder may receive a selective serotonin reuptake inhibitor (SSRI) or serotonin-norepinephrine reuptake inhibitor (SNRI). The chart below details the general adverse reactions, contraindications, and nursing interventions for SSRIs and one SNRI.

Drug	Adverse reactions		Contraindications	Nursing interventions
SSRIs • Fluoxetine (Prozac) • Paroxetine (Paxil) • Sertraline (Zoloft) • Escitalopram (Lexapro)	• Nausea • Appetite changes • Dry mouth • Headache • Nervousness • Fatigue • Suicidal behavior or ideation	• Tremor • Dizziness • Seizures • Chest pain • Skin rash • Blurred vision • Flulike symptoms	• Kidney problems • Liver problems • Diabetes mellitus • Suicidal ideation • Concurrent use of a monoamine oxidase (MAO) inhibitor	• Assess and supervise patients for suicidal ideation. • Monitor weekly for weight changes. • Monitor for safety because drug may cause dizziness.
SNRI • Duloxetine (Cymbalta)	• Nausea • Dry mouth • Somnolence • Constipation • Decreased appetite • Suicidal behavior or ideation		• Kidney problems • Liver problems • Suicidal ideation • Concurrent use of a MAO inhibitor	• Assess and supervise patients for suicidal ideation. • Monitor weekly for weight changes.

- Work on age-appropriate strategies for solving problems.
- Encourage open and appropriate expression of feelings.
- Talk about losses, what losses mean, and ways of grieving.

Outlets

- Provide physical outlets for energy and aggression (such as sports, music, or art) to help the child express feelings and develop healthy coping skills.
- Teach techniques that help the child to be assertive, speak up, and ask for what is needed.
- Have the child identify supportive people that he or she can go to when conflict or stressors are experienced and how to talk to these people about feelings and needs.

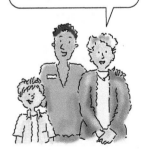

Do you have any concerns you'd like to discuss?

Quick quiz

1. What is the appropriate nursing response when the caregiver of a patient with oppositional defiant disorder asks, "will my child be cured with intervention"?
   A. "Yes, this disorder completely goes away with medication."
   B. "There is no cure for ODD so there is little intervention we can do."
   C. "I would not worry because your child will grow out of this condition."
   D. "Patients with ODD are at higher risk for conduct disorder, so intervention is important."

Answer: D. It is appropriate to notify the caregiver that patients with ODD are still at higher risk to develop conduct disorder, so intervention is important. It is inaccurate to state that the disorder completely goes away with medication, as there are no approved medications that treat ODD. It is also inaccurate to dismiss the caregiver's fear, as ODD is not necessarily something that a child will grow out of, but something that can be addressed with intervention.

2. When the nurse cares for a child with aggressive behavior related to conduct disorder, which further assessment is the **priority**?
   A. Anxiety
   B. Genetics
   C. Depression
   D. Low self-esteem

Answer: D. A child with conduct disorder struggles with low self-esteem and a low tolerance for frustration, even though he or she may attempt to portray an aggressive image. The nurse can subsequently assess for anxiety, depression, and genetic considerations.

3. The nurse is teaching the caregivers of a child with a diagnosis of ODD. What symptom of ODD will the nurse include? **Select all that apply.**
   A. Tests limits
   B. Is often annoyed
   C. Exhibits vindictiveness
   D. Deliberately tries to upset others
   E. Engages in repetitive movements
   F. Refuses to cooperate with others

Answers: A, B, C, D, F. Children with ODD engage in persistent testing of limits, are often annoyed or irritated, exhibit vindictiveness, deliberately try to upset others, and refuse to cooperate with others regardless of consequences. The child with ODD does not generally engage in repetitive movements; this behavior is closely associated with obsessive-compulsive disorder or autism.

Scoring

☆☆☆ If you answered all three items correctly, congrats! Your commitment to understanding kids is commendable!

☆☆ If you answered two correctly, pat yourself on the back! We're proud of your pediatric proficiency!

☆ If you answered one correctly, don't be sad! Review the chapter and pay close attention!

Selected references

American Academy of Child and Adolescent Psychiatry. (2018). *Conduct disorder.* https://www.aacap.org/AACAP/Families_and_Youth/Facts_for_Families/FFF-Guide/Conduct-Disorder-033.aspx

American Psychiatric Association. (2013). *Diagnostic and statistical manual of mental disorders* (5th ed.). Author.

Bonin, L. (2020). Patient education: Depression in children and adolescents (Beyond the Basics). *UpToDate.* https://www.uptodate.com/contents/depression-in-children-and-adolescents-beyond-the-basics

Burke, J. D., & Romano-Verthelyi, A. M. (2018). Oppositional defiant disorder. In M. M. Martel (Ed.), *Developmental pathways to disruptive, impulse-control and conduct disorders* (pp. 21–52). Academic Press.

Centers for Disease Control and Prevention. (2018). *Mental health conditions: Depression and anxiety.* https://www.cdc.gov/tobacco/campaign/tips/diseases/depression-anxiety.html

Centers for Disease Control and Prevention, National Centers for Injury Prevention and Control. (2020). *Web-based Injury Statistics Query and Reporting System (WISQARS)* [online]. www.cdc.gov/injury/wisqars

Children and Adults with Attention-Deficit/Hyperactivity Disorder. (2020). *Pediatric bipolar disorder.* https://chadd.org/for-parents/pediatric-bipolar-disorder/

Food and Drug Administration. (2018). *Suicidality in children and adolescents being treated with antidepressant medications.* https://www.fda.gov/drugs/postmarket-drug-safety-information-patients-and-providers/suicidality-children-and-adolescents-being-treated-antidepressant-medications

Ghandour, R. M., Sherman, L. J., Vladutiu, C. J., Ali, M. M., Lynch, S. E., Bitsko, R. H., & Blumberg, S. J. (2018). Prevalence and treatment of depression, anxiety, and conduct problems in U.S. children. *Journal of Pediatrics, 206,* 256–267.e3.

Kennedy, E., Huron, J., & Munafò, M. (2017). Substance use, criminal behaviour and psychiatric symptoms following childhood traumatic brain injury: Findings from the ALSPAC cohort. *European Child & Adolescent Psychiatry, 26*(10), 1197–1206.

Merck Manual Professional Version. (2019). *Depressive disorders.* https://www.merckmanuals.com/professional/psychiatric-disorders/mood-disorders/depressive-disorders

Mohan, L., & Ray, S. (2019). *Conduct disorder.* StatPearls Publishing.

National Council for Behavioral Health. (2019). *Understanding depression: What it is, who is at risk and where to find support.* https://www.mentalhealthfirstaid.org/2018/07/understanding-depression/

National Institute on Mental Health. (2019). *Mental illness.* https://www.nimh.nih.gov/health/statistics/mental-illness.shtml

Noordermeer, S., Luman, M., Weeda, W. D., Buitelaar, J. K., Richards, J. S., Hartman, C. A., Hoekstra, P. J., Franke, B., Heslenfeld, D. J., & Oosterlaan, J. (2017). Risk factors for comorbid oppositional defiant disorder in attention-deficit/hyperactivity disorder. *European Journal of Child & Adolescent Psychiatry, 26*(10), 1155–1164.

Orri, M., Galéra, C., Turecki, G., Boivin, M., Tremblay, R. E., Geoffroy, M. C., & Côté, S. M. (2019). Pathways of association between childhood irritability and adolescent suicidality. *Journal of the American Academy of Child & Adolescent Psychiatry, 58*(1), 99–107.

Rice, F., Riglin, L., Lomax, T., Souter, E., Potter, R., Smith, D. J., Thapar, A. K., & Thapar, A. (2018). Adolescent and adult differences in major depression symptom profiles. *Journal of Affective Disorders, 15*(243), 175–181.

Ruisch, I. H., Buitelaar, J. K., Glennon, J. C., Hoekstra, P. J., & Dietrich, A. (2018). Pregnancy risk factors in relation to oppositional-defiant and conduct disorder symptoms in the Avon Longitudinal Study of Parents and Children. *Journal of Psychiatric Research, 101*, 63–71.

Shadrina, M., Bondarenko, E., & Slominsky, P. (2018). Genetic factors in major depression disease. *Frontiers in Psychiatry, 9*, 334. https://doi.org/10.3389/fpsyt.2018.00334

Waldman, I., Rowe, R., Boylan, K., & Burke J. D. (2018). External validation of a bifactor model of oppositional defiant disorder. *Molecular Psychiatry.* https://doi.org/10.1038/s41380-018-0294-z

Williams, W. H., Chitsabesan, P., Fazel, S., McMillan, T., Hughes, N., Parsonage, M., & Tonks, J. (2018). Traumatic brain injury: A potential cause of violent crime? *The Lancet Psychiatry, 5*(10), 836–844.

Chapter 17

Substance use disorders

Just the facts

In this chapter, you'll learn:

♦ types of substance use disorders

♦ street names for commonly used substances

♦ proposed causes of substance use disorders

♦ how to assess for substance use disorders

♦ treatment and nursing interventions for patients experiencing substance use disorders and substance withdrawal.

A look at substance use disorders

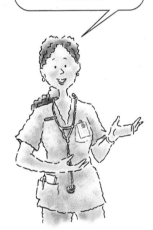

Substance use has been around for centuries.

Substance use disorder (SUD) affects people of all ages, cultures, and socioeconomic groups. People have used alcohol and other psychoactive substances—those that affect the central nervous system (CNS)—for centuries to induce changes in perception, mood, cognition, or behavior. These substances produce a state of consciousness that the user deems pleasant, positive, or euphoric.

SUDs commonly coexist with—and complicate the treatment of—other psychiatric disorders. Likewise, many people with emotional disorders or mental illness may turn to drugs and alcohol to self-medicate and help them cope.

Suspicious substances

A substance of use may be any chemical substance or preparation used therapeutically or recreationally. They are generally substances controlled by the Drug Enforcement Agency (DEA). Common substances of use include:

• alcohol
• caffeine
• cannabis (marijuana), synthetic cannabinoids such as Spice and K2
• hallucinogens—such as phencyclidine (PCP) and lysergic acid diethylamide (LSD)
• inhalants
• opioids—heroin, morphine, oxycodone, kratom and fentanyl

- sedatives, hypnotics, and anxiolytics (primarily benzodiazepines)
- stimulants—amphetamines and amphetamine-like substances, including khat
- cocaine and crack cocaine
- tobacco and inhaled nicotine
- other substances (National Institute of Drug Abuse [NIDA], 2019). Many people use a combination of substances. Drug mixing can become a very dangerous practice.

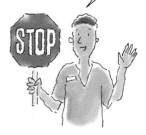

Misusing a single substance is hazardous. Mixing several substances together is especially dangerous.

The language of substance use

The language we use when treating patients with SUDs is very important. Many of the terms have changed, in order to reduce stigma. Here are some important terms and definitions you need to know to fully understand the care of individuals with SUDs.

• *Substance misuse* disorder (formally known as addiction): a primary, chronic disease of brain reward, motivation, memory, and related circuitry. Dysfunction in these circuits leads to characteristic biological, psychological, social, and spiritual manifestations. This is reflected in an individual pathologically pursuing reward and/or relief by substance use and other behaviors.

• *Craving:* an intense desire or urge for the substance that may occur at any time, but is more likely when in an environment where the drug previously was obtained or used.

• *Physical dependence:* an adaptive state that occurs as a normal physiologic response to repeated substance exposure. Physical dependence is the physiologic need to use the substance and if the individual stops taking the substance, withdrawal symptoms will occur. Physical dependence doesn't necessarily indicate substance misuse. Common substances that may lead to physical dependence requiring larger doses to get the same effect include: alcohol, benzodiazepines, methamphetamine, and all opioids including heroin, fentanyl, and oxycodone.

• *Psychological dependence:* A brain disorder and mental illness marked by a compulsive need to seek and use the substance despite the negative consequences and interference to life (e.g., work, school, home, relationships). Characterization of psychological dependence includes: impulsive and risky behaviors, continued substance seeking, and problems associated with health, legal system, financial status, and relationships.

• *Withdrawal:* an uncomfortable syndrome that occurs when tissue and blood levels of the substance decrease in a person who has used that substance heavily over a prolonged period. Withdrawal symptoms may cause the person to resume taking the substance to relieve the symptoms, thereby contributing to repeated substance use.

• *Intoxication:* a reversible, substance-specific syndrome caused by ingestion of or exposure to that substance.

• *Detoxification:* the first step in addiction treatment. The step involves managing the physical symptoms of withdrawal under medical supervision.

Consequences of substance misuse

SUDs often lead to physical dependence, psychological dependence, and usually both. With the exception of cannabis (in selected states where cannabis is legal and decriminalized), most recreational drugs are illegal and thus expose the user to other persons participating in criminal behavior, as well as possible legal consequences. Persons with SUDs may devolve into unhealthy behaviors such as poor diet, hypersomnia/insomnia, and unsafe risk-taking. Chronic substance use impairs social and occupational functioning, creating personal, professional, and financial problems. SUDs are costly not only to the individual but also the community because of the lost productivity, increased costs associated with health care, and crimes committed (Lipari & Van Horn, 2017).

Teenagers and substance use

Experimentation with substance use by preteens and teenagers is pervasive in the United States and many other countries. Greater than 40% of U.S. teenagers have tried an illicit substance at least once. In many cases, experimentation leads to SUD. In a national survey conducted in 2012, the prevalence of SUD for illicit substances in the 13 to 14 years age group is 3.4% and 15% for the 17 to 18 years age group (Bukstein, 2019). SUDs often lead to deteriorating school performance or students dropping out of school.

Which route is used?

Substances may be taken in a variety of ways to maximize effects. (See *Routes.*) Individuals may have complications associated with the substance misuse and with the route of administration.

Using the intravenous route

Using the intravenous (IV) route to inject substances or chemicals via a needle is most commonly associated with heroin use, although other substances (amphetamines, methamphetamines, and cocaine) are used. The use of the IV route can lead to life-threatening complications. (See *Complications of intravenous substance use.*)

Routes	Street names
Intramuscular injection	Muscling
Intranasal inhalation	Snorting or sniffing
Intravenous injection	Shooting up
Oral	Drinking, swallowing pills, popping
Smoking	Smoking
Subcutaneous injection	Skin popping

Complications of intravenous substance use

IV substance use can lead to numerous complications—even beyond those caused by the substances used. For example, using contaminated needles raises the risk of such infections as human immunodeficiency virus (HIV), viral hepatitis (especially hepatitis B and C), and bacterial infections. Heroin/fentanyl and cocaine may cause nephropathy. A condition called *talc granulomatosis* may occur if the drug was adulterated with an inert substance, such as talcum powder (Novick et al., 2016).

With chronic IV substance misuse, potential complications include:

- skin lesions and abscesses
- thrombophlebitis
- vasculitis
- gangrene
- endocarditis
- cardiac and respiratory arrest
- intracranial hemorrhage
- septicemia
- pulmonary emboli
- respiratory infections
- malnutrition
- gastrointestinal (GI) disturbances
- musculoskeletal dysfunction
- depression
- psychosis
- overdose
- increased suicide risk.

Terrible trips

Few people would voluntarily take a substance that is expected to cause an unpleasant experience. However, psychoactive substances often produce negative outcomes—among them, problematic behavior, "bad trips," and even long-term psychosis.

Not so street–smart

Illicit recreational substances pose added dangers. Materials used to dilute these substances can cause toxic or allergic reactions. Specific effects of recreational substances vary with the substance or substances used. Today's "heroin" and cannabis are many times stronger than the substances of 20 years ago. They may be diluted with even more dangerous substances, such as animal anesthesia agents, so potent that they can cause intoxication merely upon contact with the skin (carfentanil).

Defining the terms

According to the American Psychiatric Association (APA, 2013) substance-related disorders are divided into two groups: SUDs and substance-induced disorders. The essential feature of an SUD is a cluster of cognitive, behavioral, and physiologic symptoms indicating that the individual continues using the substance despite significant substance-related problems. SUDs can be diagnosed as mild, moderate, or severe. Substance-induced disorders are those conditions that result from the use of substances and include withdrawal, intoxication, and medication/substance-induced mental health disorders. In addition, the APA classifies gambling disorder under the substance-related and addictive disorders as gambling activates the same reward center as do substances.

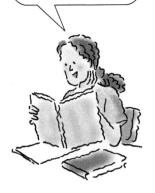

The APA classifies gambling disorder under the substance-related and addictive disorders as gambling activates the same reward center as do substances.

Defining the problem

Substance misuse is a major public health problem. Alcohol is the most common SUD in the United States (Mental Health America, 2020). Another common public health problem is nicotine use; over 34 million U.S. adults use nicotine in some form (Wang et al., 2018). Marijuana use disorder is the third most common in the United States.

In a 2017 national study, approximately 7.2% of individuals 12 and older had a diagnosable SUD within the past year. This percentage encompassed a 5.3% of individuals with alcohol use disorder (AUD) and 2.8% of individuals with an illicit SUD (Dugosh & Cacciola, 2019).

A relationship between SUDs and mental illness has been documented. For example, of the 42.1 million adults with a mental illness, 18.2% had an SUD and of those adults with SUD, 37.9% had a mental illness (Han et al., 2017).

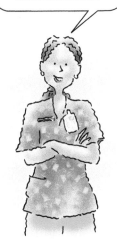

Patients with SUD have a higher risk of comorbid mental health disorders.

Causes of substance-related and addictive disorders

The exact causes of substance-related and addictive disorders aren't known but are under intensive investigation. Probable influences include genetic makeup and environmental factors (McKellen, 2017). Other factors may include personality traits, presence of other mental health disorders, pharmacologic properties of the particular substance, peer pressure, and emotional distress. Several theories explain why some individuals become substance users and why others do not.

- Genetic theories propose
  o Inherited mechanisms cause or predispose a person to substance misuse.
- Neurobiological theories propose
  o Chronic exposure to substances leads to biological and cellular adaptation.

○ Properties of some substances may exert effects on the neurotransmitter systems.

○ Individuals have an inborn deficiency of endorphins—peptide hormones that bind to opiate receptors, reducing the pain sensations and exerting a calming effect. This endorphin deficiency may heighten the sensitivity to pain and confer a greater susceptibility to narcotics use.

○ Enzymes produced by a given gene might influence hormones and neurotransmitters, contributing to the development of a personality that's more sensitive to peer pressure—including the pressure to use illicit drugs (Garmo, 2013).

• Psychobiological theories propose

○ Introducing a narcotic into the body may cause metabolic adjustments that require continued and increasing dosages to prevent withdrawal (Garmo, 2013).

• Behavioral theories propose

○ Substance misuse causes a euphoric experience that the user perceives as rewarding, which motivates the individual to keep taking the substance. The substance, then, serves as a biological reward.

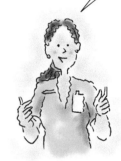

Some people take substances because of peer pressure or as part of a social ritual.

Right on cue

The stimuli and settings associated with substance use may become reinforcing in themselves—or may trigger substance craving that can lead to a relapse. Many recovering substance users change their environment in an effort to eliminate cues that could promote substance use.

• Social and psychological theories propose

○ Adolescents and young adults take substances to preserve childhood and avoid having to deal with adult conflicts and responsibilities. Many users see substances as a way to cope—however dysfunctional—with their personal and social needs and changing situational demands.

Following the crowd

In some cultures, drugs may be more available or social pressures for substance use may be stronger. Social rituals may also play a role by affecting the meaning and style of substance use adopted by a person in a given setting.

Some individuals may be endorphin deficient. This makes them more sensitive to pain—and more likely to misuse narcotics.

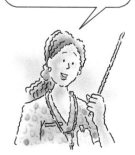

Substance use ... more than one?

When assessing a patient for SUD, establish which substances(s) are being used or have been used including the type, amount, and frequency of use. The use of one substance increases the risk of misusing other substances. Thus, it is essential that health care workers establish a trusting relationship with the patient and are nonjudgmental in interviewing the patient to gain necessary information to increase the likelihood of positive treatment outcomes. In interviewing the patient, follow the rule of most acceptable to least acceptable substance use. For example, ask about caffeine, tobacco, and alcohol use first, followed by prescription medication misuse, then marijuana, and, finally, other substances (bath salts, illicit substances) (Dugosh & Cacciola, 2019).

Alcohol-related disorders

Alcohol (ethanol) is a CNS depressant that reduces the activity of neurons in the brain. In the United States, chronic uncontrolled alcohol intake is the largest substance use problem. Alcohol consumption heightens emotions and relaxes inhibitions, causes cognitive impairment, and produces a sedative effect (Boyd, 2018).

Prevalence

AUD is a common disorder and occurs at all life stages—sometimes starting as early as elementary school age. In the United States, the 12-month prevalence of AUD has increased significantly since 2001 to 2002, especially in women, older adults, lower socioeconomic status groups, and some racial/ethnic minorities (Grant et al., 2017). Globally, the lifetime prevalence for AUD is 16% (Halgren et al., 2017).

Health hazards of alcohol abuse

Heavy alcohol intake adversely affects most body tissues, especially the liver, kidney, and brain. (See *Complications of alcohol abuse.*) Binge drinking and heavy alcohol consumption result in an increased risk of mortality (Xi et al., 2017) and has resulted in more than 2.8 million premature deaths globally (Ritchie & Roser, 2020). (See *Can alcohol kill?*)

Causes

A definitive cause of AUD hasn't been identified. Most experts believe genes play a major role in having or not having AUD. For example, in some ethnic groups, specific genes alter alcohol metabolism, which produces negative experiences (flushing, nausea, and tachycardia) resulting in less alcohol consumption. However, in other groups, alcohol consumption provides a positive experience, which may result in AUD.

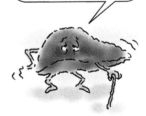

Heavy alcohol intake is rough on my buddies, the kidney and the brain and ... Ooohh ... it's especially rough on yours truly, the liver!

These research findings (among others) support a genetic influence in AUD:

- Identical twins have a higher risk of AUD than fraternal twins.
- Children of alcohol abusers have a fourfold increased risk of AUD—even if adopted at birth.

Other factors

Biochemical abnormalities, nutritional deficiencies, endocrine imbalances, and allergic responses may contribute to AUD. Psychological factors that may lead to AUD include the urge to drink alcohol to reduce anxiety or symptoms of mental illness; the desire to avoid responsibility in family, social, and work relationships; and low self-esteem.

Stress and social attitudes

Sociocultural factors include easy access to alcohol, group or peer pressure to drink, an excessively stressful lifestyle, parental alcohol use or acceptance of youth drinking, and social attitudes that approve of frequent alcohol consumption.

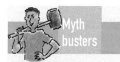

Can alcohol kill?

Don't assume that alcohol is relatively safe just because it's legal.
Myth: Alcohol intoxication doesn't directly cause death, although it can severely impair a person's functioning level.
Reality: Alcohol intoxication can be fatal if the blood alcohol level exceeds 400 mg/dL.

Complications of alcohol abuse

Alcohol damages body tissues through its direct irritating effects, through changes that occur during its metabolism, by interacting with other substances, by aggravating existing disease, or through accidents brought on by intoxication. Tissue damage can lead to a host of complications.

Cardiopulmonary complications
- Arrhythmias
- Cardiomyopathy
- Essential hypertension
- Chronic obstructive pulmonary disease
- Pneumonia
- Increased risk of tuberculosis

GI complications
- Chronic diarrhea
- Esophagitis
- Esophageal cancer
- Esophageal varices
- Gastric ulcers
- Gastritis
- GI bleeding

- Malabsorption
- Pancreatitis

Hepatic complications
- Alcoholic hepatitis
- Cirrhosis
- Fatty liver

Neurologic complications
- Alcoholic dementia
- Alcoholic hallucinosis
- Alcohol withdrawal delirium
- Korsakoff syndrome
- Peripheral neuropathy
- Seizure disorders
- Subdural hematoma
- Wernicke encephalopathy

Psychiatric complications
- Amotivational syndrome
- Depression
- Fetal alcohol syndrome
- Impaired social and occupational functioning
- Polysubstance use
- Suicide

Other complications
- Beriberi
- Hypoglycemia
- Leg and foot ulcers
- Prostatitis

Signs and symptoms

AUD is characterized by four main symptom clusters—impaired control, social impairment, risky use, and pharmacologic dynamics (APA, 2013).

- Impaired control: The individual lacks control of their use. This lack of control manifests as:
  - Taking larger amounts or over a longer period of time than intended
  - Repeated but unsuccessful attempts to cut down or stop use
  - Spending a great deal of time obtaining, using, and/or recovering from the substance
  - Having an intense desire or urge for the substance (craving)
- Social impairment: The individual progressively becomes less and less functional by:
  - Failing to fulfill major role obligations at work, school, or home
  - Continuing substance use despite having persistent or recurrent problems caused by the effects of the substance
  - Giving up or reducing important family, social, occupational, or recreational activities
- Risky use: The individual continues to use:
  - In situations in which it is physically hazardous
  - Despite knowing the negative consequences associated with substance use
- Pharmacologic dynamics
  - Tolerance
  - Withdrawal syndrome.

The patient is asked questions relating to each of the symptoms. The severity of AUD is determined by the number of symptoms present. If a patient has two or three of the symptoms, they may be diagnosed with mild AUD; four or five symptoms is moderate AUD, and severe AUD if patient has six or more of the symptoms (APA, 2013).

However, many individuals with AUD hide or deny their use and temporarily manage to maintain a functional life—which can make assessment a challenge. Nonetheless, certain physical and psychosocial symptoms suggest AUD.

For example, the patient may report minor health issues that are alcohol-related—malaise, dyspepsia, mood swings or depression, and an increased incidence of infection. Also check for poor personal hygiene and untreated injuries, such as cigarette burns, fractures, and bruises that the patient is unable to fully explain. Note an unusually high tolerance for sedatives and narcotics. Assess for signs of nutritional deficiency, including vitamin and mineral deficiencies such as low magnesium, potassium, and folic acid.

Watch for secretive behavior, which may be an attempt to hide the disorder or the alcohol supply.

Desperation tactics

When deprived of the usual supply of alcohol, a patient with AUD may seek a supply of alcohol in any form available—mouthwash, aftershave lotion, vanilla extract, hair spray, and even lighter fluid. Suspect alcohol use in a patient who buys inordinate amounts of aftershave lotion or mouthwash and does not use it in the expected way.

Denial, blame, and projection

Characteristically, a patient with AUD denies the problem—or rationalizes the problem. The patient also tends to blame others and to rationalize problem areas in their life. The patient may project feelings of anger, guilt, or inadequacy onto others to avoid confronting their illness.

Overt signs and symptoms

Overt indications of excessive alcohol use include:
- episodes of anesthesia or amnesia during intoxication (blackouts)
- violent behavior when intoxicated
- the need for daily or episodic alcohol use to function adequately
- inability to stop or reduce alcohol intake
- heavy binge drinking every weekend.

Withdrawal symptoms

A heavy drinker who stops drinking or abruptly reduces alcohol intake is likely to go through withdrawal. Symptoms begin shortly after the drinking stops and could possibly last for up to 10 days. Alcohol withdrawal is a serious condition that requires detoxification and medical treatment.

Initially, the patient experiences anorexia, nausea, anxiety, fever, insomnia, diaphoresis, agitation, tremor progressing to severe tremulousness, and, possibly, hallucinations and violent behavior. Major motor seizures and delirium tremens (DTs) may occur (Pace, 2018). (See *Assessing for alcohol withdrawal*, page 404.)

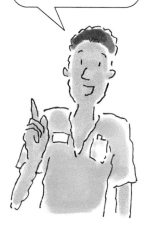

A person suffering from severe AUD with no source of alcohol may drink mouthwash, vanilla extract, or, sometimes, hand sanitizers.

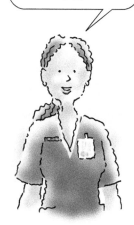

About 5% to 10% of patients with severe AUD experience alcohol withdrawal DTs.

Diagnosis

The diagnosis of AUD centers on a pattern of difficulties associated with alcohol use—*not* on the amount, duration, and frequency of alcohol consumption. In addition, various laboratory tests may suggest AUD and help evaluate for complications, such as cirrhosis of the liver.
- Individuals with a blood alcohol level of 0.01% to 0.10% may have clinical manifestations of alcohol intoxication. (See *Symptoms and treatment of alcohol intoxication*, page 405.) Although this test can't confirm AUD, it can reveal how recently the patient has been drinking—and thus when to expect withdrawal symptoms if the patient is a heavy drinker.
- Urine toxicology may uncover the use of other substance use.

Advice from the experts

Assessing for alcohol withdrawal

Alcohol withdrawal symptoms may vary from mild (morning hangover) to severe (alcohol withdrawal delirium). Formerly known as *delirium tremens* or *DTs*, alcohol withdrawal delirium is marked by acute distress brought on by drinking cessation in a person who's physically dependent on alcohol.

Signs and symptoms	Mild withdrawal	Moderate withdrawal	Severe withdrawal
Motor impairment	Inner tremulousness with hand tremor	Visible tremors; obvious motor restlessness and painful anxiety	Gross, uncontrollable shaking; extreme restlessness and agitation with intense fearfulness
Sleep disturbance	Restless sleep or insomnia	Marked insomnia and nightmares	Total wakefulness
Appetite	Impaired appetite	Marked anorexia	Rejection of all food and fluid except alcohol
GI symptoms	Nausea	Nausea and vomiting	Dry heaves and vomiting
Confusion	None	Variable	Marked confusion and disorientation
Hallucinations	None	Vague, transient visual and auditory hallucinations and illusions (commonly nocturnal)	Visual and, occasionally, auditory hallucinations, usually with fearful or threatening content; misidentification of people and frightening delusions related to hallucinatory experiences
Pulse rate	Tachycardia	Pulse 100–120 beats/minute	Pulse 120–140 beats/minute
Blood pressure	Normal or slightly elevated systolic	Usually elevated systolic	Elevated systolic and diastolic
Sweating	Slight	Obvious	Marked hyperhidrosis
Seizures	None	Possible	Common

- Serum electrolyte analysis may identify electrolyte abnormalities associated with alcohol use.
- Increased plasma ammonia level indicates severe liver disease, as in cirrhosis.
- Liver function studies may point to alcohol-related liver damage.
- Hematologic workup may identify anemia; thrombocytopenia; and increased prothrombin (PT), partial thromboplastin (PTT), and international normalized ratio (INR) times.
- Echocardiography and electrocardiography may reveal cardiac problems related to alcohol misuse such as an enlarged heart (cardiomegaly).

Diagnosis of AUD is confirmed when the patient presents with symptoms of alcohol use, resulting in a significant decrease in function.

Symptoms and treatment of alcohol intoxication

Symptoms of acute alcohol intoxication can include slurred speech, disinhibited behaviors, incoordination, nausea, vomiting, memory impairment, stupor, respiratory depression, and coma depending on the severity of the intoxication (Cowen & Su, 2018).

Acute alcohol intoxication calls for symptomatic treatment, which may involve respiratory support; fluid replacement; IV glucose to prevent hypoglycemia; correction of hypotension, hypokalemia, hypomagnesemia, and hypothermia or acidosis; and emergency measures for trauma and complications as needed.

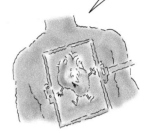

Severe AUD can cause an enlarged heart.

Treatment

Treatment is based on symptoms the patient presents with during acute withdrawal and chronic alcohol use disorder.

Managing acute withdrawal

Because abrupt alcohol withdrawal can cause death, withdrawal should take place in a monitored therapeutic setting. The patient may require IV glucose administration and administration of fluids containing thiamine and other B-complex vitamins to correct nutritional deficiencies and aid glucose metabolism.

Other treatment measures may include:
- furosemide (Lasix) to ease overhydration
- magnesium sulfate to reduce CNS irritability
- benzodiazepines, anticonvulsants, antiemetics, or antidiarrheals as needed to ease withdrawal symptoms
- antipsychotics to control hyperactivity and psychosis.

Treatment of chronic alcoholism

AUD has no known cure, and total abstinence is the only effective treatment. Management commonly involves:
- medications that deter alcohol use (as in aversion or antagonist therapy) and treat withdrawal symptoms
- measures to relieve associated physical problems
- psychotherapy, usually involving behavior modification, group therapy, and family therapy
- counseling by a Licensed Alcohol and Drug Counselor (LADC) or Masters Prepared Licensed Alcohol and Drug Counselor (MLADC) and ongoing support groups.

Antagonist therapy

Naltrexone (ReVia, Vivitrol), an opiate antagonist, may reduce alcohol craving and help prevent persons with AUD from relapsing to heavy drinking, especially when it is combined with substance use support groups or therapy. Naltrexone blocks the brain's so-called pleasure centers, reducing the urge to drink and, for many, diminishing the buzz gained from alcohol. Naltrexone can be taken orally once daily or by injection monthly.

If the patient is prescribed or using opiates, the patient must stop taking any opiates 7 to 10 days before starting naltrexone therapy. Patients taking opioids for pain control may be prescribed acamprosate (Campral).

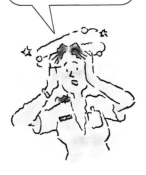

You think I look sick? This is nothing compared to what happens when someone takes alcohol and disulfiram together.

Aversion therapy

In aversion therapy, the patient receives a daily oral dose of disulfiram (Antabuse) to prevent compulsive drinking. Disulfiram impedes alcohol metabolism and increases blood acetaldehyde levels. Disulfiram can be dangerous for any patient who is not sober. Persons who drink heavily when taking disulfiram have a risk of death. Consuming alcohol even within 1 week of taking disulfiram causes an immediate and very unpleasant reaction.

The agonies of Antabuse

Signs and symptoms of a disulfiram reaction include:

- flushing
- throbbing of the neck and head
- nausea and vomiting
- headache
- shortness of breath or other respiratory difficulties
- sweating
- thirst
- chest pain
- palpitations
- tachycardia
- hyperventilation
- hypotension
- syncope
- weakness
- vertigo
- blurred vision
- confusion.

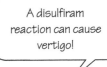

A disulfiram reaction can cause vertigo!

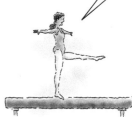

Even small quantities of alcohol, such as the amount in food sauces and cough medicines, or inhaled traces from shaving lotion or furniture varnish, may induce these symptoms.

Counseling and psychotherapy

For long-term abstinence, supportive programs that offer detoxification, rehabilitation, and aftercare—including continued involvement in sobriety support groups such as Alcoholics Anonymous (AA), Teen Challenge, SMART recovery, Women for Sobriety—are effective options. Along with individual, group, or family psychotherapy and treatment by a licensed substance use counselor, these programs improve the patient's ability to cope with stress, anxiety, and frustration and help the individual gain insight into the problems that may have led to alcohol misuse (AA, 2019).

Other types of support

Persons suffering from severe AUD commonly have lost contact with or alienated their family and friends, have a history of difficulty in maintaining jobs/unemployment, legal charges, or incarceration for driving while intoxicated. Their rehabilitation may involve significant support such as job training, sheltered workshops, sober living houses, or other supervised facilities.

Nursing interventions

For general nursing interventions during and after an episode of acute alcohol intoxication, see *General interventions for acute substance intoxication*, page 408.

These interventions may also be appropriate for the patient with AUD:

- If the patient is taking disulfiram, warn that even a small amount of alcohol (such as the amount in cough medicines, mouthwashes, and liquid vitamins) will induce an adverse reaction. Tell the patient that the longer the medication is used, the greater the alcohol sensitivity will be. Educate the patient that paraldehyde, a rarely used sedative, is chemically similar to alcohol and may provoke a disulfiram reaction.
- As appropriate, offer to arrange a visit from spiritual advisors who can help provide the motivation for a commitment to sobriety.

The A's have it

- Tell the patient about AA, a self-help group that offers emotional support from others with similar problems. Stress how this organization can provide the support needed to abstain from alcohol. Offer to arrange a visit from an AA member (AA, 2019).
- Teach the patient's family about Al-Anon and Alateen, two other self-help groups. By joining these groups, family members learn to relinquish responsibility for the individual with AUD so that they can live meaningful and productive lives. Point out that family involvement in rehabilitation also reduces family tensions.
- Refer adult children of alcoholics to the National Association for Children of Alcoholics. This organization may provide support in understanding and coping with the past.

General interventions for acute substance intoxication

Care for a patient with substance misuse starts with an assessment to determine which substance(s) the patient is using. Signs and symptoms vary with the substance and dosage.

During the acute phase of substance intoxication and detoxification, care focuses on maintaining the patient's vital functions, ensuring safety and easing discomfort.

During rehabilitation, caregivers help the patient acknowledge the substance problem and find alternative ways to cope with stress. Health care professionals can play an important role in helping patients achieve recovery and stay substance-free.

These general nursing interventions are appropriate for patients during and after acute intoxication with most types of psychoactive substances.

During an acute episode

- Continuously monitor the patient's vital signs and urine output. Watch for complications of overdose and withdrawal, such as cardiopulmonary arrest, seizures, and aspiration.
- Administer an evidence-based withdrawal scale assessment such as the Clinical Institute Withdrawal Assessment for Alcohol Revised Scale (CIWA-Ar) every 1 to 4 hours, as ordered by the health care provider, to assess for withdrawal symptoms and chart them.
- Maintain a quiet, safe environment. Remove harmful objects from the room. Institute appropriate measures to prevent suicide attempts and assaults, according to facility policy.
- Approach the patient in a nonthreatening, nonjudgmental way. Limit sustained eye contact, which may be perceived as threatening.
- Institute seizure precautions.
- As ordered, administer IV fluids to increase circulatory volume.
- Support the patient to drink large amounts of fluid or soft drinks, including giving them a small pitcher and cup.
- Administer medications, as ordered; monitor and record their effectiveness.

During drug withdrawal

- Administer medications, as ordered, to decrease withdrawal symptoms. Monitor and record their effectiveness.
- Maintain a quiet, safe environment because excessive noise may agitate the patient.

When the acute episode has resolved

- Carefully monitor and promote adequate nutrition.
- Administer medications carefully to prevent hoarding. Check the patient's mouth to ensure that they have swallowed all oral medication(s). Closely monitor visitors who might supply the patient with substances, including cigarettes.
- Coordinate with the hospital, facility social worker, or case worker to refer the patient for rehabilitation as appropriate. Provide a list of available rehab facilities, and encourage the patient to call to set up their next phase of treatment.
- Encourage family members to seek support, regardless of whether the patient seeks it. Suggest family support groups, counselors, or community mental health clinics.
- Develop self-awareness and an understanding and positive attitude toward the patient. Self-monitor your reactions to observed undesirable behaviors—commonly, psychological dependency, manipulation, anger, frustration, and alienation. Seek out support from your supervisor or nurse manager as to how to handle challenging patient behavior.
- Seek out educational opportunities regarding SUDs. The more you know, the more prepared and professional you will be.
- Set limits when dealing with demanding, manipulative behavior.

Caffeine-related disorders

Ahhhh, coffee—the quicker picker-upper!

A mild CNS stimulant, caffeine may be used to restore mental alertness when a person feels tired, weak, or drowsy. Caffeine also may confer health benefits, with many conflicting studies, and has antioxidant properties. However, when used in excess, caffeine causes uncomfortable symptoms of stimulation. Caffeine intoxication can occur with consumption of more than 250 mg of caffeine (equivalent to about 2½ cups of coffee); however, daily amounts of up to 400 mg are considered safe (Poole et al., 2017).

Age and body size influence caffeine effects. A child or a small adult may feel the effects more strongly than a large adult. Older adults are more sensitive to caffeine, feeling the effects at smaller doses, and clearing it from the body more slowly; the average half-life of caffeine for healthy adults is 5 hours, yet can range from 1.5 to 9.5 hours, depending on the individual, and tends to be cleared more slowly by the older adult.

Caffeine habit

Caffeine can be habit forming—most experts agree that some heavy caffeine users may develop caffeine tolerance. Someone who abruptly stops using caffeine may experience symptoms such as headache, fatigue, or drowsiness.

Cupboards full of caffeine

Dietary sources of caffeine include coffee, tea, chocolate, and cola drinks. Caffeine also comes in some prescription and over-the-counter (OTC) drugs. (See *Where's the caffeine?*, page 410.)

How caffeine produces its effects

Scientists aren't exactly sure how caffeine exerts its effects. A leading theory suggests that caffeine antagonizes adenosine, an inhibitory brain chemical that affects norepinephrine, dopamine, and serotonin activity. This antagonism may increase neurotransmitter levels, causing psychostimulation.

Causes

People consume caffeine for such reasons as preference of beverage, to "get going" in the morning, to relieve fatigue, or to stay awake for a particular purpose.

Risk factors for caffeine overuse or sensitivity to caffeine withdrawal aren't known. Genetic factors, such as differences in the way some people metabolize caffeine or a history of substance misuse or mood disorders, may play a role (Poole et al., 2017).

Where's the caffeine?

Common sources of caffeine include:
- coffee (brewed)—40 to 180 mg per cup
- coffee (instant)—30 to 120 mg per cup
- latte—77 mg per cup
- espresso—64 mg per ounce
- coffee, decaffeinated—3 to 5 mg per cup
- tea, brewed (American)—20 to 90 mg per cup
- tea, instant—28 mg per cup
- tea, canned iced—22 to 36 mg per 12 ounces
- cola and other soft drinks—36 to 90 mg per 12 ounces
- cola and other soft drinks (decaffeinated)—none
- cocoa—4 mg per cup
- chocolate milk—3 to 6 mg per ounce
- chocolate, bittersweet—25 mg per ounce
- energy drinks—from 10 to 150 mg per ounce.

OTC preparations that contain caffeine include Caffedrine Caplets, Enerjets, NoDoz Maximum Strength Caplets, and Vivarin. Some pain relievers, such as Excedrin and Midol, also contain caffeine. Adapted from Mayo Clinic (2020)

Signs and symptoms

Assessment findings in a patient with caffeine intoxication may include:
- tachycardia
- palpitations
- arrhythmias
- fatigue that worsens during the day
- anxiety, nervousness, irritability, and easy excitability
- exaggerated startle response
- disorganized thoughts and speech
- facial flushing
- dehydration (from caffeine's diuretic effect)
- hyperactivity
- gross muscle tremors
- restless leg syndrome (muscle cramping and twitching)
- sleep disturbances, such as insomnia or decreased sleep quality (with grogginess in the morning caused by withdrawal symptoms occurring overnight).

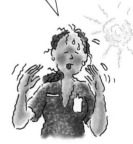

Caffeine has a diuretic effect, which may lead to dehydration.

Caffeine withdrawal symptoms

Caffeine withdrawal symptoms may occur with abrupt caffeine cessation or reduction after a long period of daily use. Withdrawal symptoms tend to be worse in heavy caffeine users (those who consume 500 mg/day or more), although people who consume as little as 100 mg/day (equivalent to one cup of coffee) may also experience discomfort. Withdrawal symptoms may start within a few hours after the time of normal caffeine consumption, reach a peak within 1 or 2 days, and persist for up to 2 weeks.

Withdrawal symptoms

Withdrawal symptoms may include:
- headache
- nausea or vomiting
- jitteriness, irritability, and anxiety
- fatigue
- drowsiness
- depression
- poor concentration or poor performance on mental tasks
- caffeine craving.

Diagnosis

Caffeine blood levels have limited use as a screening tool; most patients will honestly report their daily usage. Urine drug screening can help uncover associated substance use. Thyroid studies can rule out hyperthyroidism. No other specific tests detect caffeine-induced psychiatric disorders. Cardiac irregularities should be investigated by electrocardiogram (ECG).

The diagnosis of caffeine intoxication is confirmed when the patient presents with caffeine intoxication symptoms that are not explained by other conditions.

Treatment

Treatment for caffeine intoxication is the avoidance of caffeine in all forms. Symptoms resolve when the caffeine use stops. The patient should be monitored for caffeine withdrawal. Treatment for withdrawal is symptom based.

Nursing interventions

These nursing interventions may be appropriate for a patient with caffeine intoxication:
- Advise the patient about the expected symptoms of caffeine withdrawal and the duration of those symptoms.

- Reassure the patient that the symptoms will subside and are benign.
- If discomfort lasts more than 2 weeks, assess the patient for other disorders that cause similar symptoms and refer to primary care.

Cannabis-related disorders

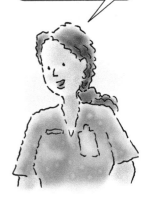

Some people consume cannabis as tea.

Cannabis is a hemp plant from which marijuana (a tobacco-like substance) and hashish (the plant's resinous secretions) are produced. Cannabis is a complex substance involving cannabinoids (tetrahydrocannabinol [THC] and cannabidiol [CBD]) and noncannabinoids (over a hundred bioactive components).

THC is the main component of cannabis that produces the psychoactive and addictive effects. Cannabis may be smoked, consumed as a tea, or mixed into foods. It is most commonly smoked in "joints" or hand-rolled cigarettes, "blunts" that are like a cigar, in water pipes known as bongs, and "vaped" by inhaling the vapor from a collection device.

Recreational and medical use of cannabis is now legal in some states. In those states, edible marijuana products are available, including gummies, brownies, candies, cookies, and drinks.

Nicknames galore

Common street names for cannabis include *pot, grass, weed, mary jane, mj, roach, reefer, joints, THC, blunt, herb, sinsemilla, smoke, boo, broccoli, ace,* and *Colombian.*

Cannabis as medicine

Medicinal use of cannabis has become more common. Cannabis is used medicinally in treating health alterations such as glaucoma, chronic pain, and epilepsy. Because of its lipophilic properties, cannabis accumulates in the adipose tissue and is slowly released. Individuals who smoke cannabis on a daily basis may have cannabis metabolites up to 30 days after the last intake, making withdrawal a slow onset.

CBD

CBD is one of the active compounds in cannabis; however, it does not produce psychoactive effects (Bridgeman & Abazia, 2017).

Prevalence

In a 2017 national study, more than 22.2 million Americans had used cannabis in the past month and more than 43% of graduating high school seniors had tried cannabis at some point, and 22% in the past month; approximately the same percentage of young adults ages 18 to 25 years used cannabis (Substance Abuse and Mental Health Services Administration [SAMHSA], 2017). Although use is relatively common in most age groups, adolescents and young adults are the most common users.

How cannabis produces its effects

The most powerful psychoactive and addictive substance in cannabis is delta-l-tetrahydrocannabinol (delta-1-THC). When marijuana is smoked, delta-1-THC rapidly passes from the lungs into the bloodstream, which carries it to the brain and other organs.

In the brain, delta-1-THC connects to cannabinoid receptors on neurons, influencing their activity. (See *The endocannabinoid system.*) It is not yet known how CBD affects the endocannabinoid system (ECS) as it works differently than delta-1-THC.

Health hazards of cannabis use

Cannabis can be addictive and may cause various adverse physiologic effects.

Respiratory effects

Marijuana smoke can harm the lungs. The smoke contains carcinogens similar to those found in tobacco smoke. Chronic and heavy cannabis use may increase the risk of chronic obstructive lung disease. Also, some studies show that respiratory tumors are more common among individuals who use marijuana habitually.

Cardiovascular effects

Acute cannabis intoxication may trigger tachycardia and orthostatic hypotension.

The endocannabinoid system

The ECS involves a complex cell-signaling system regulating such processes as: sleep, mood, appetite, learning and memory, stress, and reproduction. The body produces endogenous cannabinoid molecules that bind to endocannabinoid receptors found in the CNS (CB1 receptors) and peripheral nervous system (CB2 receptors). The activated receptor sends a signal to the ECS to take action. Specific enzymes then break down the endocannabinoids once they have activated the receptors. Although research is needed to continue exploring the specifics of the ECS, funding is difficult to secure because of federal laws associated with marijuana use.

Reproductive effects

In females, cannabis use may increase the number of anovulatory cycles. In males, it may reduce the levels of follicle-stimulating hormone, leading to a decrease in testosterone production and, possibly, testicular atrophy.

Although cannabis use has been linked to decreased sperm counts, the drug's effect on fertility remains unclear.

Other health effects

Cannabis may weaken the immune system. In very young teens, it has a profoundly negative effect on development.

Combination drug use

Marijuana may be combined with other substances, such as crack cocaine, PCP, formaldehyde, and codeine cough syrup—sometimes without the user being aware of it. These additional substances compound the risks associated with marijuana use.

Impairments associated with cannabis use

Cannabis use can result in perceptual distortions and impairments in short-term memory, learning ability, judgment, and verbal skills. Long-term use can result in marked impairment on social, family, and occupational functioning (Patel & Marwaha, 2019).

Memory and learning impairments

Marijuana's adverse impact on learning and memory can last for days or weeks after the acute drug effects wear off. Therefore, someone who smokes once a day may be functioning at a reduced intellectual level all of the time. A 25-year study following young adults found that individuals who use cannabis had cumulative, additive effects of reduced verbal memory (Auer et al., 2016).

Wasted at work

Problems at work are more common among employees who use marijuana including increased absences, tardiness, accidents, workers' compensation claims, and job turnover.

Coexisting psychiatric disorders

Marijuana use is associated with anxiety, depression, and personality disturbances. Research shows that marijuana can cause problems in daily life or worsen existing problems.

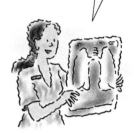

Chronic and heavy cannabis use may raise the risk of chronic obstructive lung disease and respiratory tumors.

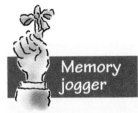

Memory jogger

WEED is a street name for cannabis—and a quick key to assessing a patient for suspected cannabis use.

Wild behavior (hallucinations, impaired cognition, paranoia, spontaneous laughter)

Euphoria

Elevated heart rate (tachycardia)

Distorted sense of time and self-perception, decreased muscle tone, dry mouth

Causes

As with other types of substance use, the exact causes of cannabis use aren't known. Suggested risk factors include:
- young age
- drug availability (influenced by geographic and cultural factors)
- coexisting alcohol use or dependence
- coexisting use of other substances.

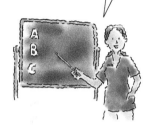

Students who regularly smoke marijuana score lower on standardized verbal and math tests.

Signs and symptoms

Assessment findings in a patient under the influence of cannabis include:
- relaxation
- euphoria
- spontaneous laughter
- feelings of well-being or grandiosity
- visual distortions and other perceptual changes
- subjective sense that time is passing more slowly than normal
- tachycardia
- dry mouth
- conjunctival redness
- drowsiness and sluggishness (or paradoxical hyperalertness)
- decreased muscle strength
- poor coordination
- increased hunger (the "munchies").

With overdose, you may detect signs or symptoms of pulmonary edema, respiratory depression, aspiration pneumonia, or hypotension.

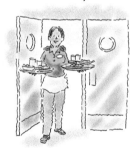

The "munchies" are but one of many telltale signs of cannabis use.

Dysphoric effects

In some people, cannabis intoxication causes a dysphoric reaction, which may manifest as:
- panic and disorientation
- paranoia
- mood swings
- altered perceptions (such as illusions or frank hallucinations)
- depersonalization
- psychotic episodes.

Findings in chronic cannabis use

Individuals who have used cannabis chronically may experience a syndrome marked by appetite changes, lack of ambition and energy, and reduced social and occupational drive (National Institutes of Health [NIH], n.d.-a).

Cannabinoid hyperemesis syndrome

With increasing use of more concentrated and potent cannabis products, emergency rooms and psychiatric units have seen a spike in patients suffering from cannabinoid hyperemesis syndrome, though the diagnosis may often be missed. Sufferers experience cyclic nausea and vomiting and may find relief from hot baths or showers. The syndrome is thought to be related to fat storage of THC compounds in individuals who have used cannabis for a long period of time and persons who may use the substance as many as three to five times daily (Schreck et al., 2018).

Withdrawal symptoms

Although withdrawal symptoms from cannabis are less severe than from other drugs, some individuals experience restlessness, irritability, appetite loss, and sleep difficulties (NIH, n.d.-a).

Diagnosis

Urine screening may reveal cannabis presence for as long as 30 days after use. The diagnosis of cannabis use disorder is confirmed when the patient presents with the symptoms associated with cannabis use disorder, resulting in a significant decrease in function.

Treatment

Acute cannabis intoxication usually resolves within 4 to 6 hours. The patient should be moved to a quiet room with minimal stimulation. Treatment is symptom based and may include comfort medications used in other withdrawal states, such as clonidine (Catapres) and hydroxyzine (Vistaril).

Treatment of withdrawal symptoms

To ease cannabis withdrawal symptoms, mirtazapine (Remeron) and quetiapine (Seroquel) have shown to be efficacious. Useful nonpharmacologic measures may include psychotherapy, exercise, relaxation techniques, and nutritional support (Brezing & Levin, 2018; Schreck et al., 2018).

Treatment of chronic cannabis use

Treatment of cannabis use disorder follows the general principles of SUDs. The goal is total abstinence from all psychoactive substances. Interventions may include psychiatric evaluation and counseling,

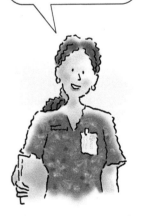

To stay off marijuana, the user must avoid all drug-related situations.

individual or group psychotherapy, occupational and family assessment, self-help groups, and lifestyle changes, such as avoiding drug-related situations (NIH, n.d.-a).

Nursing interventions

For general nursing interventions for cannabis intoxication, see *General interventions for acute substance intoxication*, page 408.

Hallucinogen-related disorders

Hallucinogens (sometimes called *psychedelic drugs*) produce hallucinations or profound distortions in the perception of reality and may also cause behavioral changes. Under the influence of hallucinogens, people see images, hear sounds, and feel sensations that seem real, but don't actually exist. Some hallucinogens also cause rapid, intense emotional swings (NIH, n.d.-a).

These agents include a wide range of substances, including LSD, ecstasy, ketamine, dextromethorphan, mescaline, and psilocybin. Most are taken orally, but some may be injected (NIH, n.d.-a). Most hallucinogens have no known medical use; however, naturally occurring hallucinogens have been used in religious rites for centuries. For example, native peoples of Mexico have used mushrooms containing psilocybin in spiritual ceremonies, and some southwest Native American tribes used peyote.

Lysergic acid diethylamide

LSD is the most potent mood- and perception-altering drug known. LSD is a synthetic substance first developed by a pharmaceutical company in 1938. Its street names include: *acid, green* or *red dragon, microdot, sugar,* and *big D*.

LSD is produced in crystalline form. The pure crystal can be crushed to a powder and mixed with binding agents to produce tablets known as *microdots* or thin gelatin squares called *windowpanes*. More commonly, it is dissolved, diluted, and applied to paper, known as *blotter acid*.

LSD has dramatic effects on the senses, causing a highly intensified perception of colors, smells, sounds, and other sensations. In some cases, sensory perceptions may blend, causing the person to "see" sounds or "hear" or "feel" colors. Hallucinations also distort or transform shapes and movements and may give rise to the perception that time is moving very slowly or that the user's body is changing shape.

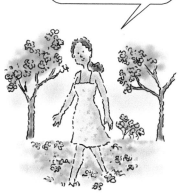

A person who has taken LSD may "see" sounds or "hear" colors.

Some call it ecstasy

Ecstasy, or 3,4-methylenedioxymethamphetamine (MDMA), is a synthetic drug with both stimulant and hallucinogenic properties. Available as capsules or tablets, it's taken orally or, rarely, injected or snorted. Street names include: *Molly, XTC, clarify, essence,* or *Adam.* The ecstasy experience is sometimes called *rolling.* Ecstasy tablets commonly contain MDMA in addition to other harmful drugs (NIH, n.d.-a).

Previously used mainly at dance clubs and raves (special music parties focused on ecstasy), ecstasy is now seen in other social settings. Its effects include distortions in time and perception and an amphetamine-like hyperactivity. Like other stimulants, it seems to have addictive potential. Depending on the dosage, acute drug effects typically last 3 to 6 hours.

Raving over ketamine

Ketamine distorts perceptions of sight and sound and produces dissociative effects—feelings of detachment from the self and the environment. It's increasingly used as a club drug and distributed at raves and parties.

For therapeutic purposes, ketamine has very few medical purposes. Currently, esketamine (Spravato) may be prescribed for patients with depression who have not responded to other treatments. Most of the ketamine used illicitly is evaporated to form a powder that's snorted, smoked, or compressed into tablets. The liquid form of the drug can be injected IV or intramuscularly (IM). Street names for ketamine include: *K, Special K, Ket, Vitamin K, Kit Kat Keller, Green, Blind Squid,* and *cat Valium* (NIH, n.d.-a).

Odorless and tasteless, ketamine can be added to beverages without being detected; also, it induces amnesia. Because of these properties, the drug sometimes is given to unsuspecting victims to aid in the commission of sexual assault ("drug rape" or date rape).

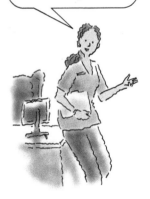

Ketamine induces amnesia and has been used as a date rape drug.

Dextromethorphan daze

Dextromethorphan, sometimes called *DXM* or *robo,* is a cough-suppressing ingredient found in some OTC cold and cough medications. The most common source of misused dextromethorphan is extra-strength cough syrup. At low doses, the drug has a mild stimulant effect and causes distorted visual perceptions. At much higher doses, it causes dissociative effects similar to those of ketamine. Effects typically last 6 hours.

Mescaline for mind alteration

Found in several cactus species (most notably, *peyote* and *San Pedro*), mescaline causes hallucinations. Mescaline "buttons" or "disks" are cut, then dried, and usually swallowed. Sometimes, the drug comes in powdered form and is taken by capsule, injection, or smoking.

Mescaline causes visual hallucinations and alters spatial perception. It can produce dizziness, vomiting, tachycardia, increased blood pressure, increased pulse and respiratory rates, sensations of warmth and cold, and headache. Effects last approximately 12 hours.

The 'shrooms of psilocybin

Psilocybin is a compound obtained from the *Psilocybe mexicana* mushroom and some types of European mushrooms. Traditionally, it was used by Mexican healers. Psilocybin can be eaten in the dried mushroom form or consumed as a white powder (NIH, n.d.-a). Effects resemble those of LSD. Used in small amounts, the drug induces relaxation and a sensation of being detached from the body. Individuals may also see brilliant arrangements of color and light. Larger doses may cause nausea; anxiety; light-headedness; sweating or chills; and numbness of the mouth, lips, and tongue.

Prevalence

Hallucinogen use is less common than alcohol, amphetamine, and cocaine use. About 12% of people in the United States have tried a hallucinogenic drug (NIH, n.d.-a).

How hallucinogens produce their effects

Hallucinogens disrupt the interaction of nerve cells and affect the functioning of serotonin, a neurotransmitter crucial to the regulation of mood, sleep, pain, emotion, and appetite.

Detecting novelty

LSD, for example, binds to and activates serotonin receptors in the brain. Drug effects are most prominent in two brain regions—the cerebral cortex (involved in mood, cognition, and perception) and the locus ceruleus, which receives sensory signals from all areas of the body and is sometimes called the brain's "novelty detector."

Disrupting neurotransmitters

Mescaline (Peyote) and psilocybin ("magic" mushrooms) are structurally similar to serotonin and produce their effects by disrupting normal functioning of the serotonin system.

Ecstasy increases levels of at least three neurotransmitters—serotonin, dopamine, and norepinephrine. By causing excess serotonin release and interfering with serotonin synthesis, ecstasy leads to serotonin depletion. A single dose of ecstasy can suppress serotonin levels for up to 2 weeks. At moderate to high doses, users may experience long-term serotonin depletion (which probably accounts for many of the drug's long-lasting behavioral effects).

Health hazards of hallucinogen use

Many hallucinogens cause unpleasant and potentially dangerous flashbacks long after the drug was used. Large doses of hallucinogens may cause seizures, ruptured blood vessels in the brain, and irreversible brain damage.

LSD intoxication may cause seizures and fatal accidents. Ketamine use can result in respiratory depression, heart rate abnormalities, heart failure, inability to move the muscles, and insensitivity to pain (which can lead to serious injury) (NIH, n.d.-a).

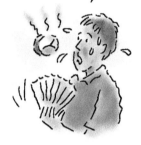

They weren't kidding when they said ecstasy might make you feel hot.

No ecstasy from these effects

Ecstasy may cause confusion, depression, sleep problems, drug craving, severe anxiety, and paranoia (during and sometimes weeks after taking the drug). Physical symptoms may include muscle tension, involuntary teeth clenching, nausea, blurred vision, rapid eye movements, faintness, and chills or sweating.

Impairments associated with hallucinogen use

Hallucinogens can cause short-term impairments in cognition, perception, mood, and communication. They may even prevent a person from recognizing reality, sometimes resulting in bizarre or dangerous behavior.

Although hallucinogens are less addictive than most psychoactive drugs, overuse can trigger psychosis in someone with a history of psychosis.

LSD psychosis

Some LSD users experience devastating psychological effects that persist after the "trip" has ended, producing a long-lasting psychosis-like state. This persistent psychosis—which may include dramatic mood swings from mania to profound depression, visual disturbances, and hallucinations—may last for years.

Bad trips and flashbacks

Many individuals who use LSD have "bad trips"—panic attacks at the height of the drug experience characterized by terrifying thoughts and nightmarish feelings of anxiety and despair. The individual may perceive real-world sensations as unreal and even frightening.

Some people who have used LSD in the past report flashbacks—spontaneous, repeated, and sometimes continuous recurrences of the sensory distortions originally produced by LSD. Flashbacks typically consist of visual disturbances, such as seeing false motion on the edges of the field of vision, bright or colored flashes, and halos or trails attached to moving objects.

Flashbacks arise suddenly—commonly without warning—a few days or more than a year after LSD use. They're most common in people who have used hallucinogens chronically or have an underlying personality disorder (although otherwise healthy people occasionally have them).

Ecstasy-related impairments

Heavy and prolonged ecstasy use has been linked to confusion, depression, sleep problems, persistent anxiety, aggressive and impulsive behavior, and selective impairment of working memory and attention. Long-term use may damage the brain's serotonin system, leading to various cognitive and behavioral disturbances, including memory impairment.

Ketamine-related impairments

Ketamine may make the user feel disconnected and out of control. Some users report a terrifying feeling of nearly total sensory detachment, described as a near-death experience.

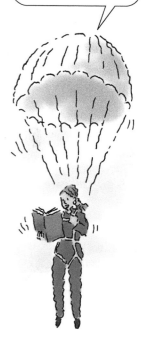

Some hallucinogen users seek to transcend the limits of the body or have a spiritual experience.

Causes

Some people take hallucinogens to enhance bodily sensations and induce sensory gratification. Under the influence of these drugs, music may sound more clear, colors may seem brighter, and sexual orgasm may feel more intense.

Unlocking the doors of perception?

Other people use hallucinogens to try to transcend the limits of the body and the time-space continuum or to have a spiritual or religious experience.

Signs and symptoms

Signs and symptoms of hallucinogen use vary with the drug used. (See *Assessing for hallucinogen use*, page 422.)

Diagnosis

The diagnosis of hallucinogen use disorder is confirmed when the patient presents with symptoms of hallucinogen use, resulting in a significant decrease in function.

Assessing for hallucinogen use

Suspect hallucinogen use if your patient has these signs and symptoms.

With LSD or mescaline

A patient under the influence of LSD or mescaline may report a sense of depersonalization, grandiosity, hallucinations, illusions, distorted perception of time and space, or mystical experiences.

GI findings include nausea, vomiting, diarrhea, and abdominal cramps. Cardiovascular findings may include arrhythmias, palpitations, tachycardia, and hypertension.

Other signs and symptoms may include:
- chills
- dizziness
- dry mouth
- fever
- sweating
- appetite loss
- hyperpnea
- increased salivation
- muscle aches.

With psilocybin

Signs and symptom of psilocybin use include:
- euphoria
- color distortions
- vivid hallucinations
- "seeing" music or "hearing" color
- dramatic mood swings and personality changes
- increases in blood pressure and body temperature.

With ecstasy

A patient under the influence of ecstasy may report or exhibit:
- distractibility
- heightened alertness
- irritability or confusion
- euphoria
- enhanced emotional and mental clarity
- increased sensitivity to touch
- enhanced sexuality
- increased energy and motor activity.
  Other common findings include:
- increased pulse rate
- elevated blood pressure
- dilated pupils
- perceptual changes
- tightened jaw muscles or jaw grinding or clenching
- increased body temperature, heavy perspiration, and dehydration.

At high doses, ecstasy may cause hallucinations, depression, paranoia, and irrational behavior (including violence).

Ketamine

Ketamine causes dissociative effects and alters visual and auditory perception. At low doses, it causes impairments in attention, learning ability, and memory. At higher doses, it may produce delirium, amnesia, impaired motor function, high blood pressure, depression, and potentially fatal respiratory problems.

Dextromethorphan

Dextromethorphan use may cause euphoria and a floating sensation, along with increased perceptual awareness and altered time perception. The patient may report tactile, auditory, or visual hallucinations. Some users experience paranoia and disorientation.

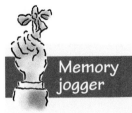

Memory jogger

When assessing a patient for suspected LSD use, think of the acronym **ACID**.

Arrhythmias and abdominal cramps

Chills

Illusions and increased salivation

Diaphoresis, depersonalization, and distortions

Treatment

Treatment measures vary with the patient's status. A patient who is dangerous to themselves or others may need to be restrained physically or chemically. Prolonged or excessive physical restraint should be avoided because it can contribute to hyperthermia and the risk of rhabdomyolysis and may exacerbate paranoia.

Cool-down phase

A patient with marked hyperthermia may require aggressive cooling measures. Benzodiazepines typically are given if the patient is anxious or agitated, or has hypertension or tachycardia. For severe hypertension or tachycardia, nifedipine (Procardia) or nitroprusside (Nitropress) may be indicated. Antiepileptics such as sodium valproate (Depakote) or diazepam (Valium) are given for seizures.

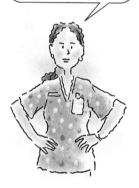

You may need to provide aggressive cooling measures if your patient has hyperthermia.

Treatment for LSD flashbacks

No established treatment exists for LSD flashbacks, although antidepressant drugs may ease symptoms. Psychotherapy may help the patient adjust to the visual distraction and ease fears that they are suffering from brain damage or a psychiatric disorder.

Nursing interventions

For nursing interventions during an acute episode or when the episode has resolved, see *General interventions for acute substance intoxication*, page 408.

Phencyclidine use disorder

A hallucinogen and dissociative drug, PCP was developed in the 1950s as an IV anesthetic; medical use has been discontinued due to neurologic effects.

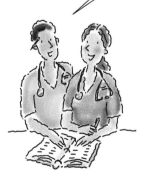

Some people call PCP the peace pill. But from what I hear, taking it is anything but peaceful.

Today, PCP is manufactured illegally in laboratories. On the street, in its pure form, it's available as tablets, capsules, and powders, and it's sold under names such as: as *angel dust, wack,* hog, *ozone, love boat, superweed, hog, peace pill, embalming fluid, elephant tranquilizer,* and *rocket fuel.* Some users ingest PCP by snorting the powder or by swallowing it in tablet form.

PCP can be snorted, smoked, injected, sprinkled on other drugs, or eaten. For smoking, it's typically applied to a leafy material, such as parsley, oregano, or marijuana. More recently, PCP has been mixed with synthetic cannabinoids to increase the high from those substances. The combined substances are called *supergrass, killer joints, or whacko tobacco.*

Numb but quarrelsome

PCP makes the person feel disconnected and out of control. It also has a numbing effect on the mind and can cause unpredictable and often violent behavior. Persons under the influence of PCP have been known to exhibit superhuman strength and be difficult to control. Repeated use may result in psychological dependence and craving (NIH, n.d.-a).

Prevalence

PCP use isn't widespread as other substances, with less than 1.3% of the population using it, and is most common among teenagers (NIDA, 2015).

How PCP produces its effects

PCP's primary sites of action are glutamate receptors known as *N-methyl-D-aspartate* (NMDA) receptors. PCP acts as an NMDA antagonist, lowering the glutamate levels in the brain.

PCP also increases levels of gamma-aminobutyric acid (GABA), an inhibitory neurotransmitter. Increased GABA levels probably explain the inhibition of pain seen in individuals who use PCP. In addition, PCP also alters the action of dopamine, which is responsible for the euphoria and "rush" associated with many psychoactive drugs (NIH, n.d.-a).

Health hazards of PCP

At low to moderate doses, PCP's physiologic effects include increased body temperature, marked rises in blood pressure and pulse, shallow respirations, flushing, and profuse sweating.

At high doses, PCP decreases blood pressure and slows the pulse and respiratory rates. Cardiac arrest, hypertensive crisis, renal failure, and seizures may occur.

Feeling no pain

Other dangerous effects include violent or suicidal behavior, seizures, decreased awareness of pain, coma, and death. However, death more commonly results from accidental injury or suicide during PCP intoxication.

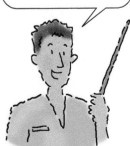

PCP sometimes causes rhabdomyolysis, a dangerous condition that may lead to kidney failure.

Causes

As with other drugs, the precise causes of PCP abuse aren't known. Some people may use PCP because it provides a feeling of strength, power, and invulnerability.

In young people, substance use commonly follows experimentation with drugs stemming from peer pressure. Risk factors for PCP use include male gender and young adulthood (ages 20 to 29 years) (NIH, n.d.-a, n.d.-b).

Signs and symptoms

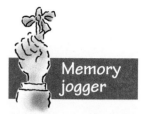

An individual under the influence of PCP may report numbness of the arms and legs and may exhibit poor muscle coordination. Psychological effects include changes in body awareness, resembling those caused by alcohol intoxication.

Other physical findings may include:
- sparse, garbled speech
- blurred vision
- blank stare
- drooling
- nausea and vomiting
- loss of balance
- dizziness
- decreased deep tendon reflexes
- fever
- gait ataxia
- nystagmus
- hyperactivity
- increased vital signs
- tachycardia.

Mental status mayhem

Mental status findings may vary greatly—even in the same person. The person may seem normal one moment, then exhibit apparent psychotic symptoms and homicidal or suicidal ideation the next.

Other mental status findings may include:
- euphoria
- amnesia
- delusions and hallucinations
- poor perception of time and distance
- distorted sense of sight, hearing, and touch
- decreased awareness of pain
- distorted body image
- excitation
- panic
- sudden behavioral changes
- violent behavior

Memory jogger

Each letter in **ANGEL DUST** stands for a sign or symptom of PCP use.

Amnesia

Nystagmus

Gait ataxia

Euphoria

Loopiness (poor perception of time and distance)

Delusions and distortions

Unpredictable effects

Sudden behavioral changes

Tachycardia

- stupor or coma
- paranoia
- disordered thinking.

Withdrawal symptoms

Research suggests that with repeated or prolonged PCP use, a withdrawal syndrome may occur when drug use is stopped. Some who use PCP experience dysphoria and an intense drug craving.

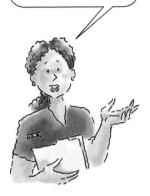

Someone with a history of prolonged PCP use may experience dysphoria and drug craving during withdrawal.

Diagnosis

The health care provider typically orders a urine drug screen if PCP use is suspected. Because PCP may cause rhabdomyolysis, serum enzyme levels (especially creatine kinase) may be useful.

The diagnosis of PCP use disorder is confirmed when the patient presents with symptoms of PCP use, resulting in a significant decrease in function.

Treatment

A patient with acute PCP intoxication should be placed in a quiet room with minimal stimulation. If the patient is violent, restraints may be needed.

Induced vomiting or gastric lavage may be performed, followed by the administration of activated charcoal if PCP was taken orally. Other drug therapy may include:

- benzodiazepines (such as diazepam [Valium]) to ease seizures, agitation, aggressiveness, psychotic symptoms, hypertension, and tachycardia
- haloperidol (Haldol) for agitation or psychotic behavior
- diuretics to force diuresis
- anticholinergic and antidiarrheal agents to relieve GI distress
- propranolol (Inderal) for hypertension or tachycardia
- nitroprusside (Nitropress) for severe hypertensive crisis
- IV fluids.

Treatment of PCP-induced psychosis

For a patient with PCP-induced psychosis, treatment must address the high risk of violence. The patient may require seclusion or restraint, and suicide and assault precautions should be instituted.

If psychosis persists, the health care provider may prescribe an antipsychotic, such as haloperidol (Haldol) or risperidone (Risperdal). The patient usually requires psychiatric follow-up care and chemical dependency treatment. Most patients with PCP-induced psychosis can be weaned from antipsychotics within 6 months.

Nursing interventions

For appropriate measures, see *General interventions for acute substance intoxication*, page 408.

Inhalant-related disorders

Inhalant use, commonly called *huffing* or *bagging*, is the deliberate inhalation of chemical vapors to attain an altered mental or physical state (usually a quick "buzz"). Individuals inhale vapors from a wide range of substances found in more than 1,000 common household products. Inhalants fall into several general categories. (See *Types of inhalants*.)

Street names for inhalants include *bang, bolt, boppers, bullet, climax, glading, gluey, hardware, head cleaner, hippie crack, kick, locker room, poor man's pot, poppers, rush,* and *snappers.*

By huff or by cuff

Inhalants are breathed in through the nose or mouth in various ways. Individuals may inhale chemical vapors directly from open containers or may huff fumes from rags soaked in a chemical substance held to the face or stuffed in the mouth.

Types of inhalants

Inhalants that are used for their psychoactive effects include aerosols, gases, nitrites, and volatile solvents.

Aerosols

Aerosol are sprays containing propellants and solvents such as toluene. Common aerosols include whipped cream canisters, spray paint, spray on deodorant, hair products, cooking sprays, and fabric protector. Silver and gold spray paint are especially popular among those who use inhalants.

Gases

Gases—substances with no definite shape or volume—include refrigerants and medical anesthetics. Individuals may inhale gases found in propane tanks, butane lighters, and air-conditioning units as well as those in such medical anesthetics as ether, chloroform, and nitrous oxide (laughing gas). The most commonly misused gas, nitrous oxide, is found in whipped cream dispensers and products that boost octane levels in racing cars.

It's also sold at raves or drug paraphernalia stores in the form of balloons or as vials called *whippets.*

Nitrites

Such chemicals as amyl nitrite, butyl nitrite, and cyclohexyl nitrite are taken mainly to enhance sexual experiences. They're available in adult bookstores and shops and over the Internet. Cyclohexyl nitrite is also found in room deodorizers. Amyl nitrite comes in mesh-covered, sealed capsules that are popped or snapped to release the vapors. Butyl nitrite is sold in small bottles.

Volatile solvents

Volatile solvents are liquids that vaporize at room temperature when left in unsealed containers. They're found in paint thinner, gasoline, correction fluid, felt-tip markers, nail polish and nail polish remover, and glue.

An aerosol may be sprayed directly into the nose or mouth. Other types of inhalants may be poured onto the collar, sleeves, or cuffs and then sniffed repeatedly.

Prevalence

Inhalant use has been increasing steadily. Low cost, easy accessibility, and rapid mood-elevating are factors that have influenced the use of inhalants. Almost 18 million people in the United States have experimented with inhalants at some time in their lives. In a 2018 survey, 9% of individuals aged 12 years or older had used an inhalant in the previous year (NIDA, 2018a).

How inhalants produce their effects

Scientists aren't sure how inhalants produce their effects. Some suggest that the inhaled substance changes the solubility of neurons' cell membranes.

Health hazards and impairments associated with inhalants

Inhalants can produce both psychological dependence and physical addiction. Chronic inhalant use may lead to serious and possibly irreversible damage to the brain, heart, liver, kidneys, and lungs. Brain damage may cause personality changes, diminished cognitive functioning, memory impairment, and slurred speech. Impaired judgment may lead to fatal injuries from motor vehicle accidents or sudden falls.

Causes

Most people who use inhalants do so because the inhalant provides a rapid euphoric effect similar to alcohol intoxication, along with loss of inhibitions. After the initial excitation, they experience drowsiness, light-headedness, and agitation.

Signs and symptoms

Assessment findings vary with the specific inhalant used. General findings may include:
- loss of muscle control
- slurred speech
- dizziness, drowsiness, or loss of consciousness
- hallucinations and delusions
- belligerence
- apathy
- impaired judgment

- drunk or disoriented demeanor
- double vision
- seizures
- nausea
- appetite loss
- red or runny nose
- watery eyes
- sores or rash around the nose or mouth
- spots or marks around the collars of shirts
- arrhythmias
- seizures.

Strong chemical odors on the breath or clothing, as well as paint or other stains on the hands, face, or clothing strongly suggest inhalant use.

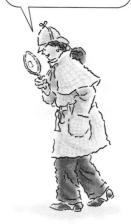

Fetch the scent detector, Watson! Chemical odors may hint at inhalant abuse.

Withdrawal symptoms

A patient undergoing inhalant withdrawal may report or exhibit excessive sweating, headache, rapid pulse, hand tremors, muscle cramps, insomnia, hallucinations, nausea, and vomiting.

Diagnosis

The diagnosis of inhalant use disorder is confirmed when the patient presents a marked impairment or distress to normal functioning such as difficulty in controlling use, greater use of the inhalant than intended, and current use of the inhalant with the desire to quit.

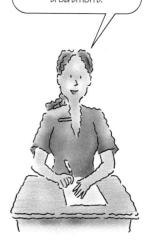

Inhalant misusers have high relapse rates. Some require up to 2 years of treatment.

Treatment

Treatment for acute inhalant intoxication is supportive and symptomatic and may include cognitive-behavioral therapy.

Other measures may include:
- fluid replacement therapy
- sedatives to induce sleep
- anticholinergics and antidiarrheal agents to relieve GI distress
- antianxiety drugs for severe agitation.

Relapse blues

Individuals who use inhalants have high relapse rates, making aftercare and follow-up extremely important. Some may require treatment in an outpatient or residential program—although few treatment programs exist specifically for inhalant users. For many users, treatment must continue for an extended period—possibly up to 2 years.

Nursing interventions

For nursing interventions during an acute episode or when the episode has resolved, see *General interventions for acute substance intoxication*, page 408.

Opioid-related disorders

Opioids are narcotics that can produce euphoria. They have a high potential for addiction. Naturally occurring opioids include morphine and codeine. Partially synthetic morphine derivatives include heroin, oxycodone, hydrocodone, hydromorphone, and oxymorphone. Synthetic opioids include fentanyl, alfentanil, levorphanol, and methadone. A plant that mimics some opiate effects is called kratom.

Opioids are used medically as analgesics. Some agents have additional uses. Codeine, for example, is used as an antitussive, opium as an antidiarrheal.

Opioids produce relaxation with an immediate "rush" but also have initial unpleasant effects, such as restlessness and nausea. With a typical dose, effects last 3 to 6 hours.

Codeine and morphine may be ingested, injected, or smoked. Heroin and fentanyl (whose street names include *junk*, *horse*, and *H*) may be injected, inhaled, or smoked. Opium (known as *O*, *ope*, or *OP*) may be ingested or smoked (NIH, n.d.-a).

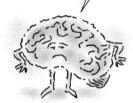

Opioid drugs stimulate opioid receptors in the brain. Injecting them IV causes an initial "rush" of pleasure.

Prevalence

Opiates may be legally prescribed and yet cause dependence that becomes addiction, and even legally prescribed opiates may cause overdose. In a 2017 national study, close to 12 million persons in the United States are misusing opiates, and most of them were using prescription medication; in contrast, an estimated 948,000 persons were using heroin (SAMHSA, 2017). More than 47,000 Americans died as a result of opiate overdose in 2016 (Centers for Disease Control and Prevention [CDC], 2017).

How opioids produce their effects

Opioids stimulate opioid receptors in the CNS and surrounding tissues. CNS effects of opioids include euphoria and sedation, followed by elation, relaxation, and then sedation or sleep.

Causes

Because of their euphoric and anxiolytic effects, opioids are strongly reinforcing agents.

Behavioral theory proposes that basic reward-punishment mechanisms perpetuate addictive behavior. Rapid development of physical dependence and a prolonged withdrawal syndrome can make abstinence difficult.

Genetic, social, and psychological factors also may play a role in opioid abuse and dependence. Opioid misuse sometimes follows the use of prescribed opioids to relieve pain. Some users are motivated by the desire to manage uncomfortable emotions, such as anxiety, guilt, and anger.

Signs and symptoms

A person who uses opioids—or other substances, for that matter—may try to hide their use from family, friends, coworkers, and health care professionals. However, even if the person isn't forthcoming, you can assess for certain telltale signs. (See *When to suspect substance misuse*, page 432.)

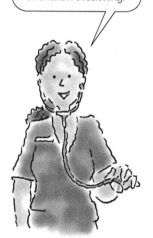

A person who has taken opioids may have respiratory depression, with slow or shallow breathing.

Signs and symptoms of opioid use include:
- constricted pupils, bloodshot eyes, and drooping eyelids
- slurred speech
- sweating
- clammy skin
- anorexia
- respiratory depression
- hypotension
- sweating
- impaired judgment
- euphoria
- drowsiness
- decreased level of consciousness
- sense of tranquility
- detachment from reality
- indifference to pain
- lack of concern
- nystagmus
- seizures
- constipation
- hemorrhoids.

Some individuals experience nausea and vomiting, hypotension, and arrhythmia. Severe opioid intoxication can lead to delirium and coma.

When to suspect substance misuse

Many individuals will try to hide or minimize their substance use. All individuals need to be assessed for substance use through a careful interview and review of their medical history, as well as a physical assessment.

History findings

History findings that suggest substance use include:
- use of a fictitious name and address
- reluctance to discuss previous hospitalizations
- seeking treatment at a medical facility across town rather than near the person's home
- history of overdose
- high tolerance for potentially addictive drugs
- history of hepatitis or HIV infection
- amenorrhea
- reports of a painful injury or chronic illness—but refusal of a diagnostic workup
- feigned illnesses, such as migraine headache, myocardial infarction, or renal colic, in an attempt to obtain certain medications
- claims of an allergy to OTC analgesics
- requests for a specific medication.

Physical findings

Physical findings that hint at substance use include:
- fever (from stimulant intoxication, withdrawal, or infection caused by IV use)
- needle marks or tracks (from IV use)
- attempts to conceal or disguise injection sites with tattoos
- use of inconspicuous injection sites, such as under the nails or tongue
- cellulitis or abscess from self-injection
- puffy hands (a late sign of thrombophlebitis or of fascial infection caused by self-injection on the hands or arms)
- dental conditions (from poor oral hygiene associated with chronic drug use)
- excoriated skin (from scratching induced by formication, a sensation of bugs crawling on the skin)
- refractory acute-onset hypertension or cardiac arrhythmias (stimulant use)
- liver enlargement, with or without tenderness (from hepatitis caused by sharing contaminated needles).

Behavioral clues

A person with opiate use disorder who is hospitalized may experience withdrawal and become uncooperative, experience mood swings, anxiety, impaired memory, sleep disturbance, flashbacks, slurred speech, depression, and thought disorders.

To obtain medication, some individuals may attempt to manipulate health care providers using ploys for sympathy, bribery, or threats. They may try to manipulate caregivers by pitting one staff member against another, or family members against staff (NIH, n.d.-a).

Tale of the tracks

With IV use, the individual may have visible needle marks or tracks, skin lesions or abscesses, soft tissue infection, and thrombosed veins. (See *Identifying IV substance use.*)

Findings in opioid withdrawal

Opioid withdrawal can be quite unpleasant. For general findings, see *Evaluating for opioid withdrawal.*

Heroin withdrawal symptoms resemble a bad case of the flu. They generally begin 12 to 14 hours after the last dose, peak within 36 and 72 hours, and may last 7 to 14 days.

Identifying IV substance use

Needle marks or tracks are an obvious sign of IV drug use. Some individuals who use IV drugs try to conceal or disguise injection sites with tattoos or by selecting an inconspicuous injection site such as under the nails.

Be aware that self-injection sometimes causes cellulitis or abscesses, especially in persons who also have AUD. Puffy hands may be a late sign of thrombophlebitis or of fascial infection caused by self-injection on the hands or arms.

Opioid overdose

With opioid overdose, auscultation may reveal bilateral crackles and rhonchi. Other cardiopulmonary findings may include pulmonary edema, respiratory depression, aspiration pneumonia, and hypotension.

Diagnosis

If opioid use disorder is suspected, the health care provider may order a serum or urine drug screen. (See *Toxicology screening*, page 434.)

For patients with clinical or historical evidence of IV drug use, the health care provider may order:

- liver function tests
- rapid plasma reagin test for syphilis
- hepatitis viral testing
- HIV testing
- lung X-rays (to check for pulmonary fibrosis).

The diagnosis of opioid use disorder is confirmed when the patient presents with symptoms of opioid use, resulting in a significant decrease in function.

Treatment

For opioid intoxication or overdose, general supportive measures include ensuring an adequate airway and ventilation (with ventilatory support if needed) and supporting cardiovascular function. Treatment with naloxone, also known as Narcan, can reverse the overdose. Today's especially potent forms of heroin may require multiple

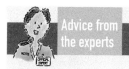

Evaluating for opioid withdrawal

Signs and symptoms of opioid withdrawal include:

- abdominal cramps, nausea, or vomiting
- anorexia
- fever or chills
- profuse sweating
- dilated pupils
- hyperactive bowel sounds
- irritability
- nausea
- panic
- piloerection (gooseflesh)
- runny nose
- tremors
- watery eyes
- yawning
- bone pain
- diffuse muscle aches
- drug craving.

administrations of naloxone to reverse overdose. (See *Naloxone for opioid reversal.*)

Other treatments depend on symptoms, the specific opioid, and administration route. If the drug was ingested, vomiting is induced or gastric lavage is performed.

IV fluids and nutritional and vitamin supplements may be given.

Withdrawal and detoxification
Treatment of withdrawal symptoms may include antidiarrheals, decongestants for runny nose, and nonopioid analgesics for pain.

Substitution strategy
For detoxification, the misused opioid usually is replaced with a drug that has a similar action but a longer duration. Opiate detoxification protocols may commonly employ one of the following substitutes: methadone, buprenorphine/suboxone, naltrexone, or codeine (less common). Gradual substitution controls withdrawal effects, reducing discomfort and associated risks. Depending on the substance, severity, form of use, and which drug the person has misused, detoxification may be managed on an inpatient or outpatient basis.

Maintenance therapy
For maintenance, the person typically receives an opioid agonist as a substitute for the misused drug. The goal of maintenance is to replace the misused drug with one that's available legally, can be taken orally, and requires only a once-daily dose.

Toxicology screening
A blood or urine screen may detect drugs that are present in concentrations above 5 µg/mL. Current methods quantitate only drugs detected in the blood.

Toxicology screening commonly is done in the emergency department or on admission. It may require a legal chain of custody in which precautions are taken to prevent anyone from tampering with the specimens.

Meds matters

Naloxone for opioid reversal

Naloxone hydrochloride (Narcan) is an opioid antagonist used to reverse the effects of opioids. It works by displacing opioids from their receptors in the CNS.

Naloxone is administered intranasally, IV, IM, or subcutaneously every 2 to 3 minutes, as needed. It rapidly reverses opioid-induced CNS depression and increases the respiratory rate within 1 to 2 minutes. Adverse effects include precipitated withdrawal symptoms such as nausea, vomiting, diaphoresis, tachycardia, CNS excitement, and increased blood pressure.

Relapse and respiratory peril
Because the opioid's duration of action may exceed that of naloxone, even a person who has apparently been revived from an overdose may later relapse into respiratory depression. Be sure to monitor respiratory rate and depth. Be prepared to provide oxygen, ventilation, and other resuscitation measures.

Buprenorphine for maintenance

Buprenorphine, in its combination formulation with naloxone (Suboxone), is prescribed as a once or twice per day sublingual tablet or strip, or a monthly injection. It is a partial agonist that does not create the level of euphoria that other opiates may cause, but it does neutralize the cravings for other opiates. Treatment with buprenorphine and concurrent psychosocial treatment have been shown to significantly reduce the risk of relapse and maintain sustained recovery (Kampman & Jarvis, 2015).

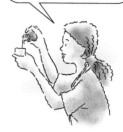

Buprenorphine, given as a sublingual tablet or strip, is a common drug used in opioid detox.

Psychotherapy

Detoxification alone, without ongoing psychosocial treatment therapy, isn't sufficient to manage a person with opioid dependence. To remain abstinence, individuals should receive standard substance use drug counseling along with cognitive-behavioral, dynamic, or group therapy. Many individuals also benefit from a personalized recovery coach, who is usually a trained and certified peer. (Some patients may prefer aversion therapy, in which aversive stimuli are paired with cognitive images of opioid use.)

Cognitive-behavioral therapy focuses on the person's thoughts and behaviors. It helps to learn specific skills for resisting drug use, as well as coping skills to reduce problems related to drug use.

Dynamic psychotherapy is based on the concept that all symptoms arise from underlying unconscious psychological conflicts. The goal is to make the person aware of these conflicts and develop better coping mechanisms and healthier ways of resolving intrapsychic conflicts.

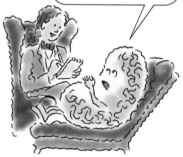

An opioid-dependent person needs psychosocial treatment therapy in addition to detox.

Group sobriety

Group therapy targets the social stigma attached to substance use. The presence of other group members who acknowledge their substance use problem has a therapeutic effect in helping the patient develop alternative methods of staying sober. (See *Reducing impaired social interaction*, page 436.)

Narcotics anonymous

Established in 1947, Narcotics Anonymous (NA) is based on principles similar to those of AA, including the progression through 12 steps of recovery. Like AA, NA has helped many individuals with substance use, offering much needed support for those attempting abstinence.

Other support groups that focus on opiate use disorder include: SMART recovery, Rational Recovery, Life Ring, and Addiction Survivors Peer Support Forum.

Advice from the experts

Reducing impaired social interaction

Impaired social interaction is common among persons who misuse substances. Appropriate nursing interventions can help the patient improve social interaction skills in both one-on-one and group settings.

• If delusions and hallucinations occur, don't focus on them. Instead, provide reality-based information and reassure the patient of safety.

• Provide additional time with the patient on each shift (besides the time spent on caregiving) to encourage social interaction. Start with one-on-one interaction and increase to group interaction when the patient's social skills indicate readiness.

• Give positive reinforcement for appropriate and effective interaction behaviors (both verbal and nonverbal). This helps the patient recognize progress and enhances feelings of self-worth.

• Assist the patient and family or close friends in progressive participation in care and therapies. This reduces feelings of helplessness and enhances the patient's feeling of control and independence.

Nursing interventions

These nursing interventions may be appropriate for a patient with acute opioid intoxication:

- Provide extra blankets or a hypothermia blanket for hypothermia.
- Reorient the patient to time, place, and person.
- Monitor breath sounds for evidence of pulmonary edema.
- Frequently monitor vital signs and cardiopulmonary status until opioids have cleared from the system.
- Monitor for withdrawal symptoms.

For other interventions during an acute episode or when the episode has resolved, see *General interventions for acute substance intoxication*, page 408.

Cocaine substance use

Cocaine, like atropine, is a tropane alkaloid. A stimulant, cocaine is one of the oldest known drugs. Coca leaves, the source of cocaine, have been ingested for thousands of years. Cocaine has few medical purposes such as local anesthesia; however, recreational use is illegal (NIDA, 2018).

Cocaine's effects occur almost immediately after a single dose and disappear within a few minutes or hours. Taken in small amounts, the drug typically makes the person feel euphoric, energetic, talkative, and mentally alert.

Cocaine may temporarily reduce the need for food and sleep. Some users find it helps them perform simple physical and intellectual tasks more quickly, although others experience the opposite effect (NIH, 2018b).

Crystal or crack

Cocaine exists in two chemical forms:

- Cocaine hydrochloride is a fine, white, crystallized powder. It's generally snorted or dissolved in water and injected, with effects lasting 15 minutes to 2 hours.
- Crack or freebase is a chunky, off-white compound that hasn't been neutralized by an acid. It's smoked after being processed with ammonia or sodium bicarbonate and water and then heated to remove the hydrochloride. Crack produces an immediate euphoric high, followed by a "down" feeling.

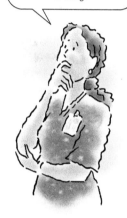

Crack produces an immediate high, followed by a "down" feeling.

By any other name ...

On the street, cocaine is known as *coke, C, snow, snowball, blow, flake, nose candy, hits, tornado, wicky stick, rock,* or *crank.* Many street dealers dilute cocaine with inert substances, such as cornstarch or sugar; others may mix it with procaine or amphetamines. Individuals also may combine cocaine powder or crack with heroin known as a "speedball."

Snorting, shooting, and rubbing

When snorted, cocaine is absorbed into the bloodstream through the nasal tissues. When injected, the drug is released directly into the bloodstream, intensifying its effects. When cocaine is smoked, the vapor is inhaled into the lungs, where it's absorbed into the bloodstream as rapidly as by injection. Cocaine also can be rubbed onto mucous membrane tissues.

Prevalence

Cocaine is used by approximately 1.9 million people (less than 1% of the population) in the United States, a figure that is lower than it was 15 years ago (SAMHSA, 2017). Globally, cocaine is used by 18.2 million people aged 15 to 65 years (Gorlick, 2019).

Health hazards of cocaine use

Cocaine use can have devastating medical consequences. Absorption of toxic amounts may cause:

- sudden death
- acute cardiovascular problems, such as arrhythmias (particularly ventricular fibrillation), tachycardia, myocardial infarction, and chest pain

- stroke
- seizures
- respiratory failure
- bowel gangrene (with cocaine ingestion).

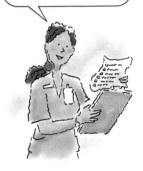

A cocaine binge can bring on paranoid psychosis—complete with auditory hallucinations.

Death-dealing duo

Combining cocaine with alcohol causes the conversion of the two drugs to cocaethylene, which has a longer duration in the brain and is more toxic than either drug alone. In fact, the mixture of cocaine and alcohol is a drug combination that may result in drug-related death more than other two-drug combinations.

Binge effects

A cocaine binge (taking the drug repeatedly and at increasingly high doses) may cause increasing irritability, restlessness, and paranoia. The result may be full-blown paranoid psychosis, in which the person loses touch with reality and experiences auditory hallucinations.

Route-related consequences

Regular cocaine snorting can lead to the loss of the sense of smell, nosebleeds, swallowing difficulty, hoarseness, and nasal septum irritation.

Fatal first use

In rare instances, sudden death can occur on the first use of cocaine or unexpectedly thereafter. Cocaine-related deaths commonly result from cardiac arrest or seizures, followed by respiratory arrest.

Impairments associated with cocaine use

Cocaine is powerfully addictive. About 10% of people who try cocaine progress to heavy use. After a person tries it, they may have trouble predicting or controlling the extent to which they will keep using it. As cocaine use continues, tolerance commonly develops. The person must take higher doses at more frequent intervals to obtain the same level of pleasure experienced with initial use (NIDA, 2018).

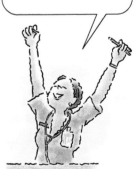

Euphoria and laughing are common effects of cocaine use.

Causes

A family history of substance use may be a risk factor for early cocaine use and rapid cocaine dependence. (See *Gathering a history*.) Some researchers attribute cocaine's addictive properties to the dopamine excess it produces; this excess may be the

Gathering a history

If your patient admits to substance use, try to determine the extent to which the substance misuse interferes with their life. Note whether the patient expresses a desire to overcome addiction.

If possible, obtain a complete substance use history. Ask which substances the patient uses, the amount used, frequency of use, and time of the last dose.

What to expect

However, you should expect incomplete or inaccurate responses. Drug-induced amnesia, a decreased level of consciousness, or lack of knowledge may distort the patient's recollection of the facts. The person may also deliberately fabricate answers to avoid arrest or downplay a suicide attempt. If necessary, interview family members and friends to fill in gaps in the history.

source of positive reinforcement and addiction. Thus, the drug's dopamine-driven "rush" reinforces repeated use.

Genetic link?

Researchers have identified a brain process that may help explain addiction to cocaine and other drugs of misuse. Studies have found that repeated cocaine exposure causes a genetic change, leading to altered levels of a specific brain protein that regulates dopamine's action (NIDA, 2018).

Signs and symptoms

In a patient under the influence of cocaine, general assessment findings may include:

- euphoria
- increased energy
- excitement
- sociability
- reduced hunger
- grandiosity
- sense of increased physical and mental strength
- decreased sensation of pain
- talkativeness or pressured speech
- good humor and laughing

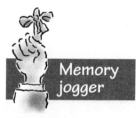

Memory jogger

CRACK clues you in to some of the symptoms of cocaine use.

Cardiotoxicity (tachycardia, ventricular fibrillation, or cardiac arrest)

Respiratory arrest

Auditory, visual, and olfactory hallucinations

Coma and confusion

Kite-like behavior (excitability, grandiosity, irritability, and psychotic symptoms)

- dilated pupils
- runny nose
- nasal congestion
- nausea and vomiting
- headache
- vertigo.

Something bugging you?

Some individuals who use cocaine experience more pronounced effects (especially with high doses). These effects include flightiness, emotional instability, restlessness, irritability, apprehension, inability to sit still, teeth grinding, cold sweats, tremors, muscle twitching, seizures, violent or bizarre behavior, and hallucinations (cocaine "bugs" or "snow lights" as well as voices, sounds, and smells). A few experience cocaine psychosis, which resembles paranoid schizophrenia.

Cardiovascular and respiratory findings

Cocaine may raise or lower the blood pressure. It may cause chest pain, tachycardia, ventricular fibrillation, or cardiac arrest. Respiratory findings may include tachypnea; deep, rapid, or labored respirations; or respiratory arrest (NIH, 2018).

Withdrawal symptoms

Cocaine withdrawal usually isn't as uncomfortable as withdrawal from other drugs. Symptoms may include:
- anxiety, agitation, and irritability
- depression
- fatigue
- angry outbursts
- lack of motivation
- nausea and vomiting
- muscle pain
- sleep disturbances—usually hypersomnia
- intense drug craving
- episodes of ST-segment elevation on ECG.

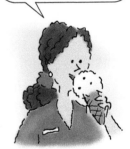

It's not cocaine I'm craving. It's ICE CREAM!

Diagnosis

The diagnosis of cocaine use disorder is confirmed when the patient presents with symptoms of cocaine use, resulting in a significant decrease in function.

Treatment

A patient with acute cocaine intoxication should receive symptomatic treatment. Cardiopulmonary resuscitation is performed, as indicated, for ventricular fibrillation and cardiac arrest. Vital signs should be monitored closely. Propranolol (Inderal) typically is given for tachycardia. Anticonvulsant medications are given for seizures. If the patient has ingested cocaine, induced vomiting or gastric lavage may be performed. If the patient has snorted cocaine, residual substance is removed from the mucous membranes. Depending on the cocaine dosage and time elapsed before admission, additional treatment may include forced diuresis and, possibly, hemoperfusion or hemodialysis.

Fluids, food, and sleep therapy

Other measures may include fluid replacement therapy and nutritional and vitamin supplements. Sedatives may be given to induce sleep, anticholinergics and antidiarrheal agents to relieve GI distress, and antianxiety drugs for severe agitation.

Withdrawal, detoxification, and rehabilitation

Treatment of cocaine dependence commonly involves detoxification, short- and long-term rehabilitation, and aftercare. The latter means a lifetime of abstinence, usually aided by participation in NA or a similar self-help group.

To ease withdrawal, useful nonpharmacologic measures may include psychotherapy, exercise, relaxation techniques, and nutritional support. Widespread cocaine use has led to extensive efforts to develop treatment programs for those who use cocaine. Cocaine use and addiction must address a variety of problems, including psychobiological, social, and pharmacologic aspects of the patient's drug abuse.

Pharmacologic approaches

Currently, there are several medications used in treating cocaine misuse, for instance, the use of high-dose vitamin preparations containing the amino acid precursors of dopamine, norepinephrine, and serotonin to address the neurotransmitter depletion. Also, the dopamine agonists bromocriptine (Parlodel) and amantadine have shown some success. Antidepressants may be prescribed to treat the mood changes that some patients experience during the early stages of cocaine abstinence. Hypnotics may be given temporarily to help the patient cope with insomnia.

A cocaine vaccination is being researched to help reduce the patient's chances of relapse. In addition, disulfiram (Antabuse) has been shown to be effective in some patients (NIDA, 2016).

Behavioral interventions

Many behavioral treatments (both outpatient and residential) have been effective in treating patients with cocaine use disorder. The treatment regimen should be tailored to the patient's individual needs, with different components added or removed as indicated. For many patients with cocaine use disorder, a treatment called *contingency management* has had positive results. This voucher-based system gives positive rewards for staying in treatment and remaining cocaine-free. Patients earn vouchers based on drug-free urine tests and can exchange them for items that promote healthy living such as joining a gym.

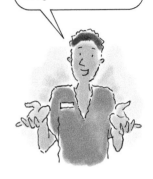

Some cocaine treatment programs give vouchers to patients who have drug-free urine tests.

Cognitive-behavioral therapy

Cognitive-behavioral coping skills therapy is a focused approach that helps cocaine addicts become abstinent. This approach strives to help patients recognize the situations in which they're most likely to use cocaine, avoid these situations, and cope more effectively with the problems and behaviors associated with drug abuse.

Therapeutic communities

Patients with more complex needs, such as coexisting mental health disorders and legal involvement, may benefit from a residential program lasting 3 to 6 months. These communities focus on returning the patient to society; some include on-site job rehabilitation and other supportive services.

Nursing interventions

For nursing interventions that may be appropriate during an acute episode or after the episode has resolved, see *General interventions for acute substance intoxication*, page 408.

Amphetamines

An amphetamine is a CNS stimulant that increases arousal; reduces fatigue; and can make a person feel stronger, more alert, and more decisive. Although they have a few medical uses (mainly in treating attention deficit hyperactivity disorder, obesity, and narcolepsy), most users take them for their stimulant or euphoric effects or to counteract the "down" feeling of alcohol or tranquilizers.

The amphetamine group includes amphetamine sulfate, methamphetamine, and dextroamphetamine. On the street, amphetamine sulfate tablets are called *bennies, grannies,* or *cartwheels.* Methamphetamine is known as *speed, meth, ice, blue, crank,* or *crystal.* Methamphetamine is more potent than amphetamines as greater amounts of the drug cross the blood-brain barrier. Dextroamphetamine sulfate may be referred to as *dexies, hearts,* or *oranges.*

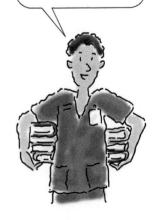

Some people take amphetamines when they have to stay up all night to cram for a test.

Pleasure rush

Amphetamines may be taken orally or by injection, snorting, or smoking. Immediately after methamphetamine is injected or smoked, the user experiences an intensely pleasurable sensation (a "rush") that lasts a few minutes. Snorting produces a longer lasting high rather than a rush, which may last up to half a day.

Individuals taking amphetamines can become addicted quickly, with rapid dose escalation. Higher doses may lead to increasing toxicity and complications.

Prevalence

An estimated 4.7 million persons (15 years of age or older) had used methamphetamine at least once in their lifetime. Use of this substance is rising and deaths have tripled since 2011 (Paulus, 2019).

How amphetamines produce their effects

Amphetamines increase the release of the neurotransmitters dopamine, norepinephrine, and serotonin into brain synapses. The "rush" or "high" experienced with these substances probably results from high levels of dopamine in the brain areas that regulate feelings of pleasure.

Detrimental to dopamine

Amphetamines may also have a neurotoxic effect, damaging brain cells that contain dopamine and serotonin. Studies suggest that over time, methamphetamine reduces dopamine levels, possibly leading to parkinsonian-like symptoms.

Health hazards of amphetamine misuse

Adverse physiologic effects of methamphetamine use include headache, poor concentration, poor appetite, dry mouth leading to tooth decay, abdominal pain, vomiting or diarrhea, sleep difficulties, paranoid or aggressive behavior, and psychosis.

Besides leading to addiction, chronic methamphetamine use can cause malignant hypertension, methamphetamine-associated cardiomyopathy, and death. Injection may damage blood vessels and cause skin abscesses. Some individuals taking methamphetamine have episodes of violent behavior, paranoia, anxiety, confusion, and insomnia. With heavy use, progressive social and occupational deterioration may occur.

Running on meth

People taking methamphetamines who become drug tolerant must take higher or more frequent doses or change their method of drug intake. In some cases, they forgo food and sleep while indulging in a form of bingeing known as a *run*, injecting methamphetamine repeatedly over several days until the drug supply runs out or the person becomes too disorganized to continue.

Hallucinations

Chronic methamphetamine use may damage the brain's frontal areas and basal ganglia. Some individuals experience a toxic psychosis that resembles paranoid schizophrenia—intense paranoia, rages, auditory hallucinations, mood disturbances, and delusions. For example, some may experience formication—the sensation of insects creeping on the skin. Psychotic symptoms may last months or years after drug use ceases.

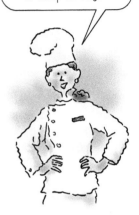

During an amphetamine binge, the user may not eat or sleep for days.

Causes

As with all types of substance use, the exact causes of amphetamine misuse are hard to identify. Some people use amphetamines in an effort to relieve fatigue, induce euphoria, or ease depression or other uncomfortable feelings.

Signs and symptoms

In a patient under the influence of amphetamines, assessment findings may include:
- euphoria
- hyperactivity and increased alertness
- diaphoresis (sweating)
- shallow respirations
- dilated pupils
- dry mouth
- exhaustion
- anorexia and weight loss
- nausea or vomiting
- tachycardia
- hypertension
- hyperthermia
- tremors
- seizures
- altered mental status, such as confusion, agitation, or paranoia
- psychotic behavior (with prolonged use).

Findings in amphetamine intoxication
Severe methamphetamine intoxication may cause the signs and symptoms listed earlier plus:
- arrhythmias
- heart failure
- subarachnoid hemorrhage

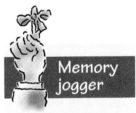

Memory jogger

SPEED helps when assessing a patient for amphetamine use.

Sweating (diaphoresis)

Psychotic behavior

Exhaustion

Everything up (hyperactive tendon reflexes, hypertension, hyperthermia, tachycardia)

Dilated pupils

Assessing for amphetamine withdrawal

During amphetamine withdrawal, the patient may exhibit or report:
* abdominal tenderness
* muscle aches
* apathy and depression
* disorientation
* irritability
* long periods of sleep
* suicide attempts (with sudden withdrawal).

* stroke
* cerebral hemorrhage
* coma
* death.

Amphetamine withdrawal symptoms

Abrupt amphetamine withdrawal may trigger CNS depression, ranging from lethargy to coma. Some patients experience hallucinations, whereas others show signs of overstimulation, including euphoria and violent behavior. (For additional withdrawal symptoms, see *Assessing for amphetamine withdrawal*.)

Diagnosis

Serum and urine drug screening may be performed if amphetamine use is suspected. Other diagnostic tests depend on the patient's symptoms. Laboratory tests may include complete blood count, metabolic panel, and serum creatinine kinase levels. In addition, an ECG may be done if the patient reports chest pain.

Synthetic stimulants, such as mephedrone, go by the street names *Plant Food* and *Bath Salts*. These drugs are not the same substance as commercially available plant food or bath salts. These newer drugs do not show up on common urine drug screens, so always consider the possibility of drug intoxication when the symptoms are present and the urine is negative (NIH, n.d.-a, n.d.-b).

Amphetamine use disorder is confirmed when the patient presents with symptoms of amphetamine use, resulting in a significant decrease in function.

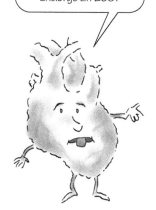

An amphetamine user who reports chest pain may undergo an ECG.

Treatment

A patient with acute amphetamine intoxication may require airway management, fluid replacement, and vigorous cooling measures. Chemical and physical restraints may be required to prevent harm to self and others. Arrhythmias may warrant cardioversion, defibrillation, and antiarrhythmic drugs. Vital signs must be monitored closely. If the drug was ingested, vomiting is induced (if the patient is conscious) or gastric lavage is performed; activated charcoal and a saline or magnesium sulfate cathartic may be given.

Other treatments are symptomatic. For example, the patient may require fluid replacement and nutritional and vitamin supplements.

Sedatives may be given to induce sleep, anticholinergics and antidiarrheal agents to relieve GI distress, and antianxiety drugs for severe agitation and symptomatic treatment of complications.

Managing drug addiction

Cognitive-behavioral therapy is commonly used to treat methamphetamine addiction. The goal of this approach is to modify the patient's thinking, expectations, and behaviors and increase the patient's ability to cope with stress.

Post-meth depression

Antidepressants may help combat the depression commonly seen in methamphetamine users who have recently become abstinent.

Rehabilitation

After withdrawal, the patient needs rehabilitation to prevent a relapse of substance use. Both inpatient and outpatient rehabilitation programs are available. They usually last a month or longer and may include individual, group, and family psychotherapy.

During and after rehabilitation, participation in a drug-oriented self-help group may be recommended as an adjunct to behavioral interventions and to promote long-term drug-free recovery.

Life after speed

Aftercare means a lifetime of abstinence, usually aided by participation in NA or a similar self-help group.

Nursing interventions

For appropriate nursing interventions during and after an episode of acute amphetamine intoxication, see *General interventions for acute substance intoxication*, page 408.

Nicotine-related disorders

One of the most commonly used addictive drugs, nicotine is the main psychoactive component found in smoke and vapor from tobacco and tobacco-derived products (cigarettes, e-cigarettes, vaping devices, cigars, and pipes). Smokeless tobacco products, such as snuff and chewing tobacco, also have a high nicotine content.

Cigarette smoking is the most prevalent form of nicotine dependence in the United States.

Tobacco dependence and withdrawal

Regular nicotine use can result in tobacco dependence and tobacco use disorder.

Most persons with tobacco dependence use tobacco regularly because they're addicted to nicotine. Although nearly 35 million smokers make a sincere attempt to quit each year, less than 7% who try to quit on their own stay abstinent for more than 1 year. Most of them relapse within a few days of trying to quit. Research has shown it may take five to seven attempts for the average person to reach sustained abstinence from tobacco.

Drawn-out withdrawal

A nicotine-dependent person who stops using nicotine experiences a withdrawal syndrome that may last a month or more. Some people have intense nicotine cravings for 6 months or longer.

Prevalence

The CDC estimates that 14% of U.S. adults are current smokers, whereas a recent report estimated that as much as 19% of all adults are tobacco product users (Wang et al., 2018). Almost all adults who use tobacco began using before the age of 18 years. Although cigarette smoking has declined dramatically over the years, rates of hookah and electronic cigarettes are rising (Camenga & Klein, 2016).

How nicotine produces its effects

Absorbed through the skin and mucosal lining of the mouth and nose or by inhalation in the lungs, nicotine activates the brain circuitry that regulates feelings of pleasure (the so-called reward pathways).

Short puffs and long draws

Nicotine can act as both a stimulant and a sedative. Small, rapid doses produce alertness and arousal, whereas long, drawn-out doses induce relaxation and sedation (NIH, n.d.-a).

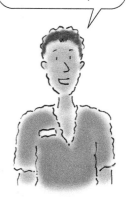

Children 5 and under are more than 5 times more likely to be hospitalized and 2.5 times more likely to have a severe outcome when exposed to e-cigarettes compared to those exposed to traditional cigarettes (Thomas Quail, 2020).

Health hazards of nicotine

Nicotine dependence has a tremendous impact in terms of illness, death, and economic costs to society. Tobacco use is one of the leading preventable causes of death in the United States. It kills more than 480,000 U.S. residents each year—more than alcohol, cocaine, heroin, homicide, suicide, car accidents, fire, and acquired immune deficiency syndrome (AIDS) combined (CDC, NIH, n.d.-a). (See *Nicotine's ugly aftermath.*)

Causes

Scientists suspect that certain genes make some people more susceptible to nicotine use disorder and cigarette smoking. Studies involving twins suggest that genes account for 50% to 70% of the risk of becoming a smoker.

Some researchers believe that as many as 50 genes are involved in nicotine use disorder. Genetic factors must be distinguished from environmental factors that contribute to smoking.

Nicotine's ugly aftermath

Tobacco use accounts for approximately one-third of all cancers. Cigarette smoking is linked to nearly 90% of all lung cancers—the leading cause of cancer deaths in both men and women. Additionally, it's associated with cancers of the mouth, pharynx, larynx, esophagus, stomach, pancreas, cervix, kidney, ureter, and bladder. Overall death rates from cancer are twice as high among smokers as nonsmokers.

Smoking also causes lung diseases, such as chronic bronchitis and emphysema, and can exacerbate asthma symptoms. It may also heighten the risk for peptic ulcers, GI disorders, maternal and fetal complications, and other disorders.

Cardiovascular disease

Smoking dramatically increases the risk of cardiovascular disease, including coronary artery disease, myocardial infarction, stroke, vascular problems, and aneurysms. Smoking accounts for nearly 20% of deaths from heart disease.

Passive smoking and its consequences

Secondhand smoke (passive smoking) causes approximately 3,000 lung cancer deaths yearly in nonsmokers and contributes to as many as 40,000 deaths from cardiovascular disease (NIH, n.d.-a).

Exposure to tobacco smoke in the home increases the severity of asthma in children and contributes to childhood asthma.

Susceptible teens

Among adolescents, risk factors for cigarette smoking include:
- use of alcohol and other drugs
- attention deficit disorder
- depression
- peer influences
- urge to experiment
- disruptive behavior
- failing to perceive the risks of smoking
- having friends who abuse substances
- having family members who smoke
- divorce or family conflict.

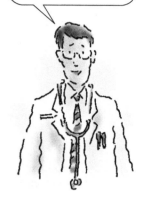

Nicotine use disorder may involve as many as 50 genes.

Signs and symptoms

Nicotine withdrawal symptoms may begin within a few hours of last use—and can quickly drive the person back to tobacco product use. Usually, symptoms peak within the first few days and subside within a few weeks. For some people, however, increased appetite and nicotine cravings last for months (NIH, n.d.-a).

Nicotine withdrawal symptoms include:
- depressed mood
- insomnia
- irritability, frustration, or anger
- anxiety
- difficulty concentrating
- restlessness
- increased appetite or weight gain
- desire for sweets
- increased coughing
- nicotine craving.

Diagnosis

The diagnosis of nicotine use disorder is confirmed when the patient presents with symptoms of nicotine use, resulting in a significant decrease in function.

Treatment

Various behavioral and pharmacologic treatments have proven to be effective in treating nicotine dependence. For patients who are motivated to quit smoking, a combination of behavioral and pharmacologic treatments can double the success rate over placebo treatments (NIH, n.d.-a).

Pharmacologic therapies for smoking cessation include nicotine replacement, antagonist therapy, aversive therapy, nicotine-mimicking agents, and non-nicotine medication. Nonpharmacologic therapies include sensory replacement and acupuncture. To remain abstinent, many patients require behavioral therapy.

Nicotine replacement
Nicotine replacement products can be used to relieve withdrawal symptoms and nicotine craving. Nicotine replacement products include

Smoking cessation
The Food and Drug Administration (FDA) has approved of seven medications to assist with smoking cessation: two non-nicotine replacement medications and five nicotine replacements. Non-nicotine medications include bupropion (Zyban) and varenicline (Chantix). Nicotine replacement therapies (NRTs) include nicotine gum, transdermal patches, nasal spray, lozenges, and inhalers (Ziedonis et al., 2017).

Behavioral treatments
Behavioral interventions can play a key role in treating nicotine addiction. Such methods help patients identify high-risk relapse situations, create an aversion to smoking, self-monitor their smoking behavior, and establish alternative coping responses. Identifying and removing environmental cues that influence the patient to smoke (such as cigarettes, lighters, and ashtrays) are crucial.

Adjunctive measures
The single most important factor in nicotine abstinence may be learning and using coping skills that aid both short- and long-term relapse prevention. Social support can also influence the outcome of a smoking cessation program. Ideally, the patient should avoid smokers and smoking environments and receive support from family and friends. (See *Improving the patient's coping skills*.)

Other helpful measures include self-help materials, educational and supportive groups, exercise, hypnosis, 12-step programs, biofeedback, family therapy, interpersonal therapy, and psychodynamic therapies.

Nursing interventions
These nursing interventions may be appropriate for a patient with nicotine use disorder:
* Teach the patient about the dangers of smoking and ways to stop.

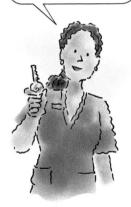

Nicotine replacement therapy has helped about 1 million people stop smoking.

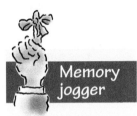

Memory jogger

During nicotine withdrawal, a patient **NEEDS CARE**.

Nervousness

Extreme fatigue

Excited cardiovascular system

Difficulty concentrating

Sleep disturbances

Cravings

Anxiety

Restlessness

Excessive appetite

Improving the patient's coping skills

Many patients who use substances exhibit ineffective coping and need help in identifying and using available support systems. To enhance your patient's coping skills, use these nursing interventions:
• Spend uninterrupted periods of time with the patient. Encourage expression of feelings; accept what is said.
• Try to identify factors that cause, exacerbate, or reduce the patient's inability to cope, such as the fear of health problems or losing a job.
• Encourage the patient to make decisions about care to increase sense of self-worth and mastery over the current situation.
• Praise the patient for making decisions and performing activities to reinforce coping behaviors.
• Encourage the patient to use support systems that can help with coping.
• Help the patient to evaluate the current situation and coping behaviors to encourage a realistic view of the crisis.
• Encourage the patient to try alternative coping behaviors. A patient in crisis tends to accept interventions and develop new coping behaviors more easily.
• Ask the patient for feedback about behaviors that seem to work. This encourages the patient to evaluate the effect of these behaviors.

- Provide emotional support for the patient's attempts to stop smoking.
- Explain how to use nicotine replacement devices and prescribed medications.
- As indicated, refer the patient to a smoking cessation program.

Sedative, hypnotic, or anxiolytic use disorder

Sedative, hypnotic, and anxiolytic drugs produce sedation, ease anxiety, and relax muscles. Most are classified as benzodiazepines. Typically, benzodiazepines act as hypnotics in high doses, anxiolytics in moderate doses, and sedatives in low doses. Besides the main indications described earlier, they're used to prevent seizures or to help patients withdraw from alcohol.

In the United States, benzodiazepines are the most widely prescribed CNS medications, with about 13 million adults taking the medication in 2013. Most of the medications are prescribed by primary care providers, and they are disproportionally prescribed to women, particularly middle aged and older adults (Agarwal &

Landon, 2019; Bachhuber et al., 2016). Because of their widespread availability, benzodiazepine misuse is common (NIH, n.d.-a). (See *Benzodiazepines from A to T.*) A total of 30.6 million adults have had a benzodiazepine prescription in the past year, or over 12% of adults in the United States (Maust et al., 2019).

Forging for drugs

Persons who misuse benzodiazepines may attempt to maintain their drug supply by getting prescriptions from several different prescribers, forging prescriptions, or buying the drugs on the street. Younger patients may buy nonpharmaceutical-grade benzodiazepines in liquid or pill form on the dark web. Street names for benzodiazepines include: Z-bars, *dolls, green and whites, roaches,* and *yellow jackets* (Mignone & Novara, 2017).

Benzodiazepines are ingested or injected. Their half-life ranges from 4 to 20 hours.

Mixed motives

Many persons become dependent on benzodiazepines insidiously, prescribed by their health care providers. An as-needed prescription for occasional anxiety may, after a year or more, lead to dependence, with the patient taking the medication three times daily and in increasing doses. Some people use benzodiazepines to get intoxicated; others take intentional or accidental overdoses. Benzodiazepines can become dangerous when combined with alcohol or opiates, causing respiratory depression, overdose, and death. Heroin users may use benzodiazepines when they can't get heroin, when they want to enhance heroin's effects, or when they're trying to stop using heroin. Individuals who use amphetamine and ecstasy may take benzodiazepines when "coming down" from a high or to induce sleep.

Prevalence

Benzodiazepine use is increasing. Approximately 13.5 million adults filled a benzodiazepine prescription in 2013. Benzodiazepines are more commonly prescribed to women (who are in general more likely to seek treatment for an anxiety complaint), and the likelihood that a woman will be prescribed a benzodiazepine increases over her lifetime. Although benzodiazepines are not recommended for use in older adults, an estimated 8% of men and 12% of women over 60 years have a persistent benzodiazepine prescription (Bachhuber et al., 2016; Tannenbaum, 2015).

How benzodiazepines produce their effects

Like alcohol, heroin, and cannabis, benzodiazepines are depressants that slow CNS activity. They work by potentiating the activity of GABA, causing sedation, relaxing muscles, easing anxiety, and having anticonvulsant properties. In the peripheral nervous system, stimulation of GABA receptors may decrease cardiac contractility and enhance perfusion (NIH, n.d.-a, n.d.-b).

Health hazards of benzodiazepines

In addition to causing tolerance and physical dependence, repeated use of large benzodiazepine doses can lead to amnesia, memory loss, hostility, irritability, and vivid or disturbing dreams. Concurrent use with alcohol or other depressants can be life-threatening.

The risky business of injection

Some people inject benzodiazepines for an enhanced "high" or to increase the effects of other drugs. This practice can lead to severe health effects, such as:

- collapsed veins
- red, swollen, infected skin
- necessity for limb amputation (because of poor circulation)
- stroke
- cardiac and respiratory arrest
- death.

Sharing needles, syringes, and other injecting equipment greatly increases the risk of contracting hepatitis and HIV.

Impairments associated with benzodiazepine use

At low to moderate doses, benzodiazepines can produce drowsiness, fatigue, lethargy, dizziness, vertigo, blurred or double vision, slurred speech, stuttering, mild impairment of memory and thought processes, feelings of isolation, and depression.

A booze-like wooziness

At high doses, these drugs may induce oversedation, sleep, or effects similar to alcohol intoxication—confusion, poor coordination, impaired memory and judgment, difficulty thinking clearly, blurred or double vision, and dizziness. Mood swings and aggressive outbursts may also occur. As the high-dose wears off, the person may feel jittery and excitable.

Benzodiazepine overdose can lead to coma. When combined with alcohol, death may occur.

Causes

Some people may have a genetic tendency toward drug dependence or misuse. Environmental factors also play a significant role. Drug availability and prescriber dispensing practices may contribute to benzodiazepine misuse.

Benzodiazepines from A to T

Benzodiazepines include:

- alprazolam (Xanax)
- chlordiazepoxide (Librium)
- clonazepam (Klonopin)
- diazepam (Valium)
- flurazepam (Dalmane)
- lorazepam (Ativan)
- midazolam (Versed)
- oxazepam (Serax)
- temazepam (Restoril)
- triazolam (Halcion).

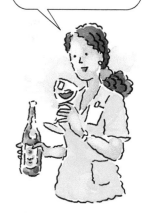

Benzodiazepines and alcohol make for a killer combination.

Signs and symptoms

A patient under the influence of benzodiazepine may exhibit:
- ataxia (poor muscle coordination)
- drowsiness
- hypotension
- increased self-confidence
- relaxation
- slurred speech.

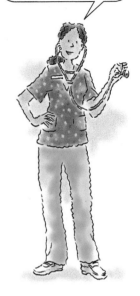

Expect low blood pressure in a patient who has taken a benzodiazepine overdose.

Findings in benzodiazepine overdose

Assessment findings in a patient with a benzodiazepine overdose may include:
- dizziness
- altered mental status, ranging from confusion and drowsiness to unresponsiveness or coma
- blurred vision
- anxiety and agitation
- nystagmus
- ataxia
- hallucinations
- slurred speech
- hypotonia (reduced skeletal muscle tone)
- weakness
- impaired cognition
- amnesia
- respiratory depression
- hypotension.

Findings in chronic use

Long-term benzodiazepine use (more than several weeks) may result in:
- drowsiness
- lack of motivation
- clouded thinking
- memory loss
- changes in personality and emotional responses
- anxiety
- irritability
- aggression
- insomnia
- disturbing dreams
- nausea
- headache
- skin rash
- menstrual problems

- sexual problems
- increased appetite
- weight gain
- increased risk of accidents (including falls in older adults).

Withdrawal symptoms

Benzodiazepine withdrawal resembles that of alcohol withdrawal and may cause seizures; benzodiazepines should not be stopped abruptly or without medical monitoring. Withdrawal symptoms may necessitate hospitalization.

Rough withdrawal

Withdrawal symptoms usually develop 1 to 4 days after the drug is stopped; however, they may arise earlier with shorter acting agents or later with longer acting agents. Symptoms can last a few weeks or months; some patients have them for 1 year—or even longer.

Withdrawal symptoms may include:
- headache
- sweating
- confusion
- seizures
- nervousness
- tension
- anxiety and panic attacks
- hypertension
- dizziness
- poor appetite
- nausea, vomiting, and abdominal pain
- inability to sleep properly
- depression
- feelings of isolation and unreality
- delirium and paranoia.

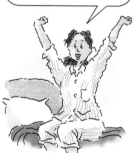

Long-term benzodiazepine use can cause insomnia.

Diagnosis

The diagnosis of benzodiazepine use disorder is confirmed if the patient presents with symptoms of benzodiazepine use, resulting in a significant decrease in function.

Treatment

Treatment of benzodiazepine intoxication depends on which drug was taken, how much, and when. The patient may need supportive care and monitoring, including cardiac monitoring, IV fluid administration, pulse oximetry, and vital sign monitoring. Respiratory depression may necessitate assisted ventilation. (See *Dealing with drug overdose.*)

Detoxification

For detoxification, single-dose activated charcoal is recommended if the patient ingested the drug within the past 4 hours. Alternatively, gastric lavage may be considered. (Ipecac is contraindicated because of the risk of CNS depression and subsequent aspiration of emesis.)

Dealing with drug overdose

Whether intentional or accidental, a drug overdose is life-threatening. In very high doses, some drugs cause CNS depression, ranging from lethargy to coma. Others cause CNS stimulation, ranging from euphoria to violent behavior.

Depending on the specific drug and the extent of damage, other symptoms of overdose may include hallucinations, respiratory depression, seizures, abnormal pupil size and response, or nausea and vomiting.

Diagnosing overdose

Arterial blood gas analysis and blood and urine screening tests help detect drug use and guide treatment.

Treatment

A patient with signs of respiratory depression receives oxygen or intubation and mechanical ventilation. The patient is attached to a cardiac monitor, and a 12-lead ECG is taken. Urine, blood, and vomitus specimens are obtained for toxicology screening. Restraints may be applied to prevent the patient from harming themselves or others.

Emergency nursing interventions

• Take appropriate steps to stop further drug absorption. If the patient ingested the drug, induce vomiting or use gastric lavage, as ordered. You may administer activated charcoal to help adsorb the substance and use a saline cathartic to speed its elimination.

• Frequently reassess your patient's airway, breathing, and circulation. Keep oxygen, suction equipment, and emergency airway equipment nearby. Be prepared to perform cardiopulmonary resuscitation, if necessary.

• When possible, find out which drug the patient took, how much, and when. Did they combine several drugs or take a drug along with alcohol? Question the patient's family, friends, or rescue personnel thoroughly.

• Watch for complications. Stay alert for shock, indicated by decreased blood pressure and a faint, rapid pulse. Reassess respiratory rate and depth, and auscultate breath sounds frequently. Know that dyspnea and tachypnea may warn of impending respiratory complications, such as pulmonary edema or aspiration pneumonia. A patient with crackles who's pale, diaphoretic, and gasping for air may have pulmonary edema. A patient with rhonchi or decreased breath sounds probably has aspiration pneumonia.

• Carefully monitor heart rate and rhythm. Because the patient's neurologic status may change as the body metabolizes the drug, frequently assess neurologic function.

• You may detect hypothermia or hyperthermia, so expect to use either extra blankets and a hyperthermia mattress or an antipyretic and a hypothermia mattress, as ordered.

• If the overdose was accidental, recommend a rehabilitation program for SUD. If it was intentional, refer the patient to crisis intervention for psychological counseling and treatment.

The only specific benzodiazepine antidote is flumazenil (Romazicon), a GABA antagonist. Given IV, flumazenil reverses sedation, memory, and psychomotor impairments and respiratory depression produced by benzodiazepines. However, it's usually reserved for severe poisoning, because it can cause withdrawal and seizures in patients with chronic benzodiazepine use (Greller & Gupta, 2018).

Treatment of chronic misuse

Treatment of chronic benzodiazepine misuse usually is done on an outpatient basis or at a drug rehabilitation center. However, patients who have been using high doses of sedatives or hypnotics have a history of withdrawal seizures or DTs, or have concurrent medical illnesses should undergo withdrawal in an inpatient setting.

Replacement therapy

The first step involves gradual reduction of the drug to prevent withdrawal and seizures. The benzodiazepine may be replaced gradually with another drug that has a similar action. A patient using benzodiazepines long-term with severe withdrawal symptoms (such as elevated vital signs or delirium) should receive an agent with a rapid onset, in doses sufficient to suppress withdrawal symptoms. IV lorazepam (Ativan) or diazepam (Valium) is commonly given for immediate results.

When stabilized, the patient is switched to an equivalent dose of an oral long-acting agent, which causes milder withdrawal symptoms. The patient is tapered off this long-acting agent slowly, over 2 to 6 months.

For mild benzodiazepine withdrawal symptoms, anticonvulsants that aren't cross-dependent with sedative-hypnotics, such as carbamazepine (Tegretol) and valproate (Depakote), have been used successfully.

Recovery phase

After withdrawal comes a prolonged recovery and rehabilitation phase in which the patient attempts to stay drug-free. The patient needs social support and involvement of family and friends during this difficult stage. A peer recovery coach can be helpful.

Rehabilitation programs are available for both inpatients and outpatients. They usually last a month or longer and may include individual, group, and family psychotherapy. During and after rehabilitation, participation in a substance use recovery self-help group may be helpful.

Nursing interventions

Nursing interventions for a patient who misuses benzodiazepine are described in *General interventions for acute substance intoxication*, page 408.

Quick quiz

1. When caring for a patient with AUD, the nurse understands that the expected effects of a disulfiram reaction include which of the following?
    A. Chest pain, chills, and hypertension
    B. Slow pulse, chills, and excitation
    C. Slow pulse, slow respiratory rate, and hypertension
    D. Chest pain, headache, and hypotension

Answer: D. A patient who consumes alcohol up to 2 weeks after taking disulfiram will experience a reaction that includes shortness of breath, chest pain, nausea, vomiting, facial flushing, headache, red eyes, blurred vision, sweating, tachycardia, hypotension, and fainting.

2. A patient admits to taking "crystal." The nurse is aware that this is a slang term for which type of drug?
    A. A depressant
    B. A stimulant
    C. A hallucinogen
    D. An antidepressant

Answer: B. "Crystal" is a street name for methamphetamine, a stimulant. Other amphetamines include amphetamine sulfate and dextroamphetamine.

3. Which assessment finding *most strongly* suggests IV substance use?
    A. Skin lesions
    B. Gastritis
    C. Tachycardia
    D. Tachypnea

Answer: A. Self-injection of drugs can cause skin lesions or abscesses.

4. To treat tachycardia induced by cocaine, the nurse will anticipate which medication to be administered?
    A. Buprenorphine
    B. Digoxin
    C. Lidocaine
    D. Propranolol

Answer: D. Propranolol is typically given to treat tachycardia caused by cocaine use.

5. When caring for a client with an opiate overdose, the nurse will anticipate which antagonist to be ordered?
    A. Disulfiram
    B. Naloxone
    C. Diazepam
    D. Bupropion

Answer: B. Naloxone (Narcan) is a narcotic antagonist that displaces previously administered narcotic analgesics from CNS receptors.

Scoring

☆☆☆   If you answered all five items correctly, mind blowing! Your comprehension of substance use has given us quite a rush.

☆☆   If you answered four items correctly, far out! One more hit of this chapter may be all you need.

☆   If you answered three or less items correctly, complete a thorough review of this chapter.

Selected references

Agarwal, S. D., & Landon, B. E. (2019, January 4). Patterns in outpatient benzodiazepine prescribing in the United States. *JAMA Network Open, 2*(1), e187399. https://doi.org/10.1001/jamaworkopen.2018.7399

Alcoholics Anonymous. (2019). https://www.aa.org/

American Psychiatric Association. (2013). *Diagnostic and statistical manual of mental disorders* (5th ed.). Author.

Auer, R., Vittinghoff, E., Yaffe, K., Kunzi, A., Kertesz, S., Levine, D., Albanese, E., Whitmer, R, Jacobs, D. R., Jr, Sidney, S., Glymour, M. M., & Pletcher, M. J. (2016). Association between lifetime marijuana use and cognitive function in middle age: The coronary artery risk development in young adults (CARDIA) study. *JAMA, 176*(3), 352–361. https://doi.org/10.1001/jamainternmed.2015.7841

Bachhuber, M. A., Hennessy, S., Cunningham, C. O., & Starrels, J. L. (2016). Increasing benzodiazepine prescriptions and overdose mortality in the United States, 1996-2013. *American Journal of Public Health, 106*(4), 686–688. https://doi.org/10.1001/10.2105/AJPH.2016.303061

Bridgeman, M., & Abazia, D. (2017). Medicinal cannabis: History, pharmacology, and implications for the acute care setting. *P & T.* 42(3), 180–188.

Brezing, C., & Levin, F. (2018). The current state of pharmacological treatments for cannabis use disorders and withdrawal. *Neuropsychopharmacology,* 43(1), https://doi.org/10.1038/npp.2017.212.

Boyd, M. (2018). *Psychiatric nursing: Contemporary practice* (6th ed.). Philadelphia, PA: Wolters Kluwer.

Bukstein, O. (2020). Substance use disorder in adolescence. *UpToDate.* https://www.uptodate.com/contents/substance-use-disorder-in-adolescents

Camenga, D., & Klein, J. (2016). Tobacco use disorder. *Child Adolescent Psychiatric Clinics of North America,* 25(3). doi: 10.1016/j.chc.2016.02.003

Centers for Disease Control and Prevention. (2017). *Understanding the epidemic.* https://www.cdc.gov/drugoverdose/epidemic/index.html

Cowen, E., & Su, M. (2018). Ethanol intoxication in adults. *UpToDate.* https://www.uptodate.com/contents/ethanol-intoxication-in-adults

Dugosh, K., & Cacciola, J. (2019). Clinical assessment of substance use disorders. *UpToDate.* https://www.uptodate.com/contents/clinical-assessment-of-substance-use-disorders

Garmo, M. (2013). Substance use disorders. In W. K. Mohr (Ed.), *Psychiatric-mental health nursing: Evidence-based concepts, skills, and practices* (pp. 619–659). Lippincott Williams & Wilkins.

Grant, B., Chou, S., Saha, T., Pickering, R., Kerridge, B., Ruan, W., Huang, B., Jung, J., Zhang, H., Fan, A., & Hasin, D. (2017). Prevalence of 12-month alcohol use, high risk drinking, and DSM-IV alcohol use disorder in the United States, 2001-2002 to 2012-2013. *JAMA Psychiatry, 74*(9), 911–923. https://doi .org/10.1001/jamapsychiatry.2017.2161

Greller, H., & Gupta, A. (2018). Benzodiazepine poisoning and withdrawal. *UpToDate.* https://www.uptodate.com/contents/benzodiazepine-poisoning-and-withdrawal

Gorlick, D. (2019). Cocaine use disorder in adults: Epidemiology, pharmacology, clinical manifestations, medical treatment, consequences, and diagnosis. *UpToDate.* https://www.uptodate.com/contents/cocaine-use-disorder- in-adults-epidemiology-pharmacology-clinical-manifestations-medical- consequences-and-diagnosis

Halgren, M., Vancampfort, D., Giesen, E., Lundin, A., & Stubbs, B. (2017). Exercise as treatment for alcohol use disorders: Systematic review and meta-analysis. *British Journal of Sports Medicine, 51*(14), 1058–1064. https://doi.org/10.1136/ bjsports-2016-096814

Han, B., Compton, W., Blanco, C., & Colpe, L. (2017). Prevalence, treatment, and un-met treatment needs of US adults with mental health and substance use dis-orders. *Behavioral Health Care, 36*(10), 1739–1747. https://doi.org/10.1377/ hlthaff.2017.0584

Kampman, K., & Jarvis, M. (2015). American Society of Addiction Medicine (ASAM) national practice guideline for the use of medications in the treatment of addiction involving opioid use. *Journal of Addiction Medicine, 9*(5), 358–367. https://doi.org/10.1097/ADM.0000000000000166

Lipari, R., & Van Horn, S. (2017). *Trends is substance use disorders among adults aged 18 or older* (The CBHSQ Report). https://www.ncbi.nlm.nih.gov/books/NBK447253/

Maust, D. T., Lin, L. A., & Blow, F. C. (2019, January 1). Benzodiazepine use and misuse among adults in the United States. *Psychiatric Services, 70*(2), 97–106.

Mayo Clinic. (2020). *Caffeine content for coffee, tea, soda and more.* http://www.mayoclinic .org/healthy-living/nutrition-and-healthy-eating/in-depth/caffeine/art-20049372

McKellen, T. (2017). Substance misuse and substance use disorders: Why do they mat-ter in healthcare. *Transactions of the American Clinical and Climatological Asso-ciation, 128*, 112–130.

Mental Health America. (2020). *Position statement 33: Substance use disorders.* https:// www.mhanational.org/issues/position-statement-33-substance-use-disorders

Mignone, M., & Novara, E. (2017). *The illegal sale of medicines on the dark net: The case of benzodiazepines and prescription drugs on Alphabay, EPS NPS Project, RISSC, Research Centre on Security and Crime, Italy.* https://www.npsproject.eu/wp- content/uploads/2017/03/NPS_Final_DarkNet-1.pdf

National Institute of Drug Abuse. (2015). *Hallucinogens and dissociative drugs.* https:// www.drugabuse.gov/publications/research-reports/hallucinogens- dissociative-drugs/

National Institute of Drug Abuse. (2016). *How is cocaine addiction treated.* https://www .drugabuse.gov/publications/research-reports/cocaine/what-treatments- are-effective-cocaine-abusers

National Institute of Drug Abuse. (2018a). *Inhalants.* https:www.drugabuse.gov/drugs- abuse/inhalants

National Institute of Drug Abuse. (2018b). *Cocaine.* https://www.drugabuse.gov/ publications/drugfacts/cocaine

National Institute of Drug Abuse. (2019). *Commonly abused drugs charts*. https://www
.drugabuse.gov/drugs-abuse/commonly-abused-drugs-charts

National Institutes of Health. (n.d.-a). *Drug facts*. http://www.drugabuse.gov/
publications/finder/t/160/DrugFacts

National Institutes of Health. (n.d.-b). *Trends & statistics*. http://www.drugabuse.gov/
related-topics/trends-statistics

Novick, T., Liu, Y., Alvanzo, A., Crews, D. C., Zonderman, A. B., Evans, M. K., & Crews,
D. C. (2016). Lifetime cocaine and opiate use and chronic kidney disease.
American Journal of Nephrology, 44(6), 447–453.

Pace, C. (2018). Alcohol withdrawal: Epidemiology, clinical manifestations, course,
assessment, and diagnosis. *UpToDate*. https://www.uptodate.com/contents/
alcohol-withdrawal-epidemiology-clinical-manifestations-course-assessment-
and-diagnosis

Patel, J., & Marwaha, R. (2019). *Cannabis use disorder*. StatPearls. www.ncbi.nlm.nih
.gov/books/NBK538131/

Paulus, M. (2020). Methamphetamine use disorder: Epidemiology, clinical manifestations,
course, assessment, & diagnosis. In A. Saxon & D. Solomon (Eds.). Retrieved
from https://www.uptodate.com/contents/methamphetamine-use-disorder-
epidemiology-clinical-manifestations-course-assessment-and-diagnosis

Poole, R., Kennedy, O. J., Roderick, P., Parkes, J., Fallowfield, J. A., & Hayes, P. C.
(2017). Coffee consumption and health: umbrella review of meta-analyses of
multiple health outcomes. *BMJ, 359*, j5024.

Ritchie, H., & Roser, M. (2020). *Alcohol consumption*. https://ourworldindata.org/alcohol-
consumption

Schreck, B., Wagneur, N., Caillet, P., Gérardin, M., Cholet, J., Spadari, M., Authier, N., &
Victorri-Vigneau, C. (2018). Cannabinoid hyperemesis syndrome: Review of
the literature and of cases reported to the French addictovigilance network.
Drug and Alcohol Dependence, 182, 27–32.

Substance Abuse and Mental Health Services Administration. (2017). *Key substance use
and mental health indicators in the United States: Results from the 2016 national
survey on drug use and health* (HHS Publication No. SMA 17-5044, NSDUH
Series H-52). Center for Behavioral Health Statistics and Quality, Substance
Abuse and Mental Health Services Administration. https://www.samhsa.gov/
data/sites/default/files/nsduh-ppt-09-2018.pdf

Tannenbaum, C. (2015). Inappropriate benzodiazepine use in elderly patients and its
reduction. *Journal of Psychiatry & Neuroscience, 40*(3), E27–E28. https://doi
.org/10.1503/jpn.140355

Thomas Quail, M. (2020). Nicotine toxicity: Protecting children from e-cigarette exposure. *Nursing, 50*(1), 44–48.

Wang, T. W., Asman, K., Gentzke A. S., Cullen, K. A., Holder-Hayes, E., Reyes-Guzman,
C., Jamal, A., Neff, L., & King, B. A. (2018). Tobacco product use among
adults—United States, 2017. *MMWR Morbidity Mortality Weekly Report, 67*,
1225–1232. https://doi.org/10.15585/mmwr.mm6744a2

Xi, B., Veeranki, S., Zhao, M., Ma, C., Yan, Y., & Mi, J. (2017). Relationship of alcohol
consumption to all cause, cardiovascular, and cancer-related mortality in U.S.
adults. *Journal of the American College of Cardiology, 70*(8), 913–922. https://
doi.org/10.1016/j.jacc.2017.06.054

Ziedonis, D., Das, S., & Larkin, C. (2017). Tobacco use disorder and treatment: New challenges and opportunities. *Dialogues in Clinical Neuroscience, 19*(3), 271–280.

Chapter 18

Neurocognitive disorders

Just the facts

In this chapter, you'll learn:

♦ mental status changes associated with older adulthood

♦ mental health disorders associated with the older adult

♦ how to recognize and provide nursing care for patients with neurocognitive disorders such as delirium, Alzheimer dementia, and other types of dementia.

A look at mental health disorders in older adults

Americans are living longer than ever before, with the vast majority surviving beyond the age of 65. Over the past 10 years, the population aged 65 and older increased from 37.8 million in 2007 to 50.9 million in 2017 (a 34% increase) and is projected to reach 94.7 million in 2060 (U.S. Department of Health and Human Services [USDHHS], 2018).

A significant number of older adults are affected by mental health disorders, including depression and anxiety, and neurocognitive disorders (NCDs), like dementia. As the life expectancy continues to rise, the number of older adults experiencing these disorders will keep growing.

Prevalence of mental illness in older adults

Approximately 13.8% of US adults aged 50 or older experienced a diagnosed mental illness in the past year (National Institute of Mental Health [NIMH], 2019a). The World Health Organization (2017) speculates that the actual rate of mental illness in this population is higher, estimating up to 15% of those aged 55 and older have some type of mental health concern. Older adults can experience the same mental illnesses as younger individuals. However, the more common mental health disorders in the older adult population are depressive and anxiety disorders, late-onset bipolar disorder, and eating disorder. Substance use disorders are also prevalent in the older adult population.

My granddaughter keeps me happy and alert. Sadly, some of my friends don't have family or friends to keep them company.

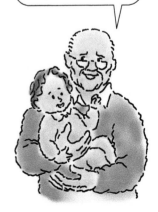

Barriers to treatment

The following may hinder the older adult from seeking treatment:

- The false belief that senility, depression, and hopelessness are natural conditions of aging.
- Reluctance to discuss psychological symptoms, dwelling instead on physical problems.
- A lack of awareness that symptoms experienced are part of a treatable mental illness.
- A preference for treatment by the primary care provider who may not readily identify mental health disorders in the older adult. Treatment of mental health disorders in older adults can be very complex even for properly trained professionals. Co-occurring medical conditions and use of multiple prescriptions complicate treatment.
- Health care system barriers:
  - High cost and insufficient insurance coverage for mental health concerns
  - Limited options and long waiting periods for care
  - Lack of trained professionals in some areas
- Lack of information about how to obtain treatment
- Stigma associated with mental health issues
- Lack of support systems.

Centers for Disease Control and Prevention. (2017). *Alzheimer's disease and healthy aging.* https://www.cdc.gov/aging/mentalhealth/depression.htm; National Council for Behavioral Health. (2019). *New study reveals lack of access as root cause for mental health crisis in America.* https://www.thenationalcouncil.org/press-releases/new-study-reveals-lack-of-access-as-root-cause-for-mental-health-crisis-in-america/

Beyond recognition?

Despite the substantial need for mental health services, older adults may not seek or readily use available resources. Only 44.4% of those identified with a mental health concern in the past year received mental health services (NIMH, 2019a). One important reason is that mental health disorders are frequently missed by health care providers, families, and even by the patient. Sometimes the symptoms are subtle, atypical, or attributed to other health issues. Older adults may assume that symptoms experienced are an inevitable part of aging, rather than symptoms of a treatable mental health disorder. Stigma and embarrassment also hinder reporting mental health concerns. Neurocognitive illnesses and mental illnesses can have overlapping symptoms, which makes an accurate diagnosis difficult. Untreated mental illness can complicate the treatment of other medical conditions like diabetes and cardiac disease. It is important for health care professionals to identify symptoms of these disorders and recognize factors that interfere with receiving adequate treatment. (See *Barriers to treatment.*)

An interprofessional approach

Comprehensive treatment for the older adult with mental health needs usually involves an interprofessional approach. This can include psychiatrists, psychologists, case managers, geropsychiatric nurses, nutritionists, and social workers with specialized training in gerontology. Gerontology is the scientific study of old age, the process of aging, and the unique problems of older people.

Community services for older adults

Community services for older adults vary from one location to another. Examples of available services may include:

- nutritional services with home delivery of meals
- transportation
- personal care services to assist with activities of daily living (ADLs)
- homemaker services
- specialized gerontology clinicals to provide health-related assessment and treatment
  - psychiatric evaluation and treatment
  - crisis intervention
  - counseling
- adult day care centers
- group homes
- case management services

- outreach—may include home evaluations
- respite care to support caregivers
- senior centers

Where to get information
- The local community mental health agency
- National Alliance on Mental Illness (local chapter)
- The Administration on Aging (AOA)—a principal agency of the USDHHS; provides services/programs to help older adults live independently in their homes and communities
- Eldercare Locator (a public service of the US Administration on Aging) to find local resources; https://eldercare.acl.gov/Public/Index.aspx

Geropsychiatric nursing

Geropsychiatric nursing is a subspecialty of psychiatric/mental health nursing that addresses the unique mental health care needs of the older adults. This area of nursing blends expertise in gerontological, psychiatric, medical-surgical, and community health nursing.

The advanced practice nurse (APRN) who specializes in geropsychiatric nursing may also:
- have prescriptive authority in some states
- provide group and individual psychotherapy
- provide education, support, and clinical consultation for nursing staff working with the mental health needs of the older adult. (See *Community services for older adults*.)

Care in the community

Multiple community-based services are available to increase the quality of life for older adults with and without mental health needs. Knowledge of and referral to local community-based resources is an essential part of patient-centered care for this population.

Support groups

Support groups give older adults a chance to discuss with peers how their conditions affect their lives. They provide an avenue to help each other by sharing workable solutions.

The linking liaison

Community liaison nurses can facilitate a smooth transition from emergency room or inpatient hospitalization to services in the community. They can provide valuable information to the intervention team and expedite rapid referral.

Assess for abuse

Elder abuse is a significant public health problem. The CDC (2017b) reports that elder abuse, including neglect and exploitation, is experienced by 1 out of every 6 to 10 people, ages 60 and older, who live at home with equal numbers in extended care facilities. This may be an underestimation because many victims are afraid to disclose or report violence. There are six types of identified maltreatment that can occur among persons over the age of 60 (CDC, 2017b).

- Physical abuse
- Sexual abuse
- Emotional abuse
- Neglect (including self-neglect)
- Abandonment
- Financial abuse

Nurses are ethically and legally required to report suspicion of elder abuse. It is essential for any nurse who treats older adults to become knowledgeable about this important public health issue and to understand the state-specific requirements and procedures for reporting.

Neurobiological changes of normal aging

As the brain ages ...

As a person gets older, changes occur in all parts of the body, including the brain. Normal aging brings certain changes in cognition or mental functioning.

Physical changes of the brain

Age-related physiologic changes in the brain include (Nichols, 2017):

- Shrinkage in certain parts of the brain, especially the prefrontal cortex and the hippocampus.
- Communication between neurons decreases because white matter is degraded or lost.
- Blood flow to the brain decreases as arteries narrow.
- Inflammation, the body's response to injury or disease, may increase in the brain.

Cognitive changes

Cognition involves the process of thinking. Reasoning and comprehension, learning, remembering, responding, and the ability to pay

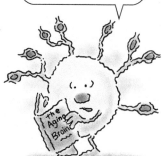

It says here that neurons shrink with age. Maybe that's why I am having trouble remembering things.

attention are all examples of cognitive skills. With advancing years, cognitive capacity declines somewhat, but important functions are spared. Age-related cognitive changes can vary significantly among individuals (Nichols, 2017).

Processing ability, complex attention, and executive functioning
Processing speed is the speed at which cognitive activity or thinking is performed as well as the speed of motor responses. There is a slowing of processing speed with normal aging.

Complex attention also tends to decline with normal aging. One example of complex attention includes being able to multitask. Another cognitive task of complex attention is the ability to selectively focus on specific information while ignoring irrelevant information (e.g., skills needed for driving).

Executive functioning is a set of processes that have to do with managing oneself and one's resources in order to achieve a goal. It includes *concept formation, abstraction, and mental flexibility. Executive functioning declines with age, especially after age 70* (Murman, 2015).

What is normal about memory?
Common cognitive concerns in the older adult frequently involve memory. Short-term memory does decline with *normal* aging. However, long-term memory shows significantly less decline. Older memories (like details about a significant event such as a wedding or birth of a child) remain intact while other memories (like remembering to take a pill in the future) decline with age (Anderson & Craik, 2017; Murman, 2015).

Additional cognitive processes that show little decline with *normal* aging include:

- Implicit memory, which is more of an automatic memory, such as remembering how to ride a bicycle.
- Procedural memory, which involves highly practiced expert skills, such as typing or playing bridge or chess.
- Ability to make new memories.
- Ability to learn new things.
- Picture recognition. (See *Using pictures and words.*)

Haven't I seen you somewhere before?

Researchers have found that aging affects *recall*, the process of bringing an experience back into consciousness without a cue. For example, a recall question might be: "What is the name of your first-grade teacher?" *Recognition*, the ability to recognize or know someone or something through remembering, is less impacted with normal aging. For example, a recognition question might be: "Is the name of your first-grade teacher Mrs. Lester?"

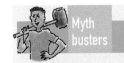

Shaking off "old people" stereotypes

Does the brain grow brittle and inflexible with age? Don't bet on it.
Myth: Older adults are slow thinking, inflexible, and unproductive.
Reality: With normal aging, intellectual functioning generally remains stable. Many older adults remain flexible in both behavior and attitude and are able to grow intellectually and emotionally.

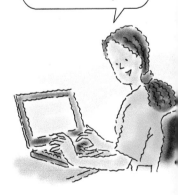

Highly practiced skills like typing and playing bridge rarely decline with age.

Advice from the experts

Using pictures and words

Aging does not seem to affect a person's ability to recognize pictures. Use pictures to help jog the memory of older adults with memory impairments.

Here are some other ways to aid memory retention:

- Choose concrete text instructions that explicitly represent material rather than those that force the patient to make subtle inferences or draw conclusions.

- Avoid irrelevant details, which can be distracting and require more mental processing.

Many of these normal age-related cognitive declines are small and do not have a big impact upon daily functioning for many older adults. One exception is the ability to drive. Because the ability to drive can decline with normal cognitive aging in some (but not all) older adults, driving presents a potential safety issue. Research shows that *cognitive retraining* can significantly improve some of these normal age-related cognitive declines including driving (Murman, 2015).

Implications for teaching

Because age-related cognitive changes can lead to *slower processing* and *slower learning*, the nurse may need to repeat new information frequently when teaching older adults. New skills and habits should be practiced repeatedly until these become automatic. Automatic and well-established skills are less likely to be completely lost at a later time.

Depression in older adults

A depressing thought ...

Clinical depression is one of the more common mental illnesses experienced by the older adult. Some estimates of major depression in older people living in the community range from less than 1% to about 5% but rise to 13.5% in those who require home health care and to 11.5% in older hospital patients (CDC, 2017a). Suicide is a significant public health issue for older adults. Those 85 years or older had the second highest rate of suicide in 2017 when compared to other age groups (NIMH, 2019b). Suicide in this age group is associated with sociocultural risk factors such as social isolation, marital status, and bereavement and clinical risk factors such as dementia, cognitive impairment, and physical illness (Conejero et al., 2018). Placement into a long-term care facility is another factor that can increase suicide risk for some individuals (Barak & Gale, 2019).

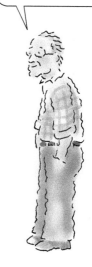

I wanted to enjoy my "golden years" ... I wonder why I am not happy?

Bereavement red flags

Bereavement can turn into a major depressive disorder. The nurse would suspect that this may be occurring if the patient experiences (Schimelpfening, 2018):

- frequent thoughts of death, especially suicide
- sense of worthlessness
- guilt about things unrelated to what prompted the grief
- pronounced slowing of psychomotor functions
- prolonged, marked functional impairment.

Not-so-harmless hallucinations
Some bereaved people hallucinate. For example, they "hear" the dead loved one's voice while trying to fall asleep or they "see" the person in a crowd. These hallucinations are common among bereaved people.

A patient who has other types of hallucinations or delusions may have a mental illness and needs to be evaluated by a health care provider.

Unlike younger patients, for some older adults with depression, sadness is not the main symptom. Instead the person may report fatigue, difficulty sleeping, or seem grumpy and irritable (NIMH, 2017a, b). Depression can also be associated with loss. The older adult may experience multiple losses such as:

- deaths of friends and loved ones loss of physical capacities
- loss of social status and/or self-esteem.

Bereavement and depression

Bereavement is a natural response to a loved one's death and causes sorrow, anxiety, crying, agitation, insomnia, and appetite loss. Grieving and depression share common characteristics. The key difference is that a grieving person stays connected to others and can periodically experience pleasure and continue to function. With depression, the person is overwhelmed by emotions and finds it difficult to cope with everyday stressors.

Woeful widows

Grief and depression can co-exist in the same individual. In fact, bereavement is an important risk factor for depression. Untreated depression can lead to disability and health impairment (including altered endocrine and immune function).

If bereavement symptoms last 2 months or more, the older adult is at risk for developing an adjustment disorder or major depressive disorder. Even when it lasts less than 2 months, bereavement should receive clinical attention because it is a highly stressful condition that increases the likelihood of mental and somatic (physical) disorders.

Guiding patients through grief

The nurse must recognize the stages and the signs and symptoms of grief to provide the most effective help. Grief is a "normal" process of reacting to a loss. Acute grief typically lasts several months up to 2 years. Prolonged grieving may persist for up to 12 years.

Grieving stages

Successful adaptation requires progressing through stages of grief. Several different theorists have described stages through which individuals advance in their progression toward resolution. It is important to note that patients don't necessarily move through the stages in an orderly way. They may experience several stages at once or may even regress.

One example of stages of grief:
1. *Numbness or protest:* feelings of shock and disbelief; the reality of the loss is not acknowledged.
2. *Disequilibrium:* there is a preoccupation with the loss, intense weeping, and anger at self and others; may also include excessive guilt associated with the loss.
3. *Disorganization and despair:* ADLs become disorganized; behavior becomes restless and aimless; fear, helplessness, social isolation, and acute loneliness are experienced.
4. *Reorganization:* person accepts or become resigned to the loss; new goals are established; there is a reinvestment in new relationships; grief becomes valued remembrances.

Pathologic grief

About 10% to 12% of bereaved individuals experience a syndrome of grief that does not resolve naturally and persists for an indefinite period with varying degrees of incapacitation. This has been labeled *complicated or prolonged grief disorder* and can have adverse long-term health effects (Malgaroli et al., 2018).

Stay alert for warning signs such as:
• intense and persistent yearning for deceased
• preoccupation with the deceased

• feelings of acute loneliness
• urge to join the deceased in death
• feelings of disbelief, anger, and ruminations about the death
• physical symptoms similar to those that the deceased person experienced
• intense reactions or avoidance of reminders of the deceased
• significant distress with negative impact upon functioning
• development of depression or symptoms of another mental illness, psychosomatic symptoms, and substance misuse.

Coping with grief

To help the patient cope with grief in a healthy manner, the nurse should:
• establish rapport and build trust
• explain the normal stages of grieving, emphasizing that a wide range of feelings and behaviors may occur
• convey a caring attitude to encourage the patient to express feelings
• discuss the patient's loss and the concrete changes that have resulted
• encourage the patient to express sadness, guilt, or anger. If the person becomes angry with you, don't get defensive
• help the patient to determine what realistic changes may need to be made
• suggest the use of more adaptive ways of coping and making concrete plans for the future
• urge the patient to review and share both good and bad memories.

Preventing complications

With early recognition of problematic symptoms, such as depression, anxiety, and suicidal thinking and behavior, complications of grieving may be averted through grief counseling.

History lessons

Issues of stigma and other patient-specific barriers to treatment can be barriers to obtaining an accurate assessment of the older adult with mental illness and neurocognitive issues. Screening tools can help with this process. The Geriatric Depression Scale (GDS) is an evidence-based, self-reporting tool that is frequently used.

Obtaining an accurate and comprehensive psychosocial and medical patient history is crucial. If the patient's cognitive status is poor, you may need to gather history information from family members or caregivers.

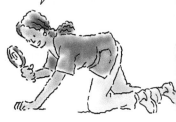

Shifting into detective mode can help you assess mental health needs for the older adult.

Treatment settings

Treatment can include medication, psychotherapy, support groups, and sociocultural supports. Ideally, a multidisciplinary team approach is used, with the patient and family helping to set goals and make decisions about treatment options.

Care settings can include acute hospitalization, partial hospitalization rehabilitation centers, long-term care facilities, and home care. Home care is one of the most common delivery settings for geropsychiatric nursing care. The nurse may also serve as the care coordinator if the patient is receiving simultaneous services from a community mental health clinic, case management agency, and community support program.

Inpatient geropsychiatric units

Acute inpatient geropsychiatric units are used to evaluate patients for suspected dementia and to stabilize aggressive or suicidal behaviors. Intervention focuses on rapid evaluation to rule out physical illness, stabilization of mood, and designing a treatment plan for the future. Inpatient stays on these units typically are brief.

Partial hospitalization

Psychiatric partial hospitalization provides intense, structured, multidisciplinary therapy for patients who have more acute needs that can be provided as an outpatient. Patients attend the program in the morning and return to the home later in the day.

Back to the real world

In a partial hospitalization program, nursing care focuses on:
* stabilizing lifestyle changes to help the patient stay well.
* preparing the patient and family to manage the patient's mental condition.
* providing the patient and family with tools for effective coping.
* The patient receives teaching about medication, stress management, and ADL management.

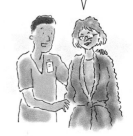

Teaching patients coping techniques is one of the things I love most about my job.

Adult day care

In some locations, adult day care centers are available for patients with chronic mental conditions. These programs provide structured activities, personal care, recreation, socialization, nutrition support, and health care. They may also include social services and caregiver support. There are specialized adult day care facilities that focus upon patients with NCDs like dementia.

Adult day care offers respite for family members and other caregivers. It may also help to postpone or avoid institutionalizing the older adult.

Community education programs

In many communities, senior centers, hospitals, and churches sponsor public education programs on mental conditions. Many institutions provide periotic-free screening for depression and anxiety.

Long-term care facilities

Older adults are at higher risk for admission to a long-term care facility because of the increase incidence of chronic conditions requiring additional care in this population. Nurses can facilitate adjustment to this new care setting by recognizing that this change in environment can be quite stressful for the older adult and by providing empathetic psychosocial support.

Obeying OBRA

Psychiatric services provided to older adults in long-term care facilities are regulated by the Omnibus Budget Reconciliation Act (OBRA) of 1987. This act and its subsequent updates mandate the

Providing acute care for hospitalized older adults

There are significant risks when older patients are admitted to the hospital.

- Delirium occurs in up to one-third of hospitalized patients over age 65.
- Bed rest increases risk for pressure injury.
- Multiple medical issues requiring multiple medical specialists makes coordination of care complicated.
- Introduction of new medications like anesthesia, pain meds, and sleep meds can lead to new-onset confusion.
- There is an increase in fall risks and other safety issues (environmental).
- Rapid deconditioning related to immobility.
- Increased potential for altered nutrition and elimination.
- Increased risk of hospital acquired infection.

- New-onset behavioral problems (like agitation) can emerge due to increase stress of hospitalization and development of delirium.

Prevention interventions:
- Avoid use of physical restraints; these are associated with increased complications.
- Provide close observation if confusion develops (use of a sitter).
- Look for beginning symptoms of more serious complications (mental status changes, vital sign changes).
- Support development of specialized geriatric hospital units with specially trained staff (Mattison, 2019).

monitoring of physical restraints and chemical restraints (psychotropic drugs) in skilled nursing facilities.

OBRA guidelines require that older nursing home residents are screened for mental health conditions. Residents with a primary mental illness are required to have access to mental health consultants to monitor patient behavior, work with the staff, and manage psychotropic medications. In 2016, there was an expansion of federal regulations. New regulations related to behavioral health include strategies to improve dementia-related care, including reduced use of psychotropic drugs, use of non-pharmacologic approaches, and person-centered dementia care practices. Increased awareness of and prevention of abuse, neglect, and exploitation of vulnerable or older adults was also added. The overall goal of these regulations was to allow the nursing home resident to maintain or attain their highest practicable physical, mental, and psychosocial well-being (Centers for Medicare and Medicaid Services [CMS], 2017).

Drug therapy

Polypharmacy, defined as the concurrent use of multiple medications, is associated with potential harm. This risk of harm may be particularly true for older adults, as age-related changes in pharmacokinetics and pharmacodynamics increase the risk of adverse drug events. Polypharmacy has been associated with decreased functional and cognitive health, and increased risk of falls, hospitalizations, and mortality. Risk of adverse drug outcomes increases with an increasing number of medications (Rieckert et al., 2018).

When considering psychotropic drugs, long-term use of antipsychotics can increase the risk of **tardive dyskinesia**, a motor disorder causing involuntary jerky movements of the face, tongue, jaws, trunk, and limbs. Taking more than one drug that depresses the central nervous system, like sedative-hypnotics, sleep medications, or pain medications, can have an additive effect increasing the risk of over-sedation, confusion, and falls in this population. Older adults are particularly vulnerable to *serotonin syndrome,* a toxic adverse drug reaction, because of the increased potential of taking two or more serotonergic drugs. Antidepressants and other psychoactive drugs have an FDA warning about an increase in suicidal thoughts.

Curbing prescriber chaos

To help ensure safe and effective drug administration, teach the patient and family to keep an up-to-date list of current medications and monitor for adverse effects and drug-drug interactions. Advise patients to inform all health care providers if taking nonprescription medications or nutritional or herbal supplements. St John's Wort is an example of an herbal supplement used for depression that interferes with the effectiveness of many medications and can cause a life-threatening reaction when used with antidepressants.

Preventing complications: Be proactive

Start low, titrate slow

Because of slower metabolism and excretion of drugs, dosages for older adults should start low and increase gradually based on the patient's tolerance and report of therapeutic benefit.

Adherence concerns

Adherence to drug treatment can present a challenge for older adults. This may be related to:

- Patients with poor vision may misread instructions or mistake one drug for another.
- Patients with cognitive impairment may not remember whether they have taken all of their doses.
- Inadequate patient teaching about the necessity or procedure for taking drugs.
- Confusion related to the need to take a large number of daily dosages, and multiple drugs taken at the same time.
- Cost of medication may prevent taking as prescribed.

Drug misuse?

Serum drug levels can be obtained to determine if the patient is taking a drug as prescribed and to identify or prevent potential toxicity. Drug misuse includes accidental or intentional taking of larger than prescribed amounts of a medication. It can also be helpful to determine if the patient is taking medication not prescribed by a health care provider or street drugs through serum drug levels. Finally, alcohol blood levels can be determined if there is suspicion of alcohol misuse. Concurrent use of alcohol and many medications increases the risk of adverse reactions.

Know your adverse effects

Many drugs taken for chronic medical conditions can cause psychiatric symptoms like anxiety and depression (NIMH, 2017a). Starting in 1991, Dr. Mark Beers and colleagues developed a list of drugs, called the "Beers List," that have a high potential to cause delirium and other harm in patients aged 65 or older. The current edition also provides a list of alternative drugs to use (American Geriatrics Society, 2015). Families and patients should be advised to use extra caution if the patient is taking one of the listed "risky" medications.

Neurocognitive disorders

A NCD can result from any condition that alters or destroys brain tissue and, in turn, impairs cerebral functioning and cognition.

According to the *Diagnostic and Statistical Manual of Mental Disorders*, 5th Edition (DSM-5) (American Psychiatric Association [APA], 2013), NCDs include delirium and major and mild NCDs. All NCDs involve potential problems in the following areas:

- Complex attention: ability to concentrate, take heed, and/or pay attention.
- Executive function: ability to plan, organize, and make decisions.
- Learning and memory: ability to remember or recall old and new things, ideas, etc. and to add to these memories (learning).
- Language: ability to name objects and to understand the meaning of a word.
- Perceptual-motor: ability to perform psychomotor tasks.
- Social cognition: perception of emotions in self and others, and reactions related to those emotions and thoughts.

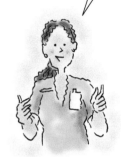

For many older patients, managing medications is a challenging juggling act.

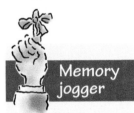

Memory jogger

To help remember the possible causes of NCDs, think of the three **Ds**:

Disease—primary brain disease

Disturbance—the brain's response to a systemic disturbance, such as a medical condition

Drugs—the brain's reaction to a toxic substance, as in substance misuse

Delirium

Delirium is one of the most commonly encountered medical conditions seen in medical practice, but is frequently overlooked. Delirium is a syndrome that is always *secondary to another condition*. Delirium is a significant risk for all hospitalized patients and nursing home residents. Older adults are at highest risk. Registered nurses (RNs) are in an ideal position to implement delirium prevention, early assessment, and treatment (American Nurses Association, 2016). Delirium is usually a transient disorder and can frequently be reversed with treatment of the underlying condition. Delirium is considered a medical emergency and requires prompt intervention to prevent irreversible damage (Halter, 2018).

Causes

Remember, delirium is always secondary to another condition. Medical conditions, substance use (intoxication and withdrawal), and medication or toxin exposure are possible causes of delirium.

Routine laboratory work such as general chemistry panel, toxicology screens, serum drug levels of known meds, and specialized radiologic tests can be used to help determine causes. Pulse oximetry, urinalysis, and electrocardiography (ECG) are other standard tests used to help determine causes.

Signs and symptoms

Delirium should be suspected when the patient presents with a sudden disturbance in consciousness (Halter, 2018). This may manifest as an inability to focus or as reduced awareness of the environment, the level of consciousness may also fluctuate. Signs and symptoms of delirium can be cognitive, behavioral, and physiologic.

Cognitive signs include:
disorientation, impairment of immediate and short-term memory, and spatial/visual ability, reduced level of consciousness, perseveration (repeating words or gestures).

Behavioral signs include:
sleep-wake cycle disturbance
hallucinations, delusion, and irritability

Physiologic signs include:
tremors, incontinence, elevated and rapidly changing vital signs (especially in alcohol withdrawal delirium).

It's an emergency!
Delirium is considered a medical emergency and requires prompt intervention to prevent long-term damage. Delirium is often undercognized! Remember, it is always due to an underlying cause (Halter, 2018).

Is it delirium?
Use the CAM
The Confusion Assessment Method (CAM) is a validated instrument for delirium detection that is designed to be used by nonpsychiatric clinicians to identify and recognize delirium quickly. Use of this tool is considered best practice in the care of older adults (Green et al., 2019).

Treatment

The first step is to determine and treat the underlying condition that precipitated the delirium. Patient safety must be maintained at all times.

Nursing interventions

There are a number of nursing interventions that can reduce some of the symptoms and complications associated with this disorder. These interventions include:

- Assess vital signs, elimination habits, and maintain food and fluid intake and pain management.
- Structure the environment to maintain stability and decrease confusion. For example, maintain lighting when appropriate so misperceptions are reduced. Turn the lights on during the day and off at night to facilitate a normal sleep/wake cycle. Reduce interruptions to sleep whenever possible and try to minimize stimulation.
- When possible assign the same nurses to minimize confusion and encourage family presence to assist with reorientation.
- Always provide orientation. Gently repeat your name and why you are present. Provide the date and time and make sure there is a clock and wall calendar in the patient's room. Patients with delirium are often very fearful and it is important to reassure the patient of their safety.
- Interventions to promote safety include frequent patient assessment to decrease the risk of falls and wandering into another patient room or away from the unit.

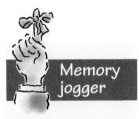

Memory jogger

Use the acronym **PILE** to help patients with cognitive impairment maintain their maximum level of functioning.

Promote "here and now" interactions.

Interact briefly but frequently.

Link conversations to meaningful topics.

Encourage self-expression.

Major and minor neurocognitive disorders

The diagnosis of major neurocognitive disorder was previously known as *dementia*. The primary feature of all NCDs is an acquired cognitive decline in one or more cognitive domains that can be observed by others and interferes significantly with ADLs. For those with *minor NCD*, there is a cognitive decline in one or more cognitive domains, but the deficits do not interfere with independence in everyday activity (APA, 2013).

Major (and minor) NCDs are further differentiated by the cause of the disorder. Major NCD due to Alzheimer disease (AD) is one example. Some other examples are NCD due to vascular disease and NCD due to Lewy body disease. There is significant cognitive decline and dementias associated with a number of other diseases such as end-stage Parkinson disease, HIV infection, Huntington disease, and substance/medication use. Each of these diseases can present as *specifiers* of minor or major NCDs (APA, 2013).

Major or mild neurocognitive disorder due to Alzheimer disease

AD is a NCDs (either major or minor, depending upon its severity) that has a subtle onset and is characterized by progressive, global impairment of cognitive functioning, memory, and personality.

There goes the memory

There is clear evidence of a decline in memory and learning plus a dysfunction of at least one other cognitive domain in AD. The course of this illness is a steady progressive, gradual decline in cognition without extended plateaus.

No safety in these numbers

In 2019, 5.8 million Americans are living with AD (Alzheimer Association [AA], 2019). Data indicate that of adults 65 years and older, 1 in 10 has AD (AA, 2019). AD affects more women than men and is the sixth leading cause of death in the United States and the leading cause of disability (AA, 2019; Gatchel et al., 2016).

Causes

No one knows exactly what causes AD. However, there are a number of known risk factors for AD. These risks include:

- Age: The number of people with AD doubles every 5 years beyond age 65. However, AD is *not* a part of normal aging. (See *Debunking dementia myths*, page 478.)
- Down syndrome: associated with early onset AD in midlife.
- Family history: having a first-degree relative with the disease increases a person's chance of developing the disease.
- Genetic factors: A specific genetic mutation causes a rare form of early onset disease.
  - apolipoprotein E (*apoE*) gene—this is a protein that helps carry cholesterol in the blood. There are three different types. One type seems to protect a person from getting the disease and another seems to increase risk (*ApoE4* gene). Research is ongoing and evolving in this area (AA, 2019).

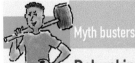

Debunking dementia myths

Misunderstandings about dementia can lead to unrealistic expectations.

Myth: Dementia is reversible if diagnosed early.
Reality: Dementia takes a progressive, deteriorating, irreversible course.
Myth: Vascular dementia isn't as serious a health problem as AD.
Reality: Vascular dementia, which is characterized by a marked disruption in cerebral blood flow with destruction of brain cells, reduces life expectancy to a greater degree than AD.

Myth: Dementia causes rapid loss of language skills.
Reality: Only the most severe forms of dementia result in aphasia and the inability to speak. Patients struggle to name objects and express themselves in middle stages of dementia and language skills continue to deteriorate as the disease progresses.

- Environmental factors: Researchers are considering infection, metals, and toxins that may trigger oxidation, inflammation, and other physiologic brain changes associated with AD (especially in people with genetic susceptibility).
- Other studies have explored such wide-ranging possibilities such as vitamin deficiencies, depression, educational level, and head injury as potential risk factors.

Biological factors in the brain

In patients with AD, brain-imaging techniques have found degenerative pathology of the brain. These include significant cortical shrinkage, hippocampus shrinkage, and enlargement of ventricles. All lobes of the brain are impacted as well as the amygdala. Impaired functioning in these brain regions leads to problems with memory, higher mental functioning, and other symptoms of this disorder, such as personality change. Neurotransmitter alterations have been noted. Abnormalities found on biopsy include neurofibrillary tangles (twisted nerve cell fibers) and a buildup of beta amyloid (a sticky protein) to form plaques (Lakhan, 2019).

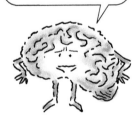

Tangles and sticky proteins—two more things that are dangerous to my brain health!

Signs and symptoms

AD can be classified into four stages including: preclinical, mild, moderate, and severe (Lakhan, 2019).

- **Preclinical AD** presents with some mild memory loss. At this stage, there are no alterations in judgment or ability to perform ADLs.

- **Mild AD** is a progression of memory loss. The person may respond to this loss of functioning with denial and depression. The following symptoms may also accompany this stage:
  - ○ Memory loss
  - ○ Confusion about the location of familiar places (getting lost begins to occur)
  - ○ Taking longer to accomplish normal daily tasks
  - ○ Trouble handling money and paying bills
  - ○ Compromised judgment often leading to bad decisions
  - ○ Loss of spontaneity and sense of initiative
  - ○ Mood and personality changes; increased anxiety.
- **Moderate AD** is a progression in memory loss where the world is quite confusing for the person. The person may respond to the confusion with anger, acting out, or inappropriate behavior. Others symptoms that can accompany this stage include:
  - ○ Increasing memory loss and confusion
  - ○ Shortened attention span
  - ○ Problems recognizing friends and family members
  - ○ Difficulty with language; problems with reading, writing, working with numbers
  - ○ Difficulty organizing thoughts and thinking logically
  - ○ Inability to learn new things or to cope with new or unexpected situations
  - ○ Restlessness, agitation, anxiety, tearfulness, wandering, especially in the late afternoon or at night (See *Is it sundowning?* page 480)
  - ○ Repetitive statements or movement; occasional muscle twitches
  - ○ Hallucinations, delusions, suspiciousness or paranoia, irritability
  - ○ Loss of impulse control (shown through behavior such as undressing at inappropriate times or places or vulgar language)
  - ○ Perceptual-motor problems (such as trouble getting out of a chair or setting the table).
- **Severe AD** is when patients lose the ability to recognize family, and sometimes themselves. Communication is grossly impaired. Death occurs from other illness (such as pneumonia) that **compounds** the advanced symptoms of AD. Other symptoms that can accompany this stage include:
  - ○ Weight loss
  - ○ Seizures, skin infections, difficulty swallowing
  - ○ Groaning, moaning, or grunting
  - ○ Increased sleeping
  - ○ Lack of bladder and bowel control
  - ○ Loss of reflexes

Is it sundowning?

Sundowning refers to a state of confusion occurring in the late afternoon and into the evening that can affect people with dementia. Symptoms of sundowning can also include anxiety, agitation, aggression, pacing, and wandering.

Tips to reduce

1. Adhere to the same schedule each day.
2. Increase daytime light.
3. Keep the patient awake and occupied during the day to facilitate sleep at night; fatigue makes sundowning worse.

4. Offer a light dinner and limit caffeine and alcohol at night.
5. Look for triggers to the behaviors.
6. Acute medical conditions such as a urinary tract infection can make sundowning worse.

Roth, E. (2016). *7 tips for reducing sundowning.* https://www.healthline.com/health/dementia-sundowning

As signs and symptoms of the disease become more obvious, the patient may look for ways to maintain self-esteem. These methods include denial, confabulation, perseveration, and avoiding questions (Halter, 2018). Confabulation is when the patient unconsciously creates stories to replace actual memories that have been lost. This is not the same as lying, which is a purposeful or conscious behavior. Perseveration occurs when the patient repeats certain phrases or behaviors. This may occur under stress and can occur in an attempt to avoid answering questions. This is an unconscious attempt at maintaining self-esteem (Halter, 2018).

Diagnosis

Numerous health concerns may be mistaken for AD. For example, depression, dementia, or NCDs and delirium can have overlapping symptoms. Up to 50% of those with AD have a concurrent depressive disorder. Delirium is a common acute co-occurring condition in hospitalized patients with dementia. Depression and dementia symptoms can look alike. All three disorders can also exist in one person at the same time, making an accurate diagnosis and effective differential treatment very challenging.

Is it depression or Alzheimer disease?

The term pseudodementia refers to the appearance of cognitive dysfunction (dementia-like) due to depression. Formal cognitive testing and screening tests and a comprehensive psychosocial assessment can help the health care provider to make a differential diagnosis. Those with depression or pseudodementia will not show evidence of significant cognitive dysfunction when tested. When depression is treated, cognitive symptoms tend to resolve.

What's the word?

Agnosia: loss of a sensory ability to recognize an object. For example, the patient does not recognize the sound of the doorbell (auditory agnosia) or recognize a glass (visual or tactile agnosia).

Aphasia: loss of language ability. This may begin as word finding difficulty. As the disease progresses vocabulary is reduced and may eventually result in babbling.

Apraxia: loss of purposeful movement. This occurs when the patient cannot perform basic tasks such as bathing or getting dressed.

Agraphia: loss of the ability to read and write.

Adapted from Halter, M. (2018). *Varcarolis' foundations of psychiatric mental health nursing* (8th ed.). Elsevier.

Is it delirium or is it Alzheimer disease?

There can be an overlapping of symptoms of delirium and AD. Differential characteristics include the following:

- Delirium has a sudden onset of symptoms; AD has a gradual onset and gradual deterioration of symptoms.
- Level of consciousness is usually altered with delirium; not dementia.
- Delirium is usually reversible; dementia shows progressive deterioration and is not reversible.

Because it is hard to obtain direct pathologic evidence of AD, diagnosis in a living patient is made by ruling out other possible causes of dementia and is based on the criteria set forth in the *DSM-5* (APA, 2013).

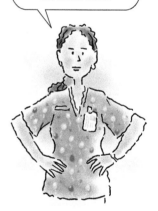

A patient can have **delirium, dementia** and **depression** all at the same time.

The full workup

Diagnostic tests that aid a health care provider in making a diagnosis include:

- Formal neuropsychological testing
- Specialized mental status exams, such as the mini-mental status examination (MMSE)
  - This exam tests cognitive skills such as attention span, problem-solving skills, counting skills, and short- and long-term memory and recall.
- Functional dementia scale, which indicates the degree of functional disability (such as ability to complete ADLs) in the person with dementia.

A comprehensive psychiatric assessment and a physical assessment including lab tests are needed to either further confirm a diagnosis of AD or exclude other possible causes for the cognitive impairment and may include:

- magnetic resonance imaging (MRI) and other brain-imaging techniques to show structural and neurologic changes common with this AD.

The clock-drawing test

The clock-drawing test is a simple and easy to use tool to screen for signs of *cognitive dysfunction* (executive functioning).

Directions:
Give the person a blank piece of paper and ask the person to draw a clock that shows the time of 10 minutes after 11.

Results:
If the person is unable to draw a clock properly, it strongly suggests cognitive impairment usually associated with dementia. Further evaluation is recommended.

Heerema, E. (2019). *How the clock-drawing test screens for dementia.* https://www.verywellhealth.com/the-clock-drawing-test-98619?print

- spinal fluid analysis, which may show increased beta-amyloid deposits.

There is promising research focusing on the development of a blood test for AD. It is believed one will be available in the next few years.

Treatment

Although no cure exists for AD, certain drugs may be prescribed in an attempt to stabilize the symptoms and slow the progression of the disease. Likewise, care strategies and activities may minimize or prevent behavioral problems. Researchers continue to look for new treatments to alter the course of the disease and improve quality of life.

Native habitat preferred

In most cases, institutional placement should be delayed until absolutely necessary. Changes in living environment can contribute to increased confusion.

Drug therapy

Drugs used to treat AD include:

- Anticholinesterase inhibitors, such as tacrine (Cognex), donepezil (Aricept), and rivastigmine (Exelon), temporarily delay the worsening of early/moderate stage symptoms. They can improve cognitive functioning slightly for some individuals by blocking the breakdown of acetylcholine in the brain.
- Memantine (Namenda) treats moderate to severe AD symptoms by blocking the action of glutamate in the brain. It may delay, but does not stop, progression of the disease.

- Namzaric is a drug that combines memantine and donepezil. Other drugs are prescribed to treat symptoms associated with AD.
- Antipsychotic agents, such as risperidone (Risperdal) and Aripiprazole (Abilify), are prescribed to calm agitated behavior and to lessen psychotic symptoms (hallucinations, delusions, paranoia). There is an FDA black box warning for use of these drugs in patients with dementia due to the higher risk of stroke and death.
- Benzodiazepines, such as alprazolam (Xanax), may be prescribed to ease anxiety. These should only be used for acute symptoms and for a short period of time. Overuse can lead to addiction and increased confusion.
- Antidepressants may be prescribed to treat depression and irritability.

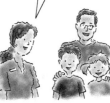

It's usually best for the patient to live at home as long as possible. However, safety concerns may necessitate a specialized long-term memory care environment.

Psychotherapy

- Supportive counseling and psychotherapy can help individuals make sense of their disease in the early stages.
- Validation therapy is a collection of nonpharmacologic techniques for those with dementia. Empathy and consideration of emotional states are emphasized in relating to patients. Although there is little evidence that helps with cognitive changes, there is some evidence of mood and behavioral improvement (Wegerer, 2019).

Preventive strategies

One comprehensive study identified a beneficial effect (as compared to controls) on cognitive performance in memory, executive functioning, and psychomotor speed from a program that included the following (Ngandu et al., 2015):

- Regular physical activity
- Healthy eating
- Cognitive training exercises
- Management of metabolic and vascular risk factors (diabetes, heart disease, hypertension, etc.).

Nursing interventions

The following nursing interventions can be useful for patients with any of the NCDs including AD.

Strive for safety

Several safety concerns exist for patients with AD and other major NCDs.

- There is a higher risk of falls.
- Patients may stop taking care of themselves.
- Patients may be resistant to care leading to unsafe conditions.

Taking steps to protect the patient from injury is imperative. Remove hazardous items or potential obstacles to help maintain a safe environment. Monitor the patient's food and fluid intake to decrease the risk for dehydration and poor nutrition. Monitor ADLs and provide assistance when needed. Facilitate sleep and rest periods. If the patient wanders, secure the environment to prevent escape. Consider use of electronic tracking devices.

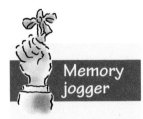

Memory jogger

How can you help keep a patient with AD safe? Just think of the word **SAFE**.

Secure the area if the patient wanders.

Arrange the room and furniture to accommodate the patient's needs.

Frequently orient the patient to time, place, and situation.

Easy access to self-care items is crucial.

Recommend routines

- Have the patient follow a regular routine, maintain normal social contacts with family and friends, and continue intellectual activities.
- Encourage the patient to see a health care provider regularly.

Soften your speech

- Speak to the patient calmly, using a soft, low-pitched voice.
- Use short, simple statements to describe what should be done.
- Minimize confusion by maintaining consistent, structured verbal, and nonverbal communication.

Affirm emotions

- If the patient discusses an event that isn't happening or people who are no longer alive, affirm the emotions without arguing or presenting reality. For example, if the person talks about a dead spouse coming to a birthday party, you might say, "Birthdays are fun" rather than presenting the information that the spouse is dead.
- If the person becomes upset, try distraction, or step away for a few minutes.

Orient often

- Add orienting material to every conversation. Frequently tell the patient your name and what you're going to do.
- Place a large clock and calendar in every room.
- Provide outdoor activities or a bed by the window.
- Redirect activities when behavior problems occur.
- Make sure patient has glasses, hearing aids, and other assistive devices as this can help with reorientation.

Stimulate to some extent

- Decrease environmental stimuli, such as noise, excessive artificial light, and television use.
- Provide frequent meaningful sensory input.
- Increase the patient's social interaction in reasonable amounts to encourage stimuli. Avoid placing the patient in large rooms with many people, such as dining rooms or group activity rooms.

Monitor medications

- Check the patient for adverse drug effects and drug interactions. Consider delirium if there is a sudden change in symptoms.
- Instruct the family to always check with the health care provider before the patient begins nonprescription agents or herbal supplements.

Offer information

- Educate the patient and family about community resources, support groups, and placement in a long-term care facility (if necessary). The Alzheimer Association is a valuable resource that provides information, care, and support for patients and families affected by Alzheimer and other dementias.
- Refer the patient to health care professionals skilled in caring for patients with AD.

Subdue stress

- Teach stress management techniques to the patient and caregivers.
- Music frequently has a calming effect.
- Provide support and education to home caregivers. Refer them to respite services as needed.
- Remind families not to take suspiciousness or angry outburst personally.
- If appropriate, refer to resources who specialize in helping the family with caregiver stress, financial pressures, and related issues.

Behavioral problems

There are several behavioral problems that commonly occur with major noncognitive disorders like AD. These can include aggression, anxiety, agitation, confusion, and depression.

To prevent some of these behaviors, it is helpful to try to determine possible causes of the behavior and then make necessary changes in the environment. Gently set limits for acting out or other inappropriate behaviors. Hallucinations, delusions, and paranoia can increase fears.

Neurocognitive disorder due to vascular dementia

In vascular dementia, blockage of blood vessels leads to brain damage and cognitive impairment.

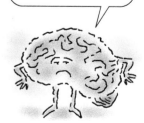

Major (and minor) NCD due to vascular dementia is the second most common type of dementia. It is caused by lack of blood flow to the brain. It can be related to atherosclerosis disease and/or stroke.

The onset of symptoms can be sudden (as with a stroke) or gradual. Stroke-related dementia often follows a "step-like" progression, rather than a gradual decline as seen with AD. There may be long periods when symptoms remain the same followed by short periods when they suddenly worsen. Early symptoms include confusion, trouble concentrating and planning, organizing and completing tasks, rather than the memory problems seen in the early stages of AD. Vision problems result and memory problems may or may not be evidenced in the mid stages of this disease. As the disease progresses, behavioral changes similar to AD are seen.

Diagnosis and treatment

Diagnostic tools used to identify AD are also useful for identifying NCD due to vascular disease.

Treatment for vascular dementia may include:

- treatment for an underlying condition (such as hypertension, high cholesterol, or diabetes), including dietary interventions, medications, and smoking cessation
- carotid endarterectomy to remove blockages in the carotid artery
- drug therapy—for example, aspirin to decrease platelet aggregation and prevent clots.

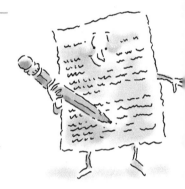

Nursing interventions

The nursing interventions for a patient with NCD due to AD apply to a patient with vascular dementia. The goal of nursing intervention is to keep the patient physically and psychologically safe.

Quick quiz

1. A 74-year-old patient admitted to the hospital with a urinary tract infection 4 days ago has developed a change in level of awareness, attempting to climb out of bed and "go home." What would the nurse suspect?

   A. Onset of delirium.
   B. Progression of Alzheimer dementia.
   C. Development of vascular dementia.
   D. Hallucinations due to hospitalization.

Answer: A. The nurse would suspect the onset of delirium associated with the underlying infection. Delirium is marked by an acute onset and begins with acute changes in behavior and level of awareness. Alzheimer dementia and vascular dementia occur gradually but with a continuous decline. Hallucinations can occur with delirium and are not a normal occurrence with hospitalization.

Assessing the patient's ability to count months backward can help to diagnose vascular dementia.

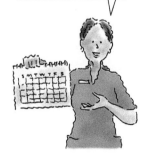

2.   A patient with AD is pointing to a clock and asks the nurse, "What is that?" How will the nurse document this behavior?
   A.   The patient is exhibiting confabulation.
   B.   The patient is experiencing agnosia.
   C.   The patient has developed aphasia.
   D.   The patient has perseveration.

Answer: B. Agnosia is an inability to recognize familiar items. The nurse would document that the patient is experiencing agnosia and then use direct statements to describe the patient interaction. The patient is not exhibiting confabulation (creation of stories in place of memories), aphasia (loss of language), or perseveration (repetition of phrases or behaviors).

3.   What does the nurse recognize as a normal response to aging?
   A.   A decrease in executive function after age 70
   B.   A decline in implicit memory after age 60
   C.   An inability to learn new things after age 65
   D.   A decreased ability to make new memories after age 70

Answer: A. *Executive functioning* is a set of processes that have to do with managing oneself and one's resources in order to achieve a goal. It includes *concept formation, abstraction, and mental flexibility. Executive functioning declines with age, especially after age 70. A decline in implicit memory, an inability to learn new things, and a decreased ability to make new memories are not normal responses to aging.*

4.   A patient has recently lost her husband aged 54 years. What nursing assessment data would indicate complicated grief or depression versus normal grieving?
   A.   The patient cries and talks about her husband.
   B.   The patient reports, "sometimes I think I hear him calling my name."
   C.   The patient states, "I just want to join him."
   D.   The patient is somewhat disorganized in daily life.

Answer: C. An urge to join the deceased in death is a warning sign of complicated grief or depression. Normal grieving involves crying and talking about the lost loved one. It is normal for the loved one to "hear" the loved one or "see" them in a crowd. A degree of disorganization in daily life is normal following the death of a loved one, as a new pattern or life rhythm has not yet been established.

5.   A patient with AD is talking about his deceased spouse as though she is alive. Which is the appropriate nursing response?
   A.   "You wife died 10 years ago."
   B.   "Tell me about your wife that died."
   C.   "Let's go to the common room and talk to our friends."
   D.   "I would like to talk with your wife too."

Answer: C. It is important to engage with the patient and work to re-direct versus presenting repeatedly that the spouse is dead. With AD, the patient will likely not remember that the spouse has died and tell the patient repeatedly can be traumatic and cause undue upset.

Scoring

☆☆☆ If you answered all five items correctly, marvy! Your mastery of older adults' mental health is magnificent!

☆☆ If you answered three or four items correctly, mazel tov! Your knowledge of mental disorders is maturing quite nicely.

☆ If you answered fewer than three items correctly, don't be melancholic! Just read the chapter again—your working memory is bound to improve.

Selected references

Alzheimer's Association. (2018) *Alzheimer's disease facts and figures. Alzheimer's dementia, 14*(3), 367–429. https://www.alz.org/facts/overview.asp

Alzheimer's Association. (2019). *Alzheimer's disease facts and figures. Alzheimer's dementia.* https://www.alz.org/media/documents/alzheimers-facts-and-figures-2019-r.pdf

American Geriatrics Society 2015 Beers Criteria Update Expert Panel. (2015). American Geriatrics Society 2015 updated Beers criteria for potentially inappropriate medication use in older adults. *Journal of the American Geriatrics Society, 63*(11), 2227–2246. https://doi.org/10.1111/jgs.13702

American Nurses Association. (2016). *Delirium: A nurse's primer.* https://www.nursingworld.org/~4afe6a/globalassets/practiceandpolicy/innovation—evidence/deliriumprimer20160517rev2.pdf

American Psychiatric Association. (2013). *Diagnostic and statistical manual of mental disorders* (5th ed.). Author.

Anderson, N. C., & Craik, F. I. M. (2017). 50 years of cognitive aging theory. *Journals of Gerontology: Series B, 72*(1), 1–6. https://doi.org/10.1093/geronb/gbw108

Barak, Y., & Gale, C. (2019). Suicide in long-term care facilities—The exception or the norm? *JAMA, 2*(6), e195634. https://doi.org/10.1001/jamanetworkopen.2019.5634

Centers for Disease Control and Prevention. (2017a). *Alzheimer's disease and healthy aging.* https://www.cdc.gov/aging/mentalhealth/depression.htm

Centers for Disease Control and Prevention. (2017b). *Elder abuse prevention, National Center for Prevention and Control.* https://www.cdc.gov/features/elderabuse/index.html

Centers for Medicare and Medicaid Services. (2017). *National partnership to improve dementia care in nursing homes & quality assurance and performance improvement (QAPI).* https://www.cms.gov/Outreach-and-Education/Outreach/NPC/Downloads/2017-06-15-Dementia-Care-Presentation.pdf

Conejero, I., Olié, E., Courtet, P., & Calati, R. (2018). Suicide in older adults: current perspectives. *Clinical Interventions in Aging, 13*, 691–699. https://doi.org/10.2147/CIA.S130670

Gatchel, J. R., Wright, C. I., Falk, W. E., & Trinh, N.-H. (2016). Dementia. In T. A. Stern, M. Fava, T. E. Wilens, & J. F. Rosenbaum (Eds.), *Massachusetts General Hospital comprehensive clinical psychiatry* (2nd ed., pp. 184–197). Elsevier.

Green, J. R., Smith, J., Teale, E., Collinson, M., Avidan, M. S., Schmitt, E. M., Inouye, S. K., & Young, J. (2019). Use of the confusion assessment method in multi-centre delirium trials: Training and standardization. *BMC Geriatrics, 19*, 107. https://doi.org/10.1186/s12877-019-1129-8

Halter, M. (2018). *Varcarolis' foundations of psychiatric mental health nursing* (8th ed.). Elsevier.

Heerema, E. (2019). *How the clock-drawing test screens for dementia.* https://www.verywellhealth.com/the-clock-drawing-test-98619?print

Lakhan, S. (2019). Alzheimer disease clinical presentation. *Medscape.* https://emedicine.medscape.com/article/1134817-clinical#b4

Malgaroli, M., Maccallum, F., & Bonanno, G. A. (2018). Symptoms of persistent complex bereavement disorder, depression, and PTSD in a conjugally bereaved sample: A network analysis. *Psychological Medicine, 48*(14), 2439–2448. https://doi.org/10.1017/S0033291718001769

Mattison, M. (2019). Hospital management of older adults. *UpToDate.* https://www.uptodate.com/contents/hospital-management-of-older-adults

Murman, D. L. (2015). The impact of age on cognition. *Seminars in Hearing, 36*(3), 111–121. https://doi.org/10.1055/s-0035-1555115

National Council for Behavioral Health. (2019). *New study reveals lack of access as root cause for mental health crisis in America.* https://www.thenationalcouncil.org/press-releases/new-study-reveals-lack-of-access-as-root-cause-for-mental-health-crisis-in-america/

National Institute of Mental Health. (2017a). *Depression and older adults.* https://www.nia.nih.gov/health/depression-and-older-adults

National Institute of Mental Health. (2017b). *How the aging brain affects thinking.* https://www.nia.nih.gov/health/how-aging-brain-affects-thinking

National Institute of Mental Health. (2019a). *Mental health information: Mental Illness.* https://www.nimh.nih.gov/health/statistics/mental-illness.shtml

National Institute of Mental Health. (2019b). *Suicide.* https://www.nimh.nih.gov/health/statistics/suicide.shtml

Ngandu, T., Lehtisalo, J., Solomon, A., Levälahti, E., Ahtiluoto, S., Antikainen, R., Bäckman, L., Hänninen, T., Jula, A., Laatikainen, T., Lindström, J., Mangialasche, F., Paajanen, T., Pajala, S., Peltonen, M., Rauramaa, R., Stigsdotter-Neely, A., Strandberg, T., Tuomilehto, J., … Kivipelto, M. (2015). A 2 year multidomain intervention of diet, exercise, cognitive training, and vascular risk monitoring versus control to prevent cognitive decline in at-risk elderly people (FINGER): A randomised controlled trial. *Lancet, 385*(9984), 2255–2263.

Nichols, H. (2017, August 19). What happens to the brain as we age? *Medical News Today.* https://www.medicalnewstoday.com/articles/319185.php#1

Rieckert, A., Trampisch, U. S., Klaaßen-Mielke, R., Drewelow, E., Esmail, A., Johansson, T., Keller, S., Kunnamo, I., Löffler, C., Mäkinen, J., Piccoliori, G., Vögele, A., & Sönnichsen, A. (2018). Polypharmacy in older patients with chronic diseases: a cross-sectional analysis of factors associated with excessive polypharmacy. *BMC Family Practice, 19*(1), 113. https://doi.org/10.1186/s12875-018-0795-5

Roth, E. (2016). *7 tips for reducing sundowning.* https://www.healthline.com/health/dementia-sundowning

Schimelpfening, N. (2018). *Grief vs. depression: Which is it?* https://www.verywellmind.com/grief-and-depression-1067237

U.S. Department of Health and Human Services. (2018). *2018 profile of older Americans.* Administration on Aging, Administration for Community Living, U.S. Department of Health and Human Services.

Wegerer, J. (2019). *Empathy for Alzheimer's: The validation method.* https://www.alzheimers.net/2013-11-07/validation-method-for-alzheimers/

World Health Organization. (2017). *Mental health of older adults.* https://www.who.int/news-room/fact-sheets/detail/mental-health-of-older-adults

Chapter 19

Personality disorders

Just the facts

In this chapter, you'll learn:

◆ major features of personality disorders

◆ proposed causes of personality disorders

◆ assessment findings and nursing interventions for patients with personality disorders

◆ recommended treatments for patients with personality disorders.

A look at personality disorders

Your personality defines who you are and how you relate to others. A personality disorder occurs when behavior patterns and relationship patterns become maladaptive. Personality disorders affect the way a person perceives the environment and impacts the person's cognition, behavior, and interactions with others. Many who have a personality disorder have inadequate coping mechanisms and may have trouble dealing with everyday stresses. "By definition, a personality disorder is an enduring pattern of thinking, feeling, and behaving" that is not consistent with the cultural norms (American Psychiatric Association [APA], 2013, p. 647). These patterns are generally inflexible and create some degree of impairment in every area of life.

Currently, the APA (2013) recognizes 10 different personality disorders. These disorders are then clustered into three groups based on similarities. In this chapter, an overview of personality disorders will be discussed as well as specifics related to each cluster of disorders.

Cluster A

Behavior is odd or eccentric (paranoid, schizoid, schizotypal personality disorders).

Cluster B

Behavior is emotional and dramatic (antisocial, borderline, histrionic, narcissistic personality disorders).

Cluster C

Behavior is fearful or anxious (avoidant, dependent, obsessive-compulsive personality disorders).

Stress, symptoms, and sequelae

Personality disorders are often overlapping with other psychiatric disorders. In addition, it is common for individuals to experience a co-occurring personality disorder from another cluster.

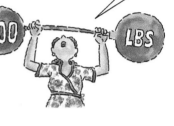

Severe personality disorders impose a hefty financial and emotional burden.

Mild symptoms of personality disorder may have little effect on a person's social, family, or work life. However, when symptoms get worse—as they commonly do during times of increased stress—the disorder can seriously interfere with emotional, psychological, social, and occupational functioning. Severe symptoms may result in hospitalization, poor work performance, and lost productivity. Their emotional toll—unhappiness, domestic violence, child abuse, imprisonment, and even suicide—is equally staggering.

Relationship woes

People with personality disorders have trouble in their relationships with others. The expectation is that people will adjust to the person with personality disorder. When others don't or can't adjust, the person with the disorder may become angry, frustrated, depressed, or withdrawn. This sets up a vicious cycle of interaction in which the person with the disorder persists with their maladaptive behavior until their needs are met, which can further anger those around them. (See *Can a personality be changed?*)

Common features

To one degree or another, most people with personality disorders share the following features:

* disturbances in self-image

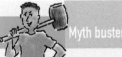

Myth busters

Can a personality be changed?

Relationship problems may arise if the patient's family and friends don't understand the nature of personality disorders.

Myth: If someone with a personality disorder seems normal, that means he or she is capable of changing behavior.

Reality: With a personality disorder, personality traits are fixed and not conducive to change. Yet with a mild personality disorder, the patient's behavior seems normal, so friends and family may assume he or she can easily change behavior. When the patient doesn't change, they may think that he or she is not willing to—when the problem is that he or she *can't.*

Culture and personality disorders

Before concluding that a patient has a personality disorder, always consider his or her cultural, ethnic, and religious background. According to the *Diagnostic and Statistical Manual of Mental Disorders*, 5th Edition (*DSM-5*), the patient's signs and symptoms must deviate markedly from the expectations of his or her culture to qualify for the diagnosis of a personality disorder (APA, 2013).

Skirting the stereotypes
Avoid stereotyping patients. Individuals within a culture—or even within a particular family—may vary widely in personality traits and emotional expression.

- inappropriate range of emotions
- poor impulse control
- maladaptive ways of perceiving themselves, others, and the world
- long-standing problems in personal relationships, ranging from dependency to withdrawal
- reduced occupational functioning, ranging from compulsive perfectionism to intentional self-sabotage.

All in the mix

These common features mix together to create pervasive patterns of behavior that differ markedly from the norms of the patient's cultural or ethnic background. (See *Culture and personality disorders*.)

Demographic dynamics

Personality disorders are relatively common, affecting an estimated 12% of the U.S. population (Volkert et al., 2018). Gender plays a role in their prevalence. For example, antisocial and obsessive-compulsive personality disorders are more common in men, whereas borderline, dependent, and histrionic personality disorders are more prevalent in women.

Age and intensity

Personality disorders are lifelong conditions with an onset in adolescence or early adulthood. Some personality disorders, such as antisocial and borderline, tend to grow less intense in middle age and late life, whereas other disorders (most notably obsessive-compulsive and schizotypal) tend to become exaggerated.

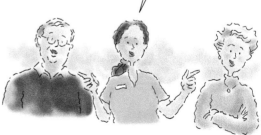

More women have borderline and dependent personality disorders, whereas more men have antisocial personality disorder.

Causes

No one knows the exact cause of personality disorders. Most likely, they represent a combination of genetic, biological, social, psychological, developmental, and environmental factors.

Chain of influence

Genetic factors influence the biological basis of brain function as well as basic personality structure. In turn, personality structure affects how a person responds to and interacts with life experiences and the social environment. Over time, each person develops distinctive ways of perceiving the world and of feeling, thinking, and behaving.

Out-of-control emotions

Some researchers suspect that poor regulation of the brain circuits that control emotion increases the risk for a personality disorder—when combined with such factors as abuse, neglect, or separation.

For a biologically predisposed person, the major developmental challenges of adolescence and early adulthood (such as separation from the parents, identity, and independence) may trigger a personality disorder. Perhaps this explains why personality disorders usually emerge during those years.

Psychodynamic theories

Psychodynamic theories propose that personality disorders stem from deficiencies in ego and superego development. These deficiencies may relate to mother-child relationships highlighted by unresponsiveness, overprotectiveness, or early separation.

Social theories

According to social theories, personality disorders reflect the responses that a person learns through the processes of reinforcement, modeling, and aversive stimuli. When even low levels of stress occur, chronic trauma or long-term stressors may create new neurochemical pathways. As a result, the person "acts out" old patterns of behaviors.

Evaluation

A patient with a suspected personality disorder should undergo a physical examination to rule out an underlying physical or organic cause for the symptoms. (See *Personality changes and physical illness*.)

Personality changes and physical illness

Be aware that a personality change may be the first sign of a serious neurologic, endocrine, or medical illness—which may be reversible if detected early.

For example, a patient with a frontal lobe tumor may show changes in personality and motivation, even though the results of a neurologic assessment are otherwise negative. Such problems should be ruled out before the patient is diagnosed with a personality disorder. The *DSM-5* includes an additional personality disorder: personality change because of another medical condition, which is a personality disorder that is directly caused by a medical condition and has physiologic effects, for example, frontal lobe injury (APA, 2013).

A psychological evaluation can exclude other psychiatric disorders—or it may suggest additional ones. Psychological tests, such as the Minnesota Multiphasic Personality Inventory-2 (MMPI-2) and the Millon Clinical Multiaxial Inventory-III (MCMI-III), may support or guide the diagnosis. In addition, toxicology screening may be warranted because intoxication with certain substances can mimic the features of a personality disorder.

Diagnosis

The diagnostic process is virtually the same for all personality disorders. Each disorder has specific criteria determined by the APA that the patient must meet in order to be diagnosed (APA, 2013). The key to diagnosis is enduring patterns of behavior. In other words, a personality disorder doesn't develop overnight and it isn't diagnosed overnight. Providers are looking for patterns of behavior. Some patients meet the criteria for multiple personality disorders, making diagnosis a particular challenge. As nurses, we frequently see these patients for other health problems. However, the nursing diagnosis will often focus on the underlying behaviors.

Approach to treatment

Personality disorders are among the most challenging psychiatric disorders to treat—partly because, by definition, a personality is an integral part of what defines the individual and his or her self-perceptions. "No sharp division exists between normal and abnormal personality functioning. Instead, personalities are viewed on a continuum from normal at one end to abnormal at the other. Many of the same processes involved in the development of a 'normal' personality are responsible for the development of a personality disorder" (Boyd, 2018, p. 487). Rather than aiming for a cure, treatment

Diagnostic criteria: General personality disorder

These general criteria from the *DSM-5* apply to all patients with personality disorders. However, each particular disorder has additional criteria that further define and distinguish the disorder.

Criteria

A. An enduring pattern of inner experience and behavior that deviates markedly from the expectations of the individual's culture. This pattern is manifested in two (or more) of the following areas:
1. Cognition (i.e., way of perceiving and interpreting self, other people, and events)
2. Affectivity (i.e., the range, intensity, lability, and appropriateness of emotional response)
3. Interpersonal functioning
4. Impulse control

B. The enduring pattern is inflexible and pervasive across a broad range of personal and social situations.

C. The enduring pattern leads to clinically significant distress or impairment in social, occupational, or other important areas of functioning.

D. The pattern is stable and of long duration, and its onset can be traced back at least to adolescent or early adulthood.

E. The enduring pattern is not better explained as a manifestation or consequence of another mental disorder.

F. The enduring pattern is not attributable to the physiologic effects of a substance (e.g., a drug of abuse, a medication) or another medical condition (e.g., head trauma).

typically focuses on enhancing the patient's coping skills, solving short-term problems, and building relationship skills through psychotherapy and education.

The road to rapport

Traditionally, long-term psychotherapy has been the treatment of choice. Effective psychotherapy always requires a trusting relationship with the therapist. Each disorder presents unique challenges in developing a lasting relationship between a patient and a provider.

Adjunctive medication

Today, many patients also receive drugs to relieve associated symptoms, such as acute anxiety or depression. However, drugs should be used only as an adjunct to psychotherapy—not as a cure for the personality disorder.

Cluster A personality disorders

Behavior is characterized as odd or eccentric and includes: paranoid, schizoid, and schizotypal personality disorders.

Paranoid personality disorder

Paranoid personality disorder is marked by a distrust of other people and a constant, unwarranted suspicion that others have sinister motives. Patients with this disorder place excessive trust in their own knowledge and abilities. They search for hidden meanings and hostile intentions in everything that others say and do.

Conspiracy theorists

The paranoid personality is quick to challenge the loyalties of friends and loved ones. Many patients with this disorder seem cold and distant. They shift blame to others and carry long grudges. Because they tend to drive people away, they have few friends—which only bolsters their suspicions of a conspiracy against them.

Prevalence

The prevalence of paranoid personality disorder is estimated at 2.3% to 4.4% of the general population. In clinical samples (and possibly in the general population as well), the disorder is more common in males (APA, 2013).

Causes

The specific cause of paranoid personality disorder is unknown. Its higher incidence in families with a schizophrenic member suggests a possible genetic influence. As children, these individuals are prone to temper outburst and can be difficult to manage. They are often perceived as odd by other children and may be teased as a result (APA, 2013; Boyd, 2018). The person with paranoid personality may lack friends and develop social anxiety (Halter, 2018).

Signs and symptoms

The hallmarks of paranoid personality disorder are suspicion and distrust of others' motives. Other signs and symptoms include:
- refusal to confide in others
- inability to collaborate with others
- hypersensitivity
- inability to relax (hypervigilance)
- need to be in control
- self-righteousness
- detachment and social isolation
- poor self-image

- sullenness, hostility, coldness, and detachment
- humorlessness
- anger, jealousy, and envy
- bad temper, hyperactivity, and irritability
- lack of social support systems.

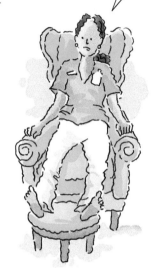

Keep calm and relax.... Someone with paranoid personality disorder may be unable to relax.

Treatment

Few patients with paranoid personality disorder seek treatment on their own. When they do, health care providers may have difficulty establishing a rapport because of these patients' suspicious, distrustful nature. The challenge is to engage the patient in a collaborative working relationship based on trust.

Psychotherapy

Individual psychotherapy is preferred over group therapy because of the patient's suspicious nature. The most effective psychotherapy for a paranoid patient takes a simple, honest, businesslike approach rather than an insight-oriented approach. It focuses on the current problem that brought the patient to therapy. As therapy progresses, the patient may begin to trust the therapist more and, eventually, start to disclose some of the paranoid ideations.

Pharmacologic therapy

Some health care providers recommend medication for patients with paranoid personality disorder. There is not one drug used to treat paranoid personality disorder. It is important to note that these medications are for symptom control.

- antipsychotic drugs such as olanzapine (Zyprexa) or risperidone (Risperdal) to treat severe agitation or delusional thinking
- antidepressants such as selective serotonin reuptake inhibitors (SSRIs; e.g., fluoxetine [Prozac]) to treat irritability, anger, and obsessional thinking.

Doubts about medications

A patient with paranoid personality disorder may distrust medications and, in particular, may resent the suggestion that he or she needs an antipsychotic agent. For this reason, some health care providers delay considering medication until the patient asks about it or until the symptoms warrant the risk of use. Drug therapy should be limited to the briefest course possible. The patient should receive thorough teaching about possible adverse effects so he or she does not get more suspicious if these occur.

Nursing interventions

These nursing interventions may be appropriate for a patient with paranoid personality disorder:

- Use a straightforward, honest, professional approach rather than a casual or friendly approach.
- Offer persistent, consistent, and flexible care.
- Provide a supportive, nonjudgmental environment in which the patient can safely explore their feelings.
- Establish a therapeutic relationship by actively listening and responding.

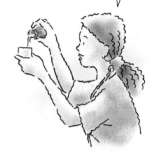

The paranoid patient may distrust medications—especially if they cause adverse effects.

Don't get too personal

- Avoid inquiring too deeply into their life or history unless it's relevant to clinical treatment.
- Don't challenge the patient's paranoid beliefs. Such beliefs are delusional and aren't reality based, so it's useless to argue with them from a rational point of view.
- Avoid situations that may threaten the patient's autonomy.
- Be aware that the patient may not respond well to interviewing. (See *Guidelines for an effective interview,* page 500.)

You call that funny?

- Use humor and sarcasm cautiously. A paranoid patient may misinterpret a remark that was meant to be humorous.
- Encourage the patient to take part in social interactions. This provides exposure to others' perceptions and realities and helps to promote social skill development.
- Help the patient identify negative behaviors that interfere with relationships so they can see how their behavior affects others.
- Encourage the expression of feelings, self-analysis of behavior, and accountability for actions.

Distance yourself

- Recognize the patient's need to be physically and emotionally distant.
- Avoid a defensive attitude and arguments with paranoid patients.
- Assess the patient's coping skills. Teach effective strategies to alleviate stress and reduce anxiety.
- Teach patients about prescribed medications.
- Encourage the patients to continue therapy for optimal therapeutic results.

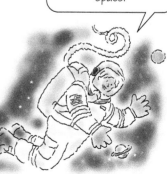

Give the patient adequate personal space.

Guidelines for an effective interview

You may have difficulty establishing a rapport with a patient with a personality disorder. These guidelines may be helpful:

- Start the interview with a broad, empathetic statement: "You look upset; what seems to be bothering you today?"
- Explore normal behaviors before discussing abnormal ones: "What do you think helps you to cope with the pressures of your job?"
- Phrase questions sensitively to ease the patient's anxiety: "Things were going well at home and then you became depressed. Tell me about that."
- Ask the patient to clarify vague statements: "Explain to me what you mean when you say, 'They're all after me.'"

- If the patient rambles, help him or her focus on the most pressing problem: "You've talked about several problems. Which one bothers you the most?"
- Interrupt a nonstop talker as tactfully as possible: "I appreciate the information you're giving me. Can I ask...?"
- Express empathy toward a tearful, silent, or confused patient who has trouble describing a problem: "I realize it's difficult for you to talk about this."

Schizoid personality disorder

The hallmarks of schizoid personality disorder are detachment, social withdrawal, indifference to others' feelings, and a restricted emotional range in interpersonal settings. People with this disorder are commonly described as loners, with solitary interests and occupations and no close friends. Typically, they maintain a social distance even from family members and seem unconcerned about others' praise or criticism.

They want to be left alone

Most people with this disorder function adequately in everyday life but don't develop many meaningful relationships. Although they fare poorly in groups, they may excel in positions where they have minimal contact with others. (See *What's in a name?*)

Prevalence

Schizoid personality disorder affects 3.1% to 4.9% of the general population. More males are affected than females and they also experience higher impairments associated with the disorder (APA, 2013). Some people with schizoid personality disorder also have additional personality disorders, most commonly schizotypal, paranoid, or avoidant personality disorder.

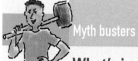

What's in a name?

Psychiatric disorders with similar names such as schizophrenia and/or schizotypal don't necessarily share common traits.

Myth: Schizoid personality disorder is similar to schizophrenia.
Reality: People with schizoid personality disorder don't have schizophrenia. (*Schizotypal* personality disorder, on the other hand, does share certain features with schizophrenia.) Unfortunately, because the names sound alike, people with schizoid personality may be misunderstood.

Causes

As with the other personality disorders, the exact cause of schizoid personality disorder is not known. Some researchers think it may be inherited. Other possible causes may include:
- a sustained history of isolation during infancy and childhood
- cold or grossly deficient early parenting.

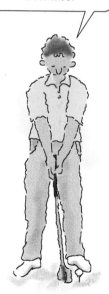

Some people might call me lonely, but I truly prefer solitary activities.

Signs and symptoms

Assessment of a patient with schizoid personality disorder may reveal:
- emotional detachment
- inability to experience pleasure
- lack of strong emotions and little observable change in mood
- indifference to others' feelings, praise, or criticism
- avoidance of activities that involve significant interpersonal contact
- little desire for or enjoyment of close relationships
- no desire to be part of a family
- strong preference for solitary activities
- little or no interest in sexual experiences with another person
- lack of close friends or confidants other than immediate family members
- shyness, distrust, and discomfort with intimacy
- loneliness
- feelings of utter unworthiness coexisting with feelings of superiority
- self-consciousness and feeling ill at ease with people.

Treatment

For general diagnosis of personality disorders, see page 496. Someone with schizoid personality disorder isn't likely to seek treatment unless he or she is under great stress. Additionally, treatment poses a challenge because of the patient's initial inability or lack of desire to form a relationship with a therapist or other health care professional.

In search of a solitary niche

Treatment goals include:

- helping the patients find the most comfortable solitary niche and cultivate satisfying hobbies that allow them to be on their own
- decreasing their resistance to change
- reducing patients' social isolation and improving their social interaction
- enhancing patients' self-esteem.

Individual psychotherapy

Individual psychotherapy should be short term, focusing on solving the patient's immediate concerns or problems. Generally, long-term psychotherapy for the schizoid patient has a poor outcome and isn't recommended.

Developing a rapport and trusting therapeutic relationship with this patient is usually a slow, gradual process. To avoid confrontations, the therapist should make every effort to help the patient feel secure and acknowledge the patient's boundaries.

Fears and fantasies

When the patient opens up, he or she may reveal fantasies, imaginary friends, and fears of unbearable dependency. The patient may also fear growing dependent on the therapist and prefer to remain in fantasy and withdrawal. The therapist should bring such feelings into proper focus.

Support, not smothering

Stability and support for the patient are essential—but the therapist must take care not to smother and should expect and tolerate some acting-out behaviors.

Cognitive therapy

Cognitive restructuring may be useful in dealing with illogical thoughts that impede the patient's coping ability and functioning. In this technique, the patient learns to identify his or her own patterns of thought, emotion, and behavior and then works to change thinking patterns to benefit overall mental health.

Group therapy

Initially, group therapy isn't a good treatment choice because most schizoid patients can't tolerate being in a social group. However, a patient who's graduating from individual therapy with adequate social skills may be able to tolerate group therapy. Supportive group members can help the patient overcome fears of closeness and feelings of isolation.

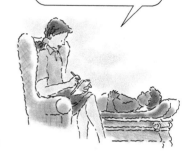

The therapist should expect some acting-out behaviors in a schizoid patient.

People who don't need people

In a group therapy session, patients with schizoid personality disorder are usually quiet, seeing little or no reason for social interaction. The group leader should expect this behavior and not pressure them into participating more fully until they are ready. Also, the leader should protect them from criticism by other group members. Eventually, if the group can tolerate their silence, these patients may participate more.

Self-help support groups

Self-help support groups can play an important role in promoting healthier social relationships, enhanced functioning, greater ability to cope with unexpected stressors, and reducing fears of closeness and feelings of isolation. Within the group, the patients can try out new coping skills and learn that social attachments don't have to happen with rejection or fear.

Pharmacologic therapy

Drug therapy isn't warranted if patients are comfortable with their symptoms. However, medications may be prescribed if these patients have an overlapping psychiatric disorder such as major depressive disorder or need relief from other acute symptoms. Patients with psychotic ideations may benefit from low-dose treatment with an antipsychotic, such as olanzapine (Zyprexa) or risperidone (Risperdal). Generally, long-term drug treatment is avoided.

Nursing interventions

The following nursing interventions may be appropriate for patients with schizoid personality disorder:

- Respect the patients' need for privacy and slowly build a trusting therapeutic relationship so that they find more confidence than fear in relating to you.
- Offer persistent, consistent, and flexible care. Take a direct, involved approach to gain the patients' trust.

No crowding allowed
- Recognize the patient's need for adequate personal space.
- Remember that they need close human contact but can become overwhelmed by too much contact.

Time, space, and social skills
- Give the patients plenty of time to express their feelings. Keep in mind that pushing these patients to talk before they are ready may cause them to withdraw.
- Teach the patients social skills and reinforce appropriate behavior.
- Encourage patients to express their feelings, analyze their own behaviors, and take accountability for their actions.
- Avoid defensive behavior and arguments with schizoid patients.

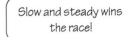

Slow and steady wins the race!

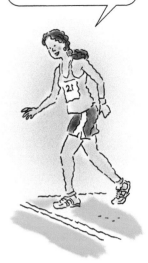

Schizotypal personality disorder

Schizotypal personality disorder is marked by a pervasive pattern of social and interpersonal deficits, along with acute discomfort with others. People with this disorder have odd thought and behavioral patterns. This disorder is a more advanced form of the schizoid disorder but not as advanced as the diagnosis of schizophrenia (Boyd, 2018).

During times of extreme stress, some patients also have cognitive or perceptual disturbances—although these psychotic symptoms aren't as fully developed as in schizophrenia. Any psychotic episode is short-lived, resolving with the use of an appropriate antipsychotic drug.

Figures of speech
Patients with schizotypal personality disorder commonly exhibit eccentric behaviors and have trouble concentrating for long periods. Their mannerisms and dress may be peculiar and their speech may be unusual—overly elaborate, vague, metaphorical, and hard to follow.

Is there a schizophrenic link?
In the *DSM-5*, "schizotypal disorder is identified as both a personality disorder and the first of the schizophrenia spectrum disorders, which are, in general, listed from least to most severe" (Halter, 2018, p. 455). The patients may have magical thinking, strange fantasies, odd beliefs (such as thinking they have extrasensory abilities), unusual perceptions and bodily illusions, social isolation, and paranoid ideas. However, unlike patients with schizophrenia, people with schizotypal personality disorder are not psychotic. "A major difference between this disorder and schizophrenia is that people with schizotypal personality disorder can be made aware of their

misinterpretations of reality. Schizophrenia results in a far stronger grip on delusions" (Halter, 2018, p. 455).

Party of one

Typically, these patients have severe social anxiety—usually because they are paranoid about others' motivations. They may relate to others in a stiff or inappropriate way or fail to respond to normal interpersonal cues. Although some people with this disorder marry, most have no more than one person they relate to closely.

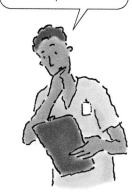

Schizotypal personality disorder is similar to schizophrenia but without the psychotic component.

Prevalence

Schizotypal personality disorder is found in about 3.9% of the general population and is slightly more common in men than in women (APA, 2013). "This disorder has a relatively stable course, with only a small proportion of individuals going on to develop schizophrenia or another psychotic disorder" (APA, 2013, p. 657). About 30% to 50% of patients with schizotypal personality disorder also have major depression. A large number have an additional personality disorder, especially paranoid, borderline, or avoidant personality disorder.

Causes

Schizotypal personality disorder as part of the schizophrenia spectrum does have a genetic link, as there is a higher incidence of the disorder among first-degree relatives with schizophrenia (APA, 2013; Halter, 2018). Environmental factors (such as severe stress) may determine whether schizotypal personality disorder or schizophrenia manifests. Abnormalities in brain structure, function, chemistry, and physiology similar to schizophrenia have been found in individuals with schizotypal disorder, such as reduced cortical volume (Halter, 2018).

Psychological and cognitive theories

Psychological and cognitive explanations for schizotypal personality disorder focus on deficits in attention and information processing. These patients perform poorly on tests that assess continuous performance tasks, which require the ability to maintain attention on one object and to look at new stimuli selectively.

Signs and symptoms

Assessment findings in patients with schizotypal personality disorder may include:
- odd or eccentric behavior or appearance
- belief that others are out to get them

- odd beliefs or magical thinking
- unusual perceptual experiences, including bodily illusions
- vague, circumstantial, metaphorical, overly elaborate, or stereotypical speech or thinking
- unfounded suspicion of being followed, talked about, persecuted, or under surveillance
- inappropriate or apathetic affect
- lack of close relationships other than with immediate family members
- social isolation
- excessive social anxiety that doesn't go away
- a sense of feeling different and the inability to easily fit in with others.

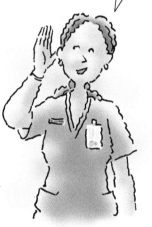

The schizotypal patient may speak in a vague, metaphorical, or elaborate way.

Diagnosis and treatment

General diagnostic parameters for all personality disorders are discussed in page 498. Treatment options for patients with schizotypal personality disorder include individual psychotherapy, family therapy, group therapy, cognitive-behavioral therapy, self-help measures, and medications. The patients may also benefit from social skills training and other behavioral approaches that emphasize the basics of social interactions.

Psychoanalytic intervention focuses on defining ego boundaries. Cognitive-behavioral therapy attempts to help the patients interpret their odd beliefs and teach them valuable coping and interpersonal skills.

Avoid challenges

Initially, individual therapy is usually preferred. A warm, supportive, patient-centered approach helps establish rapport. The therapist should avoid directly challenging the patient's delusional or inappropriate thoughts.

Group suspicion

Group therapy may be considered when these patients make progress in individual therapy. However, patients with this disorder may have trouble tolerating a group because they are mistrustful and suspicious.

Pharmacologic therapy

Antipsychotic agents, such as risperidone (Risperdal), may be used to treat psychotic symptoms; they're usually given in low doses. SSRIs have also been effective in some cases.

Nursing interventions

These nursing interventions may be appropriate for patients with schizotypal personality disorder:

- Offer the patients persistent, consistent, and flexible care. Take a direct, involved approach to promote the patients' trust.
- Know that these patients are easily overwhelmed by stress. Give them plenty of time to make difficult decisions.
  - ○ Give the patient space and respect their need for social isolation.
  - ○ Provide careful assessment so as not to overlook other psychological or medical issues.

The patient likes me, can't stand you

- Be aware that these patients may relate unusually well to certain staff members but not at all to others.
- Recognize the patient's need for physical and emotional distance.

Social skills and self-analysis

- Teach the schizotypal patients social skills and reinforce appropriate behaviors.
- Encourage the patient's expression of feelings, self-analysis of behaviors, and accountability for actions.
- Avoid defensive behavior and arguments with schizotypal patients.

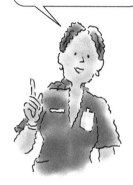

The schizotypal patient may relate well to you but not your colleagues—or vice versa.

Cluster B personality disorders

Behavior is characterized as emotional and dramatic and includes: antisocial, borderline, histrionic, and narcissistic personality disorders.

Antisocial personality disorder

The highlight of antisocial personality disorder is chronic antisocial behavior that violates others' rights or generally accepted social norms. This disorder predisposes a person toward criminal behavior. This pattern of behavior has been referred to as *psychopathy* or *sociopathy* (APA, 2013).

Other features of this disorder include impulsivity, egocentricity, disregard for the truth, and aggression. The antisocial person can't tolerate boredom and frustration. They are reckless, irritable, and unable to maintain consistent, responsible functioning at work, at school, or as a parent. They lack remorse and exhibit few, if any, feelings. (See *Insight into antisocial personality disorder*, page 508.)

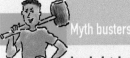

Insight into antisocial personality disorder

Do you think you understand the antisocial personality? Think again.

Myth: Most people with antisocial personality disorder are powerful and are always "out for number 1."

Reality: Patients with antisocial personality disorder see themselves as victims. They seek revenge and don't accept responsibility for their actions.

Crime and politics

Although individuals with antisocial personality disorder are the most common among people who get into trouble with the law, antisocial personality disorder also occurs in milder forms. Examples include the spouse who continually cheats and the con artist who scams others out of their money.

Prevalence

In the general population, the prevalence of antisocial personality disorder is about 0.2% to 3.3%. In prison populations, it may be higher than 70% (APA, 2013). Many of the people with this disorder have a history of arrest and issues with the law.

Antisocial personality disorder affects more males than females. However, there has been some concern that this disorder is underdiagnosed in women because of the "emphasis on aggressive items" in the diagnostic criteria (APA, 2013, p. 662). This diagnosis is not used for children. A conduct disorder in a teenager may lead to an antisocial personality diagnosis after the patient is 18 years old.

Causes

Genetic and biological factors may influence the development of antisocial personality disorder. Biological factors include:

1. Low levels of serotonin and dopamine hyperfunction have been implicated in antisocial personality disorder and may contribute to disinhibition, poor impulse control, aggressive behavior, and substance abuse (Halter, 2018).
2. Genetic factors may be involved. Twin studies point to a predisposition to Antisocial Personality Disorder (APD). The traits of aggressive-disregard, or violent tendencies with lack of regard to others, and disinhibition, or a lack of concern for consequences, are two dimensions of genetic risk.

> Poor serotonin regulation in certain brain regions may factor into antisocial personality disorder.

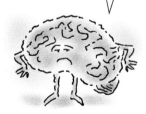

3. Reduced autonomic activity and developmental or acquired abnormalities in the prefrontal brain systems could account for impulsive behavior with aggressive tendency and emotional distance.

Risk factors

Other possible causes or risk factors include attention deficit hyperactivity disorder, large families, and childhood exposure to the following conditions:
- substance abuse
- criminal behavior
- physical or sexual abuse
- neglectful or unstable parenting
- social isolation
- transient friendships
- low socioeconomic status.

Signs and symptoms

Patients with antisocial personality disorder have a long-standing pattern of disregarding the rights of others as well as societal values. Other assessment findings may include:
- repeatedly performing unlawful acts
- reckless disregard for their own safety or the safety of others
- deceitfulness
- lack of remorse
- consistent irresponsibility
- power-seeking behavior
- destructive tendencies
- impulsivity and failure to plan ahead
- superficial charm
- manipulative nature
- inflated, arrogant self-appraisal
- irritability and aggressiveness
- inability to maintain close personal or sexual relationships
- disconnection between feelings and behaviors
- substance abuse.

Diagnosis

The patient with antisocial personality disorder rarely seeks evaluation or treatment on his or her own. Much more commonly, the patient is mandated by the court or pressured by family members to seek help.

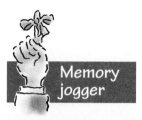

Memory jogger

Each letter in **ANTISOCIAL** stands for a feature of antisocial personality disorder.

Abuses substances (some patients)

No satisfying interpersonal relationships

Tends to manipulate others

Irresponsible and exploitative

Social norms are disregarded

Obnoxious toward others (no sense of guilt, shame, or remorse)

Cold and callous

Intimidates others

Argumentative

Legal problems

Not all criminals qualify

Because not all criminals have antisocial personality disorder, the health care provider must differentiate this condition from simple criminal activity, adult antisocial behavior, or other behaviors that don't justify the personality disorder as a diagnosis. Formal psychological testing, as with the MMPI-2, may prove invaluable. (See *Personality and projective tests.*)

The official diagnosis of antisocial personality disorder is confirmed if the patient meets the diagnostic criteria in the *DSM-5*. See general diagnostic information related to all personality disorders on page 496 for more information.

Treatment

Working with patients with antisocial disorder can be challenging because they seem to neither show nor feel emotions, especially guilt after doing something wrong. For therapy to be effective, they need help in drawing the connection between their feelings and behaviors.

Psychotherapy is the usual treatment of choice. Options include individual psychotherapy, group therapy, family therapy, and self-help support groups. If needed, the patients should also undergo drug or alcohol rehabilitation.

Individual psychotherapy

Many patients with antisocial personality disorder are mandated to have therapy, sometimes in a forensic or prison setting.

In a confined setting, therapy should focus on alternative life issues, such as:
- goals the patients can pursue after their release from custody
- improvement in social or family relationships
- learning new coping skills.

In an outpatient setting, therapy should focus on discussing the patients' antisocial behavior and lack of feelings, as well as addressing other mental health issues.

Ultimatums are unwise

Threats are never an appropriate motivating factor for any type of treatment and are least effective in antisocial patients who have been mandated by the courts to have therapy. Instead of threatening to report the patient's lack of motivation to the courts or the prison warden, the therapist should try to help the patients find good reasons to want to work on their problems—for example, avoiding more jail time or further trouble with the law.

Personality and projective tests

Personality and projective tests elicit patient responses that provide insight into mood, personality, or psychopathology. These tests include the Beck Depression Inventory (BDI), draw-a-person test, MMPI-2, sentence completion test, and thematic apperception test.

Beck Depression Inventory
A self-administered, self-scored test, the BDI asks patients to rate how often they experience symptoms of depression, such as poor concentration, suicidal thoughts, guilt feelings, and crying. Questions focus on cognitive symptoms, such as impaired decision-making, and physical symptoms such as appetite loss.

The sum of 21 items gives the total, with a maximum possible score of 63. A score of 11 to 16 indicates mild depression; a score above 17 indicates moderate depression.

You may help patients complete the BDI by reading the questions—but be careful not to influence their answers. Instruct patients to choose the answer that describes them most accurately.

If you suspect depression, a BDI score above 17 may provide objective evidence of the need for treatment. To monitor the patient's depression, repeat the BDI during the course of treatment.

Draw-a-person test
In the draw-a-person test, the patient draws a human figure of each sex. The psychologist interprets the drawing systematically and correlates the interpretation with diagnosis. The draw-a-person test also provides an estimate of a child's developmental level.

Minnesota Multiphasic Personality Inventory-2
The MMPI-2 is a structured paper-and-pencil test that provides a practical way to assess personality traits and ego function in adolescents and adults. Most patients who read English need little assistance in completing it. The MMPI—the original version of this test—was developed at the University of Minnesota and introduced in 1942. The Minnesota Multiphasic Personality Inventory-2-Restructured Form (MMPI-2-RF) was released in 2008, with 338 questions. It takes about 1 hour to complete (Ben-Porath & Tellegen, 2008).

Questions are designed to evaluate the thoughts, emotions, attitudes, and behavioral traits that comprise personality.

A psychologist translates the patient's answers into a psychological profile and then combines the profile with data gathered from the interview. Test results shed light on the patient's coping strategies, defenses, personality strengths and weaknesses, sexual identification, and self-esteem. The MMPI-2 may also identify certain personality disturbances or mental deficits caused by neurologic problems.

A patient's test pattern may strongly suggest a diagnostic category. If the results reveal a risk of suicide or violence, monitor the patient's behavior. If they show frequent somatic complaints indicating possible hypochondriasis, evaluate the patient's physical status. If the complaints lack medical confirmation, help the patient explore how these symptoms may signal emotional distress.

Sentence completion test
In the sentence completion test, the patient completes a series of partial sentences. A sentence might begin, "When I get angry, I ...." The response may reveal the patient's fantasies, fears, aspirations, or anxieties.

Thematic apperception test
In the thematic apperception test, the patient views a series of pictures depicting ambiguous situations and then tells a story describing each picture. The psychologist evaluates these stories systematically to help analyze the patient's personality, particularly regarding interpersonal relationships and conflicts.

Emotional breakthrough

Intensive psychoanalytic approaches aren't indicated for patients with an antisocial personality disorder. Instead, therapy should focus on reinforcing appropriate behaviors, helping patients gain greater access to their feelings, and helping them make connections between their actions and feelings.

These patients may be unfamiliar with their feelings associated with various emotional states, such as depression. Getting them to experience these feelings is crucial. In fact, experiencing intense affect usually is a sign of progress in these patients.

Keeping confidences

A therapeutic relationship can occur only when the patients and the therapists establish a solid rapport and the patients can trust the therapists implicitly. However, fears about confidentiality may pose an obstacle to the patients' trust. (See *Confidentiality in criminal cases.*)

For example, if the patients were mandated to have therapy, the therapists must report on their progress. Although this can be done in a way that doesn't reveal specific details about the content of the therapy, the patient may be suspicious and distrustful of their therapist—especially at first.

To ease the patient's fear, caregivers should honestly disclose what they'll reveal to the courts. In time, these patients can learn that what they say in therapy won't necessarily become common knowledge.

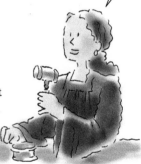

Judges see the consequences of antisocial personality disorder all too often.

Consequences, not conscience

If the patient is morally and ethically deficient, dwelling on this problem may bring little progress. A better approach is to try to have the patient face up to the consequences of his or her behavior. Eventually, this may motivate the patient to continue with therapy.

Group therapy

After the patient is able to overcome the initial fears of joining a group, they may find group therapy beneficial. Ideally, the group should consist exclusively of people with antisocial personality disorder. In such a group, the patient has a greater reason to contribute and share. However, the group leader must make sure that the group doesn't become a how-to course in criminal behavior or a forum to brag about criminal exploits. For this disorder, group therapy provides the benefit of allowing others to validate or challenge the patient's view or perspective.

Confidentiality in criminal cases

If you're caring for a patient who has been mandated by the courts to have treatment, you may be required by law to disclose confidential patient information to the authorities. Some laws create an exemption to the privilege doctrine in criminal cases, which gives the courts access to all essential information.

Even in states where neither a law nor an exemption to the law exists, the court may find an exemption to the privilege doctrine in criminal cases.

Family therapy

Family therapy can help the family understand the patient's antisocial behavior. Open discussion should be encouraged—especially regarding confusion, guilt, and temptation to make restitution for the patient's criminal acts and the frustrations of being with someone who's ill but resists treatment.

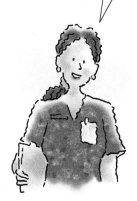

The group leader must make sure that the group doesn't become a forum for patients to brag about their criminal exploits.

Inpatient care

Although patients with antisocial personality disorder rarely require inpatient hospital care, they may be hospitalized for treatment of a crisis or major depression. Inpatient programs may be intensive and expensive and rarely sought out by patients themselves.

To maintain treatment gains, the patients need to have community follow-up and support by the hospital staff or professionals or, possibly, a self-help support group after discharge.

Specialized treatment programs

Specialized treatment programs are available for patients with antisocial personality disorder. For example, a program at Patuxent Institution in Jessup, Maryland, uses a strict behavioral approach and is based on treatment progress. Research is ongoing to determine the long-term effectiveness of this approach. Anger management is also a beneficial component of therapy for this disorder. Patients with this disorder are impulsive and have aggressive tendencies, which can be a difficult combination. Teaching these patients how to express their anger in nonviolent ways is important and for many patients is a priority intervention (Boyd, 2018).

Pharmacologic therapy

Although research doesn't support using medications to treat antisocial personality disorder directly, medications may be given to treat disorganized thinking, stabilize mood swings, or ease the acute symptoms of concurrent psychiatric disorders. For patients who are willing to take medication, lithium carbonate has been found to reduce threatening behavior and serves as a mood stabilizer (Black, 2019).

Nursing interventions

These nursing interventions may be appropriate for a patient with antisocial personality disorder:

- Keep in mind that the patient may seem charming and convincing.
- Using a straightforward, matter-of-fact approach, set limits on acceptable behavior. Encourage and reinforce positive behavior. (See *Setting limits effectively.*)
- Clearly convey your expectations of the patient as well as the consequences if he or she fails to meet them.

Managing manipulative behavior

- Anticipate manipulative efforts. Help the patients identify such behaviors so that they can learn that other people aren't just extensions of themselves.
- Expect the patient to refuse to cooperate in an effort to gain control.
- Establish a behavioral "contract" to communicate to the patient that other behavioral options are available.
- Hold the patient responsible for their behavior to promote the development of a collaborative relationship.

No-struggle zone

- Avoid power struggles and confrontations, as this maintains the opportunity for therapeutic communication.
- Avoid defensive behavior and arguments.
- When teaching, engage the patient in a discussion and try to guide the discussion to the key points. A lecture approach will not work, as these patients enjoy challenging "rules." Approach learning with a sense of humor and use creative and thought-provoking questions in the discussion (Boyd, 2018).

Anger alert

- Observe the patient for physical and verbal signs of agitation.
- Help the patient manage their anger.
- Teach the patient social skills and reinforce appropriate behavior.
- Encourage the patient to express feelings, analyze behavior, and be accountable for their actions.

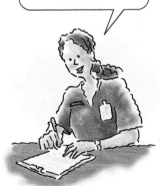

You may have to draw up a behavioral "contract" with a patient who has antisocial personality disorder.

Setting limits effectively

In a therapeutic setting, placing limits on behavior gives these patients a sense of security and self-control. It also communicates caring on the part of the staff. Limit-setting establishes boundaries, for example, that the patient may not hurt others or destroy property. It also helps the nurse avoid getting angry and frustrated with the patient and increases the effectiveness of the therapeutic relationship. The patients benefit from developing a sense of responsibility for their actions.

To set effective limits, follow these guidelines:

Choosing battles wisely
• Choose your battles wisely by setting limits only as needed.
• Set limits when you first sense that the patient is violating others' rights. Don't tolerate this behavior for several days and then attempt to set limits.
• Avoid using limits as punishment or retaliation. Don't set limits only when you're angry or under stress because this will hurt your efforts to build a therapeutic relationship.
• Let the patients express their feelings about what the limits mean to them. They may perceive them as a message that you no longer like them or may feel increased anxiety because they are not used to external controls.

Focusing on behavior
• Establish limits strictly for the patient's *behavior*, not their feelings. If the patients overstep the limits, convey that although you don't accept this behavior, you accept them as a person. If instead you focus on such feelings as anger, the patients may sense that their emotions are unacceptable.
• Make sure that the patients know exactly what behavior you expect.
• Apply the rules consistently and, when possible, offer alternatives to unacceptable behavior.

Ensuring consistency
• Inform other staff members of the limits you've set. Otherwise, patients who are manipulative may try to split the staff into factions that they can pit against one another.
• Apply the same principles when working with the patients' families. Many patients come from families that have had little success in establishing discipline. Explain to them that rules may be enforced in a way that communicates love, caring, and acceptance.

Borderline personality disorder

"The essential feature of borderline personality disorder is a pervasive pattern of instability of interpersonal relationships, self-image, and affects and marked impulsivity that begins by early adulthood and is present in a variety of contexts" (APA, 2013, p. 663). Although people with this disorder may experience it in various ways, most find it hard to distinguish reality from their own misperceptions of the world. Their emotions overwhelm their cognitive functioning, creating many conflicts with others. Alternating extremes of anger, anxiety, depression, and emptiness is common in patients with borderline disorder. However, intense bouts of these emotions typically last only hours or at most a day.

Fluctuations and flip-flops

Distortions in cognition and sense of self can lead to frequent changes in long-term goals, jobs and career plans, friendships, values, and even gender identity.

The patient may see himself or herself as fundamentally bad or unworthy. The patient may feel misunderstood, mistreated, bored, and empty, with little idea of who they really are as a person.

People with borderline personality disorder tend to act impulsively without considering the consequences. Impulsive behaviors may include promiscuity, substance abuse, and eating or spending binges. Outbursts of intense anger may lead to violence, which are easily triggered when others criticize or thwart their impulsive acts. Some even have brief psychotic-like experiences.

All or nothing at all

Persons with borderline personality disorder tend to have intense and stormy relationships, alternating between a black and white view of others. Their perceptions of family members and friends may shift suddenly from great admiration and love to intense anger and dislike.

For example, they may adore and idealize another person—but when a slight separation or conflict occurs, they may switch unexpectedly to the other extreme and angrily accuse that person of not caring for them.

Called *splitting*, this tendency to view others as either heroes or villains is a defense mechanism meant to protect these patients from the perception of dangerous anxiety and intense affects. However, instead of offering real protection, splitting leads to destructive behavior and turmoil.

Rejection blues

With borderline personality comes extreme sensitivity to rejection. The patient may react with anger and distress to even mild separations from loved ones, such as vacations, business trips, or a sudden change in plans.

Self-injury

To escape from their inner turmoil, they may resort to self-destructive behaviors, such as self-jury (cutting or burning themselves), substance abuse, eating disorders, and suicide attempts. These symptoms commonly are triggered by fear of abandonment.

Prevalence

Borderline personality disorder affects 1.6% to 5.9% of the general population, about 10% of psychiatric outpatients, nearly 20% of psychiatric inpatients, and approximately 6% in primary care settings. It is three times more common in females (about 75%) than in males (APA, 2013).

Age and stability

The disorder usually begins in early childhood and peaks in adolescence and early adulthood. It can take a tumultuous course, resulting in the high use of health care resources by patients in their late teens and 20s. However, by their 30s and 40s, up to 60% of patients achieve some stability in their work and personal life (although significant areas of dysfunction usually remain).

Borderline personality disorder commonly overlaps with other personality disorders, as well as bipolar disorder, depression, anxiety disorders, posttraumatic stress disorder, and substance abuse.

Causes

The precise cause of borderline personality disorder is unknown, but several theories are being investigated. Because it's five times more common in first-degree relatives of people who have it, researchers suspect genetics may play a role.

Biological factors may involve:
- dysfunction in the brain's limbic system or frontal lobe
- decreased serotonin activity
- increased activity in alpha-2-noradrenergic receptors.

Early losses and abuse

Prolonged separation from their parents; other major losses early in life; and physical, sexual, or emotional abuse or neglect seem to be more common in patients with this disorder than in the general population. In a recent systematic review, sexual abuse was found to play a major role in borderline personality disorder, particularly in women (Ferreira et al., 2018).

Signs and symptoms

Major signs and symptoms of borderline personality disorder fall into four main categories: unstable relationships, unstable self-image, unstable emotions, and impulsivity. Symptoms are most acute when the patients feel isolated and without social support, causing them to make frantic efforts to avoid being alone.

Assessment findings may include:

- a pattern of unstable and intense interpersonal relationships
- splitting (viewing others as either extremely good or extremely bad)
- intense fear of abandonment, as displayed by clinging and distancing maneuvers
- rapidly shifting attitudes about friends and loved ones
- desperate attempts to maintain relationships
- unstable perceptions of relationships, with estrangement over ordinary disagreements
- manipulation, as in pitting people against one another
- limited coping skills
- dissociation (separating objects from their emotional significance)
- transient, stress-related paranoid ideation or severe dissociative symptoms
- inability to develop a healthy sense of oneself
- uncertainty about major issues, such as self-image, identity, life goals, sexual orientation, values, career choices, or types of friends
- imitative behavior
- rapid, dramatic mood swings, from euphoria to intense anxiety to rage, within hours or days
- acting-out of feelings instead of expressing them appropriately or verbally
- inappropriate, intense anger or difficulty controlling anger
- chronic feelings of emptiness
- unpredictable self-damaging behavior, such as driving dangerously, gambling, sexual promiscuity, overeating, spending, and abusing substances
- self-destructive behaviors, such as physical fights, recurrent accidents, self-injury, and suicidal gestures.

Diagnosis and treatment

Standard psychological tests may reveal a high degree of dissociation in a patient with borderline personality disorder. The diagnosis is confirmed if the patient meets the criteria in the *DSM-5*.

Treatment of borderline personality disorder may involve:

- individual psychotherapy
- group therapy
- family therapy

- milieu therapy
- alcohol and drug rehabilitation as indicated.

Psychotherapy

Psychotherapy is usually the treatment of choice for this disorder. Although borderline personality disorder can be hard to treat, individual and group therapy are at least partially effective for many patients.

The patients' unstable relationships and intense anger can cause difficulty in establishing a therapeutic relationship with health care professionals. They may fail to respond to therapeutic efforts and may make considerable demands on the caregiver's emotional resources, especially when suicidal behaviors are prominent.

Sign on the dotted line

In the past, patients who were considered suicidal were asked to commit to a safety contract indicating that they would not harm themselves. However, evidence shows this does not actively reduce suicide and may create a false sense of security (Schreiber & Culpepper, 2019). Suicidal potential should be carefully assessed and monitored throughout the entire course of treatment. Patients at high risk for suicide may require medications and hospitalization.

Borderlines with boundaries

A structured therapeutic setting is important. The borderline patient may try to test limits, so the therapist must set boundaries for the relationship when therapy begins. Everyone involved in the care should maintain these boundaries consistently. Some patients have had success with a psychosocial treatment called *dialectical behavior therapy* (DBT). (See *Dialectical behavior therapy*, page 520.)

Other types of psychotherapy

Therapies that focus on social learning theory and conflict resolution may also be used to treat borderline personality disorder. However, these solution-focused therapies may neglect the patient's core problems, such as difficulty expressing appropriate emotions and problems forming emotional attachments to others because of faulty cognitions.

Hospitalization

Long-term care in a hospital setting is rarely appropriate. However, during an episode of acute depression or another crisis, the patient may be seen in a hospital emergency department, an inpatient unit, or a local community health center.

Dialectical behavior therapy

A psychosocial treatment called DBT—developed specifically to treat borderline personality disorder—has proven effective in helping patients cope with the disorder.

In this comprehensive approach, the patients are taught to better control their life and emotions through self-knowledge, emotional regulation, and cognitive restructuring.

Treatment modes

DBT involves four primary modes of treatment:
- individual therapy
- group skills training
- telephone contact with the therapist
- therapist consultation (Skodol, 2018).

Individual therapy sessions

The main work of therapy occurs in individual therapy sessions. (The therapist may add group therapy and other treatment modes as appropriate.) Between sessions, patients are offered telephone contact with their therapists to give them help and support in applying the skills they are learning to real-life situations and to help them avoid self-injury.

Therapeutic hierarchy

In individual therapy sessions, goals are addressed according to the following hierarchy:

- decreasing suicidal behaviors
- decreasing behaviors that interfere with therapy
- decreasing behaviors that interfere with the quality of life
- increasing behavioral skills
- decreasing behaviors related to posttraumatic stress
- improving self-esteem
- individual goals negotiated with the patient.

Skills training

Skills training is carried out in a group setting. In the group, patients learn:
- core mindfulness skills (meditation-like techniques)
- interpersonal effectiveness skills
- emotion modulation skills (ways of changing distressing emotional states)
- distress tolerance skills (techniques for coping with the emotional states that can't be changed for the time being).

Because hospital visits are costly, the patient should be encouraged to find additional social support within the community from such sources as:
- telephone or personal contact with their health care providers
- self-help support groups (including those available through the Internet)
- crisis hotlines.

Partial hospitalization and day treatment programs

Partial hospitalization and day treatment programs provide a safe environment offering support, feedback, and structure for a short time or during the day. Patients usually return home in the evening.

Diminishing dependency

During times of increased stress or difficulty coping, partial hospitalization treatment may be more appropriate than inpatient

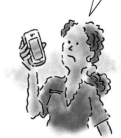

Crisis hotlines and self-help groups are good alternatives to hospitalization for a borderline patient.

Milieu therapy

Whether it takes place in the hospital or in a community setting, milieu therapy uses the patient's setting or environment to help him or her overcome social anxiety as well as receive feedback from peers. If your patient is undergoing this type of therapy, the following guidelines may be helpful.

Patient preparation

Explain the purpose of milieu therapy to the patient. Tell the patient what you expect of them and explain how they can participate in the therapeutic community. Orient the patient to the routines of the community, such as the schedule for various activities, and introduce him or her to other patients and staff.

Monitoring and aftercare

Regularly evaluate the patient's symptoms and therapeutic needs. Oversee activities, encouraging the patient to keep a schedule typical of life outside the hospital. Also, encourage the patient to interact with others so that they do not become withdrawn or feel secluded. Point out the importance of respecting others and their environment.

Home care instructions

If the patient eventually returns to the outside community, encourage them to keep follow-up appointments with their therapist.

hospitalization. Also, the patient is less dependent on others to solve problems. Milieu therapy is another option. (See *Milieu therapy*.)

Pharmacologic therapy

There are currently no medications approved by the U.S. Food and Drug Administration (FDA) for the specific treatment of borderline personality disorder. Medications can be used to control symptoms and improve overall quality of life. Antidepressants, such as SSRIs, can help decrease impulsivity and self-destructive behavior. Anticonvulsants and lithium can also be used for mood regulation and emotional lability. Opioid receptor antagonist, such as naltrexone (Revia), is used to reduce self-injuring behaviors (Halter, 2018).

Overdose alert

Dosages should be kept low and the patients should be under psychosocial intervention. Also, prescriptions must be closely monitored because the patients may overdose impulsively if they have an adequate drug supply.

Nursing interventions

These nursing interventions may be appropriate for patients with borderline personality disorder:

- Encourage the patients to take responsibility. Don't try to rescue them from the consequences of their actions (except suicidal and self-injuring behaviors).

- Convey empathy and support, but don't try to solve problems they can solve.
- Maintain a consistent approach in all interactions with these patients and ensure that other team members use the same approach.
- Avoid sympathetic, nurturing responses.

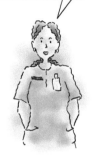

Make sure to set appropriate expectations for social interactions.

Manipulation and expectation

- Recognize behaviors that patients with borderline personality disorder use to manipulate people so that the nurse can avoid unconsciously reinforcing these behaviors.
- Set appropriate expectations for social interactions and praise the patient when they meet these expectations.
- To promote trust, respect the patients' personal space.

Staff subjects

- Be aware that the patients may idealize some staff members and devalue others.
- Don't take sides in the patients' disputes with staff members.
- Avoid defensiveness and arguing.
- Try to limit patients' interactions to assigned staff in order to decrease splitting behaviors. Know that using only a few consistent staff members helps maintain consistent treatment.

Cheek checks

- If the patient is taking medications, monitor for "cheeking" (holding medications in the cheek) or hoarding of medications for overdose at a later time.
- Encourage the patients to express their feelings, analyze their behaviors, and be accountable for their actions.

Skills expansion

- Help the patient develop problem-solving skills.
- Review and encourage relaxation techniques.
- Encourage the patients to start an exercise regimen. Exercise promotes stability by decreasing mood swings and aiding the release of anger.

Histrionic personality disorder

Histrionic personality disorder is characterized by a pattern of emotionally driven behaviors and overt attention seeking. People with this disorder are drawn to momentary excitements and fleeting adventures.

Those with histrionic disorder can be charming, dramatic, and expressive. However, they are also easily hurt, vain, demanding, capricious, excitable, self-indulgent, and inconsiderate. The words and feelings they express seem shallow and simulated, not real or deep. As a result, they often come across as manipulative and phony. Despite their emotional responsiveness, their emotions may shift instantly from rage to friendliness.

"Look at me!"

Their style of speech is excessively impressionistic, if not downright theatrical, and their gestures are exaggerated. They use grandiose language to describe everyday events and value words more for their emotional content than for their factual accuracy.

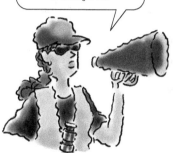

With histrionic personality disorder, the drama is always on!

People with histrionic personality disorder need to be the center of attention at all times. They place great emphasis on physical appearance, often dressing provocatively and behaving seductively. Consumed with superficialities, they devote little time or attention to their internal lives.

Chameleon effect

With limited self-knowledge, they may have no sense of who they are, aside from their identification with others. They may change their attitudes and values depending on the views of significant others. (See *Watching the watchers*, page 524.)

Exaggerations and embellishment

People with histrionic personality disorder may exaggerate their illnesses to gain attention, interrupt others so that they can dominate the conversation, and seek constant praise. They exaggerate friendships and relationships, believing that everyone loves them. They consider friendships and relationships to be far more intimate than they are.

From fairytale to nightmare

Because they don't view others realistically, people with histrionic personality disorder have trouble developing and sustaining satisfactory relationships. Typically, their relationships start out as ideal and end up as disasters. They idealize the significant other early in the relationship and may see the connection as more intimate than it really is.

Watching the watchers

Patients with histrionic personality disorder rarely gain an understanding of others. Instead, they devote their intense observation skills to determining which behaviors, attitudes, or feelings are most likely to win others' admiration and approval. Essentially, they watch other people watch them.

Because of their limited understanding of how others feel, they tend to see their relationships as closer or more significant than they really are. They don't realize when they're being humored or placated by someone who has lost patience with their constant need for attention and their inability to relate in an honest way.

If others start to pull back from the incessant demands, the histrionic person becomes dramatic and demonstrative in an attempt to bind the other person to the relationship. To avoid rejection, they may resort to crying, coercion, temper tantrums, assault, and suicidal gestures.

Despite their attempts to bind others to them, the individuals with histrionic personality disorder often lack fidelity and loyalty.

Prevalence

Histrionic personality disorder affects an estimated 1.84% of the general population. Although more commonly diagnosed in women, it may be just as common in men (APA, 2013). Without treatment, the disorder can lead to social, occupational, and functional impairments. However, many people function at a high level and succeed at work (although frequent disruption of intimate relationships is common). Histrionic personality disorder commonly coexists with somatic symptom disorder, conversion disorder, and major depressive disorder.

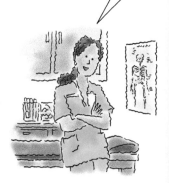

The histrionic person can be dramatic, seductive, and have an overwhelming desire for attention.

Causes

The cause of histrionic personality disorder is not known. Certain character traits, such as egocentricity, are associated with a predisposition to this disorder (Halter, 2018).

Signs and symptoms

Assessment of a patient with histrionic personality disorder may reveal:
- constant craving for attention, stimulation, and excitement
- intense affect
- shallow, rapidly shifting expression of emotions

- vanity
- flirting and seductive behavior
- overinvestment in appearance
- exaggerated, vague speech
- self-dramatization
- impulsivity
- exhibitionism
- suggestibility and impressionability
- egocentricity, self-indulgence, and lack of consideration for others
- intolerance of frustration, disappointment, and delayed gratification; impatience
- somatic (physical) preoccupations and symptoms
- angry outbursts and tantrums
- sudden enraged, despairing, or fearful states
- intense anger toward people viewed as withholding
- divisive, manipulative behavior
- intolerance of being alone
- dread of growing old
- demanding and manipulative nature
- use of alcohol or drugs to quickly alter negative feelings
- depression
- suicidal gestures and threats.

When assessing a patient for histrionic personality disorder, keep in mind that the expression of emotion and interpersonal behavior can vary widely across cultures, gender, and age groups (APA, 2013).

Diagnosis and treatment

No specific tests can diagnose histrionic personality disorder; however, personality and projective tests can be helpful. If the patient has somatic concerns, physiologic disorders must be ruled out. The official diagnosis of histrionic personality disorder is confirmed if the patient meets the criteria in the *DSM-5*.

Individuals with histrionic personality disorder rarely seek treatment unless a crisis occurs or a situational factor causes functional impairments and ineffective coping. Psychotherapy is the treatment of choice.

Psychotherapy

Psychotherapy focuses on solving problems in the patients' life rather than producing long-term personality changes. Individual therapy is preferred over group or family therapy because a group environment may trigger the patients' dramatic, attention-seeking behaviors. For this reason, self-help support groups are not recommended.

While establishing a rapport and trust with the patient, the therapist must avoid a dependent situation with a needy patient who may see the therapist as their rescuer.

Insight

Insight-oriented and cognitive approaches aren't especially effective because histrionic patients have little capacity or inclination to examine their unconscious motives and thoughts. Instead, therapists should try to help the patients view their interactions objectively and explore and clarify patients' emotions.

Let's get real

Patients with histrionic personality disorder may use mechanisms such as suppression, disavowal, denial, and avoidance to block information that could cause emotional distress. In addition, these patients have difficulty focusing and are easily distracted. Therapists should focus on the issues that the patient is avoiding and work to keep the patient engaged in a reality-based environment.

Serious about suicide

The patient should be assessed regularly for suicidal potential, and suicidal thoughts and plans should be taken seriously. "The actual risk of suicide is not known, but clinical experience suggests that individuals with this disorder are at increased risk for suicidal gestures and threats to get attention and coerce better caregiving" (APA, 2013, p. 668).

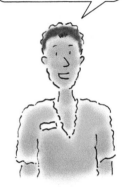

A histrionic patient may try to block out distressing information.

Pharmacologic therapy

Medications usually aren't indicated for histrionic personality disorder; however, they may relieve associated symptoms, such as anxiety or depression. In a crisis, the patients may seek drugs for self-destructive or harmful purposes. Also, they may respond to the adverse effects of medications with intense, dramatic overreactions.

Nursing interventions

These nursing interventions may be appropriate for a patient with histrionic personality disorder:
- Give the patient choices in care options and incorporate his or her wishes into the treatment plan as much as possible. Increasing the patient's sense of self-control may lower his or her anxiety.
- Be aware that the patient will want to "win over" the caregiver and—at least initially—will be responsive and cooperative.

Role modeling

- Teach the patient appropriate social skills and reinforce appropriate behavior.
- Help the patient learn to think more clearly and base his or her reactions on reality.
- Promote the expression of feelings, self-analysis of behavior, and accountability for actions.
- Encourage warmth, genuineness, and empathy.

Crisis management

- Teach stress-reducing techniques, such as deep breathing and an exercise regimen.
- Help them manage crisis situations and feelings.
- Monitor the patient for suicidal thoughts and behavior.

Narcissistic personality disorder

The hallmarks of narcissistic personality disorder are self-centeredness, self-absorption, and an inability to empathize with the effects of one's behavior on others. A person with this disorder takes advantage of people, using them without regard for their feelings. They have an inflated sense of self and an intense need for admiration.

Image control

The narcissists try to maintain an image of perfection and invincibility to prevent others from discovering their weaknesses and imperfections. However, beneath the image are insecure individuals with low self-esteem.

Superior species?

The narcissists expect to be recognized as superior. Preoccupied with fantasies of brilliance and unlimited success or power, they believe that they are special and entitled to favored treatment. They expect others to comply with their wishes automatically and believe they should associate only with other special or high-status people. Many narcissists are driven and achievement oriented.

Shattered illusions

The narcissists' illusion of greatness may be shattered by a threat to their ego from:
- physical illness
- loss of a job
- loss of a relationship
- feelings of emptiness and depression despite material wealth and success.

Such threats trigger panic. They feel their world is falling apart and their lives are unraveling.

Prevalence

Narcissistic personality disorder ranges between 0% and 6.2% in the general population. It affects about three times as many males as females (APA, 2013).

Although it develops by early adulthood, this disorder may not be identified until middle age when the person experiences the sense of a loss of opportunity or faces personal limitations. Many people with narcissistic personality disorder also have histrionic or borderline personality disorder.

Causes

The exact cause of narcissistic personality disorder is unknown. A psychodynamic theory proposes that it arises when a child's basic needs go unmet.

Signs and symptoms

In patients with narcissistic personality disorder, assessment findings may include:

- arrogance or haughtiness
- self-centeredness
- unreasonable expectations of favorable treatment
- grandiose sense of self-importance
- exaggeration of achievements and talents
- preoccupation with fantasies of success, power, beauty, brilliance, or ideal love
- manipulative behavior
- constant desire for attention and admiration
- lack of empathy
- lack of concern for those they offend
- exploiting others to achieve their own goals
- rage, shame, or humiliation in response to criticism.

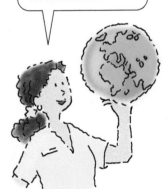

A patient with narcissistic disorder thinks the world revolves around them.

Diagnosis and treatment

The patient should undergo psychological evaluation and personality and projective testing. However, just like most personality disorders, there is not one specific test to diagnose narcissistic personality disorder. Multiple assessments and patterns of behavior are assessed and compared to the diagnostic criteria. The official diagnosis is confirmed if the patient meets the criteria in the *DSM-5*.

Most patients with narcissistic personality disorder seek treatment only in a crisis and terminate it as soon as their symptoms ease. Those who don't terminate treatment may be seeking help for depression or interpersonal difficulties.

Long-term psychotherapy is the treatment of choice because it helps establish a strong alliance between the patient and the therapist. Therapy should focus on making small, not large, changes in personality traits.

Pulling away the pedestal

The goals of therapy include placing the patients' exaggerated self-importance in perspective, helping them develop empathy, and teaching them how to handle slights and rejections without feeling extremely threatened.

Group therapy tends to be ineffective because these patients typically dominate the group. Other participants in the group may tire of hearing about the narcissistic accomplishments and talents. If or when they are being criticized by other participants in the group, they are likely to drop out of the group therapy.

Inpatient therapy

Hospitalization may be necessary for a patient with severe symptoms, such as self-destructive behavior and poor reality testing. However, hospitalization should be brief, with treatment specific to the particular symptoms.

Milieus for weak egos

Patients with little motivation for outpatient treatment, chronic destructive acting-out, and chaotic lifestyles may need longer therapy. Inpatient programs can offer intensive milieu therapy, individual psychotherapy, family involvement, or a specialized residential environment. Such treatment may be appropriate for patients with severe ego weakness, helping them to improve their self-concept.

Nursing interventions

The following nursing interventions may be appropriate for patients with narcissistic personality disorder:

- Convey respect and acknowledge the patient's sense of self-importance so that they can reestablish a coherent sense of self. However, don't reinforce their pathologic grandiosity or their weakness.
- Focus on positive traits or on the feelings of pain, loss, or rejection.

Don't play a judge

- If the patient makes unreasonable demands or has unreasonable expectations, tell them in a matter-of-fact way that they are being unreasonable. However, remain nonjudgmental because a critical attitude may make the patient even more demanding and difficult. Don't avoid the patient, as this could increase their maladaptive attention-seeking behaviors.
- Avoid defensive behavior and arguments with patients with narcissistic personality disorder.
- Offer persistent, consistent, and flexible care. Take a direct, involved approach to develop a trusting provider relationship.
- Teach the patients social skills and reinforce appropriate behaviors.

Cluster C personality disorders

Cluster C personality disorders include those that are characterized by anxious or fearful behavior. Cluster C disorders include: avoidant, dependent, and obsessive-compulsive personality disorders.

Avoidant personality disorder

Avoidant personality disorder is marked by feelings of inadequacy, extreme social anxiety, social withdrawal, and hypersensitivity to the opinions of others. People with this disorder have low self-esteem and poor self-confidence. They dwell on the negative and have difficulty viewing situations and interactions objectively. To rationalize their avoidance of new situations, they exaggerate the potential difficulties involved. They may create fantasy worlds to substitute for the real one.

Wallflower syndrome

The avoidant person yearns for social interaction but the fear of being rejected or embarrassed in front of others is a daily obstacle. In fact, many times they are not willing to enter into social relationships without the assurance of uncritical acceptance. They even seek out jobs that require little contact with others.

Prevalence

In the adult general population, avoidant personality disorder has a prevalence estimated at 2.4%, affects males and females equally, and develops by early adulthood (APA, 2013). It is common to see additional psychiatric diagnoses with avoidant personality disorder. One of the more common is dependent personality disorder. When the patient with avoidant personality finds someone whom they can trust, he or she may become very attached to the point of dependence (APA, 2013).

Causes

As with most personality disorders, there is no clear cause of avoidant personality disorder. The primary psychosocial cause seems to center on parental rejection and the feelings of abandonment as a child (Halter, 2018). There is also suggestion of biological predisposition to anxiety in social situations, creating a genetic relation with social anxiety disorder (Halter, 2018).

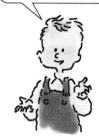

Being belittled as a child makes me want to avoid the world.

Genetic and biological theories

Avoidant personality disorder is closely linked to temperament. Some evidence suggests that a timid temperament in infancy may predispose a person to developing avoidant personality disorder later in life (Halter, 2018).

Information overload

The inherited tendency to be shy may result from overstimulation or an excess of incoming information. The patient can't cope with the excess information and withdraws in defense. Inability to cope with the information overload may stem from a low autonomic arousal threshold. Research suggests that in people with this disorder, certain structures in the brain's limbic system may have a lower threshold of arousal and a more pronounced response when activated.

Environmental factors

Some experts believe that significant environmental influences during childhood, such as rejection by the parents or peers, lead to the full development of avoidant personality disorder. (See *The rejected child*, page 532.)

Signs and symptoms

Patients with avoidant personality disorder may exhibit or report:
- shyness, timidity, and social withdrawal
- behavior or appearance that is used to drive others away
- reluctance to speak or, conversely, overtalkativeness
- constant mistrust or wariness of others
- testing of others' sincerity
- difficulty starting and maintaining relationships
- perfectionism
- rejection of people who don't live up to impossibly high standards
- limited emotional expression
- tenseness and anxiety

The rejected child

Normal, healthy infants may encounter varying degrees of parental rejection. In those who subsequently develop avoidant personality disorder, the amount of rejection seems to be particularly intense or frequent.

Particular types of parental rejection can alter a child's attitude and behavior in a way that predisposes him or her to developing avoidant personality disorder later in life. For example, if a parent is aloof or critical when the child expresses positive emotions, the child might learn to spare himself or herself the anguish by keeping positive feelings to himself or herself.

Likewise, if the child is repeatedly told that it's bad to feel angry, they might swear off relationships to avoid the intermittent feelings of dissatisfaction or anger that occur in nearly all close relationships.

Peer rejection

Repeated social interactions expose a person to potential rejection over a sustained period. Such rejection can wear down self-esteem. After humiliation and rejection by peers, a person may begin to criticize himself or herself.

Feelings of loneliness and isolation worsen with these harsh self-judgments. Deepening feelings of personal inferiority and self-worthlessness contribute to social withdrawal.

Rejection by peers seems to validate rejection by the parents. When a child can't turn to parents, peers, or even himself or herself for gratification or validation, they retreat—and avoidant personality disorder may result.

- low self-esteem
- feelings of being unworthy of successful relationships
- self-consciousness
- loneliness
- reluctance to take personal risks or to engage in new activities
- frequent escapes into fantasy, such as by excessive reading, watching TV, or daydreaming.

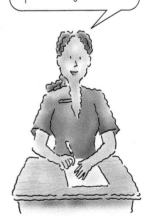

Personality and projective tests can help determine if a patient has avoidant personality disorder.

Diagnosis and treatment

No specific tests can diagnose avoidant personality disorder. The patient should undergo a psychological evaluation, along with personality and projective tests. The diagnosis is confirmed if the patient meets the criteria in the *DSM-5*.

People with avoidant personality disorder rarely seek treatment unless something goes wrong in their lives to indicate that they are not coping adequately. High-functioning patients may need psychotherapy only, whereas others benefit from a combination of medication and psychotherapy.

The goals of treatment are to:
- enhance self-esteem
- improve social interaction and increase confidence in interpersonal relationships

- desensitize the reaction to criticism
- decrease resistance to change
- improve coping
- achieve cognitive restructuring
- develop appropriate affect and expression of emotions.

Psychotherapy

Individual psychotherapy is the preferred treatment. It is the most effective when it is short term and focused on solving specific life problems. As patients successfully progress through individual therapy, group therapy may be considered.

All's well that ends well

Establishing a solid therapist-patient relationship may be difficult, and the patient may terminate therapy early. However, a successful ending to the relationship is important because it reinforces for the patient the possibility of new relationships.

Self-help support groups

Although self-help support groups can be effective for patients with avoidant personality disorder, such groups may be difficult to find. Additionally, patients with this disorder are likely to avoid groups because of their social anxiety.

Pharmacologic therapy

Medications may be prescribed as an adjunct to psychotherapy when patients have moderate to severe functional impairments. For many individuals with avoidant personality, serotonin-based antidepressants such as sertraline (Zoloft) may be helpful (Sadock & Sadock, 2015). If the patient feels disconnected from his or her emotions, medications may interfere with effective psychotherapeutic management.

Nursing interventions

These nursing interventions may be appropriate for patients with avoidant personality disorder:

- Offer persistent, consistent, and flexible care. Take a direct, involved approach to gain trust.
- Be aware that the patient may become dependent on the few staff members that they feel they can trust. Monitor for signs of dependency, and encourage self-care.
- Assess the patient for signs of depression because social impairment increases the risk of mood disorders.

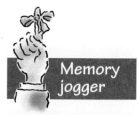

Memory jogger

For an easy way to remember the signs and symptoms of avoidant personality disorder, think of AVOIDANT.

Anxious and angry with oneself because of the lack of meaningful relationships

Very socially withdrawn

Often feels lonely and unwanted

Intensely shy

Desires close relationships but has difficulty developing and sustaining them

Awkward and uncomfortable in others' company

No natural optimism or positive regard for oneself

Terrified by the fear of rejection

Advice from the experts

Basic requirements for relaxation

According to Dr. Herbert Benson (1975), the Harvard professor who first described the relaxation response, four basic elements are needed to elicit this response:

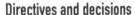

- a quiet environment that's free from distraction
- a sound, process, or image to dwell on, such as breathing or a mantra (such as that used in transcendental meditation)

- a passive attitude in which the mind is cleared of thoughts and images
- a comfortable position that can be kept easily for at least 20 minutes.

Advance warning

- Make sure that the patient knows about upcoming procedures in plenty of time to adjust because they don't handle surprises well.
- Inform the patient when you will and will not be available if they need assistance.

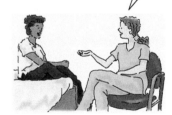

I'm glad you trust me to care for you, but you need to be involved in your care, too.

Directives and decisions

- Initially, give the patient explicit directives rather than asking them to make decisions. Then gradually encourage him or her to make easy decisions. Continue to provide support and reassurance as their decision-making ability improves.
- Avoid actions that foster dependency.
- Encourage the expression of feelings, self-analysis of behavior, and accountability for actions.
- Teach the patient relaxation and stress management techniques to help him or her cope in times of stress and manage his or her anxiety level. (See *Basic requirements for relaxation*.)

Dependent personality disorder

Dependent personality disorder is characterized by an extreme need to be taken care of, which leads to submissive, clinging behavior and fear of separation or rejection. People with this disorder let others make important decisions for them and have a strong need for constant reassurance and support. To elicit caregiving, they engage in dependent behavior. Feeling helpless and incompetent, they comply passively

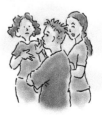

A basic requirement for relaxation? I'm thinking a week at the beach.

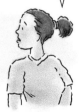

and transfer responsibility to others. In fact, they seek others to dominate and protect them. Some stay in abusive relationships and are willing to tolerate mistreatment.

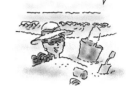

I'm clingy, I have trust issues, I get jealous. All because I don't feel good enough.

Replacement therapy

When the breakup of a romantic relationship is imminent, individuals with dependent personality disorder may become suicidal. After a close relationship ends, they urgently seek another relationship as a source of care and support.

People who need people

These behaviors arise from the perception that they can't function adequately without others. They crave attention and validation and may repeatedly request attention to their complaints. The complaints can be simple or complex in nature such as their overall lifestyle, social relationships, meaning in life, or medical problems.

That worthless feeling

Overly sensitive to disapproval, people with dependent personality disorder often feel helpless and depressed. They belittle their own abilities and are racked with self-doubt. They take criticism and disapproval as proof that they are worthless. They are likely to avoid positions of responsibility. If their job requires independent initiative, they may suffer occupational impairments.

Prevalence

In mental health clinics, dependent personality disorder is among the most frequently reported personality disorders. In the general population, its prevalence is about 0.49% to 0.6%. It affects more females than males, but some reports suggest that there is a comparable prevalence between the genders (APA, 2013). Individuals who suffered chronic physical illness in childhood are more prone to develop dependent personality disorder (Sadock & Sadock, 2015).

Many patients with dependent personality disorder have an additional personality disorder—most commonly borderline, histrionic, or avoidant.

Causes

The exact cause of dependent personality disorder is not known. Because it tends to run in families, it may involve a genetic component.

Dictators and coddlers

According to some experts, authoritarian or overprotective parenting may lead to high levels of dependency. These parenting styles may cause these children to believe that they cannot function without others' guidance and protection and that the way to maintain relationships is to give in to others' demands.

Signs and symptoms

Assessment findings in a patient with dependent personality disorder may include:

- submissiveness
- self-effacing, apologetic manner
- low self-esteem
- lack of self-confidence
- lack of initiative
- incompetence and a need for constant assistance
- intense need to be loved in a stable long-term relationship
- anxiety and insecurity, especially when deprived of a significant relationship
- feelings of pessimism, inferiority, and unworthiness
- hypersensitivity to criticism
- in females, little need to overtly control or compete with others
- clinging, demanding behavior
- use of cajolery, bribery, promises to change, and even threats to maintain key relationships
- fear and anxiety over losing a relationship or being alone
- dependence on a number of people, any one of whom could substitute for the other
- difficulty making everyday decisions without advice and reassurance
- avoidance of change and new situations
- exaggerated fear of losing support and approval.

Somatically speaking . . .

A patient with dependent personality disorder may also present with somatic complaints, such as fatigue and lethargy, as well as tension, anxiety, or depression.

Diagnosis and treatment

The patient should undergo a psychological evaluation and psychological and projective tests, as indicated. If somatic concerns are present, medical evaluation and diagnostic testing should be completed to rule out any underlying medical conditions. The diagnosis of dependent personality disorder is confirmed if the patient meets the criteria in the *DSM-5*.

Although patients with this disorder frequently attend outpatient mental health clinics, they rarely seek treatment for dependency or help in making decisions. Instead, they typically complain of anxiety, tension, or depression.

Psychotherapy

Psychotherapy is the treatment of choice. Promoting autonomy and self-efficacy is the overriding treatment goal.

Clinging vine

The most effective approach is short-term therapy that focuses on helping the patient solve specific life problems. Long-term therapy is contraindicated because it only reinforces a dependent relationship with the therapist. (However, some degree of dependency is bound to develop no matter the length of therapy.)

Individual and group therapy may be helpful, although the patient may use a group setting to find new dependent relationships.

After-hours attention

The patient may be very needy with the therapist and seek tremendous reassurance and attention—especially between therapy sessions. At the start of therapy, the therapist should set boundaries as to how the treatment will be conducted, including such issues as appropriate times to contact the therapist between sessions.

Final endings

Termination of therapy is an important issue because it is a test of how effective the therapy has been. The therapist should set goals for therapy and make it clear to the patient that when they attain these goals, therapy will end.

Behavioral approaches

A patient with dependent personality disorder can benefit from such behavioral approaches as assertiveness training. Treatment may include behavior modification using assertiveness techniques.

Self-help support groups

Self-help support groups allow patients with dependent personality disorder to share their experiences and feelings as well as put to use their newly learned skills. However, a support group shouldn't be the sole treatment for this disorder because it may encourage dependent relationships.

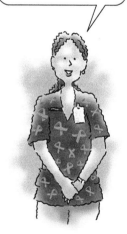

For a dependent patient, long-term therapy only reinforces a dependent relationship with the therapist.

Pharmacologic therapy

The health care provider may prescribe medications to treat associated symptoms, such as low energy, fatigue, and depression. Some patients respond well to antidepressants. In a crisis, benzodiazepine antianxiety drugs such as alprazolam (Xanax), lorazepam (Ativan), or clonazepam (Klonopin) may be prescribed. However, because the patient may abuse these agents, their use should be limited and monitored.

Nursing interventions

The following nursing interventions may be appropriate for patients with dependent personality disorder:

- Offer persistent, consistent, and flexible care. Take a direct, involved approach to develop a trusting relationship.
- Give the patients as much opportunity to control their treatment as possible. Offer options and allow them to choose, even if they choose all of them.
- Verify the patient's approval before initiating specific treatment.
- Try to limit caregivers to a few consistent staff members to increase the patient's sense of security.

Encourage dependent patients to plan their own meals, balance their own checkbook, and pay bills on their own.

Deter dependency

- Deter actions that promote dependency on caregivers.
- Encourage activities that require decision-making (such as balancing a checkbook, planning meals, and paying bills) to promote autonomy.
- Help the patient establish and work toward goals to foster a sense of autonomy.
- If the patient has physical concerns, don't minimize or dismiss—but don't encourage either. Use a simple, matter-of-fact approach.

Aim for assertiveness

- Help the patient express his or her ideas and feelings assertively.
- Be aware that outwardly, the patient may seem overly compliant, with suggestions for treatment. However, they may fail to make real gains in therapy because his or her adherence to treatment plans may be superficial.

Monitor medications

- Teach the patient about prescribed medications, including exactly what each medication is prescribed for.
- Emphasize that there are no magical drug effects.
- Monitor the patient to make sure that they are not abusing medication. If the patient is receiving benzodiazepines, check for signs and symptoms of psychological dependence.

Obsessive–compulsive personality disorder

Obsessive-compulsive personality disorder is marked by a desire for perfection and order at the expense of openness, flexibility, and efficiency. The person with this disorder sees the world as black and white. Along with perfectionism comes relentless anxiety about not getting things perfect. The patient with obsessive-compulsive personality disorder places a great deal of pressure on himself or herself and those around him or her. Mistakes are viewed as unacceptable and the patient with this disorder may have a constant sense of righteous indignation and feel anger and contempt for anyone who disagrees with him or her.

My way or the highway

Patients with this disorder view their methods as the only right way; all other ways are wrong according to their view. Their inflexibility extends to interpersonal relationships, as well as daily routines. A lifelong pattern of rigid thinking may lead to poor social skills.

Controlling nature

Those with obsessive-compulsive personality disorder have an overwhelming need to control the environment. They may force themselves and others to follow rigid moral principles and conform to extremely high standards of performance. Conscientious, scrupulous, and inflexible about morality, ethics, and value, they insist on literal compliance with authority and rules.

Indecisive impasse

In their effort to avoid being wrong, they may suffer severe procrastination and indecisiveness because they cannot determine with certainty which choice is correct. They may have trouble even starting a task because of their need to sort out the priorities correctly. Their symptoms may cause extreme distress and interfere with occupational and social functioning. (See *A confusing similarity*, page 540.)

Prevalence

Obsessive-compulsive personality disorder affects about 2.1% to 7.9% of the general population. It is one of the most common personality disorders in the general population. About twice as many males as females are diagnosed with this disorder (APA, 2013). Incidence may be higher among the oldest children in a family and among people whose occupations require attention to detail and methodical perseverance.

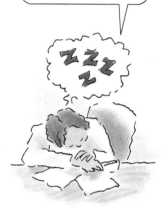

The patient with obsessive-compulsive personality disorder is all bound up in self-imposed rules and regulations.

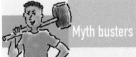

A confusing similarity

Although the two disorders have almost identical names, obsessive-compulsive personality disorder and obsessive-compulsive disorder share little in common.

Myth: Obsessive-compulsive personality disorder is the same thing as obsessive-compulsive disorder.
Reality: Obsessive-compulsive disorder is an anxiety disorder characterized by obsessions and compulsions.

In contrast, obsessive-compulsive *personality* disorder is marked by a constant striving for perfection and control. Obsessions and compulsions aren't a part of the personality disorder because the patient's preoccupation with orderliness isn't intense enough to be considered an obsession.

Causes

Genetic and developmental factors may play a role in the development of this disorder.

Psychodynamic theories view the patient's needing control as a defense against feelings of powerlessness or shame. Individuals diagnosed with obsessive personality disorder often experienced harsh discipline during childhood (Sadock & Sadock, 2015).

Signs and symptoms

A patient with obsessive-compulsive personality disorder may describe his or her symptoms in a logical way, attaching little emotion to any physical discomfort. Assessment findings commonly include:
- behavioral, emotional, and cognitive rigidity
- perfectionism
- severe self-criticism
- indecisiveness
- controlling manner
- difficulty expressing tender feelings
- poor sense of humor
- cool, distant, formal manner
- solemn, tense demeanor
- emotional constriction
- excessive discipline
- aggression, competitiveness, and impatience

- bouts of intense anger when things stray from the patient's idea of how things "should be"
- difficulty incorporating new information into his or her life
- psychosomatic complaints
- hypochondriasis
- sexual dysfunction
- chronic sense of time pressure and inability to relax
- indirect expression of anger despite an apparent undercurrent of hostility
- hoarding of money and other possessions
- preoccupation with orderliness, neatness, and cleanliness
- scrupulousness about morality, ethics, or values
- signs and symptoms of depression
- physical complaints (commonly stemming from overwork).

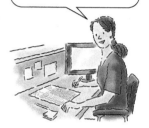

A patient with obsessive-compulsive personality disorder may show signs of indecisiveness.

Diagnosis and treatment

The patient should undergo a psychological evaluation, including personality and projective tests. The diagnosis of obsessive-compulsive personality disorder is confirmed if the patient meets the criteria in the *DSM-5*.

Typically, people with obsessive-compulsive personality disorder seek treatment only if they are depressed, unproductive, or under extreme stress—circumstances that tax their limited coping skills. Treatment usually involves individual psychotherapy, possibly in conjunction with medication.

Psychotherapy

Effective psychotherapeutic treatment centers on short-term symptom relief and support for existing coping mechanisms (with new ones taught as therapy progresses). Long-term work on changing the personality is unrealistic because the inherent nature of obsessive-compulsive personality disorder makes it especially resistant to change.

Down to business

The therapist should discuss the nature of the disease process and explain typical treatments in a businesslike, factual manner rather than give vague impressions. When patients accept the treatment regimen, they are likely to adhere to it rigorously and strive to be a good patient. They are conscientious, honest, motivated, and hardworking.

Ideally, therapy should replace skills that aren't working with new skill sets, examine social relationships, and identify feeling states. Proper identification and realization of feelings can help produce changes in the patient's life.

Focus on feelings

Because the patients with obsessive-compulsive personality disorder are likely to be out of touch with their emotions, the therapist should lead them away from describing situations, events, and daily happenings. A better approach is to have them express how these events make them feel. Having these patients keep a daily journal of feelings can help them remember how they felt at any given time. Cognitive approaches rarely work with these patients because they are likely to use this type of therapy as a means for verbally attacking the therapist or otherwise taking the focus off himself or herself.

Group therapy

The patients may find group therapy intolerable because of the social contact necessary in healthy group dynamics. In fact, group members may ostracize these patients if they point out their deficits and incorrect ways of doing things.

Pharmacologic therapy

SSRIs are approved by the FDA for use in obsessive-compulsive disorder, which is the more severe form of this disorder. "Clomipramine (Anafranil) may help reduce the obsessions, anxiety, and depression associated with this disorder" (Halter, 2018, p. 458).

Nursing interventions

These nursing interventions may be appropriate for patients with obsessive-compulsive personality disorder:

- Offer persistent, consistent, and flexible care. Take a direct, involved approach to gain trust.
- Let the patient control his or her own treatment plan by giving choices whenever possible.
- Maintain a professional attitude. Avoid informality; these patients want strict attention to detail.

Don't get too close

- Recognize the need for adequate personal space.

Pay attention!

- Be prepared for long monologues centering on the patient's goals and ambitions and reasons why family members, friends, and work subordinates need to be rigidly controlled. Try to remain attentive.

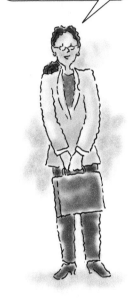

A businesslike approach is best if your patient has obsessive-compulsive personality disorder.

- Use tolerance and ordinary kindness when dealing with these patients. Remember that they are used to causing exasperation in others but do not fully understand why.
- Avoid defensive behavior and arguments with patients with obsessive-compulsive personality disorder.

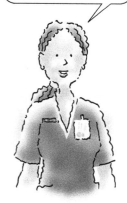

Try to be attentive even if your patient rambles on about others' faults.

No-pressure tactics

- Don't brush aside issues that the patient thinks are important in an effort to get on with affective issues. Pressuring the patient to focus prematurely on emotions will alienate him or her.
- If appropriate, encourage the patient to record his or her feelings in a journal.
- Remember that the patient's defensive structure (which makes him or her seem arrogant and argumentative) is a cover for his or her vulnerability to shame, humiliation, and dread.

Teaching topics

- Teach the patients social skills and reinforce appropriate behaviors.
- Teach them about prescribed medication.
- Encourage them to continue therapy for optimal results.

Quick quiz

1. Which personality disorder is characterized primarily by mistrust?
   A. Paranoid personality disorder.
   B. Antisocial personality disorder.
   C. Dependent personality disorder.
   D. Schizotypal personality disorder.

Answer: A. Paranoid personality disorder is characterized by an extreme distrust of others. Patients with this disorder avoid relationships in which they aren't in control or have the potential of losing control.

2. What is the treatment of choice for patients with most personality disorders?
   A. Group therapy.
   B. Individual psychotherapy.
   C. Self-help support groups.
   D. Inpatient therapy.

Answer: B. Individual psychotherapy is usually the treatment of choice for patients with personality disorders.

3.   In which personality disorder can ideas of reference and magical thinking occur?
   A.   Borderline personality disorder.
   B.   Schizotypal personality disorder.
   C.   Schizoid personality disorder.
   D.   Histrionic personality disorder.

Answer: B. Schizotypal personality disorder is marked by ideas of reference, odd beliefs, or magical thinking, among other features.

4.   What behavior is a hallmark of borderline personality disorder?
   A.   Irresponsibility.
   B.   Reckless disregard for others.
   C.   Impulsivity.
   D.   Unlawful behavior.

Answer: C. Impulsivity is the most prominent characteristic of borderline personality disorder.

5.   The nurse is caring for a patient with dependent personality disorder who reports physical concerns. How would the nurse respond?
   A.   Overlook the symptoms.
   B.   Encourage the patient to talk about his or her symptoms.
   C.   Disregard symptoms until emotional issues have been explored.
   D.   Explore symptoms in a matter-of-fact way.

Answer: D. The nurse should explore the patient's symptoms in a matter-of-fact way. Although physical complaints should be evaluated promptly, caregivers shouldn't encourage the patient to talk about them.

6.   Which personality disorder is reflected in a patient who is preoccupied with details and lists?
   A.   Histrionic personality disorder.
   B.   Obsessive-compulsive personality disorder.
   C.   Schizotypal personality disorder.
   D.   Narcissistic personality disorder.

Answer: B. Obsessive-compulsive personality disorder is marked by a preoccupation with details, lists, rules, and schedules.

Scoring

☆☆☆   If you answered all six items correctly, take a bow! We won't hold it against you if you're feeling a bit narcissistic right now.

☆☆   If you answered four or five items correctly, you certainly don't need to be rescued. You're right on the borderline between good and excellent.

☆   If you answered fewer than four items correctly, don't get histrionic. Just cling to this chapter a little longer.

Selected references

American Psychiatric Association. (2013). *Diagnostic and statistical manual of mental disorders* (5th ed.). Author.

Ben-Porath, Y., & Tellegen, A. (2008). *The Minnesota multiphasic personality inventory-2 restructured form (MMPI-2-RF)*. https://www.upress.umn.edu/test-division/MMPI-2-RF

Benson, H. (1975). *The relaxation response*. HarperCollins.

Black, D. (2019). Treatment of antisocial personality disorder. *UpToDate*. https://www.uptodate.com/contents/treatment-of-antisocial-personality-disorder

Boyd, M. (2018). *Psychiatric nursing: Contemporary practice* (6th ed.). Lippincott Williams & Wilkins.

Ferreira, L. F., Pereira, F. H., Benevides, A. M., & Melo, M. C. (2018). Borderline personality disorder and sexual abuse: A systematic review. *Psychiatry Research, 262*, 70–77. https://doi.org/10.1016/j.psychres.2018.01.043

Halter, M. (2018). *Varicolis' foundation of psychiatric mental health nursing: A clinical approach* (8th ed.). Elsevier.

Personality. (n.d.). In *Merriam-Webster's online dictionary*. http://www.merriam-webster.com/dictionary/personality

Sadock, B. J., & Sadock, V. A. (2015). *Synopsis of psychiatry* (11th ed.). Lippincott Williams & Wilkins.

Schreiber, J., & Culpepper, L. (2019). Suicidal ideation and behavior in adults. *UpToDate*. https://www.uptodate.com/contents/suicidal-ideation-and-behavior-in-adults

Skodol, A. (2018). Psychotherapy for borderline personality disorder. *UpToDate*. https://www.uptodate.com/contents/psychotherapy-for-borderline-personality-disorder

Townsend, M. (2014). *Psychiatric mental health nursing: Concepts of care in evidence-based practice* (8th ed.). F.A. Davis.

Volkert, J., Gablonski, T., & Rabung, S. (2018). Prevalence of personality disorders in the general adult population in Western countries: Systematic review and meta-analysis. *The British Journal of Psychiatry, 213*(6), 709–715. https://doi.org/10.1192/bjp.2018.202

Appendices and index

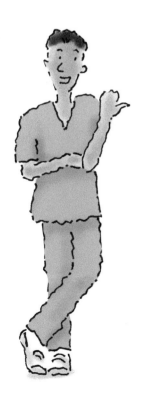

Practice makes perfect

1. The nurse is collaborating with a patient diagnosed with obsessive-compulsive disorder (OCD) to develop holistic treatment options. Which nursing intervention is appropriate? **Select all that apply.**
    A. Practice deep breathing.
    B. Engage in guided imagery.
    C. Avoid exposure to stressors.
    D. Participate in individual and group therapy sessions.
    E. Complete exposure and response prevention (ERP) therapy.

2. A patient with OCD believes that children will die if praying every 20 minutes per hour does not occur. The nurse understands that this compulsive behavior is rooted in what need?
    A. Receipt of affirmation
    B. Decrease in physical pain
    C. Reduction of anxiety and fear
    D. Desire to receive gratification

3. The nurse is caring for a patient who reports having an obsession about hitting people. Which nursing intervention is the priority?
    A. Perform a self-evaluation.
    B. Provide a safe environment.
    C. Help the patient identify specific triggers.
    D. Use an interprofessional approach to care.

4. The nurse is caring for a patient that is dangerously underweight who refuses to eat any food other than apples, stating "other foods are poison." Which nursing response is appropriate?
    A. "Other food is really good for you."
    B. "What makes you feel other foods are poison?"
    C. "You have so much to live for, so you need to eat."
    D. "Can you understand that your beliefs are killing you?"

5. The nurse is caring for a patient with body dysmorphic disorder who recently had a fourth rhinoplasty, stating "my nose just didn't look right." What assessment data does the nurse anticipate collecting at this time?
    A. Reluctance to look at the postsurgical nose
    B. Satisfaction with the nose's appearance after the fourth surgery
    C. Acceptance of the health team's recommendation for no more surgery
    D. Desire to continue seeking future interventions to enhance appearance

6. Which verbal assessment tool will the nurse choose to assess a patient for hoarding disorder? **Select all that apply.**
    A. Life Event Checklist (LEC)
    B. Hoarding Rating Scale (HRS) (verbal tool)
    C. Saving Inventory-Revised (SIR) (verbal tool)
    D. Clutter Image Rating Scale (CIRS) (picture-based tool)
    E. Patient Health Questionnaire 9 (PHQ-9)

7. A patient's spouse reports that the patient has been collecting fast food containers that have become a clutter and hazard in their home; the patient states that this is "not a problem" How does the nurse document the patient's understanding of this behavior?
    A. Poor insight
    B. Flight of ideas
    C. Magical thinking
    D. Healthy recycling habits

8. The caregiver of a 9-year-old patient expresses a disbelief in childhood depression. What is the appropriate nursing response?
    A. "I must say that I agree with you."
    B. "Research is mixed regarding whether childhood depression exists."
    C. "Children may experience depression."
    D. "Why do you think children can't have depression?"

9. A caregiver tells the nurse that a 5-year-old patient has difficulty talking with other children when playing. Which disorder does the nurse anticipate?
    A. Language disorder
    B. Speech sound disorder
    C. Childhood-onset fluency disorder
    D. Social (pragmatic communication) disorder

10. A caregiver requests that the health care provider assess a 2-year-old patient for attention-deficit hyperactivity disorder (ADHD). What is the appropriate nursing response?
    A. "I can schedule the appointment for you now."
    B. "Children aged 4 and older can be evaluated."
    C. "Why do you think your child has ADHD?"
    D. "Caregiver and teacher input determine the ADHD diagnosis."

11. A 12-year-old patient with ADHD who started taking atomoxetine (Strattera) 2 weeks ago reports feeling no better and describes ongoing feelings of inattentiveness. What is the appropriate nursing response?
    A. "It will take up to 4 weeks for the effect to be noticed."
    B. "Have you spoken to your health care provider about this problem?"
    C. "It is likely that you will need a different type of drug to treat ADHD."
    D. "Let's speak to your provider about increasing the dose of your medicine."

12. The nurse is teaching a female patient who plans to become pregnant about risk factors associated with intellectual disability. What teaching will the nurse provide? **Select all that apply.**
    A.   Avoid environmental toxins.
    B.   Cut down on alcohol consumption.
    C.   Consume less leafy green vegetables.
    D.   Attend all prenatal check-ups as scheduled.
    E.   Plan ahead for how the baby will be cared for after birth.

13. Which nursing intervention is appropriate when caring for a patient with dissociative identity disorder? **Select all that apply.**
    A.   Establish clear boundaries.
    B.   Establish trusting relationship.
    C.   Monitor for suicidal ideation.
    D.   Help patient uncover subconscious causes of trauma.
    E.   Identify emotions that occur while patient is under stress.

14. What is the priority nursing intervention when the nurse begins to care for a patient found walking on the side of a road with no memory of how they got there?
    A.   Establish a trusting relationship.
    B.   Test for the presence of substances.
    C.   Complete a physical assessment.
    D.   Obtain a complete medical history.

15. Which patient statement does the nurse identify that is associated with derealization?
    A.   "Time is moving in slow motion."
    B.   "I am a giant."
    C.   "I feel like I am outside my body watching myself."
    D.   "I am the president of the United States."

16. A patient who has been experiencing continuous conflict with a coworker comes to the clinic reporting ongoing abdominal pain. When all diagnostic testing is negative, which origin does the nurse anticipate?
    A.   Manipulation
    B.   Constipation
    C.   Primary gain
    D.   Family stressors

17. A patient with somatic symptom disorder reports taking off work at least 3 days weekly due to headaches. Which term would the nurse associate with this behavior?
    A.   Primary gain
    B.   Manipulation
    C.   Secondary gain
    D.   Hypochondriacism

18. The nurse is caring for a patient with somatic symptom disorder who has visited the emergency department daily for the past week for chest pain. Which assessment question is appropriate when the patient reports chest pain today? **Select all that apply.**
    A. "Can you rate your pain on a scale of 1 to 10?"
    B. "Are you using any prescription or illicit drugs?"
    C. "Do you have a history of anxiety or depression?"
    D. "Why are you returning to the emergency department again?"
    E. "Do you have a way to pay for the visits you've had this week?"

19. The nurse is caring for a patient with conversion disorder who reports being unable to move the left side of the body. Which assessment finding during the neurologic examination does the nurse anticipate? **Select all that apply.**
    A. Normal pupillary responses
    B. Lack of pupillary responses
    C. Tendon reflexes on the left side
    D. Lack of tendon reflexes on the left side
    E. Tendon reflexes on the right side
    F. Lack of tendon reflexes on the right side

20. When assessing a newly admitted patient with schizophrenia, which assessment data will the nurse document a negative symptom? **Select all that apply.**
    A. Asociality
    B. Delusions
    C. Blunted affect
    D. Hallucinations
    E. Poor motivation
    F. Disorganized speech

21. While pacing the room, a patient with rapid and tangential speech reports being followed by the FBI and seeing bugs crawling over the walls. Which diagnosis does the nurse anticipate will be made by the health care provider?
    A. Schizophrenia
    B. Bipolar disorder
    C. Delusional disorder
    D. Schizoaffective disorder

22. Which patient statement demonstrates that nurse teaching about clozapine has been effective? **Select all that apply.**
    A. "I should check my blood glucose levels daily."
    B. "It is important to have my labs drawn regularly."
    C. "This medication will help me with my manic symptoms."
    D. "If I miss the morning dose, I can take it with my bedtime dose."
    E. "When getting out of bed in the morning, I should stand up slowly."
    F. "If I can't sit still and become extremely restless, I should call my provider."

23. A patient with schizophrenia states, "the devil keeps telling me I am going to burn in hell." What is the appropriate nursing response?
    A. "Don't be silly, the voices aren't real; it's all in your head."
    B. "Would you like some medication to make the devil go away?"
    C. "The devil told me you are going to heaven because you have been a good person."
    D. "The voices must be scary for you. What you hear is part of your illness; it is not real."

24. Which drug order will the nurse question for a patient admitted with schizoaffective disorder?
    A. Oxybutynin
    B. Olanzapine
    C. Paliperidone
    D. Lamotrigine

25. A patient with schizophrenia reports to the emergency room stating, "my head itches and bugs are crawling into my brain." What is the priority nursing response?
    A. Assess the patient for head lice.
    B. Offer medication to help the patient feel more relaxed.
    C. Allow the patient to wash hair to address the itching sensation.
    D. Reorient to reality and explain that bugs are a somatic delusion.

26. A patient hospitalized in an inpatient psychiatric unit states that all meals taste sour and rotten. How will the nurse document this type of hallucination?
    A. Tactile
    B. Auditory
    C. Olfactory
    D. Gustatory

27. The nurse is caring for a patient whose family reports have a history of promiscuous behavior, charging $10,000 on credit cards for designer merchandise and not taking medication as prescribed. Which diagnosis does the nurse anticipate when logging into the electronic health record?
    A. Bipolar I disorder
    B. Bipolar II disorder
    C. Cyclothymic disorder
    D. Major depressive disorder

28. The nurse is teaching a patient about newly prescribed lithium. Which patient statement requires further teaching?
    A. "I will plan to have frequent bloodwork done at the laboratory."
    B. "My usual fluid intake is 2,800 mL per day, so that should be OK."
    C. "I will eat a diet that is rich in vitamins and minerals from plants and fruits."
    D. "Vomiting and dizziness should disappear in a few days after starting the medicine."

29. While the nurse leads a group session, a patient with mania becomes disruptive by interrupting others who are trying to participate. What is the nurse's appropriate action?
    A. Ignore the behavior.
    B. Allow the patient with mania to speak.
    C. Set limits and ask the patient to not interrupt.
    D. Have the patient with mania leave the group immediately.

30. A patient with cyclothymia is experiencing a hypomanic phase. Which patient statement does the nurse identify that reflects this phase? **Select all that apply.**
    A. "I feel hopeless."
    B. "I have so much energy."
    C. "My thoughts are racing."
    D. "It's hard to sit still in class."
    E. "I've lost interest in things I used to enjoy."
    F. "I am sleeping a lot more than usual at night."

31. A patient with bipolar disorder paces around the unit, bangs on the door demanding to leave, and becomes verbally threatening to others. What is the priority nursing intervention?
    A. Administer medication to decrease agitation.
    B. Clear the unit and ask other patients to go to their rooms.
    C. Escort the patient to the seclusion room for decreased stimulation.
    D. Inform the patient that only a health care provider can give an order for discharge.

32. Which drug order will the nurse question when caring for a patient with cyclothymic disorder?
    A. Sertraline
    B. Verapamil
    C. Lamotrigine
    D. Valproic acid

33. The caregiver of a 2-year-old reports that the toddler does not want to cuddle with the caregiver, other than at select times such as after naptime, before bedtime, or after a bath. What nursing response is appropriate?
   A. "It is important to talk to the provider about testing for autism."
   B. "Why do you think there is something wrong with your child?"
   C. "The child is at high risk for developing oppositional defiant disorder."
   D. "This is a normal developmental expectation, as the child develops independence."

34. When teaching the caregivers of a child with oppositional defiant disorder, which caregiver statement requires further teaching? **Select all that apply.**
   A. "Medication will make this condition go away."
   B. "We will establish boundaries regarding behavior."
   C. "It may be helpful for our child to talk about feelings of anger."
   D. "There will be appropriate consequences when limits are exceeded."
   E. "We will acknowledge our child's good behavior when it happens."

35. The nurse is admitting a 14-year-old patient who fights constantly with family, has been noted to inflict pain upon the family dog, and has run away from home three times. Which priority assessment question will the nurse ask of the caregiver? **Select all that apply.**
   A. "Do you know how tall your child is?"
   B. "How much did the child weigh at birth?"
   C. "Are your child's vaccinations up to date?"
   D. "Did you experience any birth complications?"
   E. "Does your child have a history of head injuries?"

36. Which statement by the caregiver of a 15-year-old child with a major depressive disorder reflects understanding of the plan of care provided by the nurse?
   A. "My child probably is just feeling a little bit down."
   B. "I will watch my child for signs or symptoms of suicidal ideation."
   C. "After a month of medication, my child won't need to take anything."
   D. "Effects of this drug should start within a couple of days of taking it."

37. The nurse is collaborating with a patient with female sexual interest/arousal disorder. Which action will the nurse encourage the patient to do? **Select all that apply.**
   A. Practice squeeze play.
   B. Engage in sexual fantasies.
   C. Self-administer vasodilator agents.
   D. Reduce stressors through lifestyle changes.
   E. Participate regularly in group therapy sessions.

38. The nurse is caring for a patient who reports an inability to control pedophilic behaviors at home. Which nursing intervention is the priority?
   A. Participate in group therapy.
   B. Urge to try new coping strategies.
   C. Refer to professional psychological counseling.
   D. Ask if he or she has access to children at home or locally.

39. A patient tells the nurse that he has had difficulty achieving and maintaining a rigid penis during sexual activity for the past 9 months. Which sexual dysfunction does the nurse anticipate?
   A. Erectile dysfunction
   B. Delayed ejaculation
   C. Premature ejaculation
   D. Male hypoactive sexual desire disorder

40. A patient discontinued taking a medication that was causing medication-induced sexual dysfunction 2 days ago. The patient reports seeing no improvement in sexual function. Which is the appropriate nursing response?
   A. "It may take 1 to 2 weeks for you to see improvement."
   B. "Discuss this with your health care provider as soon as possible."
   C. "Begin taking the medication again as it isn't helping your sexual function."
   D. "It may be likely that you have other causes affecting your sexual function."

41. Which patient statement demonstrates that nursing teaching about sildenafil has been effective? **Select all that apply.**
   A. "I may get back pain and a headache."
   B. "My lab values should be taken every 6 months."
   C. "I will need to change positions slowly while taking this medication."
   D. "I need to seek medical treatment if my erection lasts longer than 4 hours."
   E. "If I have vision loss, I should call my provider and avoid taking the medication."

42. A patient is at high risk for suicide. Which treatment will the nurse anticipate as a priority?
    A. Behavioral therapy
    B. Group cognitive therapy
    C. Monoamine oxidase inhibitors (MAOIs)
    D. Selective serotonin reuptake inhibitors (SSRIs)

43. A patient at a health clinic tells the nurse, "I'm so depressed." Using the SADPERSONS Scale, the nurse assesses that the patient has a score of 8. Which action would the nurse take first?
    A. Educate about sleep routine.
    B. Encourage inpatient therapy.
    C. Prepare for electroconvulsive treatments.
    D. Administer prescribed SSRIs.

44. A patient with major depressive disorder is prescribed an SSRI and a tricyclic antidepressant (TCA). Which teaching will the nurse include in the patient's plan of care? **Select all that apply.**
    A. Report thoughts of harming yourself.
    B. Encourage a follow-up visit after 2 months of drug therapy.
    C. Avoid foods or fluids that contain tyramine, caffeine, or tryptophan.
    D. Continue to take the medications daily even if you are feeling better.
    E. It may take several medication adjustments before you are feeling like yourself.

45. A nurse is teaching a patient about to undergo electroconvulsive therapy (ECT). Which patient statement requires further teaching?
    A. "I may receive oxygen during the treatment."
    B. "I need to fast for 6 to 8 hours before the treatment."
    C. "I can leave in my dentures throughout the procedure."
    D. "I will feel the electrical current for only 30 seconds to 1 minute."

46. A nurse is caring for a patient with major depressive disorder. Which intervention will the nurse include in the patient's plan of care? **Select all that apply.**
    A. Encourage fluid intake.
    B. Offer small, frequent meals.
    C. Assist the patient with personal hygiene.
    D. Plan activities for times when the patient's energy level peaks.
    E. Allow the patient to have several hours of privacy during the day.

47. A nurse is caring for a patient with substance use disorder. Which sign/symptom will the nurse monitor for as a complication from long-term IV substance misuse?
    A. Fever and chills
    B. Urinary retention
    C. Peripheral edema
    D. Shortness of breath with exertion

48. A nurse is caring for a patient with diaphoresis, agitation, and violent behaviors relating to alcohol withdrawal. Which action will the nurse take first?
    A. Encourage fluids and monitor output.
    B. Educate family members about Al-Anon.
    C. Assess vital signs and level of consciousness.
    D. Approach the patient in a nonthreatening manner.

49. A nurse is caring for a patient who is prescribed disulfiram. Which symptom will the nurse teach regarding a disulfiram reaction? **Select all that apply.**
    A. Flushing
    B. Chest pain
    C. Diaphoresis
    D. Hallucinations
    E. Severe diarrhea

50. A nurse is caring for a patient who is experiencing sudden amphetamine withdrawal. Which action will the nurse take?
    A. Monitor liver enzymes.
    B. Apply a hyperthermia blanket.
    C. Provide one-to-one observation.
    D. Encourage the patient to stay awake.

51. A nurse is teaching a group of laypersons in the community about marijuana (cannabis). Which layperson statement indicates a need for further teaching?
    A. "Marijuana is safer to use than opiates."
    B. "Marijuana smoke can harm the lungs."
    C. "Cannabis use does not affect judgment or coordination."
    D. "Cannabidiol (CBD) does not give the person a 'high' when smoked or eaten."

52. After a rape, a patient is diagnosed with posttraumatic stress disorder (PTSD). When developing a plan of care, which action will the nurse implement first?
    A. Assist patient in recalling the details of the violent act.
    B. Administer medications prescribed by the health care provider.
    C. Promote an environment that is conducive to establishing a trusting relationship.
    D. Teach the patient coping skills such as deep breathing, relaxation techniques, and meditation.

53. A young child is found wandering the hospital alone. A nurse approaches the toddler and asks, "Where is your mommy?" The child responds, "I don't know, but I can go to your house." What does this child's response demonstrate?
   A. Exhibitionism
   B. Social isolation or withdrawal
   C. A potential lack of bonding as an infant
   D. Normal growth and development behavior

54. A patient with adjustment disorder was admitted yesterday and has not been out in the dining room for meals. Which nursing response is appropriate?
   A. "Where would you like to eat your dinner this evening?"
   B. "If it makes you feel comfortable, I will bring your dinner tray to your room."
   C. "Let me walk with you to the dining room and I will sit with you while you eat."
   D. "You will start to feel better if you get out of your room and eat with the other patients."

55. A patient with a history of panic attacks says, "I feel trapped after I have a panic attack." The nurse understands that the patient is experiencing which fear?
   A. Loss of control
   B. Loss of identity
   C. Loss of maturity
   D. Loss of memory

56. A nurse is creating a plan of care for a patient with acute stress disorder following a catastrophic event where others died. Which nursing intervention will the nurse include?
   A. Avoid discussing the stressful event.
   B. Teach bonding or attachment activities.
   C. Help the patient to identify feelings associated with survivor's guilt.
   D. Educate the patient on how to respond the next time the event happens.

57. A nurse is caring for a patient during a panic attack. Which nursing action is appropriate?
   A. Teach the patient about the causes of panic attacks.
   B. Ask close-ended questions during the panic attack.
   C. Encourage the patient to participate in group therapy.
   D. Ensure the environment is safe and secure for the patient.

58. A patient with frequent panic attacks states, "My health care provider said I needed cognitive restructuring. Is this going to hurt?" Which nursing response is appropriate?
    A. "Yes, it will be uncomfortable for 30 to 60 seconds during the treatment."
    B. "No, it will not hurt but it may cause you to have a headache afterward."
    C. "Yes, however, it will make your panic attacks go away after five treatments."
    D. "No. It is about teaching you how to think differently about the panic attacks."

59. A patient has been prescribed alprazolam. Which statement will the nurse make to the patient?
    A. "Avoid drinking grapefruit juice."
    B. "It may take 6 to 8 weeks for improvement."
    C. "Monitor your blood pressure everyday."
    D. "If you miss a dose, double the next dose."

60. A patient with frequent panic attacks is talking with the nurse. Which patient statement indicates the patient is improving?
    A. "I can control my anxiety."
    B. "I no longer have any guilt feelings."
    C. "I take my medications daily as prescribed."
    D. "I am starting to think about what triggers my panic attacks."

61. A nurse is caring for a patient with generalized anxiety disorder and who is currently experiencing anxiety. Which nursing action is appropriate? **Select all that apply.**
    A. Stay with the patient.
    B. Use distraction techniques.
    C. Dim lights, reduce noise, avoid crowds.
    D. Assist the patient through guided imagery.
    E. Administer antianxiety medication as prescribed.

62. A nurse is reviewing laboratory values for a patient with anorexia nervosa. Which lab value requires the nurse to take action first?
    A. Leukopenia
    B. Hypokalemia
    C. Decreased hemoglobin
    D. Elevated blood urea nitrogen

63. A nurse is assessing a patient newly diagnosed with anorexia nervosa. Which assessment finding will the nurse anticipate? **Select all that apply.**
   A. Hallucinations
   B. Cold intolerance
   C. Rapid weight gain
   D. Distorted body image
   E. Obsession with food

64. Which assessment finding for a patient with anorexia nervosa does the nurse identify that may require inpatient therapy?
   A. Heart rate 58
   B. Temperature 102.5 °F
   C. Body mass index 10
   D. Systolic blood pressure 98

65. A patient who has anorexia nervosa is on a behavior modification approach to support weight gain. Which assessment will the nurse make to ensure the weight is accurate when weighing the patient? **Select all that apply.**
   A. Anticipate a weight gain of 1 to 3 lb per week.
   B. Weigh before breakfast, after voiding, using the same scale.
   C. Observe the patient for any additional clothing when weighing.
   D. Allow the patient to weigh themselves and maintain a weight log.
   E. Encourage the patient to avoid drinking large amounts of fluids before weighing.

66. Which assessment finding will the nurse anticipate for a patient with bulimia nervosa?
   A. Muscle atrophy
   B. Body mass index below 20
   C. Emaciated body appearance
   D. Persistent sore throat and heartburn

67. The nurse is assessing a patient who reports a diagnosis of a personality disorder. Which patient statement causes the nurse to question the diagnosis?
   A. "I was acting odd for a few weeks and my psychiatrist diagnosed me with a personality disorder."
   B. "I have paranoid personality disorder that makes me suspicious of others."
   C. "Sometimes I misinterpret humor because I am suspicious of people."
   D. "I was mandated by the court to be here for treatment."

68. The nurse is caring for a patient with antisocial personality disorder. What signs and symptoms would the nurse anticipate? **Select all that apply.**
    A. Impulsive behavior
    B. Destructive behavior
    C. Aggressive speech
    D. Attempts to manipulate interactions
    E. Lack of strong emotions
    F. Feelings of unworthiness

69. A patient with antisocial personality disorder has been mandated by the court to receive therapy. Which nursing statement is appropriate?
    A. "Anything you say here is confidential."
    B. "The law protects your confidentiality related to mental health care."
    C. "I will be reporting your progress to the courts."
    D. "If you do not cooperate with me, I will need to report to the court."

70. The nurse is caring for a patient with borderline personality disorder. Which nursing action is appropriate?
    A. Initiate a safety contract.
    B. Allow freedom in the treatment setting.
    C. Assess for self-injury and suicidality.
    D. Refer the patient for solution-based therapy.

71. The nurse is caring for a group of patients in an inpatient psychiatric unit. Which patient would the nurse suspect has the diagnosis of histrionic personality disorder?
    A. A patient who is withdrawn and unable to focus on others.
    B. A patient who is manipulative and seeking ways to control others.
    C. A patient with a grandiose presentation and flair for drama.
    D. A patient who is enraged in response to criticism.

72. The nurse is caring for a patient who is in the midst of transitioning from a natal sex male named Chris to a transgender woman named Christie. How will the nurse address the patient?
    A. "Hello Chris, it's good to see you today."
    B. "Christie, I'm going to be your nurse."
    C. "My name is Nurse Jake, how may I address you?"
    D. "I'm not sure whether to call you Chris or Christie."

73. The nurse is caring for a patient who lost his spouse 4 months ago. Which signs would alert the nurse to anticipate a diagnosis of complicated grief or grief disorder?
    A. Disorganization in the activities of daily living.
    B. A feeling of disbelief that they still cannot believe the spouse is gone.
    C. An urge to join the deceased in death.
    D. Hearing the loved one's voice while trying to fall asleep.

74. The nurse is teaching a patient's family about delirium. Which teaching will the nurse include? **Select all that apply.**
    A. Delirium is always caused by another condition.
    B. Delirium does not go away.
    C. Delirium comes on suddenly and can affect the level of consciousness.
    D. Delirium can cause tremors and incontinence.
    E. Delirium only affects physiologic behavior, not cognitive response.

75. The nurse is caring for a patient who was recently diagnosed with Alzheimer's disease (AD). Which patient statement requires nursing education?
    A. "At least we caught it early so it will improve with treatment."
    B. "I knew my risk was higher since my mother also had AD."
    C. "I guess this is why it takes me longer to do my normal daily tasks."
    D. "I will take the memantine (Namenda) daily to slow the disease progression."

76. The nurse is teaching a group of teens about the importance of adequate rest. What teaching will the nurse include?
    A. Teens need less sleep than their adult parents.
    B. The average teen needs 10 hours of sleep.
    C. Teens have four stages of sleep.
    D. Rapid eye movement (REM) sleep is often decreased in the teenager.

77. The nurse is caring for a patient with obstructive sleep apnea (OSA). What signs of OSA would the nurse expect? **Select all that apply.**
    A. Snoring
    B. Priapism
    C. Depression
    D. Irritability
    E. Memory problems

78. The nurse is caring for a patient with hypersomnolence disorder. What symptoms would the nurse anticipate? **Select all that apply.**
    A. Suddenly falling asleep during activity
    B. Excessive sleepiness on a daily basis
    C. Napping during the day
    D. Short periods of sleep at night
    E. Early awakening with difficulty falling asleep

79. The nurse is teaching a patient with insomnia sleep hygiene. What teaching will the nurse include?
    A. "Watch television in your bed to help you get comfortable."
    B. "Try to go to bed at the same time each night."
    C. "Make sure your bedroom is warm to promote sleep."
    D. "Exercise right before bed to help you release energy."

80. A patient with gender dysphoria states, "My gender identity is female." How will the nurse interpret this statement?
    A. The patient's assigned gender is female.
    B. The patient experiences gender as female.
    C. The patient is a transgendered female.
    D. The patient's natal sex is male.

Answers

CN: –Client Needs Category

CNS: —Client Needs Subcategory.

NOTE: There are no CNSs for the CN of Psychosocial Integrity. (CNS is only applicable to Safe and Effective Care Environment, and Physiological Integrity.)

CL: —Cognitive Level

1. *Correct answers:* A, B, D, E. Rationale: Deep breathing and guided imagery can help the patient decrease an anxiety reaction to stressors. Individual and group therapy, and ERP therapy are evidence-based interventions that can help patients with OCD. Patients should not be encouraged to avoid exposure to stressors, but rather should be encouraged to participate in ERP.
CN: Psychosocial Integrity; CL: Application.

2. *Correct answer:* C. Rationale: Compulsions are intended to reduce a patient's anxiety or fear, or to prevent a dreaded occurrence from happening.
CN: Psychosocial Integrity; CL: Understanding.

3. *Correct answer:* B. Rationale: Safety is always the priority when caring for any patient.
CN: Psychosocial Integrity; CL: Application.

4. *Correct answer:* B. Rationale: By using an open-ended question, the nurse has effectively used therapeutic communication to allow the patient to express concerns or fears. Stating that food is good, that the patient has much to live for, or insinuating that the patient's beliefs are unfounded or unhealthy is nontherapeutic and nonproductive.
CN: Psychosocial Integrity; CL: Application.

5. *Correct answer:* D. Rationale: Evidence suggests that patients who seek expensive and body-altering treatments do not feel better, and sometimes feel worse, about their appearance following modification. Patients with body dysmorphic disorder continually assess their appearance. These individuals are not likely to accept the health care provider's recommendations, nor to be satisfied with the surgical outcome.
CN: Psychosocial Integrity; CL: Application.

6. *Correct answers:* B, C. Rationale: The HRS and SIR are verbal tools that can be used by the nurse to assess a patient for hoarding disorder. The CIRS can be used to assess for hoarding disorder, but this is a picture-based tool—not a verbal one. The LEC is used to assess for trauma, and the PHQ-9 is used to assess for depression.
CN: Psychosocial Integrity; CL: Application.

7. *Correct answers:* A. Rationale: Individuals with hoarding disorder often have poor insight regarding their behaviors. Flight of ideas includes a rapid shifting of topics that are only loosely associated with each other. Magical thinking is exhibited when a patient believes that his or her actions influence outcomes of events. Collections that become a hazard are not reflective of healthy recycling practices.
CN: Psychosocial Integrity; CL: Application.

8. *Correct answer:* C. Rationale: Children do experience depression and can be diagnosed with this condition. Research is not mixed about the reality of childhood depression. Asking the caregiver "why" is nontherapeutic and increases the likelihood that the caregiver may become defensive.
CN: Psychosocial Integrity; CL: Application.

9. *Correct answer:* D. Rationale: Social (pragmatic communication) disorder involves ongoing difficulty in social use of verbal and nonverbal communication.
CN: Psychosocial Integrity; CL: Understanding.

10. *Correct answer:* B. Rationale: Children as young as 4 can be evaluated for ADHD. Normal childhood development prior to the age of 4 can be mistaken for ADHD. Asking the caregiver "why" they think the child has ADHD can be perceived as demanding an answer, which may elicit a defensive response from the caregiver. Although caregiver and teaching input are important, these alone do not determine an ADHD diagnosis.
CN: Psychosocial Integrity; CL: Understanding.

11. *Correct answer:* A. Rationale: It can take 3 to 4 weeks for the effects of atomoxetine (Strattera) to be felt, so the patient should continue taking the medication until at least that time. Although speaking to the health care provider can be helpful, the same information will be conveyed, so the nurse will intervene first to provide teaching. At this time, a different medication or increasing the dose is not necessary until the full therapeutic effects of this drug can be evaluated after 3 to 4 weeks.
CN: Physiological Integrity; CNS: Pharmacological and Parenteral Therapies; CL: Application.

12. *Correct answers:* A, D, E. Rationale: Intellectual disability has been correlated to environmental toxins, maternal consumption of alcohol and drugs, maternal disease, and severe social deprivation. The nurse will teach the patient to avoid exposure to environmental toxins and to eliminate (not just cut down on) drinking, and to attend all prenatal check-ups because maternal disease can be identified and treated early. Planning ahead for caregiving ensures that the child will receive the necessary social interaction. The patient should not cut down on leafy green vegetables, as these provide important nutrients.
CN: Physiologic Integrity; CL: Application.

13. *Correct answers:* A, B, C, E. Rationale: Nurses can assist patients with dissociative identity disorder by establishing boundaries in the midst of a therapeutic relationship, monitoring for suicidal ideation, and identifying emotions that the patient experiences when under stress. Helping the patient uncover subconscious causes of trauma is the role of a trained therapist or health care provider, not the nurse.
CN: Psychosocial Integrity; CL: Application.

14. *Correct answer:* A. Rationale: A patient found wandering with no memory is likely to be frightened. The nurse needs to first establish a therapeutic relationship of trust; then, a medical history and physical assessment can be performed and subsequent testing can take place.
CN: Psychosocial Integrity; CL: Application.

15. *Correct answer:* A. Rationale: Derealization takes place when the patient's awareness of personal surroundings is altered or lost. Depersonalization occurs when a patient believes something about himself or herself that is not accurate. Stating that one is a president or important figure is an example of grandiose delusion.
CN: Psychosocial Integrity; CL: Application.

16. *Correct answer:* C. Rationale: Primary gain is defined as the unconscious psychological conflict causing physical symptoms. The anxiety is converted to physical symptoms decreasing the level of anxiety. Constipation is a medical diagnosis that has been ruled out

in the scenario. Secondary gain is the benefit of avoiding a stressor. Family stress is not mentioned in the scenario and so it does not apply. Patients with somatic symptom disorder experience true distress; they do not engage in purposeful manipulation.
CN: Psychosocial Integrity; CL: Application.

17. *Correct answer:* C. Rationale: Secondary gain is defined as the benefit or advantage coming from having a certain symptom. Primary gain is the relief of the unconscious psychological conflict, wish, or need that is causing the physical symptom. Patients with somatic symptom disorder experience true distress; they do not engage in purposeful manipulation nor are they considered to be hypochondriac.
CN: Psychosocial Integrity; CL: Application.

18. *Correct answers:* A, B, C. Rationale: The patient with somatic symptom disorder must be treated equally and fairly, without bias, just like any other patient. It is appropriate to gather a full medical and psychosocial history from the patient. It is inappropriate to ask why the patient is returning, because the question "why" can be perceived as nontherapeutic, which can elicit a defensive reply. It is inappropriate to ask if the patient has a way to pay for his or her visits, as this is not the nurse's concern.
CN: Psychosocial Integrity; CL: Application.

19. *Correct answers:* A, C, E. Rationale: The patient with conversion disorder usually has normal and expected anatomic and physiologic responses. The nurse anticipates that the patient will have normal pupillary responses, as well as visible tendon reflexes on the left and right sides of the body.
CN: Psychosocial Integrity; CL: Understanding.

20. *Correct answers:* A, C, E. Rationale: Negative symptoms in a patient with schizophrenia include poor motivation, asociality, and blunted affect. Hallucinations, delusions, and disorganized speech are positive symptoms.
CN: Psychosocial Integrity; CL: Understanding.

21. *Correct answer:* D. Rationale: Hallucinations, delusions, and mania behaviors are consistent with schizoaffective disorder.
CN: Psychosocial Integrity; CL: Understanding.

22. *Correct answers:* B, E, F. Rationale: Orthostatic hypotension is a common side effect of antipsychotic medications, so it is important to stand up slowly from a lying position. Labs should be drawn regularly to monitor white blood cell counts for signs of agranulocytosis. Restlessness (akathisia) is a side effect to an antipsychotic drug and a symptom of EPS (extrapyramidal symptoms) that should be reported to the provider. This medication does not require daily blood glucose

monitoring. Clozaril is an antipsychotic, not an antimania drug. A missed dose of clozaril should not be taken with a subsequent dose.
CN: Physiological Integrity; CNS: Pharmacological and Parenteral Therapies; CL: Analysis.

23. *Correct answer:* D. Rationale: It is important to acknowledge the patient's symptoms and fears, while educating them about symptoms of their illness. Telling the patient to not be silly minimizes the patient's experience. It does not help to state that the voices are in the patient's head, without providing further information. Providing medication may be helpful, but it does not address the patient's statement of concern. The nurse should not acknowledge the voice as being real.
CN: Psychosocial Integrity; CL: Application.

24. *Correct answer:* A. Rationale: The nurse will question the order for oxybutynin, which is a bladder relaxant drug; it is not a drug that treats schizoaffective disorder. Paliperidone, lamotrigine, and olanzapine are used to treat schizoaffective disorder.
CN: Physiological Integrity; CNS: Pharmacological and Parenteral Therapies; CL: Application

25. *Correct answer:* A. Rationale: The nurse must always assess the patient for physical concerns as well as psychiatric symptoms. The nurse's first action will be to determine whether the patient has head lice. If lice are found, the nurse can begin a treatment plan in conjunction with the health care provider to address this problem. If no lice are found, it can be reasonably determined that the patient is experiencing a hallucination. Other actions can take place after determining that the patient does not have a physiologic problem.
CN: Physiologic Integrity; CNS: Reduction of Risk Potential; CL: Application.

26. *Correct answer:* D. Rationale: Gustatory hallucinations are sensations or tastes that are not real. Olfactory hallucinations are smells that are not present. Tactile hallucinations occur when the patient feels something that is not present. Auditory hallucinations are sounds or voices that are not real.
CN: Psychosocial Integrity; CL: Application.

27. *Correct answer:* A. Rationale: These behaviors are all symptoms of bipolar I disorder. The nurse will not make the diagnosis; rather, the nurse anticipates this is the patient's diagnosis because there is a history of these behaviors. Bipolar II disorder, cyclothymic disorder, and major depressive disorder are not characterized by manic behaviors such as promiscuity or spending recklessly.
CN: Psychosocial Integrity; CL: Understanding.

28. *Correct answer:* A. Rationale: Vomiting and dizziness are serious side effects and could be a sign of lithium toxicity. It's important to notify the provider immediately if these symptoms occur. Frequent blood work is necessary to monitor lithium blood levels. Eating a

well-balanced diet and consuming fluid intake between 2,500 mL and 3,000 mL per day are appropriate guidelines for patients taking lithium.

CN: Physiological Integrity; CNS: Pharmacological and Parenteral Therapies; CL: Application

29. *Correct answer:* C. Rationale: It is important to set clear limits when managing patients with manic behaviors. Asking the patient to leave the group may agitate the patient and does not allow the patient to benefit from the group experience. Ignoring the behaviors or allowing the patient to interrupt others reinforces negative behaviors.

CN: Psychosocial Integrity; CL: Application.

30. *Correct answers:* B, C, D. Rationale: Increased energy, restlessness, and racing thoughts are examples of symptoms that appear in the hypomanic phase of cyclothymic disorder. Hypersomnia, hopelessness, and loss of interest are symptoms that occur within the depressive phase.

CN: Psychosocial Integrity; CL: Application.

31. *Correct answer:* B. Rationale: Ensuring the safety of others takes priority over everything else. Once the unit is cleared, staff can then initiate crisis intervention, which may involve medication administration and/or seclusion. Informing the patient that discharge from the hospital requires a health care provider's order can be done after all other actions are taken.

CN: Psychosocial Integrity; CL: Analysis.

32. *Correct answer:* A. Rationale: The nurse will question the order for sertraline, as this is an antidepressant that can induce mania. All other drugs listed can be used in the treatment of a patient with cyclothymic disorder.

CN: Physiologic Integrity; CNS: Pharmacologic and Parenteral Therapies; CL: Application.

33. *Correct answer:* D. Rationale: Children between 18 months and 3 years old begin to see themselves as a separate person from the caregiver. The child is still showing affection at the times it is desired, so this is a normal developmental occurrence. The child is not demonstrating signs of autism, nor is the child at risk for development of oppositional defiant disorder. Asking "why" the caregiver thinks there is something wrong with the child does not address their concern and is nontherapeutic.

CN: Psychosocial Integrity; CL: Application.

34. *Correct answer:* A. Rationale: Medication does not make oppositional defiant disorder go away; it is used to manage symptoms. Therefore, this statement needs further teaching. Establishing boundaries regarding behavior, allowing the child to talk about feelings of anger, administering appropriate consequences for exceeding limits,

and acknowledging the child's good behavior demonstrate appropriate understanding of this condition and do not require further teaching.
CN: Psychosocial Integrity; CL: Analysis.

35. *Correct answers:* B, D, E. Rationale: The child's symptoms are reflective of conduct disorder. Risk factors for the development of conduct disorder include neurologic damage caused by low birth weight or birth complications. A history of head trauma has also been shown to increase risky behaviors. These questions should therefore be asked as the priority. Asking about the child's height and vaccination status is not the priority and should be asked after the priority questions are answered.
CN: Psychosocial Integrity; CL: Analysis.

36. *Correct answer:* B. Rationale: Antidepressant medication has a black box warning to indicate that adolescents may experience suicidal ideation as a result of taking this type of drug. The caregiver has demonstrated understanding by indicating that the child will be monitored for such. Further teaching is needed if the caregiver says the child just feels down, because major depressive disorder is a mood disorder; it is not a feeling. Further teaching is also needed if the caregiver believes only 1 month of medication is needed; generally, the patient will take medication for 6 to 12 months before discontinuation is considered. Further teaching is also needed if the caregiver believes that the drug effects will start within a few days of taking it; most antidepressants take 7 to 14 days to begin therapeutic effect.
CN: Physiological Integrity; CNS: Pharmacological and Parenteral Therapies; CL: Application.

37. *Correct answers:* B, D. Rationale: Engaging in sexual fantasies increases erotic thoughts and can result in sexual interest. Reducing stressors through lifestyle changes can help the patient to increase sexual interest/arousal. Male patients, not females, with erectile dysfunction are encouraged to practice squeeze play and may be prescribed vasodilators for self-injection. Individual therapy and couples therapy are evidence-based treatments for female sexual interest/arousal disorder, but group therapy is not recommended.
CN: Psychosocial Integrity; CL: Application.

38. *Correct answer:* D. Rationale: Identification of children in harm's reach in the patient's environment is the most important safety intervention. The nurse can complete other interventions after addressing the safety of children as the priority.
CN: Psychosocial Integrity; CL: Application.

39. *Correct answer:* A. Rationale: Erectile dysfunction involves the patient's inability to achieve or maintain an erect penis for

penetration. Infrequent, absence, or a delay in ejaculation is known as delayed ejaculation. Premature ejaculation involves the patient's inability to control the ejaculatory reflex during sexual activity, causing an ejaculation to occur prior to or within 1 minute of penetration. A recurrent deficient or absent sexual or erotic thoughts, fantasies, or desire for sexual activity is a manifestation of male hypoactive sexual desire disorder.
CN: Psychosocial Integrity; CL: Understanding.

40. *Correct answer:* A. Rationale: It takes longer than 2 days for some medications to be fully metabolized and excreted from the body and for the body to resume premedicated function. The patient will be educated that it may take 1 to 2 weeks for sexual function to return after discontinuing the medication. Discussing the concerns with the provider may be beneficial; however, this is a concern the nurse can address without a delay. The patient will be given the same information by the provider. The patient should not be told to restart the medication without talking with their provider. The nurse can conduct a discussion with the patient about other contributors in sexual dysfunction, but this should only take place after the medication side effect is addressed.
CN: Physiological Integrity; CNS: Pharmacological and Parenteral Therapies; CL: Application.

41. *Correct answers:* A, C, D, E. Rationale: Side effects of sildenafil (Viagra) include gastrointestinal (GI) upset, headache, back pain, dizziness, one or both eye vision loss, blurred vision, priapism (erection lasting longer than 4 hours), rash, or stuffy or runny nose. Medical attention is needed and the patient should stop taking the medication if priapism or vision changes occur. Lab values associated with sildenafil are not necessary.
CN: Physiological Integrity; CNS: Pharmacological and Parenteral Therapies; CL: Application.

42. *Correct answer:* D. Rationale: The nurse will anticipate the patient being treated with SSRIs and psychotherapy. MAOIs and group cognitive therapy are not recommended as a priority. The nurse will also need to monitor the patient closely as it may take 1 to 2 weeks for medications to be effective.
CN: Physiological Integrity; CNS: Pharmacological and Parenteral Therapies; CL: Analysis.

43. *Correct answer:* B. Rationale: When a patient scores 7 to 10 on the SADPERSONS scale, the patient is at high risk for suicide and should be encouraged to have inpatient therapy. Although inpatient care may include ECT, SSRIs, and education on a sleep routine, inpatient care is needed to closely monitor the patient and keep the patient safe from harming themselves or others.
CN: Psychosocial Integrity; CL: Application.

44. *Correct answers:* A, B, D, E. Rationale: A patient taking an SSRI and/or a TCA needs to report thoughts of suicide or harming oneself or others, as this is an adverse effect. A patient taking any SSRIs or TCAs will be encouraged to follow up with the prescribing provider for reevaluation of medications and dosages and to continue taking medications as prescribed. The patient will need to know that it may take several medication adjustments to find the optimal effectiveness. Patients taking MAOIs—not TCAs and SSRIs—need to avoid foods with tyramine, caffeine, and tryptophan.
CN: Physiological Integrity; CNS: Pharmacological and Parenteral Therapies; CL: Application.

45. *Correct answer:* C. Rationale: Patients preparing to undergo ECT will need to void and remove dentures, contact lenses, glasses, and other items. The patient will need to fast for 6 to 8 hours prior to treatment. Patient teaching will include that the electrical current lasts 30 to 60 seconds and that the patient may receive oxygen during the treatment.
CN: Psychosocial Integrity; CL: Application.

46. *Correct answers:* A, B, C, D. Rationale: Patients who have major depressive disorder may require assistance with personal hygiene and eating/feeding. Offering small, frequent meals may not be as overwhelming to the patient as a full meal. Encouraging fluid intake helps to prevent constipation, a common complication of depression. Patients will participate more in activities when energy levels are high. Patients will be encouraged to socialize (not be isolated) and join in activities during the day to facilitate healing.
CN: Psychosocial Integrity; CL: Application.

47. *Correct answer:* A. Rationale: Gangrene is a complication of long-term IV substance misuse and may present as fever and chills. Peripheral edema, shortness of breath with exertion, and urinary retention are not directly related to complications for a patient with long-term IV substance misuse unless other conditions are comorbid.
CN: Physiological Integrity; CNS: Reduction of Risk Potential; CL: Application.

48. *Correct answer:* D. Rationale: Although all of the nursing actions are appropriate for a patient who is having alcohol withdrawal presenting with agitation and violent behavior, it is important to approach the patient in a nonthreatening manner to avoid further agitation and possible injury to the patient and health care team members.
CN: Psychosocial Integrity; CL: Application.

49. *Correct answers:* A, B, C. Rationale: A patient taking disulfiram for alcohol aversion therapy will have a disulfiram reaction if the patient drinks alcohol. A disulfiram reaction results in flushing,

diaphoresis, and chest pain. Severe diarrhea and hallucinations are not usual manifestations of a disulfiram reaction.
CN: Physiological Integrity; CNS: Pharmacological and Parenteral Therapies; CL: Application.

50. *Correct answer:* C. Rationale: With sudden amphetamine withdrawal, the patient may attempt suicide requiring one-to-one observation or frequent rounding to ensure patient safety. The patient may sleep for a long period of time (does not need to be encouraged to stay awake) and may require cooling blankets (not hyperthermia blankets). Liver enzymes do not need to be monitored unless other conditions warrant it.
CN: Psychosocial Integrity; CL: Application.

51. *Correct answer:* C. Rationale: Marijuana (cannabis) contains over 100 chemicals, two of which are delta-9-tetrahydrocannabinol (THC) and CBD. THC causes the "high" sensation for the person smoking or eating the THC; CBD does not incite the "high." Marijuana smoke can harm the lungs, yet marijuana is safer to use than opiates. The statement, "Cannabis use does not affect judgment or coordination" is incorrect and further teaching is needed.
CN: Psychosocial Integrity; CL: Understand.

52. *Correct answer:* C. Rationale: Establishing a trusting relationship is necessary for the patient to feel comfortable in relating the traumatic experience, accepting medications as prescribed, and participating in using new coping skills.
CN: Psychosocial Integrity; CL: Application.

53. *Correct answer:* C. Rationale: Disinhibited social engagement disorder (DSED) is a pattern of behavior where a child actively approaches and interacts with unfamiliar adults. DSED affects children in their first years of life due to insufficient caregiving. DSED is not a normal growth and development behavior.
CN: Psychosocial Integrity; CL: Application.

54. *Correct answer:* C. Rationale: It is natural for a patient with an adjustment disorder to have challenges acclimating to a new routine. Encouraging the patient to resume normal activities in the appointed location of the dining room assists the patient in coping with the situation. Offering self helps build a trusting relationship with the patient. Telling the patient that eating in a new location will foster better feelings does not address the patient's underlying disorder. The patient will be encouraged to be part of the therapeutic milieu rather than eating alone, or choosing where to eat.
CN: Psychosocial Integrity; CL: Application.

55. *Correct answer:* A. Rationale: Individuals who fear loss of control during a panic attack commonly make statements about feeling trapped, getting hurt, or having little or no personal control over their situations.
CN: Psychosocial Integrity; CL: Application.

56. *Correct answer:* C. Rationale: Nursing interventions for a patient with acute stress disorder include encouraging the patient to discuss the stressful event to validate the situation was beyond the person's control and encouraging the patient to identify feelings of survivor guilt, inadequacy, or blame. Bonding or attachment activities are not appropriate for patients with acute stress disorder.
CN: Psychosocial Integrity; CL: Application.

57. *Correct answer:* D. Rationale: During a panic attack, the patient may feel like they are dying, going crazy, or losing control. Ensuring them that they are in a safe and secure environment will assist in decreasing anxiety. Teaching the patient about their causes of panic attacks, asking the patient close-ended questions, or encouraging the patient to participate in group therapy does not assist the patient in reducing anxiety during an actual panic attack. However, after the patient's environment has been secured, teaching the patient about their causes of panic attacks and encouraging the patient to participate in group therapy may be helpful.
CN: Psychosocial Integrity; CL: Analysis.

58. *Correct answer:* D. Rationale: Cognitive restructuring through cognitive behavioral therapy can be helpful for patients who worry that their panic attacks mean they are going crazy or are about to have a heart attack. This method teaches the patient to replace negative thoughts with more realistic, positive ways of viewing the attacks.
CN: Psychosocial Integrity; CL: Application.

59. *Correct answer:* A. Rationale: Patients taking alprazolam will be educated to avoid drinking grapefruit juice during therapy, as this can potentiate the effects of the drug. Patients will also be educated that if they miss a dose, skip the dose, and resume the normal schedule (do not double the dose). This drug does not require daily blood pressure monitoring. Alprazolam begins to work very quickly; it does not take 6 to 8 weeks to notice improvement.
CN: Physiological Integrity; CNS: Pharmacological and Parenteral Therapies; CL: Application.

60. *Correct answer:* A. Rationale: A patient who states "I can control my anxiety" shows improvement. Taking medications daily as prescribed indicates the patient is adherent to medication treatments yet does not demonstrate improvement. The statement "I am starting to think about what triggers my panic attacks" indicates the patient is taking the first step in being able to control the panic attack, but does not demonstrate improvement yet. Guilt is not always associated with panic attacks; it is much more likely to manifest in patients with acute traumatic stress disorder to PTSD.
CN: Psychosocial Integrity; CL: Application.

61. *Correct answers:* A, B, C, D, E. Rationale: Nursing interventions for a patient experiencing anxiety include staying with the patient during the episode, using distraction techniques, reducing

environmental stimuli, assisting the patient through guided imagery, and administering antianxiety medications as prescribed.
CN: Psychosocial Integrity; CL: Application.

62. *Correct answer:* B. Rationale: Hypokalemia can result in cardiac arrhythmias, electrocardiograph changes such as nonspecific ST intervals, T-wave changes, and cardiac arrest. Leukopenia places the patient at risk for infection. Decreased hemoglobin indicates anemia. An elevated blood urea nitrogen may indicate renal dysfunction.
CN: Physiological Integrity; CNS: Pharmacological and Parenteral Therapies; CL: Analysis.

63. *Correct answer:* B, D, E. Rationale: The patient with anorexia nervosa will have multiple findings such as cold intolerance, distorted body image, obsession with food and weight, amenorrhea, and emaciated appearance. The nurse would not anticipate hallucinations nor rapid weight gain as findings for a patient with anorexia nervosa.
CN: Psychosocial Integrity; CL: Application.

64. *Correct answer:* C. Rationale: A patient with anorexia nervosa requires inpatient therapy for a heart rate consistency below 50, temperature below 97 °F, body mass index below 16, and/or systolic blood pressure below 90. This patient's heart rate and systolic blood pressure do not indicate the need for inpatient treatment; the temperature can be managed in the outpatient setting as this is likely related to infection, not to anorexia nervosa.
CN: Physiological Integrity; CNS: Reduction of Risk Potential; CL: Application.

65. *Correct answer:* B, C. Rationale: Assessments relating to an accurate weight include weighing before breakfast, after voiding, using the same scale, and observing the patient for any additional clothing when weighing. Encouraging the patient to avoid drinking large amounts of fluids is important, however; it is not an assessment. Patients who have anorexia nervosa need to be weighed by a health care worker to ensure an accurate weight. Anticipating a weight gain of 1 to 3 lb is appropriate for the weight plan, however; it is not an assessment.
CN: Physiological Integrity; CNS: Physiological Adaptation; CL: Application.

66. *Correct answer:* D. Rationale: Patients with bulimia nervosa generally have a normal body weight or are slightly overweight, calluses or scarring on the back of the hands from inducing vomiting, and persistent sore throat and heartburn from vomited stomach acids. Muscle atrophy, emaciated body appearance, and a body mass index below 20 are findings associated with anorexia nervosa.
CN: Physiological Integrity; CNS: Physiological Adaptation; CL: Application.

67. *Correct answer:* A. Rationale: Personality disorders are diagnosed based on an enduring pattern of behavior (APA, 2013). As such, acting odd for a few weeks would not cause a diagnosis of a

personality disorder. This would cause the nurse to question the accuracy of the patient's report as well as the accuracy of the diagnosis.
CN: Psychosocial integrity; CL: Application.

68. *Correct answers:* A, B, C, D. Rationale: The patient with antisocial personality disorder has a pattern of disregarding the rights of others as well as societal norms. Signs include: impulsive behavior, deceitfulness, lack of remorse, destructive behavior, aggressive speech and behavior, manipulative behavior with consistent irresponsibility. They often show strong emotions and have an inflated sense of self versus feelings of unworthiness.
CN: Psychosocial Integrity; CL: Application.

69. *Correct answer:* C. Rationale: To establish a therapeutic relationship it is best to let the patient know upfront that progress regarding the patient's therapy will be reported to the court. This can often be done in a manner that protects private details; however, confidentiality in court-mandated therapy is not always protected. Threats to tell the court about behavior are never an appropriate motivational approach.
CN: Psychosocial Integrity; CL: Application.

70. *Correct answer:* C. Rationale: The patient with borderline personality disorder may resort to self-destructive behavior to escape inner turmoil. Suicidal potential should be carefully assessed and monitored throughout the entire course of treatment. Safety (or suicide contracts) is not effective in preventing self-destructive behavior. Firm boundaries and structure are required in the treatment setting and dialectical behavior therapy is the treatment of choice for these patients.
CN: Psychosocial Integrity; CL: Application.

71. *Correct answer:* C. Rationale: The patient with histrionic personality disorder is often charming and overdramatic. This patient will attempt to be the center of attention, often presenting in a grandiose fashion with a flair for drama and self-expression.
CN: Psychosocial Integrity; CL: Application.

72. *Correct answer:* C. The nurse will always introduce himself or herself, and if there is a question about which name a patient prefers, then ask the patient how they prefer to be addressed. The nurse will not assume that the patient wants a certain name. It is unprofessional to state that the nurse does not know how to properly greet a patient.
CN: Psychosocial Integrity; CL: Application.

73. *Correct answer:* C. Rationale: An urge to join the deceased in death is a sign of complicated grief that indicates pathologic grief beyond the normal stages of grief. A feeling of shock and disbelief, disorganization in activities of daily living, as well as hearing the loved one's voice are all considered normal responses to a significant loss.
CN: Psychosocial Integrity; CL: Application.

74. *Correct answers:* A, C, D. Rationale: Delirium is a syndrome that is always secondary to another condition, meaning it is caused by something else. Treating the underlying condition generally stops the delirium. Signs and symptoms of delirium can be physiologic, behavioral, and cognitive. These signs can include tremors, incontinence, and a sudden change in behavior or consciousness.
CN: Physiological Integrity; CNS: Physiological Integrity; CL: Application.

75. *Correct answer:* A. Rationale: AD treatment is not a cure. Drugs can be used to temporarily delay progression or slow the disease progression. However, treatment will not improve existing deficits or prevent the slow, gradual progression of the disease. This statement requires further education from the nurse.
CN: Physiological Integrity; CNS: Pharmacological and Parenteral Therapies; CL: Application.

76. *Correct answer:* B. Rationale: Preadolescents and teens need approximately 10 hours of sleep. Teens require more sleep than their parents who are young and middle-aged adults. Teens (like all people) have five sleep stages. REM sleep is not decreased in the teenager.
CN: Physiologic Integrity; CNS: Physiologic Adaptation; CL: Application.

77. *Correct answers:* A, C, D, E. Rationale: The patient with OSA has an upper airway that becomes blocked during sleep, which impedes airflow. This can cause snoring. The disruption in sleep pattern can lead to depression, irritability, and memory problems. OSA is associated with impotence, not priapism (which is a painful, persistent erection of the penis).
CN: Physiologic Integrity; CNS: Physiologic Adaptation; CL: Application.

78. *Correct answers:* B, C. Rationale: Hypersomnolence disorder is a condition of excessive sleepiness and difficulty awakening on a daily basis. Symptoms include excessive sleepiness during the day, napping during the day, long periods of sleep at night (8 to 12 hours), difficulty awakening in the morning.
CN: Physiologic Integrity; CNS: Physiologic Adaptation; CL: Application.

79. *Correct answer:* B. Rationale: Sleep hygiene incorporates elements that promote sleep, which include going to bed at the same time each night, using the bed only for sleep and sex, making sure the bedroom is cool and dark, and exercising in the evening, not right before bed.
CN: Physiologic Integrity; CNS: Physiologic Adaptation; CL: Application.

80. *Correct answer:* B. Rationale: Gender identity is the way a person feels inside and how they experience gender. This may or may not correlate with the recorded sex at birth.
CN: Psychosocial Integrity; CL: Knowledge.

abreaction: verbalization of a repressed memory, idea, or emotion

abuse: self-administration of any drug in a culturally disapproved manner that causes adverse consequences

acetylcholine: a neurotransmitter in the autonomic nervous system

acting out: repeatedly performing actions without weighing the possible results of those actions

addiction: a behavioral pattern of drug abuse characterized by overwhelming involvement with the use of a drug (compulsive use), the securing of its supply, and a strong tendency to relapse after discontinuation

age-related cognitive decline (ARCD): deficits in memory that do not significantly impact daily function; also called *age-associated cognitive decline*

Alzheimer disease: a progressive, degenerative disorder that attacks the brain's nerve cells, or neurons, resulting in loss of memory, thinking and language skills, and behavioral changes

ambivalence: coexisting, strong positive and negative feelings, leading to emotional conflict

amphetamine: stimulant drugs used to increase alertness, relieve fatigue, and feel stronger and more decisive; used for euphoric effects or to counteract the "down" feeling of tranquilizers or alcohol

anhedonia: a diminished capacity to experience pleasure; may be reflected by a lack of interest in activities, with substantial time spent in purposeless activity

antisocial personality disorder: a pervasive lack of remorse or lack of exhibiting feelings that leads to a total disregard for the rights of others

asociality: a lack of interest in relationships

assigned gender: the genitalia that is present at birth. Also called "sex". "biological sex", or "natal sex"

attention level: ability to concentrate on a task for an appropriate length of time

aversion therapy: application of a painful stimulus that creates an aversion to the obsessed thought leading to the undesirable behavior

avoidant personality disorder: negativity, poor self-esteem, and issues surrounding social interaction; difficulty looking at situations and interactions in an objective manner

Beck Depression Inventory: a tool that helps diagnose depression and determine its severity

blunted affect: a flattening of emotions in which the person's face may appear immobile with poor eye contact and lack of expressiveness

body dysmorphic disorder: preoccupation with an imagined or an actual slight defect in physical appearance

borderline personality disorder: a pattern of instability or impulsiveness in a person's mood, interpersonal relationships, self-esteem, self-identity, behavior, and cognition; originates in early childhood

clang association: words that rhyme or sound alike used in an illogical,

nonsensical manner—for example, "It's the rain, train, pain."

cocaine: a narcotic and stimulant that may be ingested, injected, sniffed, or smoked to obtain its effects

cognition: conscious mental activities: the activities of thinking, understanding, learning, and remembering

cognitive assessment scale: measures orientation, general knowledge, mental ability, and psychomotor function

comorbidity: the existence of two disorders, occurring together in a person

compensation: hiding a weakness by stressing too strongly the desirable strength

comprehension: the ability to understand, retain, and repeat material

compulsion: a preoccupation that's acted out, such as constantly washing one's hands

concept formation: testing the patient's ability to think abstractly

concrete thinking: inability to form or understand abstract thoughts

confabulation: unconscious filling of gaps in memory with fabricated facts and experiences

conversion disorder: disorder in which patients resolve psychological conflicts through the loss of a specific physical function; examples include paralysis, blindness, or the inability to swallow; patients exhibit symptoms that suggest a physical disorder, but evaluation and observation can't determine a physiologic cause

delusions: false ideas or beliefs accepted as real by the patient; somatic illness, depersonalization, and delusions of grandeur, persecution, and reference are common in schizophrenia

dementia: description of a group of symptoms affecting memory, thinking, and social abilities severely enough to interfere with daily functioning

denial: protecting oneself from unpleasant aspects of life by refusing to perceive, acknowledge, or deal with them

dependence: the physiologic state of neuroadaptation produced by repeated administration of drug, necessitating continued administration to prevent the appearance of the withdrawal syndrome

dependent personality disorder: an extreme need to be taken care of that leads to submissive, clinging behavior and fear of separation

depersonalization: a persistent or recurrent feeling that one is detached from one's own mental processes or body

depression: a mood disorder that causes a persistent feeling of sadness and loss of interest

derailment: speech that vacillates from one subject to another; the subjects are unrelated; ideas slip off the track between clauses

derealization: the persistent or recurrent feeling of detachment from other persons, objects, or their surroundings

displacement: misdirecting pent-up feelings toward something or someone that's less threatening than that which triggered the response

dissociation: separating objects from their emotional significance

dyspareunia: painful sexual intercourse; although it occurs in both sexes, it is more common in women

echolalia: meaningless repetition of words or phrases

echopraxia: involuntary repetition of movements observed in others

exhibitionism: exposing one's sex organs and genitalia to strangers; classified as a form of paraphilia

fantasy: creation of unrealistic or improbable images to escape from daily pressures and responsibilities

fetishism: sexual attraction and arousal an individual feels in relation to a specific object, body part, context, or situation, which is used to achieve sexual gratification; classified as a form of paraphilia

flat affect: unresponsive range of emotion, possibly an indication of schizophrenia or Parkinson disease

flight of ideas: rapid succession of incomplete and poorly connected ideas

flooding: a frequent full-intensity exposure, possibly through the use of imagination, to an object that triggers a symptom; produces extreme discomfort

fluid intelligence: a form of intelligence defined as the ability to solve novel problems

focusing: a technique in which the nurse assists the patient in redirecting attention toward something specific, especially if the patient is vague or rambling

frotteurism: touching or rubbing against a nonconsenting or unaware person to achieve sexual satisfaction

fugue: travel away from home with no memory of what happened on these trips

functional dementia scale: measures orientation, affect, and the ability to perform activities of daily living

gender: a social construct of categorization

gender: the behaviors, attitudes, and feelings that are culturally and socially compatible with a person's biological sex

Gender dysphoria: a descriptive term reflecting the conflict that occurs when there is an incongruence between a person's physical or assigned natal sex and the gender with which the person identifies

Gender expression: the way that a person chooses to express gender in public; all external behaviors and socially defined characteristics, such as dress, haircut, clothing, social mannerisms, speech, and behavior

gender identity: the way the person feels inside, and how they experience gender. This may or may not correlate with their recorded sex at birth

Gender nonconforming: behaviors not typical of individuals of the same assigned gender in a specific society

geropsychiatry: a discipline focused on the special needs of older adults with mental health concerns and psychiatric/substance misuse disorders

global deterioration scale: assesses and stages primary degenerative dementia based on orientation, memory, and neurologic function

grief: the normal process of reaction to a loss

hallucinations: false sensory perceptions with no basis in reality; usually visual or auditory, hallucinations also may be olfactory (smell), gustatory (taste), or tactile (touch)

hallucinogens: drugs that produce behavioral changes that are often multiple and dramatic; no known medical use

histrionic personality disorder: a pervasive pattern of excessive emotionality and attention-seeking; often begins in early adulthood and may be present in a variety of contexts

hypochondriasis: misinterpretation of the severity and significance of physical signs or sensations or the fear of contracting a disease; leads to the preoccupation with having a serious disease, which persists despite medical reassurance to the contrary; significant distress or impairment in functioning occurs

ideas of reference: misinterpreting acts of others in a highly personal way

identification: unconscious adoption of the personality, characteristics, attitudes, values, and behavior of another person

illusions: false sensory perceptions with some basis in reality; for example, a car backfiring mistaken for a gunshot

immature defense mechanisms: internal reactions to threats such as idealizing or devaluating others, projecting, and acting out

implicit memory: information that can't be brought to mind but can be seen to affect behavior

implosion therapy: a form of desensitization; requires repeated exposure

(that increases in graduated levels) to a highly feared object, requires strong interpersonal support or anxiolytic medication

inappropriate affect: inconsistency between expression (affect) and mood (e.g., a patient who smiles when discussing an anger-provoking situation)

incoherence: incomprehensible speech

intellectualization: hiding feelings about something painful behind thoughts; keeping opposing attitudes apart by using logic-tight comparisons

introjection: adopting someone else's values and standards without exploring whether or not they actually fit; often responds to "should" or "ought to"

lability of affect: rapid, dramatic fluctuation in the range of emotion

loose associations: not connected or related by logic or rationality

magical thinking: belief that thoughts or wishes can control other people or events

magnetoencephalography: measures the brain's magnetic field

Minnesota Multiphasic Personality Inventory: helps assess personality traits and ego function in adolescents and adults

modeling: provides a reward when the patient imitates the desired behavior

narcissistic personality disorder: projecting an image of perfection and personal invincibility because of a fear of personal weakness and imperfection; often projecting an inflated sense of self to hide low self-esteem

negative reinforcement: involves the removal of a negative stimulus only after the patient provides a desirable response

neologisms: distorted or invented words that have meaning only for the patient

nonverbal communication: eye contact, posture, facial expression, gestures, clothing, affect, silence, and other body movements that can convey a powerful message

obsessions: intense preoccupations that interfere with daily living

obsessive-compulsive personality disorder: a lack of openness and flexibility in daily routines as well as in interpersonal relationships and expectations; a preoccupation with orderliness and perfectionism; treatment options that don't fit in with the patient's cognitive schema will be rejected quickly

opiates: narcotics and depressants used medicinally to relieve pain but have a high potential for abuse

paranoid personality disorder: extreme distrust of others and an avoidance of relationships in which the person isn't in control or has the potential of losing control

paraphilia: objects or behaviors that sexually arouse and stimulate an individual—the person frequently becomes dependent on that object or behavior in order to achieve sexual gratification

pedophilia: having sex or engaging in sexual activity with a minor

pharmacodynamics: the drug's effect on its target organ

phencyclidine or PCP: a hallucinogen that produces behavioral changes that are often multiple and dramatic; flashbacks may occur long after use

phobia: an irrational and disproportionate fear of objects or situations

positive reinforcement: increase of the likelihood of a desirable behavior being repeated by promptly praising or rewarding the patient when performing it

poverty of speech: diminution of thought reflected in decreased speech and terse replies to questions, creating the impression of inner emptiness

priapism: a painful and prolonged erection

processing capacity: understanding text, making inferences, and paying attention, which all depend on working memory capability

projection: displacement of negative feelings onto another person

prospective memory: remembering things that one needs

punishment: discouraging of problem behavior by inflicting a penalty, such as temporary removal of a privilege

rationalization: substitution of acceptable reasons for the real or actual reasons motivating behavior

reaction formation: conduct in a manner opposite from the way the person feels

recent memory: an event experienced in the past few hours or days

regression: return to an earlier developmental stage

remote memory: ability to remember events in the more distant past, such as birthplace or high school days

repression: unconsciously blocking out painful thoughts

response prevention: a form of behavior therapy that may require hospitalization as well as family involvement to be effective

schizoid personality: a pervasive pattern of detachment from social relationships and restricted range of expression of emotions in interpersonal settings

schizotypal personality disorder: a pervasive pattern of social and interpersonal deficits marked by acute discomfort with, and reduced capacity for, close relationships, as well as by cognitive or perceptual distortions and eccentricities of behavior; begins in early adulthood and is present in a variety of contexts

self-efficacy: a personality measure defined by the ability to organize and execute actions required to deal with situations likely to happen in the future

sex: a person's biological sex of being male, female, or intersex based on anatomy, chromosomes, and sex organs

sexual dysfunction: a broad term that includes disorders of sexual desire, sexual arousal, orgasmic disorders, and sexual pain disorders

sexual masochism: deriving sexual gratification through being physically and/or emotionally abused

sexual sadism: achieving sexual gratification by causing others pain through the use of cruelty and emotional and/or physical abuse

shaping: initially rewards any behavior that resembles the desirable

one; then, step by step, the behavior required to gain a reward becomes progressively closer to the desired behavior

sharing impressions: a communication technique in which the nurse attempts to describe the patient's feelings and then seeks corrective feedback from the patient

somatization disorder: experiencing multiple signs and symptoms that suggest a physical disorder, but no verifiable disease or pathophysiologic condition exists to account for them

sublimation: transforming unacceptable needs into acceptable ambitions and actions; for instance, a person can funnel anger and resentment into an obsession to excel in a lucrative career

substance abuse: a maladaptive pattern of substance use coupled with recurrent and significant adverse consequences

substance dependence: physical, behavioral, and cognitive changes resulting from persistent substance use

substance intoxication: the development of a reversible substance-specific syndrome due to the ingestion of or exposure to a substance

tardive dyskinesia: a neurologic syndrome characterized by repetitive, involuntary, purposeless movements caused by the long-term use of certain drugs called *neuroleptics*

thematic apperception test: test in which, after seeing a series of pictures that depict ambiguous situations, the patient tells a story describing each picture

thought blocking: sudden interruption in the patient's train of thought

thought stopping: method that breaks the habit of fear-inducing anticipatory thoughts; to stop unwanted thoughts by saying the word *stop* and then focus attention on achieving calmness and muscle relaxation

tolerance: an increased need for a substance or need for an increased amount of the substance to achieve an effect

Transgender: one whose sense of gender does not match the biological and anatomic sex; typically, the individual may have feelings of having been born into the wrong body

undoing: trying to superficially repair or make up for an action without dealing with the complex effects of that deed; also called *magical thinking*

voyeurism: the act of obtaining sexual gratification while secretly observing others engaged in such activities as sex, intimate acts, or undressing

withdrawal: becoming emotionally uninvolved by pulling back and being passive

word salad: illogical word groupings; the extreme form of loose associations; for example, "She had a star, barn, plant."

working memory: the part of the brain that enables not paying attention to irrelevancies

INDEX

Note: Page numbers followed by i refers to an illustration; t refers to a table.